Techniques in Cartilage Repair Surgery

Asode Ananthram Shetty
Seok-Jung Kim • Norimasa Nakamura
Mats Brittberg
Editors

Techniques in Cartilage Repair Surgery

Springer

EUROPEAN SOCIETY OF SPORTS TRAUMATOLOGY, KNEE SURGERY AND ARTHROSCOPY
ESSKA

Editors
Asode Ananthram Shetty, MD, PhD, MCh, FRCS Ed., FRCS Eng., FRCS Orth
Department of Minimally Invasive Surgery, Faculty of Health and Social Sciences
Canterbury Christ Church University
Chatham Maritime
Kent, UK

Faculty of Stem Cell Research and Regenerative Medicine
NITTE University
Mangalore, India

Seok-Jung Kim, MD, PhD, FRCS
Department of Orthopaedic Surgery
Uijeongbu St. Mary's Hospital
College of Medicine
The Catholic University of Korea
Gyeonggi-do
Korea, Republic of (South Korea)

Faculty of Stem Cell Research and Regenerative Medicine
NITTE University
Mangalore, India

Norimasa Nakamura, MD, PhD
Institute for Medical Science in Sports
Osaka Health Science University
Osaka
Japan

Center for Advanced Medical Engineering and Informatics
Osaka University
Suita
Osaka
Japan

Mats Brittberg, MD, PhD
Cartilage Research Unit
Department of Orthopaedic
University of Gothenburg
Kungsbacka
Sweden

Region Halland Orthopaedics
Kungsbacka Hospital
Kungsbacka
Sweden

ESSKA ASBL
Centre Médical
Fondation Norbert Metz
76, rue d'Eich
1460 Luxembourg
Luxembourg

ISBN 978-3-642-41920-1 ISBN 978-3-642-41921-8 (eBook)
DOI 10.1007/978-3-642-41921-8
Springer Heidelberg New York Dordrecht London

Library of Congress Control Number: 2014934310

Printed on acid-free paper

Springer is part of Springer Science+Business Media (www.springer.com)

Foreword

It is a privilege for me to write the Foreword for this excellent text which covers all current techniques for repair of articular cartilage. A great deal has happened since we first described successful transplantation of viable chondrocytes into joint surfaces of animals with normal and papain arthritic joints in 1971. This laid the foundations of the present-day widespread acknowledgement of the requirement for this repair and also the application of such cellular techniques to the human patient. After some years of experimenting with various matrices to support the formation of hyaline cartilage, Brittberg et al. published the pivotal report of the results of isolated articular chondrocyte grafts in human knees which led to the development of ACI (autologous chondrocyte implantation) and many other studies over the years involving various methods to regenerate the unique hyaline cartilage structure of joints after the loss of osteochondral and chondral fragments.

In essence, the vital question is whether cells from the subchondral bone marrow or elsewhere in the haematopoietic system can transform into hyaline cartilage permanently or whether transplantation of differentiated chondrocytes is necessary to achieve this. Persuasive reports on microfracture and stem cell grafts suggest, but have not proven, this despite genetic manipulation of the cells or stimulation of cell division differentiation and proliferation by growth factors. To date, the longest and largest follow-up of successful results for treatment of osteochondral defects has been with ACI and MACI (matrix assisted chondrocyte implantation). It appears definite that isolated cells, free from matrix, are essential for perfect cartilage regeneration. However, no method has yet been shown to be effective for a prolonged period of time or in established osteoarthritis.

Nevertheless, the ACI/MACI method is two-stage, time consuming and expensive, and involves two operations with a long rehabilitation period. Clearly, a one-stage procedure with rapid rehabilitation is required so that overall the treatment is quicker, cheaper and as effective as ACI/MACI.

This excellent book, with its internationally famous faculty, addresses all these problems, describing in detail the current techniques, the pros and cons of each method, accompanied by visionary theories for the future. Thus the basic science, the experimental and the clinical results of the whole range of methods available, is covered. The long-term goal is not only the curing of pain and healing of acute osteochondral injuries, but the prevention of osteo-arthritis which affects 50 % of the population over 60 in the Western world and is a major cause of disability and healthcare expenditure for the future. This book provides many of the clues and hopes for that future.

London, UK

George Bentley, MB, ChM, DSc, FRCS, FRCS(E), FMedSci

Preface

It is 55 years since Pridie described the drilling technique for the treatment of cartilage defects and 26 years since the first human chondrocyte implantation was done. Yet we are still looking for the perfect cartilage repair and regeneration method. However, when you realise that cartilage takes over 20 years to mature into adult cartilage tissue, you begin to appreciate that cartilage treatment is indeed a difficult task.

There is no single treatment for all types of cartilage injuries. First of all, we need to define what a local cartilage defect is, as opposed to an osteoarthritic lesion. Also, where does the transition begin when we have pre-osteoarthritic cartilage? Secondly, is it possible to use only intrinsic derived repairs with or without augmentations with scaffolds or should we also use extrinsic repairs with manipulated cells to improve the repair? Thirdly, do we need to have a different philosophy when treating other joint besides the most treated joint, the knee joint?

These are the questions that this book tries to answer in the different chapters: from the histology and biology of cartilage repair with different biological repair alternatives available today. Finally, but not least, the extremely important post-operative rehabilitation is also presented.

Unfortunately, we do not have a perfect regeneration solution in this book, but there are several interesting tools in the cartilage toolbox that are put forward in the different chapters.

After reading this book, we hope that you can feel more comfortable when treating your future patients with cartilage defects and be able to offer the patient a larger number of alternatives for size, location and quality of surrounding cartilage.

Each chapter has been edited by a specialist who has experience and expertise in different types of cartilage repair, cartilage radiology and cartilage repair rehabilitation. All the described knowledge in this book will help surgeons and others involved in cartilage repair to take better care of their patients. Hopefully this will benefit the patient with much improved treatment and care.

On behalf of the editors,

Kungsbacka, Sweden — Mats Brittberg, MD, PhD

Contents

Editorial Assistants

Vishvas A. Shetty, MBBS, MCh Department of Minimally Invasive Surgery, Faculty of Health and Social Sciences, Canterbury Christ Church University, Kent, UK

David Stelzeneder, MD, PhD Department of Orthopaedics, Medical University of Vienna, Vienna General Hospital, Vienna, Austria

Neha Shetty, MSc, MBA The Business School, Faculty of Health and Social Sciences, Canterbury Christ Church University, Kent, UK

Contributors

Wataru Ando, MD, PhD Department of Orthopaedics, Kansai Rosai Hospital, Amagasaki, Hyogo, Japan

Knut Beitzel Department of Trauma and Orthopedic Surgery, Berufsgenossenschaftliche Unfallklinik Murnau, Murnau, Germany

Ágnes Berta, MD, MSc, M Res Department of Orthopaedics, Uzsoki Hospital, Budapest, Hungary

Department of Traumatology, Semmelweis University, Budapest, Hungary

P. Bilagi Kent Knee Unit, Spire Alexandra Hospital, Impton lane, Chatham, Kent, UK

T. Bonanzinga II Orthopaedic and Traumathologic Clinic - Biomechanics Lab, Rizzoli Orthopaedic Institute, Bologna, Italy

Timothy W.R. Briggs Royal National Orthopaedic Hospital, Stanmore, London, UK

Institute of Orthopaedic and Musculoskeletal Science, University College London, London, UK

Mats Brittberg, MD, PhD Cartilage Research Unit, Orthopaedic Department, University of Gothenburg, Kungsbacka, Sweden

Region Halland Orthopaedics, Kungsbacka Hospital, Kungsbacka, Sweden

M.O. Brix Department of Orthopaedics, Medical University of Vienna, Vienna, Austria

D. Bruni II Orthopaedic and Traumathologic Clinic - Biomechanics Lab, Rizzoli Orthopaedic Institute, Bologna, Italy

William Bugbee, MD Division of Orthopaedic Surgery, Scripps Clinic, La Jolla, CA, USA

Department of Orthopaedic Surgery, University of California, San Diego, La Jolla, CA, USA

Jaskarndip Chahal, MD, MSc, FRCSC University of Toronto Orthopaedic Sports Medicine (UTOSM), Toronto Western Hospital and Women's College Hospital, Toronto, ON, Canada

Brian J. Cole, MD, MBA Division of Sports Medicine, Rush University Medical Center, Chicago, IL, USA

Tommy S. de Windt, MD Department of Orthopaedics, University Medical Center Utrecht, Utrecht, GA, The Netherlands

S. Domayer Orthopaedic Rehabilitation Center SKA Zicksee, St. Andrä am Zicksee, Austria

Christoph Erggelet, MD, PhD Center for Biologic Joint Surgery, University of Freiburg Medical Center Freiburg/Germany, Zurich, Switzerland

Department for Orthopaedic Surgery and TraumatologyAlbert-Ludwigs-University Medical Center, Freiburg, Germany

M. Faimali Royal National Orthopaedic Hospital, Stanmore, London, UK

G. Filardo Biomechanics Laboratory, II Orthopaedic Clinic, Rizzoli Orthopaedic Insitute, Bologna, Italy

P.D. Gikas Royal National Orthopaedic Hospital, Stanmore, London, UK

Institute of Orthopaedic and Musculoskeletal Science, University College London, London, UK

Alberto Gobbi, MD Orthopaedic Arthroscopic Surgery International, OASI Bioresearch Foundation Gobbi NPO, Milan, Italy

A. Grassi II Orthopaedic and Traumathologic Clinic - Biomechanics Lab, Rizzoli Orthopaedic Institute, Bologna, Italy

Florian Halbwirth, MA Center for Regenerative Medicine and Orthopedics, Department for Biomedicine and Health, Danube University Krems, Austria

László Hangody, MD, PhD, DSc Department of Orthopaedics, Uzsoki Hospital, Budapest, Hungary

Department of Traumatology, Semmelweis University, Budapest, Hungary

Paul Hayden, BSc, MRCP, FRCA, DICM, FFICM Department of Anaesthesia and Critical Care, Medway NHS Foundation Trust, Kent, UK

James H.P. Hui Department of Orthopaedic Surgery, University Orthopaedic, Hand and Reconstructive Microsurgery Cluster, National University Health System, Singapore

Andreas B. Imhoff Department of Orthopaedic Sports Medicine, Technical University Munich, Munich, Germany

L. Johnston Royal National Orthopaedic Hospital, Stanmore, London

Chan Kwon Jung, MD, PhD Department of Hospital Pathology, College of Medicine, The Catholic University of Korea, Seoul, Republic of Korea

Sara Jurek, MD Santa Monica Orthopaedic and Sports Medicine Group, Santa Monica, CA, USA

Richard W. Kang, MS, MD Departments of Sports Medicine and Shoulder Surgery, Hospital for Special Surgery, New York, USA

Georgios Karnatzikos, MD Orthopaedic Arthroscopic Surgery International, OASI Bioresearch Foundation Gobbi NPO, Milan, Italy

Seok-Jung Kim, MD, PhD, FRCS Department of Orthopedic Surgery, Uijeongbu St. Mary's Hospital, College of Medicine, The Catholic University of Korea, Gyeonggi-do, Republic of (South Korea)

Faculty of Stem Cell Research and Regenerative Medicine, NITTE University, Mangalore, India

Ludwig Kohn Department of Orthopaedic Sports Medicine, Technical University Munich, Munich, Germany

Elizaveta Kon NAno-BIotechnology Laboratory, III Orthopaedic Clinic, Codivilla-Putti Research Center, Rizzoli Orthopaedic Institute, Bologna, Italy

Anup Kumar, MD Department of Orthopaedics, India Institute of Medical Sciences, Patna, Bihar, India

Derrick Lam Yong Loo Lin School of Medicine, National University of Singapore, Singapore

Ping Law Tissue Engineering and Cell Therapy (GMP) Laboratory, National University Health System, Singapore

Joel Lee Department of Orthopaedic Surgery, University Orthopaedic, Hand and Reconstructive Microsurgery Cluster, National University Health System, Singapore

Thomas Luksch, MD, MSc Department of Orthopedic, Hospital Krems, Austria

Richard Ma, MD Departments of Sports Medicine and Shoulder Surgery, Hospital for Special Surgery, New York, USA

Bert Mandelbaum, MD Santa Monica Orthopaedic and Sports Medicine Group, Santa Monica, CA, USA

Sureshbabu Manivannan Department of Orthopaedic Surgery, University Orthopaedic, Hand and Reconstructive Microsurgery Cluster, National University Health System, Singapore

M. Marcacci II Orthopaedic and Traumathologic Clinic - Biomechanics Lab, Rizzoli Orthopaedic Institute, Bologna, Italy

Andrew McCaskie, MB ChB, MMus, MD, FRCS, FRCS (T&O) Division of Trauma and Orthopaedic Surgery, Department of Surgery, Cambridge University, Cambridge University Hospitals NHS Foundation Trust, Cambridge, UK

Stéphane Méthot, PhD Piramal Life Sciences, Bio-Orthopaedic Division, Laval (QC), Canada

G.M. Marcheggiani Muccioli II Orthopaedic and Traumathologic Clinic - Biomechanics Lab, Rizzoli Orthopaedic Institute, Bologna, Italy

M. Mumme Center for Orthobiologics and Cartilage Repair, Schulthess Clinic Zurich, Zurich, Switzerland

Norimasa Nakamura, MD, PhD, FRCS Institute for Medical Science in Sports, Osaka Health Science University, Osaka, Japan

Center for Advanced Medical Engineering and Informatics, Osaka University, Osaka, Japan

Stefan Nehrer, MD Center for Regenerative Medicine and Orthopedics, Department for Biomedicine and Health, Danube University Krems, Austria

M.P. Neri II Orthopaedic and Traumathologic Clinic - Biomechanics Lab, Rizzoli Orthopaedic Institute, Bologna, Italy

M. Nitri II Orthopaedic and Traumathologic Clinic - Biomechanics Lab, Rizzoli Orthopaedic Institute, Bologna, Italy

Delia A. Pais, BA Departments of Sports Medicine and Shoulder Surgery, Hospital for Special Surgery, New York, USA

F. Perdisa NAno-BIotechnology Laboratory, II Orthopaedic Clinic, Rizzoli Orthopaedic Insitute, Bologna, Italy

Alberto Restrepo, MD Piramal Life Sciences, Bio-Orthopaedic Division, Laval (QC), Canada

James B. Richardson, MBChB, FRCS, MD Institute of Orthopaedics, Institute of Science and Technology in Medicine (Keele University), Robert Jones and Agnes Hunt Orthopaedic Hospital, Oswestry, Shropshire, UK

Sally Roberts, PhD Department of ARC/TORCH Building, Robert Jones and Agnes Hunt Orthopaedic Hospital and Institute of Science and Technology in Medicine (Keele University), Oswestry, Shropshire, UK

Daniel B.F. Saris, MD, PhD Department of Orthopaedics, University Medical Center Utrecht, Utrecht, GA, The Netherlands

Reconstructive Medicine, MIRA Institute for Technical Medicine & Biomedical Engineering, University of Twente, Enschede, The Netherlands

Asode Ananthram Shetty, MD, PhD, MCh, FRCS Ed., FRCS Eng., FRCS Orth Department of Minimally Invasive Surgery, Faculty of Health and Social Sciences, Canterbury Christ Church University, Chatham Maritime, Kent, UK

Faculty of Stem Cell Research and Regenerative Medicine, NITTE University, Mangalore, India

Vishvas A. Shetty, MBBS, MCh Department of Minimally Invasive Surgery, Faculty of Health and Social Sciences, Canterbury Christ Church University, Chatham Maritime, Kent, UK

Kazunori Shimomura, MD, PhD Department of Orthopaedics, Osaka University Graduate School of Medicine, Suita, Osaka, Japan

Matthew S. Shive, PhD Piramal Life Sciences, Bio-Orthopaedic Division, Laval (QC), Canada

Mohammed Shukrimi Department of Orthopaedic Surgery, University Orthopaedic, Hand and Reconstructive Microsurgery Cluster, National University Health System, Singapore

Clint Soppe, MD Santa Monica Orthopaedic and Sports Medicine Group, Santa Monica, CA, USA

William D. Stanish, MD Department of Surgery, Dalhousie University, Halifax (NS), Canada

Matthias Reinhard Steinwachs, PD Dr. med. Center for Orthobiologics and Cartilage Repair, Schulthess Clinic Zurich, Zurich, Switzerland

Department of Orthopedics and Trauma Surgery, University Hospital Freiburg, Freiburg, Germany

S. Trattnig High Field MR Centre, Department of Biomedical Imaging and Image-guided Therapy, Medical University of Vienna, Vienna, Austria

Victor Valderrabano, MD, PhD Orthopaedic Department, University Hospital of Basel, Basel, Switzerland

A. Visani II Orthopaedic and Traumathologic Clinic - Biomechanics Lab, Rizzoli Orthopaedic Institute, Bologna, Italy

B. Waibl Center for Orthobiologics and Cartilage Repair, Schulthess Clinic Zurich, Zurich, Switzerland

Matthew Wichman, MD Santa Monica Orthopaedic and Sports Medicine Group, Santa Monica, CA, USA

Martin Wiewiorski, MD Orthopaedic Department, University Hospital of Basel, Basel, Switzerland

Riley J. Williams III , MD Departments of Sports Medicine and Shoulder Surgery, Hospital for Special Surgery, New York, USA

Keng Lin Wong Department of Orthopaedic Surgery, University Orthopaedic, Hand and Reconstructive Microsurgery Cluster, National University Health System, Singapore

Hideki Yoshikawa, MD, PhD Department of Orthopaedics, Osaka University Graduate School of Medicine, Suita, Osaka, Japan

S. Zaffagnini II Orthopaedic and Traumathologic Clinic - Biomechanics Lab, Rizzoli Orthopaedic Institute, Bologna, Italy

Part I

Introduction

The History of the Treatment of Cartilage Injuries

1

Mats Brittberg

Contents

M. Brittberg, MD, PhD
Cartilage Research Unit, Orthopaedic Department, University of Gothenburg, Kungsbacka, Sweden

Region Halland Orthopaedics, Kungsbacka Hospital, Kungsbacka, Sweden
e-mail: mats.brittberg@telia.com

1.1 Introduction

There is a direct correlation between the ability of a tissue for repair after trauma and the tissue turnover rate. Adult articular cartilage has an extremely slow metabolic rate and thus a very low ability to repair itself after injury. In the edge of a cartilage injury, there is some mitotic activity to be noticed early after a trauma, but it is not strong enough to repair the defect. Principally, the initial amount of cells that can take part in the repair events is of major importance.

In a mesenchymal tissue, there are primitive prechondrocytes/stem cells that during beneficial conditions can differentiate into the cells of the injured tissue. The repair of the mesenchymal tissue is dependent of the local availability of these chondrogenic cells, and the ultimate goal for all types of treatments of a cartilage defect must be to deliver and activate high densities of these stem cells into the injured site.

The different types of treatment that are mentioned below ultimately produce and/or deliver different types of repair cells that are thought to in the end of differentiation lineage to appear as mature chondrocytes producing a more or less differentiated hyaline articular cartilage.

A.A. Shetty et al. (eds.), *Techniques in Cartilage Repair Surgery*,
DOI 10.1007/978-3-642-41921-8_1, © ESSKA 2014

1.2 Shaving, Abrasion or Debridement of Fibrillated Cartilage

Burman et al. [20] reported a reduced disability in degenerative arthritic patients following arthroscopic lavage which was attributed to the removal of mechanical irritants in the joint.

The concept of shaving or debriding of fibrillated cartilage, mostly superficially situated, is to remove the irregularities of the lesion to get a smooth stable articular surface. This procedure was first described by Haggart [37] and Magnuson [57]. They removed all intra-articular abnormalities, such as abnormal synovial membrane, osteophytes, torn menisci and degenerative fibrillated cartilage, and performed a so-called house cleaning of the joint. The technique has been used in open debridement as well as in transarthroscopic procedures, mainly as a 'shaving' technique.

A postoperative temporary relief of pain is often seen but no signs of cartilage repair. The combination of debridement and joint irrigation and lavage could give an effect by eliminating cartilage debris that could cause inflammation, synovitis. However, the value of this treatment is uncertain [10], and as in most studies regarding the treatment of injured cartilage, the diagnosis has been osteoarthritis and the studied group consisted of elderly patients in nonrandomised studies [18]. It has also been shown that the success of the arthroscopic debridement correlates inversely with the severity of the disease, and thus, patients with a mild disease improved the most, particularly when a coexisting meniscal tear was treated [1].

1.3 Drilling, Resection or Abrasion of Subchondral Bone Plate

Pridie in 1959 [78] introduced drilling of the bare exposed subchondral bone to stimulate fibrocartilaginous ingrowth from the vascular bone marrow. Different ways to achieve resurfacing via an opening of the subchondral bone marrow cavity have been tried. Ficat et al. [31] described the spongialisation, a resection of the entire subchondral bone plate in chondromalacic patellas, and reported 79 % of good to excellent results in their patients. Steadman suggested that an awl should be used instead of a high-speed drill bit. The awl creates a rough surface around the fractured bone plate which according to Steadman will give a better blood clot formation [87, 88, 91]. Johnson [44] introduced the transarthroscopic abrasion arthroplasty where the sclerotic exposed subchondral bone was excised 1–3 mm with a motorised burr to reach intracortical vascularity. The resulting fibrin clot formation is protected with non-minor weight bearing for 2 months.

Evidence exists that the above described techniques will produce a repair mainly consisting of fibrocartilaginous tissue. Despite this, several authors describe an improvement in the patients' symptoms [32, 43, 44]. It is to note that the follow-up times in most studies have been short, and it has been difficult to compare the treated groups due to lack of common descriptions of the cartilage lesions, single cartilage lesion, or generalised OA. Furthermore, there is a marked lack of randomised controlled studies.

Buckwalter and Mow [19] claimed that arthroscopic abrasion arthroplasties and debridements may provide temporary relief of symptoms in selected patients when performed by surgeons with considerable experience in cartilage handling. Salisbury and McMahon [82] discussed the role of abrasion arthroplasty in cartilage resurfacing. In a knee with a degenerative meniscal lesion, the forces that dislocate the meniscal flap may often create a damage on the adjacent condylar weight-bearing cartilage area, and the lesion can be debrided after resection of the meniscal flap. This would be a localised area that can be treated by the surgeon in two ways: either accepting the debrided defect now with stable edges or abrade the base of the lesion to get a bleeding bony surface. Salisbury and McMahon [82] state that debridement alone will give reduction in symptoms like locking, catching and effusions for a while but by time the decrease in meniscal load sharing will lead to a gradual cartilage degeneration also of the surrounding cartilage. To what extent an abrasion arthroplasty could hinder such a progress is not known. The filling up of the defect might stabilise the edges of the defect, but there is doubt that the fibrocartilage tissue repair after abrasion will stand against wear for a prolonged time. The abrasion arthroplasty however was suggested to be used for small chondral defects. The results of an extended abrasion arthroplasty as a treatment for widespread unicompartmental or multicompartmental OA have been more unpredictable and disputable [13, 18]. Dandy [24, 25] has suggested that lesions less than 1 cm^2 could be treated by abrasion arthroplasties or spongialisation while larger defects could be treated by drilling leaving cortical bridges.

Steadman et al. [89] have presented that over a 7- to 17-year follow-up period (average, 11.3 years), patients 45 years and younger who underwent the microfracture procedure for full-thickness chondral defects, without associated meniscus or ligament pathology, showed statistically significant improvement in function and indicated that they had less pain. However, Kreuz et al. [52] found that the clinical results after microfracture of full-thickness cartilage lesions in the knee are age dependent. Deterioration begins 18 months after surgery and is significantly pronounced in patients aged older than 40 years. The best prognostic factor was found to be a patient age of 40 or younger with defects on the femoral condyles.

Mithoefer et al. [62] in 2009 made a systematic review of published papers on microfracture. Their conclusion was that microfracture provides effective short-term functional improvement of knee function, but not enough data are available on its long-term results. Weaknesses of the technique include limited hyaline repair tissue, variable repair cartilage volume and possible functional deterioration.

Today, there is an increased interest to use augmentation techniques for bone marrow stimulation operations. One of the first was carbon fibre rods and pads [14, 15]. Other such augmentation techniques are AMIC [8], osteochondral synthetic plugs [21] and different collagen scaffolding materials [72].

1.4 Osteochondral Allo- and Autografting Techniques

1.4.1 Allografts

In osteochondral grafting techniques, the cartilage defect area and underlying bone are replaced with a matching articular graft that has been harvested either as an allograft from an organ donor or as an autograft.

The limited source of autologous grafts has led to an interest in allografts. The chondrocyte has transplantation antigens [30], but the surrounding cartilage matrix is protective against immunological reaction [55]. Allografts have therefore been tried clinically both in fresh and frozen preparations. A lot of experience has the transplantation unit in Toronto [61]. They have shown that the chondrocytes were found to be viable up to 92 months after transplantation. The use of an osteochondral graft with bone thickness less than 1 cm was of importance prior to or simultaneously with the implantation of the graft as well as it is essential to correct joint malalignment prior to or simultaneously with graft transplantation [99]. In the beginning, the indications for allografting were not clearly defined, and the early results of the technique consist of a wide variety of patients. By time it has been found that best results are achieved in patients of young age with post-traumatic defects and before the onset of degenerative changes. In many of the allografted patients, a complimentary realignment was also needed [17]. Long-term results after allografting of post-traumatic defects have been reported by the Toronto group with success rates of 75 % at 5 years, 64 % at 10 years and 63 % at 14 years. Best results are with patients <60 years of age and with traumatically induced defects of the articular surface in the knee joint [58].

Important to ensure long-term survival of the allografts is that the subchondral bone support must be maintained. However, studies have shown that the subchondral bone sometimes is resorbed and that 75 % of the failures of cryopreserved grafts were due to subchondral necrosis [59]. Advantages are that large selections of donors are available and that fresh as well as frozen allografts can be used. The frozen grafts could be more cartilage structural changed and have lower concentrations of proteoglycans [90]. The frozen grafts make it possible to use it for elective reconstructive surgery while one may have the time to examine the grafts for diseases. The grafts also have the advantage that they have the structure of the normal cartilage, and they can be prepared to fit exactly the size of the defect to be treated. Disadvantages are a risk for immunologic reactions and disease transmission. The bone component gives rise to an immunological response [54]. Instead autologous osteochondral grafting has advantages: reliability of bony union, a high survival rate of grafted cartilage and no risk for disease transmission. Gross et al. [36] have found that with a stable osseous graft base, the hyaline cartilage portion of the allograft can survive and function for 25 years or more.

1.4.2 Autografts

Wagner [96] and Muller [64] in Germany used a part of the posterior femoral condyle as an autogenic graft. Yamashita et al. (1985) used an autogenic graft from the anterior aspect of the medial femoral condyle, and Outerbridge et al. [70] used part of the patella to treat osteochondral defect of the knee in ten patients who were followed for 6 and a half years. Function was improved and symptoms were alleviated in all the patients. Matsusue and associates 1993 [60] described an interesting alternative technique in which multiple autologous osteochondral grafts were harvested as cylinders from the lateral wall of the patellar groove, non-weight-bearing area.

Hangody and Kárpáti [39] described their new method of operation used in cases of severe cartilage damage of the superficial articular surface of the patella and of the weight-bearing surface of the knee. It has similarities to the Matsusue technique [60]. Authors harvested from the non-weight-bearing articular surface of the femur cartilaginous-osseous cylinders for the supply of the defects of the weight-bearing surface and the cartilaginous defects of the patella. This was the first description of the so-called mosaicplasty technique in 14 patients.

1.5 Periosteal and Perichondral Resurfacing (Soft Tissue Arthroplasty)

Another way to deliver a new cell population to the cartilage defect site is to use periosteal and perichondral implantations. Both of these tissues consist of a certain amount of multipotential mesenchymal stem cells with the ability of cartilaginous metaplasia. They have subsequently been used to resurface cartilage defects but with varying success. The results in different studies are difficult to compare since the methods used vary considerably as well as the properties of the experimental grafting materials.

1.5.1 Periosteum

In most of the repair studies, the periosteal grafting was combined with an opening of the subchondral space permitting cells from the marrow to invade the defects. The number of these pluripotential stem cells seems to decline drastically in the mature periosteum compared to in an immature periosteal graft, and O'Driscoll and Keeley [67] showed that adult periosteum regenerated a repair tissue in adult rabbits that had only 15 % type II collagen compared for 93 % in the adolescent group. This is important to consider since in most studies of periosteal grafting, the animals have been adolescent, and the grafting procedures have been combined with an opening into the bone marrow cavity containing pluripotent mesenchymal cells, the number of which also decreases steadily with age.

Poussa et al. [77] found that periosteum transplanted as a free graft in the rabbit knee joint formed a cartilaginous body without any bone formation. Rubak et al. [81] used periosteum to treat cartilage defects in the rabbit knee with success, and the repair was described as hyaline-like. Similar animal studies regarding the chondrogenic potential of the periosteum have been made by Salter and O'Driscoll and co-workers [67, 68]. They have studied the periosteum as a free graft in the joint and as graft for the repair of rabbit trochlear groove defects as well as for rabbit full-thickness patellar chondral defects. They developed the concept of continuous passive motion for resurfacing with periosteal grafts and were able to show that there was a significant higher degree of chondrogenesis in the grafts in continuous passive motion knees compared to immobilised knees [68, 69]. They also showed that the results were dependent on the orientation of the graft and the age of the animal. Grafting with the cambium layer, rich in mesenchymal multipotential stem cells with osteochondrogenic potential, facing into the joint resulted in the best repair compared to those with the cambium layer facing towards the subchondral bone. The repair quality was also better in adolescent animals compared to adult animals. The repair could withstand wear up to 1 year post-surgery without any deterioration of the grafted tissue [67].

Vachon et al. [93] used periosteal autografts for repair of large osteochondral defects in 10 horses aged 2–3 years old. In each horse, osteochondral defects measuring 1.0×1.0 cm^2 were created bilaterally on the distal articular surface of each radial carpal bone. Control and experimental defects were drilled. Periosteum was harvested from the proximal portion of the tibia and was glued into the defects, using a fibrin adhesive. Control defects were glued, but were not grafted. Sixteen weeks after the grafting procedure, the quality of the repair tissue of control and grafted defects was assessed biochemically. All biochemical variables were compared with those of normal equine articular cartilage taken from the same site in another group of clinically normal horses. The biochemical composition of repair tissue of grafted and nongrafted defects was similar, but clearly differed from that of normal articular cartilage.

In clinical studies, Niedermann et al. [65] presented five patients with osteochondral defects that were treated with periosteal resurfacing with an excellent result. The defects were drilled subchondrally prior to grafting, and the grafts were fixed with fibrin glue. Hoikka et al. [41] treated 13 patients (mean age 36 years) with patellar chondral defects with free periosteal grafts and followed them for a mean 4 years. The cambium layer faced the subchondral bone, and the periosteum was sutured or glued into the defect. Eleven patients reached what was called an acceptable level post-surgery. Korkkala and Hukkanen [51] used free, autogenous periosteal grafts to treat six patients, three with acute traumatic patellar cartilage lesions and three with local sclerotic osteochondritis of the medial femoral condyle. The treatment resulted in satisfactory results with symptomatic amelioration, 14–59 months after the procedures. Fourteen patients with osteochondritis dissecans of the femoral condyle (mean size 4 cm^2) treated with periosteal transplantation were reviewed by Angermann and Riegels-Nielsen in 1994 [4]. The patients were followed for 1 year, and then 43 % were free of symptoms. In 29 % of the patients, defect was reduced in size radiographically while 64 % were unchanged.

1.5.2 Perichondrium

Tizzoni as early as in 1878 [92] described the chondrogenic potential of perichondrium. Skoog et al. [84] described the potential for the cells in the perichondrium to produce neocartilage with the potential to repair cartilage defects. This evoked an interest for the perichondrium, and several animal studies have been done to confirm the chondrogenic potential of the perichondrium [29, 48, 83]. Homminga et al. [42] treated pure chondral lesions in young rabbits with the epiphyses still open with perichondrium and noted hyaline-like repair on the grafted areas. They also found that it might be important to leave the subchondral bone intact while it could play an important role in preventing cartilage degeneration and referred to the studies of Radin and Rose [79].

Amiel et al. [2] reconstructed full-thickness cartilage defects in the rabbit knee with rib perichondrium and noted that the differentiation of this basic tissue into a hyaline repair was dependent on extrinsic influences emanating from the environment. They suggested that the presence of motion, low oxygen tension and absence of vascularity could favour hyalinisation of the repair.

However, despite the initially promising results from periosteal and perichondral graftings, the long-term durability of these grafts still remains uncertain as have shown by Engkvist [27] when they resurfaced patellar cartilage defects in the dogs with perichondrium. Two to eight months post-surgery, the repair was of hyaline character, but between 12 and 17 months post-surgery, the graft tissue degenerated leaving areas of exposed bone bare. However, it is important to notice that the results in long-term follow-ups are dependent of the site that has been treated.

Regarding the beneficial results with periosteum and continuous passive motions, few results regarding CPM and perichondrium have been reported. Kwan et al. [53] reported that CPM did not improve the quality of the repair tissue when evaluated 1 year post-surgery compared to free cage activity.

The clinical use of perichondrium to resurface cartilage defects was first described for the wrist and finger joints in human patients [28, 71]. Homminga et al. [42] used autologous costal perichondrium to treat 30 chondral knee defects in patients with mean age of 31. Twenty-five patients were evaluated by arthroscopy 1 year post-surgery; 14 patients were re-evaluated at 2 years postoperatively when it was found that 27 of 30 defects had healed with a tissue resembling cartilage. Three biopsies showed a hyaline-like morphology. However, later on, Beckers et al. [7] reported on high frequencies of loosening of the perichondral grafts sometimes due to calcification of the graft. In the patella, the results were worse if the defect had previously been drilled. The results were better in young persons, mean age 27 years in the success group compared to 34 years in the failure group. They concluded that the perichondral grafts should be used for osteochondritis dissecans and early post-traumatic cartilage defects in young persons.

Also other authors have found that perichondral resurfacing seems to be more successful in fairly young patients with post-traumatic defects of the articular cartilage [83].

Vachon et al. [94] compared the repair effect of perichondral and periosteal grafts on cartilage defects in 6 young horses (2–4 years old). Periosteal autografts were obtained from the medial aspect of the proximal portion of the tibia, and perichondral autografts were obtained from the sternum. Using arthroscopic visualisation, each autograft was placed as a loose body into 1 tarsocrural joint in the horse. The animals were hand-walked daily, starting the day after surgery, for a total of 6 h/week for 8 weeks. Eight weeks after autograft implantation, radiographs were taken of each tarsocrural joint and were interpreted with regard to mineralisation in the transplanted autografts. Grafts were then surgically removed and examined macroscopically and microscopically for viability, size and production of chondroid tissue. All autografts appeared viable, and most showed evidence of growth. Neochondrogenesis was observed in 5 of 6 periosteal grafts and in 1 of 6 perichondral grafts. Furthermore, the amount of chondroid tissue produced in periosteal autografts was significantly greater than that produced in the 1 perichondral graft. The chondroid tissue produced by periosteal autografts had morphologic and matrix staining properties similar to those of hyaline cartilage.

A common finding both in animals and in humans is that the grafts produce the best results in young individuals and in traumatic defects. The fact that the number of potential repair cells in any graft declines steadily with age could be one explanation of these effect.

1.6 Chondrogenic Cell Transplantation

It is possible to differentiate between two types of repair with cells; Intrinsic repair means a replication of chondrocytes from the area adjacent to the defect site, while extrinsic repair consists of a metaplasia of chondrocytes from other cell types such as connective tissue stem cells, i.e. subchondral marrow cells and synovial cells [86].

Cell transplantation has for a long time been explored as an alternative to other types of repair methods. The cells could be harvested autologously or as allografts from a healthy part of the donor tissue, isolated, expanded in vitro and finally implanted into the defect site in high densities. Pure chondrocytes, epiphyseal or mature, allogeneic or autologous, as well as other types of mesenchymal cells have been used.

In 1965 Smith [85] perfected the isolation of chondrocytes, and chondrocytes were thereafter able to be grown using standard culture methods. Chestermann and Smith [22] isolated chondrocytes from rabbit cartilage, and those cells were then transplanted into cartilage defects in the humerus of adult sister rabbits. The defects healed but no hyaline cartilage was found. Bentley and Greer [11] transplanted isolated articular cartilage chondrocytes and epiphyseal chondrocytes from young rabbits to cartilage defects on adult rabbits of the same inbreed. A nice repair with hyaline-like neocartilage was described in more than 50 % of the defects.

Green [35] reported a significant better repair after heterologous chondrocyte transplantation of chondral lesions of the rabbit knee. Autoradiography confirmed that the implanted isolated chondrocytes were responsible for the repair, and three generations of transplanted chondrocytes could be identified by the decrease in intensity in nuclear labelling.

Bentley et al. [12] transplanted isolated epiphyseal chondrocytes as allografts into rabbit knee tibial drill holes. Cells were pipetted into the defects with a success rate of 47 % of the defects repaired. Aston and Bentley [5] compared allografts of intact cartilage, isolated chondrocytes and cultured chondrocytes from the epiphyseal growth plate and articular surface from immature rabbits inserted into full-thickness defects in mature rabbits. Both intact articular cartilage and intact epiphyseal growth plates induced significantly better repair versus controls. Cultured chondrocytes also produced a significantly better repair than when the defects were left ungrafted in arthritic joints.

Yoshihashi [98] studied isolated articular chondrocytes in comparison with normal articular cartilage and used chondrocytes that were released by enzymatic digestion from slices of articular cartilage taken from 8-week-old white rabbits. The isolated cells were inoculated in a large number into a 0.28-cm2 stainless cylinder on a Millipore filter. After 12 h these chondrocytes were layered by gravity onto the Millipore filter and were cultured in the same medium during 7 days. Subsequently the cell aggregate was transferred to an organ culture system and was fed every other day. Aggregates of cells were sampled at 1, 2, 4, 8 and 12 weeks in culture for morphological and biochemical studies. The results obtained were as follows: After 1 week in culture, deposition of metachromatic matrix was observed under a light microscope only at the periphery of the aggregate of cells. Matrix formation in the whole aggregate occurred after 2 weeks in culture. The tissue reformed in this culture consisted of metachromatic hyaline cartilage like matrix and chondrocytes within lacunae but for cells at the surface arranged in a tangential flattened layer. The collagen in this tissue was of type II mixed with a very small amount of type I. The tissue reconstituted in vitro by freshly isolated chondrocytes had characteristics of hyaline cartilage except over the surface. Compared with normal articular cartilage, the cells in this tissue were distributed more randomly, and the intercellular hyaline matrix was poor under a light microscope, and collagen fibrils in the matrix observed under an electron microscope were much thinner than those of normal articular cartilage. This method provides a tissue culture model of cartilage organisation.

Wakitani and associates 1994 [97] implanted osteochondral progenitor cells from the periosteum and bone marrow cells-mesenchymal stem cells into the femoral condyle cartilage defects of rabbit knees. Those cells were preferred opposed to chondrocytes because they were said to be capable of a broader range of chondrogenic expression and that they may recapitulate the embryonic lineage transitions originally involved in the formation of joint tissue. No difference between the bone marrow cells and the periosteum-derived cells was seen, and the best scores were seen at 4 weeks. At 12 weeks, the subchondral bone plate was restituted. There was a gap between the host cartilage and the neocartilage, but the underlying bone was almost completely united with that of the host.

Goldberg and Caplan [33] compared implantation of mature chondrocytes, so-called committed, with mesenchymal stem cells for the repair of full-thickness defects in the femoral condyles of adult rabbits. Both cell types repaired the defect with a hyaline-like neocartilage. However, the mesenchymal stem cell repair had a more hyaline-like morphology and cartilage zonal characteristics than the repair from the committed chondrocytes. They hypothesised that the open subchondral bone releases host-derived bioactive factors like different growth factors and cytokines that could influence the biologic properties of the mesenchymal stem cells but not of the already differentiated chondrocytes.

Robinson et al. [80] implanted chondrocytes derived from chick embryos into defects of articular surfaces of young and old adult chickens. The embryonic chondrocytes underwent an accelerated ageing process in the old chickens implying that the maturation stages within the implant were shorter in the old animals leading to a shorter healing time.

The above reported cell transplantations have been allografts. The chondrocyte has transplantation antigens, and these cells can theoretically participate in immunological reactions. The cartilage matrix acts as a protective barrier [30]. Kawabe and Yoshinao [45] studied the immune responses to reparative tissue formed by allogeneic growth plate chondrocyte implants. The neocartilage yielded by implantation of these cells into cartilage defects of adult rabbits looked very good in the beginning but began to degenerate 2–3 weeks after implantation partially because of humoral immune response but also because of cell-mediated cytotoxicity. Host lymphocytes were seen around the allograft at 2–12 weeks.

Noguchi and associates 1995 [66] compared allografted chondrocytes with autografts that were cultured in a collagen gel and transplanted into osteochondral defects in knee joints of inbred rats. At 12 weeks 100 % of the autografts had healed successfully while only 50 % of the allograft was healed. At 26 and 52 weeks, all defects except one had healed, and there was no significant difference in the success rate between the groups.

Using the knee joints of adult rabbits, Peterson et al. [74] and Grande and co-workers [34] examined the effect of autologous chondrocytes grown in vitro on the healing rate of chondral defects not penetrating the subchondral bone plate. To determine whether any of the reconstituted cartilage resulted from the chondrocyte graft, an experiment was conducted involving grafts with chondrocytes that had been labelled prior to grafting with a nuclear tracer. Results were evaluated using both qualitative and quantitative light microscopy. Macroscopic results from grafted specimens displayed a marked decrease in synovitis and other degenerative changes. In defects that had received transplants, a significant amount of cartilage was reconstituted (82 %) compared to ungrafted controls (18 %). Autoradiography on reconstituted cartilage showed that there was labelled cells incorporated into the repair matrix [34].

In a randomised animal study, Brittberg et al. [16] used adult New Zealand rabbits which were transplanted autologously with harvested and in vitro cultured chondrocytes into patellar chondral lesions that had been made previously and were 3 mm in diameter, extending down to the calcified zone. Healing of the defects was assessed by gross examination, light microscope and histological-histochemical scoring at 8, 12 and 52 weeks. Chondrocyte transplantation significantly increased the amount of newly formed repair tissue compared to that found in control knees in which the lesion was solely covered by a periosteal flap.

Brittberg et al. [14, 15] transferred the rabbit ACI technology to be used in humans with the first patient operated on in October 1987. Autologous chondrocyte implantation (ACI) has then since the first patient was operated on been performed in more than 30,000 patients throughout the world with up to 20 years of follow-up [76].

Peterson et al. reported a retrospective analysis on the first 100 patients treated with ACI, follow-up ranging between 2 and 9 years [75]. Twenty-three of 25 (92 %) patients with isolated femoral condyle chondral lesions had successful outcomes, while 16 of 18 (89 %) patients with osteochondral defects had good to excellent results. Sixty-seven percent success was found in patients with multiple chondral lesions or salvage (one third of the patients had lesions involved bipolar lesions). Peterson et al. [73] also published their long-term durability biomechanical data showing a 96 % durability factor with the first 62 consecutive patients treated at 2 years and then again at 7.5 years. The clinical outcomes remained constant (80 % good to excellent results at 2 years and 78 % at 7.5 years) and second-look arthroscopies did not show signs of tissue breakdown [73].

Minas [63] have reported their results on 235 patients treated with autologous chondrocyte implantation and have had an 87 % success rate over a 6-year period. The Cartilage Registry Report [3], an international multicenter observational assessment of patients treated with ACI, has revealed by patient assessment that 78 % of all defects treated with ACI had improvement, while 81 % of isolated femoral condyle defects had improved. Clinician evaluations have shown a 79 % improvement for all lesions and an 85 % improvement in femoral condyle lesions. The most common adverse event reported with ACI is intra-articular adhesions (2 %). The other most common adverse events include detachment/delamination of graft (1.4 %), hypertrophic tissue (1.3–17 %) and catching/popping (1.0 %), with the overall adverse event rate and safety profile less than 7 %.

Peterson et al. [76] did a long-term follow-up on 224 of 341 patients who replied to their posted questionnaires. The mean cartilage lesion size was 5.3 cm (2). Ten to 20 years after the implantation (mean, 12.8 years), 74 % of the patients reported their status as better or the same as the previous years. There were 92 % who were satisfied and would have the ACI again. The Lysholm, Tegner-Wallgren and Brittberg-Peterson scores were improved compared with the preoperative values. The average Lysholm score improved from 60.3 preoperatively to 69.5 postoperatively, the Tegner from 7.2 to 8.2 and the Brittberg-Peterson from 59.4 to 40.9. At the final measurement, the KOOS score was on average 74.8 for pain, 63 for symptoms, 81 for activities of daily living (ADL), 41.5 for sports and 49.3 for quality of life (QOL). The average Noyes score was 5.4. Patients with bipolar lesions had a worse final outcome than patients with multiple unipolar lesions. The presence of meniscal injuries before ACI or history of bone marrow procedures before the implantation did not appear to affect the final outcomes. The age at the time of the operation or the size of lesion did not seem to correlate with the final outcome.

The second generation of ACI appeared when the periosteum was exchanged with a resorbable collagen membrane. Most published results with that technique have been published by Professor Bentley's group at Stanmore. Recently, in 2012, they presented a minimum of 10 years follow-up with the second-generation ACI, C-ACI in a randomised study versus mosaicplasty [9]. The mean age of the patients at the time of surgery was 31.3 years (16–49). The lesions had a mean size for the ACI group being 440.9 mm^2 and the mosaicplasty group being 399.6 mm^2. Patients were assessed using the modified Cincinnati knee score and the Stanmore-Bentley Functional Rating system. The number of patients whose repair had failed at 10 years was 10 of 58 (17 %) in the ACI group and 23 of 42 (55 %) in the mosaicplasty group ($p<0.001$). The functional outcome of those patients with a surviving graft was significantly better in patients who underwent ACI compared with mosaicplasty ($p=0.02$) (Fig. 1.1).

The third-generation ACI consists of either cells grown on the surface of a membrane-like MACI or cells grown within a scaffold. Macmull et al. [56] have compared treatment of patella cartilage lesions with either second-generation ACI (C-ACI) or third-generation ACI with MACI. They found that excellent and good results were achieved in 40 % of C-ACI patients and in 57 % of the MACI patients. Filardo et al. (2011) have so far the longest follow-up with a third-generation AC, the Hyalograft C. Thirty-four knees affected by symptomatic OCD grade III or IV on the ICRS scale were treated and prospectively evaluated at 12 and 24 months of follow-up and at a final mean 6 ± 1 years of follow-up. The mean age at treatment was 21 ± 6years. The average size of the defects was

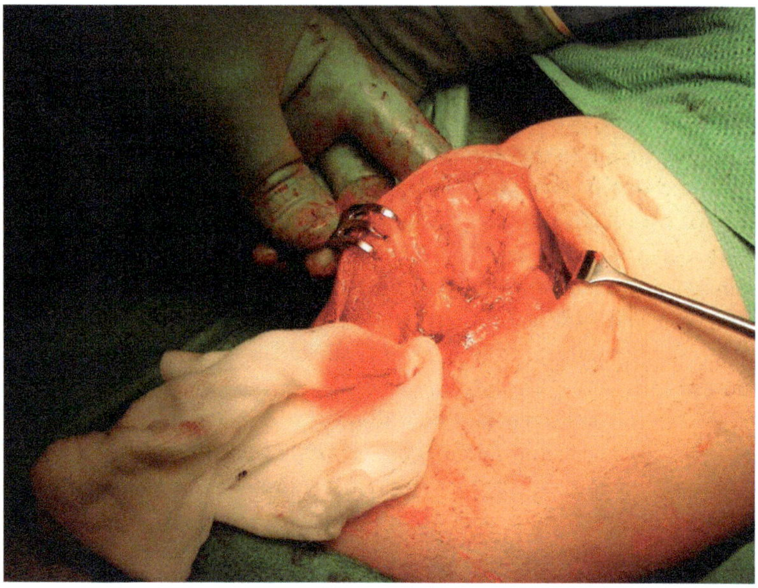

Fig. 1.1 A 2nd-generation ACI with cells in suspension implanted in under a collagen membrane on a patella cartilage defect

3 ± 1 cm^2. Patients were evaluated with IKDC, EQ-VAS and Tegner scores, and statistically significant improvement in all scores was observed after the treatment. The IKDC subjective score improved from 38 ± 13 to 81 ± 20, and 91 % of the knees were rated as normal or nearly normal in the objective IKDC at the final evaluation. To note was that a better outcome was obtained in men, sport-active patients and for smaller lesions. The use of cells in scaffolds opens up the possibility to use arthroscopic implantations. Kon et al. [49, 50] interestingly found that despite a similar success in returning to competitive sport, microfracture allowed an initial faster recovery but deteriorated over time, whereas arthroscopic autologous chondrocyte implantation delayed the return of high-level male soccer players to competition but offered more durable clinical results.

The first randomised study with autologous chondrocytes was published in 2004 [47]. There were no differences between patients operated on with ACI and patients operated on with microfracture. In 2007, the 5 years results were published from the same group [46]. Both methods provided satisfactory results in 77 % of the patients at 5 years. There was no significant difference in the clinical and radiographic results between the two treatment groups and no correlation between the histological findings and the clinical outcome.

The most recent randomised papers show a different outcome. Basad et al. [6] compared the clinical outcomes of patients with symptomatic cartilage defects treated with a third-generation ACI, matrix-induced autologous chondrocyte implantation (MACI) or microfracture (MF). Sixty patients were included (40 MACI, 20 MF) and were followed up 8–12, 22–26 and 50–54 weeks postoperatively with outcome measures as the Tegner, Lysholm and ICRS scores. The difference between baseline and 24 months postoperatively for both treatment groups was significant for the Lysholm, Tegner, patient ICRS and surgeon ICRS scores (all $P<0.0001$). However, MACI was significantly more effective over time (24 months vs. baseline) than MF according to the Lysholm ($P=0.005$), Tegner ($P=0.04$), ICRS patient ($P=0.03$) and ICRS surgeon ($P=0.02$) scores. Vanlauwe et al. presented their 5-year follow-up results of patient in a randomised study with autologous chondrocytes implantation (1st-generation ACI, characterised chondrocytes implantation, CCI) compared with microfracture (MF) [95]. At 5 years after treatment, clinical outcomes for CCI and MF were comparable. In the early treatment group, CCI obtained statistically significant and clinically relevant better results than MF. Delayed treatment resulted in less predictable outcomes for CCI.

1.7 Implantation of Stem Cells

The most recent trend is to use mesenchymal stem cells instead of cultured chondrocytes. As the majority of work with mesenchymal stem cell-derived articular cartilage repair has been carried out in vitro and in animal studies, more work still has to be done before this technique can be used for clinical purposes. However, Haleem et al. [38] tested autologous BM-MSCs that were culture expanded, placed on platelet-rich fibrin glue intraoperatively and then transplanted into 5 full-thickness cartilage defects of femoral condyles of five patients and covered with an autologous periosteal flap. Patients were evaluated clinically at 6 and 12 months by the Lysholm and Revised Hospital for Special Surgery Knee (RHSSK) scores and radiographically by x-rays and magnetic resonance imaging (MRI) at the same time points. Repair tissue in two patients was rated arthroscopically after 12 months using the International Cartilage Repair Society (ICRS) Arthroscopic Score. All patients' symptoms improved over the follow-up period of 12 months. Average Lysholm and RHSSK scores for all patients showed statistically significant improvement at 6 and 12 months postoperatively ($P<0.05$). There was no statistically significant difference between the 6 and 12 months postoperative clinical scores ($P=0.18$). ICRS arthroscopic scores were 8/12 and 11/12 (nearly normal) for the two patients who consented to arthroscopy. MRI of three patients at 12 months postoperatively revealed complete defect fill and complete surface congruity with native cartilage, whereas that of two patients showed incomplete congruity.

1.8 The Future

The future will be focusing on using either progenitor cells found within the cartilage tissue or mesenchymal stem cells with chondrogenic properties. We will see more of one stage procedures making use of cell-free scaffolds allowing ingrowth of mesenchymal stem cells from the subchondral bone. Promising such techniques are carbon fibre resurfacing [16, 26], cartilage fragment technology [23], multilayered biocomposites [49, 50] and the use of thermo gels as augmented bone marrow stimulations [40].

In this book, the reader will find a wide variety of cartilage repair techniques, some described in this historical chapter and some new thrilling techniques.

References

1. Aichroth PM, Patel DV, Moyes ST (1991) A prospective review of arthroscopic debridement for degenerative joint disease of the knee. Int Orthop 15:351–355
2. Amiel D, Coutts RD, Abel M, Stewart W, Harwood F, Akeson WH (1985) Rib perichondrial grafts for the repair of full thickness articular cartilage defects. A morphological and biochemical study in the rabbits. J Bone Joint Surg 67A:911–920
3. Anderson AF, Browne JE, Erggelet C et al (2001) Cartilage repair registry, vol 7. Genzyme Biosurger, Cambridge, pp 1–7
4. Angermann P, Riegels-Nielsen P (1994) Osteochondritis dissecans of the femoral condyle treated with periosteal transplantation. A preliminary clinical study of 14 patients. Orthopaedics 2:425–428
5. Aston JE, Bentley G (1986) Repair of articular surfaces by allografts of articular and growth-plate cartilage. J Bone Joint Surg 68B:29–34
6. Basad E, Ishaque B, Bachmann G, Stürz H, Steinmeyer J (2010) Matrix-induced autologous chondrocyte implantation versus microfracture in the treatment of cartilage defects of the knee: a 2-year randomised study. Knee Surg Sports Traumatol Arthrosc 18(4):519–527
7. Beckers JMH, Bulstra SK, Kuijer R, Bouwmeester SJM, van der Linden AJ (1992) Analysis of the clinical results after perichondral transplantation for cartilage defects of the human knee. Abstracts from the 19th symposium of the ESOA-Joint Destruction and osteoarthritis, Nordwijkerhout, Netherlands, p 157
8. Benthien JP, Behrens P (2011) The treatment of chondral and osteochondral defects of the knee with autologous matrix-induced chondrogenesis (AMIC): method description and recent developments. Knee Surg Sports Traumatol Arthrosc 19(8):1316–1319
9. Bentley G, Biant LC, Vijayan S, Macmull S, Skinner JA, Carrington RW (2012) Minimum ten-year results of a prospective randomised study of autologous chondrocyte implantation versus mosaicplasty for symptomatic articular cartilage lesions of the knee. J Bone Joint Surg Br 94(4):504–509
10. Bentley G, Dowd G (1984) Current concepts of etiology and treatment of chondromalacia patellae. Clin Orthop 189:209–228

11. Bentley G, Greer RB 3rd (1971) Homotransplantation of isolated epiphyseal and articular cartilage chondrocytes into joint surfaces of rabbits. Nature 230(5293): 385–388
12. Bentley G, Smith AV, Mukerjhee R (1979) Isolated epiphyseal chondrocyte allografts into joint surfaces. Ann Rheum Dis 37:449–458
13. Bert JM (1993) Role of abrasion arthroplasty and debridement in the management of osteoarthritis of the knee. Rheum Dis Clin North Am 19:725–739
14. Brittberg M, Faxén E, Peterson L (1994) Carbon fiber scaffolds in the treatment of early knee osteoarthritis. A prospective 4-year follow-up of 37 patients. Clin Orthop Relat Res 307:155–164
15. Brittberg M, Lindahl A, Nilsson A, Ohlsson C, Isaksson O, Peterson L (1994) Treatment of deep cartilage defects in the knee with autologous chondrocyte transplantation. N Engl J Med 331(14):889–895
16. Brittberg M, Nilsson A, Lindahl A, Ohlsson C, Peterson L (1996) Rabbit articular cartilage defects treated with autologous cultured chondrocytes. Clin Orthop Relat Res 326:270–283
17. Brooks PJ (1994) Role of osteochondral transplantation in the treatment of joint surface defects. Sports Med Arthrosc Rev 2:59–64
18. Buckwalter JA, Lohmander S (1994) Operative treatment of osteoarthritis: current practice and future development. J Bone Joint Surg 76A:1405–1418
19. Buckwalter JA, Mow VC (1994) Cartilage repair in osteoarthritis. In: Moskowitz RW, Howell DS, Goldberg VM, Mankin HJ (eds) Osteoarthritis. Diagnosis and medical/ surgical management, 2nd edn. WB Saunders Company, Philadelphia, pp 71–108
20. Burman MS, Finkelstein H, Mayer L (1934) Arthroscopy of the knee joint. J Bone Joint Surg 16:255–268
21. Carmont MR, Carey-Smith R, Saithna A, Dhillon M, Thompson P, Spalding T (2009) Delayed incorporation of a TruFit plug: perseverance is recommended. Arthroscopy 25(7):810–814
22. Chestermann PJ, Smith AU (1968) Homotransplantation of articular cartilage and isolated chondrocytes. J Bone Joint Surg 50B:184–197
23. Cole BJ, Farr J, Winalski CS, Hosea T, Richmond J, Mandelbaum B, De Deyne PG (2011) Outcomes after a single-stage procedure for cell-based cartilage repair: a prospective clinical safety trial with 2-year follow-up. Am J Sports Med 39(6):1170–1179
24. Dandy D (1992) Chondral and osteochondral lesions of the femoral condyle. In: Aichroth PM, Dilworth Cannon W, Patel DV (eds) Knee surgery. Current practice. Martin Dunitz, London, pp 443–449
25. Dandy D (1987) Arthroscopic management of the knee, 2nd edn. Churchill Livingstone, Edinburgh, p 191
26. de Windt TS, Concaro S, Lindahl A, Saris DB, Brittberg M (2012) Strategies for patient profiling in articular cartilage repair of the knee: a prospective cohort of patients treated by one experienced cartilage surgeon. Knee Surg Sports Traumatol Arthrosc 20(11): 2225–2232
27. Engkvist O (1979) Reconstruction of patellar articular cartilage with free autologous perichondrial grafts. Scand J Plast Reconstr Surg 13:361–369
28. Engkvist O, Johansson SH (1980) Perichondral arthroplasty: a clinical study in twenty-six patients. Scand J Plast Reconstr Surg 14:71–87
29. Engkvist O, Ohlsén L (1979) Reconstruction of articular cartilage with free autologous perichondral grafts. An experimental study in rabbits. Scand J Plast Reconstr Surg 13:269–274
30. Elves MW (1974) A study of the transplantation antigenes on chondrocytes from articular cartilage. J Bone Joint Surg 56B:178–185
31. Ficat RP, Ficat C, Gedeon PK, Toussaint JB (1979) Spongialization: a new treatment for diseased patellae. Clin Orthop 144:74–83
32. Friedman MJ, Berasi DO, Fox JM, del Pizzo W, Snyder SJ, Ferkel RD (1984) Preliminary results with abrasion arthroplasty in the osteoarthritic knee. Clin Orthop 182:200–206
33. Goldberg VM, Caplan AI (1994) Cellular repair of articular cartilage. In: Kuettner KE, Goldberg VM (eds) Osteoarthritic disorders. American Academy of Orthopedic Surgery, Monterrey, pp 357–364
34. Grande DA, Pitman MI, Peterson L, Menche D, Klein M (1989) The repair of experimentally produced defects in rabbit articular cartilage by autologous chondrocyte transplantation. J Orthop Res 7:208–218
35. Green WT (1977) Articular cartilage repair, behaviour of rabbit chondrocytes during tissue culture and subsequent allografting. Clin Orthop 124:237–250
36. Gross AE, Kim W, Las Heras F, Backstein D, Safir O, Pritzker KP (2008) Fresh osteochondral allografts for posttraumatic knee defects: long-term follow-up. Clin Orthop Relat Res 466(8):1863–1870
37. Haggart GE (1941) Surgical treatment of degenerative arthritis of the knee joint. J Bone Joint Surg 22B:717
38. Haleem AM, Singergy AA, Sabry D, Atta HM, Rashed LA, Chu CR, El Shewy MT, Azzam A, Abdel Aziz MT (2010) The clinical use of human culture-expanded autologous bone marrow mesenchymal stem cells transplanted on platelet-rich fibrin glue in the treatment of articular cartilage defects: a pilot study and preliminary results. Cartilage 1(4): 253–261
39. Hangody L, Kárpáti Z (1994) New possibilities in the management of severe circumscribed cartilage damage in the knee. Magy Traumatol Ortop Kezseb Plasztikai Seb 37(3):237–243
40. Hoemann CD, Hurtig M, Rossomacha E, Sun J, Chevrier A, Shive MS, Buschmann MD (2005) Chitosan-glycerol phosphate/blood implants improve hyaline cartilage repair in ovine microfracture defects. J Bone Joint Surg Am 87(12):2671–2686
41. Hoikka VEJ, Jaroma HJ, Ritsilä VA (1990) Reconstruction of the patellar articulation with periosteal grafts. Acta Orthop Scand 61:36–39
42. Homminga G, Bulstra SK, Bouwmeester PSM, van der Linden AJ (1990) Perichondral grafting for

cartilage lesions of the knee. J Bone Joint Surg 72B:1003–1007
43. Insall J (1974) The Pridie debridement operation for osteoarthritis of the knee joint. Clin Orthop 101:61–67
44. Johnson LL (1986) Arthroscopic abrasion arthroplasty. Historical and pathologic perspective: present status. Arthroscopy 2:54–59
45. Kawabe N, Yoshinao M (1991) The repair of full thickness articular cartilage defects. Immune responses to reparative tissue formed by allogeneic growth plate chondrocyte implants. Clin Orthop 268:279–293
46. Knutsen G, Drogset JO, Engebretsen L, Grøntvedt T, Isaksen V, Ludvigsen TC, Roberts S, Solheim E, Strand T, Johansen O (2007) A randomized trial comparing autologous chondrocyte implantation with microfracture. Findings at five years. J Bone Joint Surg Am 89(10):2105–2112
47. Knutsen G, Engebretsen L, Ludvigsen TC, Drogset JO, Grøntvedt T, Solheim E, Strand T, Roberts S, Isaksen V, Johansen O (2004) Autologous chondrocyte implantation compared with microfracture in the knee. A randomized trial. J Bone Joint Surg Am 86-A(3):455–464
48. Kon M, de Visser AC (1981) A poly(HEMA) sponge for restoration of articular cartilage defects. Plast Reconstr Surg 67(3):288–294
49. Kon E, Delcogliano M, Filardo G, Busacca M, Di Martino A, Marcacci M (2011) Novel nano-composite multilayered biomaterial for osteochondral regeneration: a pilot clinical trial. Am J Sports Med 39(6):1180–1190
50. Kon E, Filardo G, Berruto M, Benazzo F, Zanon G, Della Villa S, Marcacci M (2011) Articular cartilage treatment in high-level male soccer players: a prospective comparative study of arthroscopic second-generation autologous chondrocyte implantation versus microfracture. Am J Sports Med 39(12):2549–2557
51. Korkkala O, Hukkanen H (1991) Autogenous osteo-periosteal grafts in the reconstruction of full thickness joint surface defects. Int Orthop 15:233–237
52. Kreuz PC, Erggelet C, Steinwachs MR, Krause SJ, Lahm A, Niemeyer P, Ghanem N, Uhl M, Südkamp N (2006) Is microfracture of chondral defects in the knee associated with different results in patients aged 40 years or younger? Arthroscopy 22(11): 1180–1186
53. Kwan MK, Woo SL-Y, Amiel D et al (1987) Neocartilage generated from rib perichondrium: a long-term multidisciplinary evaluation. Trans Orthop Res Soc 12:277
54. Langer FL, Czitrom AA, Pritzker KPH, Gross AE (1975) The immunogenicity of fresh and frozen allogeneic bone. J Bone Joint Surg 57A:216
55. Langer F, Gross AE (1974) The immunogenicity of allograft articular cartilage. J Bone Joint Surg 56A:297–304
56. Macmull S, Jaiswal PK, Bentley G, Skinner JA, Carrington RW, Briggs TW (2012) The role of autologous chondrocyte implantation in the treatment of symptomatic chondromalacia patellae. Int Orthop 36: 1371–1377
57. Magnuson PB (1941) Joint debridement, surgical treatment of degenerative arthritis. Surg Gynecol Obstet 73:1–9
58. Mahomed MN, Beaver RJ, Gross AE (1992) The long-term success of fresh, small-fragment osteochondral allografts used for intra-articular post-traumatic defects in the knee joint. Orthopaedics 15:1191–1199
59. Mankin HJ, Fogelson FS, Trasher A (1976) Massive resection and allograft transplantation in the treatment of malignant tumours. N Engl J Med 294:1247–1255
60. Matsusue Y, Yamamuro T, Hiromichi H (1993) Case report. Arthroscopic multiple osteochondral transplantation to the chondral defect in the knee associated with anterior cruciate ligament disruption. Arthroscopy 9:318–321
61. McDermott AG, Langer F, Pritzker KP, Gross AE (1985) Fresh small-fragment osteochondral allografts. Long-term follow-up study on first 100 cases. Clin Orthop Relat Res 197:96–102
62. Mithoefer K, McAdams T, Williams RJ, Kreuz PC, Mandelbaum BR (2009) Clinical efficacy of the microfracture technique for articular cartilage repair in the knee: an evidence-based systematic analysis. Am J Sports Med 37(10):2053–2063
63. Minas T (2001) Autologous chondrocyte implantation for focal chondral defects of the knee. Clin Orthop Relat Res 391(Suppl):S349–S361
64. Muller W (1978) Osteochondritis dissecans. In: Hastings DW (ed) Progress in orthopaedics surgery. Springer, New York, p 135
65. Niedermann B, Boe S, Lauritzen J, Rubak JM (1985) Glued periosteal grafts in the knee. Acta Orthop Scand 56:457–460
66. Noguchi T, Oka M, Fujino M, Neo M, Yamamuro T (1994) Repair of osteochondral defects with grafts of cultured chondrocytes. Comparison of allografts and isografts. Clin Orthop 302:251–258
67. O'Driscoll SW, Keeley FW (1988) Durability of regenerated articular cartilage produced by free autogenous periosteal grafts in major full thickness defects in joint surfaces under the influence of continuous passive motion. J Bone Joint Surg 70A: 595–606
68. O'Driscoll SW, Keeley FW, Salter RB (1986) The chondrogeneic potential of free autogenous periosteal grafts for biological resurfacing of major full thickness defects in joint surfaces under the influence of continuous passive motion. J Bone Joint Surg 68A:1017–1035
69. O'Driscoll SW, Salter RB (1984) The induction of neochondrogenesis in free intra-articular periosteal autografts under the influence of continuous passive motion. J Bone Joint Surg 66A:1248–1257
70. Outerbridge HK, Outerbridge AR, Outerbridge RE (1995) The use of lateral patellar autologous graft for the repair of a large osteochondral defect in the knee. J Bone Joint Surg 77A:65–72

71. Pascaldi P, Engkvist O (1979) Perichondrial wrist arthroplasty in rheumatoid patients. Hand 11:184–190
72. Panseri S, Russo A, Cunha C, Bondi A, Di Martino A, Patella S, Kon E (2011) Osteochondral tissue engineering approaches for articular cartilage and subchondral bone regeneration. Knee Surg Sports Traumatol Arthrosc 20(6):1182–1191
73. Peterson L, Brittberg M, Kiviranta I, Akerlund EL, Lindahl A (2002) Autologous chondrocyte transplantation. Biomechanics and long-term durability. Am J Sports Med 30(1):2–12
74. Peterson L, Menche D, Grande D, Pitman M (1984) Chondrocyte transplantation; an experimental model in the rabbit. In: Transactions from the 30th annual meeting Orthopaedic Research Society, Atlanta, 7–9 Feb 1984. Palatine III, Orthopaedic Research Society, p 218
75. Peterson L, Minas T, Brittberg M, Nilsson A, Sjögren-Jansson E, Lindahl A (2000) Two- to 9-year outcome after autologous chondrocyte transplantation of the knee. Clin Orthop Relat Res 374:212–234
76. Peterson L, Vasiliadis HS, Brittberg M, Lindahl A (2010) Autologous chondrocyte implantation: a long-term follow-up. Am J Sports Med 38(6):1117–1124
77. Poussa M, Rubak J, Ritsilä V (1981) Differentiation of the osteochondrogenic cells of the periosteum in chondrotrophic environment. Acta Orthop Scand 52:235–239
78. Pridie KH (1959) A method of resurfacing osteoarthritic knee joints. J Bone Joint Surg 41B:618–619
79. Radin EL, Rose RM (1986) Role of subchondral bone in the initiation and progression of cartilage damage. Clin Orthop Relat Res 213:34–40
80. Robinson D, Halperin N, Nevo Z (1989) Fate of allogeneic embryonal chick chondrocytes implanted orthotopically as determined by the host's age. Mech Ageing Dev 50:71–80
81. Rubak J (1982) Reconstruction of articular cartilage defects with free periosteal grafts. An experimental study. Acta Orthop Scand 53:175–180
82. Salisbury RB, Mc Mahon MR (1994) Joint debridement and abrasion arthroplasty for degenerative joint disease of the knee joint. In: Parisien SJ (ed) Current techniques in arthroscopy. Current Medicine, Philadelphia, pp 147–167
83. Seradge H, Kutz JA, Kleinert HE, Lister GD, Wolff TW, Atasoy E (1984) Perichondral resurfacing arthroplasty in the hand. J Hand Surg 9A:880–886
84. Skoog T, Ohlsén L, Sohn A (1972) Perichondral potential for cartilaginous regeneration. Scand J Plast Reconstr Surg 6:123–125
85. Smith AV (1965) Survival of frozen chondrocytes isolated from cartilage of adult animals. Nature 205:782–784
86. Sokoloff L (1974) Cell biology and the repair of articular cartilage. J Rheumatol 1:1–10
87. Steadman R (1992) Chondral defects in athletes. The 5th Annual Panther Sports Medicine symposium, Pittsburgh, pp 2–4
88. Steadman JR, Rodkey WG, Briggs KK, Rodrigo JJ (1999) The microfracture technic in the management of complete cartilage defects in the knee joint. Orthopade 28(1):26–32, German
89. Steadman JR, Briggs KK, Rodrigo JJ, Kocher MS, Gill TJ, Rodkey WG (2003) Outcomes of microfracture for traumatic chondral defects of the knee: average 11-year follow-up. Arthroscopy 19(5):477–484, Review
90. Stevenson S, Li XQ, Martin B (1991) The fate of cancellous and cortical bone after transplantation of fresh and frozen tissue-antigen-matched osteochondral allografts in dogs. J Bone Joint Surg 73A: 1143–1156
91. Suh JK, Scherping S, Marui T, Steadman JR, Woo S-LY (1995) Basic science of articular cartilage injury and repair. In: Sledge SL (ed) Operative techniques in sports medicine. Management of osteochondral injuries. WB Saunders Company, Philadelphia, pp 78–86
92. Tizzoni G (1878) Sulla istologica normale e patologica delle cartilagini ialini. Arch Sci Med 2:27–102
93. Vachon AM, McIlwraight CW, Keeley FW (1991) Biochemical study of repair of induced osteochondral defects of the distal portion of the radial carpal bone in horses by use of periosteal autografts. Am J Vet Res 52:328–332
94. Vachon AM, McIlwright CW, Trotter GW, Nordin RW, Powers BE (1989) Neochondrogenesis in free intra-articular, periosteal and perichondrial autografts in horses. Am J Vet Res 50:1787–1794
95. Vanlauwe J, Saris DB, Victor J, Almqvist KF, Bellemans J, Luyten FP, TIG/ACT/01/2000&EXT Study Group (2011) Five-year outcome of characterized chondrocyte implantation versus microfracture for symptomatic cartilage defects of the knee: early treatment matters. Am J Sports Med 39(12):2566–2574
96. Wagner H (1964) Operative behandlung der osteochondrosis dissecans der kniegelenkes. Z Orthop 98:333–355
97. Wakitani S, Goto T, Pineda SJ, Toung RG, Mansour JM, Caplan AI, Goldberg VM (1994) Mesenchymal cell-based repair of large, full thickness defects of articular cartilage. J Bone Joint Surg 76A:579–592
98. Yoshihashi Y (1983) Tissue reconstitution by isolated articular chondrocytes in vitro. Nihon Seikeigeka Gakkai Zasshi 57:629–641
99. Zukor DJ, Gross AE (1989) Osteochondral allograft reconstruction of the knee. Part 1: a review. Am J Knee Surg 2:139–149

Articular Cartilage: Histology and Physiology

2

Chan Kwon Jung

Contents

C.K. Jung, MD, PhD
Department of Hospital Pathology,
College of Medicine,
The Catholic University of Korea,
Seoul 137-701, Republic of Korea

2.1 Cartilage

Adult cartilage lacks blood vessels, lymphatics, and nerves and has three types: hyaline cartilage, fibrocartilage, and elastic cartilage. Hyaline cartilage is the most widespread cartilage and found in the nose, larynx, trachea, bronchus, ribs, and articular surfaces of bones. The surface of hyaline cartilage is surrounded by the perichondrium, a transitional zone between cartilage and the surrounding connective tissue, but articular cartilage lacks the perichondrium. The perichondrium consists of two layers: an outermost fibrous layer and the innermost chondrogenic cell layer. Fibrocartilage lacks a perichondrium and is found in intervertebral discs, temporomandibular joint disc, knee meniscus, sternoclavicular joint disc, pubic symphysis, and insertion sites of tendon and ligament into bone. The fibrocartilage has great tensile strength. Elastic cartilage is covered by the perichondrium and found in the external ear, auditory tube, and epiglottis. The specialized matrix of the elastic cartilage has flexibility and the ability to retain its original shape after an applied force.

2.2 Articular Cartilage

Articular surfaces, at the ends of the long bones, are covered by hyaline cartilage. The articular cartilage is the highly specialized connective tissue that provides a lubricated surface for movable joints and facilitates the load transmission

A.A. Shetty et al. (eds.), *Techniques in Cartilage Repair Surgery*,
DOI 10.1007/978-3-642-41921-8_2, © ESSKA 2014

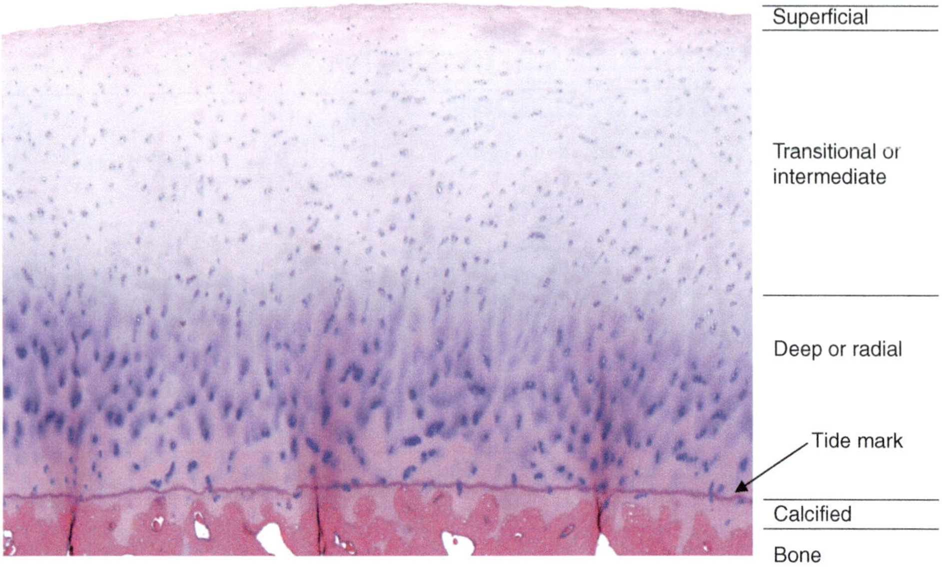

Fig. 2.1 A section of a normal articular surface shows four zones of articular cartilage: superficial, transitional (intermediate), deep (radial), and calcified zone. Tidemark is a distinct basophilic line which separates the deep zone from the calcified zone

and distribution with a low coefficient of friction. The hyaline cartilage consists of chondrocytes, type 2 collagen, and extracellular matrix including water, proteoglycans, glycoproteins, and lipids [1]. Chondrocytes contain glycogen, lipids, a well-developed RER, and Golgi apparatus and synthesize fibers and extracellular matrix. Chondrocytes occupy small spaces within the extracellular matrix called lacunae. Each lacuna is usually occupied by a single chondrocyte, but it may contain two or more cells.

As articular cartilage is avascular, alymphatic, and aneural tissue, oxygen and nutrients are supplied to the chondrocytes by diffusion predominantly from the synovial fluid [2]. Articular cartilage thickness and cell density varies from joint to joint, and in humans it is thickest over ends of femur and tibia, ranging from 2 to 4 mm.

Articular cartilage has four horizontal layers based on the cell morphology and structure of the extracellular matrix: the superficial, transitional, deep, and calcified cartilage zones (Fig. 2.1) [1, 3]. The arrangement of chondrocytes and collagen fibers varies among the layers. Cell density is highest at the superficial layer and decreases with increasing distance from the articular surface [2].

- Superficial or tangential layer: It is responsible for sliding movement and lubrication and makes up about 10–20 % of the articular cartilage. This zone has two collagen layers: thin fibrillary lamina splendens without cells and cellular layer with flattened chondrocytes. The most superficial part (lamina splendens) consists of a sheet of small fibrils with no chondrocytes, and the fine fibrils are arranged parallel to the articular surface. The cellular layer consists of small flattened chondrocytes and collagen fibers orientated tangentially to the articular surface. The proteoglycan content is lowest.
- Transitional, intermediate, or middle layer: It is responsible for transition between the shearing forces of superficial layer and compression forces in the layers, makes up 40–60 % of the cartilage, and is composed of slightly larger, round chondrocytes surrounded by extracellular matrix. The collagen fibers are thick and arranged randomly, and the proteoglycan content is highest. The chondrocytes are spherical.

- Deep, radial, or radiate layer: It makes up approximately 30 % of the articular cartilage and responsible for distribution of loads and resistance of compression. Large chondrocytes are usually grouped in radial columns and arranged perpendicular to the surface. The cell density is lowest among four layers. Collagen fibrils are arranged perpendicular to the articular surface. This zone contains the highest content of proteoglycan and the lowest content of water.
- Layer of calcified cartilage: The calcified zone is clearly separated from the deep zone by a tidemark (Fig. 2.1). It is responsible for bone anchorage and composed of round chondrocytes located in uncalcified lacunae. The collagen fibrils are arranged perpendicular to the articular surface. Collagen fibrils penetrate from the deep zone through calcified cartilage into subchondral bone.

2.3 Chondrocytes

Chondrocytes vary in shape, number, and size depending on the location of the articular cartilage. They are round or polygonal but flattened in the superficial zone. Chondrocytes synthesize and maintain the extracellular matrix.

2.4 Extracellular Matrix Zone

The extracellular matrix consists of the pericellular, territorial, and interterritorial regions based on proximity to the chondrocytes, different matrix composition, collagen fibril diameter, collagen fibril orientation, and noncollagenous protein content and organization.

Pericellular matrix is a thin rim of the matrix closest to chondrocytes and entirely surrounds chondrocytes. It is rich in proteoglycans and noncollagenous proteins and also contains nonfibrillar collagen type VI.

Territorial matrix envelops the pericellular matrix and is present throughout the articular cartilage. It surrounds a cluster of chondrocytes or isolated chondrocytes (Fig. 2.2). The collagen fibrils are arranged in a crisscross pattern surrounding chondrocytes.

Interterritorial matrix makes up more than 90 % and is not integrated with chondrocytes. Chondrocytes in the transitional and deep layers of the articular cartilage are well integrated with their territorial matrices (Fig. 2.2). The interterritorial matrix has collagen fibrils of greater diameter than the territorial matrix. The collagen fibrils are oriented parallel to the articular surface in the superficial zone, randomly in the transitional zone, and perpendicular in the deep zone.

Wet weight of cartilage contains mainly water (60–80 %) and macromolecules (20–40 %) including collagens, proteoglycans, and noncollagenous proteins. Collagens contribute 50–60 % of the dry weight of cartilage, and proteoglycans contribute 30 % of the dry weight.

2.5 Proteoglycans

Proteoglycans are macromolecules and composed of a protein core and glycosaminoglycan carbohydrate chains covalently attached to this core. These chains may be composed of more than 100 monosaccharides and extend out from the protein core. Proteoglycans contain a lot of negative charges that attract positively charged sodium ions, so the high osmotic pressure attracts water molecules between the proteoglycan aggregates [4].

2.6 Water

Water is the most abundant component of articular cartilage (65–80 %) [4]. The proteoglycan aggregates are swollen by the water and enable cartilage to withstand compressive loads. The majority of water is contained within the intrafibrillar space made by the collagen and proteoglycan matrix, and small percentage is contained within the intracellular space and the pore space of the matrix [3].

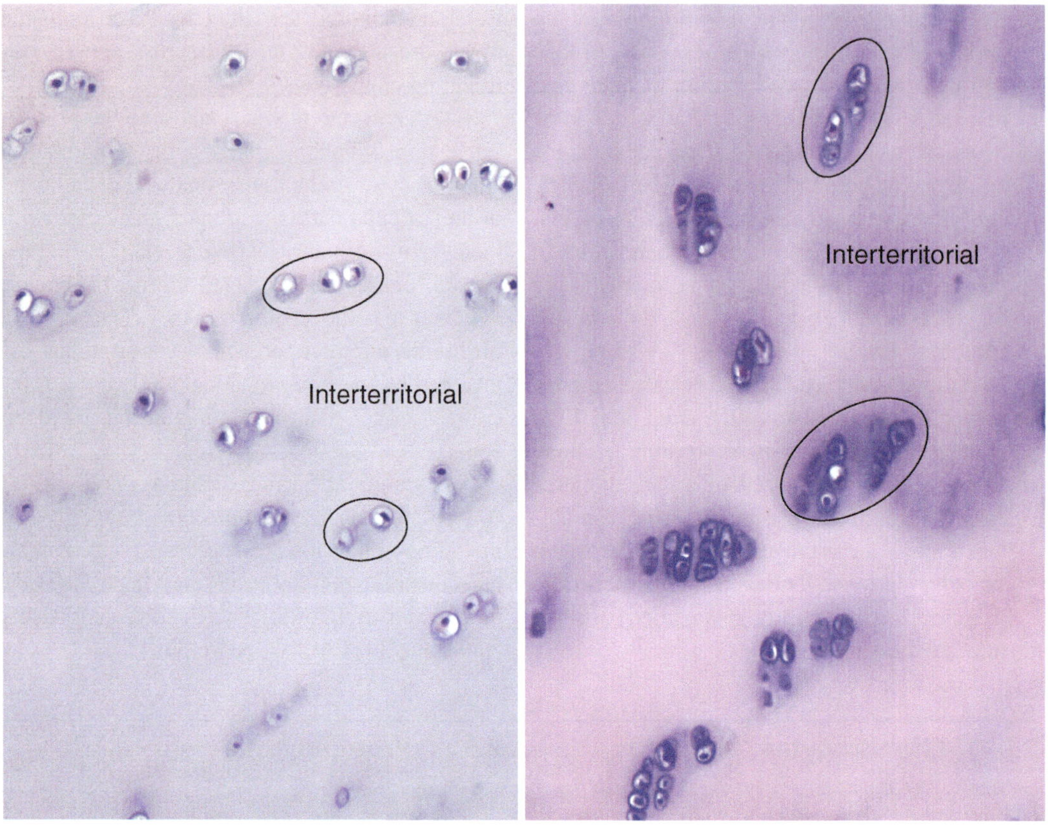

Fig. 2.2 Encircled areas representatively show the territorial matrix of the transitional (*left*) and deep (*right*) zones of articular cartilage. The interterritorial matrix lying between the territorial matrices is the matrix that is not integrated with any chondrocyte

2.7 Collagens

The solid component of articular cartilage is composed predominantly of collagen fibril networks intertwined with proteoglycan aggregates. At least 14 types of collagen have been identified, but type II collagen represents 90–95 % of the collagen fibrils [3].

2.8 Noncollagenous Proteins and Glycoproteins

These molecules appear to play a role in the organization and maintenance of the macromolecular structure of the extracellular matrix and in response to arthritis and osteoarthritis although their specific function has not been fully understood [1, 3].

2.9 Cartilage Degeneration

Cartilage in osteoarthritis shows softening, fibrillation, erosion, and ulceration grossly. Microscopical features of osteoarthritis include cartilage clefts and breakdown, loss of the cartilage layers, necrosis, chondrocyte cloning, and a duplication of the tidemark (Fig. 2.3) [5].

2.10 Cartilage Regeneration

As cartilage is avascular and aneural, articular cartilage lacks the intrinsic ability to regenerate completely after injury or disease to loss of tissue and formation of a defect. Thus, damaged cartilage is not replaced with functional tissue.

Many techniques including marrow stimulation and cartilage replacement with allograft or

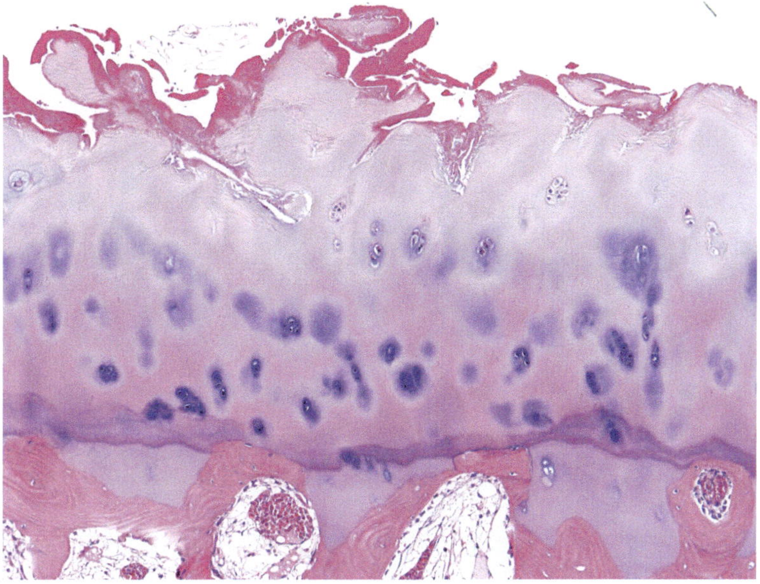

Fig. 2.3 The degenerated articular cartilage shows surface fibrillation, fissuring, clefts, and thinning of the layers

autograft have been used for cartilage repair, but none of them has been able to heal the damaged cartilage completely [6, 7].

References

1. Huber M, Trattnig S, Lintner F (2000) Anatomy, biochemistry, and physiology of articular cartilage. Invest Radiol 35(10):573–580
2. Zhou S, Cui Z, Urban JP (2004) Factors influencing the oxygen concentration gradient from the synovial surface of articular cartilage to the cartilage-bone interface: a modeling study. Arthritis Rheum 50(12):3915–3924
3. Sophia Fox AJ, Bedi A, Rodeo SA (2009) The basic science of articular cartilage: structure, composition, and function. Sports Health 1(6):461–468
4. Pearle AD, Warren RF, Rodeo SA (2005) Basic science of articular cartilage and osteoarthritis. Clin Sports Med 24(1):1–12
5. Mankin HJ (1982) The response of articular cartilage to mechanical injury. J Bone Joint Surg Am 64(3):460–466
6. Huey DJ, Hu JC, Athanasiou KA (2012) Unlike bone, cartilage regeneration remains elusive. Science 338(6109):917–921
7. Marcacci M, Filardo G, Kon E (2013) Treatment of cartilage lesions: what works and why? Injury 44(Suppl 1):S11–S15

Treatment Algorithm for Articular Cartilage Repair of the Knee: Towards Patient Profiling Using Evidence-Based Tools

3

Tommy S. de Windt and Daniel B.F. Saris

Contents

T.S. de Windt, MD
Department of Orthopaedics,
University Medical Center Utrecht,
85000, 3508, GA Utrecht, The Netherlands
e-mail: t.s.dewindt@umcutrecht.nl

D.B.F. Saris, MD, PhD (✉)
Department of Orthopaedics,
University Medical Center Utrecht,
85000, 3508, GA Utrecht, The Netherlands

Reconstructive Medicine, MIRA Institute
for Technical Medicine and Biomedical Engineering,
University of Twente, Enschede, The Netherlands
e-mail: d.saris@umcutrecht.nl

Abbreviations

ACI Autologous chondrocyte implantation
AMZ Anteromedialization
MF Microfracture
OA Osteoarthritis
OAT Osteochondral autologous transplantation

3.1 Introduction

The management of patients with articular cartilage defects continues to pose significant challenges to orthopedic surgeons worldwide. The evolution in diagnostic and treatment modalities or "technovolution" [15, 50] in cartilage repair of the last decade as well as the increase in physical demands has rapidly increased the number of patients seeking a solution for their cartilage defect. The challenge for physicians lies in the decision-making process where timing and selection of the procedure are of paramount importance. Current cartilage repair techniques include

A.A. Shetty et al. (eds.), *Techniques in Cartilage Repair Surgery*,
DOI 10.1007/978-3-642-41921-8_3, © ESSKA 2014

nonoperative strategies; debridement; marrow stimulation methods such as microfracture (MF), drilling, and abrasion; and transplantation methods such as autologous chondrocyte implantation (ACI) and osteochondral autologous or allograft transplantation [6]. In clinical practice, these techniques are selected based on algorithms that are derived from previous (randomized controlled) trials and long-term cohort studies. However, strong (comparative) evidence to support one single algorithm is lacking [9, 19, 34]. Furthermore, there is a variance in treatment selection between different expert centers based on healthcare availability and surgeon preference. Taking this into account, it is difficult for the surgeon to make an evidence-based decision for the individual patient. This chapter seeks to explore the current evidence for treatment selection and provides tools for daily clinical practice as well as an updated comprehensive evidence-based treatment algorithm.

3.2 General Indications and Contraindications for Cartilage Repair

When assessing a patient suspected of having a cartilage defect, identifying concomitant knee (ligament) injuries is crucial as subsequent treatment of these injuries may provide symptom relief and improve the joint homeostasis [67]. Furthermore, symptoms following knee injury may not be related to the cartilage defect. Nonoperative treatment including physiotherapy and anti-inflammatory medication (NSAIDS) along with (sports) activity and dietary modification can be considered as primary treatment options, especially for smaller defects with normal joint function and limited physical demands [75]. However patients are frequently referred to specialized centers with long-standing complaints, and symptom to treatment delay is known to negatively influence treatment outcome [16, 45, 56, 76]. In fact, the average patient suitable for cartilage repair had 2.1 prior treatments which again are potential impediments for clinical outcome [21, 36, 64]. Therefore, careful interpretation of a patient's history and early and accurate diagnostics are needed before determining the treatment modality of choice. Furthermore, body mass index, mechanical alignment, occupation, sports participation, responsiveness, and rehabilitation are important factors to take into consideration in the decision-making process [14]. Patients with degenerative joints, particularly older patients, can be treated with steroid injections, viscosupplementation, and physiotherapy. Of these, patients with a desire to maintain certain (sport) activities can be counselled in terms of expectations to decide whether or not a salvage procedure and subsequent rehabilitation program is viable. In general, surgery should be reserved for patients with grade III to IV full-thickness cartilage defects where conservative treatment has failed or has a limited probability of success. In these, timing of surgery should be considered an important parameter. Obesity, smoking, and meniscal and/or ligamentous injury are relative contraindications, although strong supporting evidence is lacking [25].

3.3 Indicators for Treatment

3.3.1 Defect Size

Once an (osteo)chondral defect has been identified, the current literature suggests (postdebridement) defect size to be an important indicator for treatment selection. In randomized controlled trials comparing autologous transplantations with MF, both Knutsen et al. and Gudas et al. found inferior clinical outcome after MF for defects larger than 4 and 2 cm^2, respectively [29, 39]. This was corroborated by prospective studies of Asik et al., Mithoefer et al., and Steadman et al. who found similar size thresholds that reduced clinical outcome of MF after a mean of 2–11 years [2, 56, 72]. Fortunately, the clinical outcome after ACI or osteochondral autologous transplantation (OAT) has not been found to correspond to defect size. However, defects greater than 4 cm^2 seem to respond better to ACI than

OAT [10]. In a more recent randomized controlled trial, the histological and functional outcomes of ACI were also significantly better than those for MF in defects averaged 2.5 cm^2 [68]. Although a single size threshold is difficult to identify, the literature suggests that defects greater than 2–3 cm^2 should be treated with more complex transplantation procedures, and MF nor other treatments are useful in defects larger than 4 cm^2. Indeed, one systematic review concluded that defects larger than 2.5 cm^2 should be treated with ACI or OAT [7]. Here, again, individual decision making is considered to be important as relative defect size and depth (i.e., in comparison to the femoral condyle) and the extent to which the local homeostasis has been disturbed vary between patients [67].

3.3.2 Age

A variety of studies reported that patients under 30 years of age benefit more from cartilage repair in terms of clinical outcome when compared to older patients [2, 16, 38, 43]. Conversely, a recent randomized controlled trial in patients aged 18–50 years did not find correlation between age and clinical outcome [76]. In fact, several other studies did not find correlation between age and treatment success [17, 23, 65]. One study demonstrated low failure rates in patients 45 years and older, while another study showed no difference in clinical outcome after ACI in patients 40 years and older compared to younger patients [40, 60]. Overall, there is insufficient and inconclusive data to support age as primary indicator for treatment selection.

3.3.3 Patient Activity

Patient activity can be considered an important indicator for treatment selection in cartilage repair. A randomized controlled trial demonstrated that more active patients (as indicated by the Tegner score) achieved superior clinical results, regardless of treatment type [38]. In a 5-year follow-up study, Kon et al. found ACI to be more durable in terms of (sport related) activity compared to MF [41]. The superior histomorphometric and histologic scores found for ACI compared to MF and a higher return to sports rate further suggest ACI to be a better option for active patients [54, 68]. Interestingly, deterioration in sports activity has been observed after MF, possibly due to poor repair morphology, defect fill, and peripheral integration [54]. Nevertheless, MF has been found to be effective in different high-impact (professional) sports such as American football and soccer [56, 73].

3.4 Treatment Selection for Patients with Smaller Defects

Debridement can be considered as initial treatment for defects <2 cm^2 in less demanding patients especially for defects found incidentally during arthroscopy and in mild to moderate osteoarthritis (OA) [1, 66]. Randomized controlled trials in patients with OA have shown that arthroscopic debridement has no advantage over optimal physical and medical care [37, 58]. Although debridement of small defects can provide symptom relief in terms of pain and catching and locking, the response to treatment of these defects as well as their natural history remains unpredictable [18, 22, 71]. Both MF and OAT are generally considered good options for smaller (<2–3 cm^2) defects. OAT may be indicated in deep osteochondral defects of up to 2 cm^2. In defects 2–3 cm^2, MF or ACI is usually preferred over OAT based on the possible risk of donor-site morbidity. However, the bone portion also influences treatment choice. Although strong supporting evidence is lacking, donor-site morbidity may lead to pain, tissue deterioration, and a decline in knee function [32, 46]. In contrast, in a case series following 112 patients, Paul et al. found no influence of the size or number of donor grafts on clinical outcome [63]. Concerning smaller defects, more complex procedures such as ACI are generally reserved for high demand and revision cases as marrow-stimulating techniques seem less reliable in these instances [17, 54].

3.5 Treatment Selection for Patients with Larger Defects

For larger (>3 cm^2) defects, both ACI and allograft transplantation have shown good to excellent results. As a randomized controlled comparison between these interventions is lacking, local availability and surgeon and patient preference will still largely determine the treatment of choice. For ACI, good to excellent clinical outcome has been reported up to 20 years in 70–90 % of patients with defects >3 cm^2 [25, 65]. An advantage of allograft transplantation might be that it permits treatment of relatively large defects, particularly when there is accompanying bone loss [25]. Shasha and colleagues found an 85 % femoral condylar graft survival rate at 10 years and a 65 % graft survival rate after failed tibial plateau fractures [28, 70]. Bugbee et al. demonstrated an 86 % success rate after allograft transplantation for unipolar defects averaged 8.2 cm^2 while 54 % of bipolar defects were rated good to excellent [13]. In like manner, Beaver et al. found a higher failure rate for bipolar defects [5]. Other factors that were reported to reduce clinical outcome after allograft transplantation include primary osteoarthritis and malalignment [6]. Interestingly, Ossendorf et al. recently demonstrated good midterm results after ACI in 51 patients with large and complex articular defects [61]. In their cohort, kissing lesions had similar results as single defects indicating that ACI might be a safer treatment modality for this category. If for larger defects deeper than 8–10 mm, allograft transplantation is not feasible, the ACI sandwich technique can be a viable option. Barlett et al. used a sandwich technique with two matrix-induced ACI (MACI) membranes and a bone graft in deep osteochondral defects (mean 5.2 cm^2, range 2.2–8.0) and found good to excellent 1-year results in all eight patients treated [4].

3.6 Treatment Selection for Patients with Defects in the Patellofemoral Joint

The limited healing capacity and the frequently occurring abnormalities in the extensor mechanism make defects in the patella a considerable challenge. For these defects, MF has been found to have limited effect on clinical outcome, deteriorating after 18–36 months [44]. OAT also seems less promising for patellar defects. Although Hangody et al. reported good results in 19 of 26 patients after OAT, patellofemoral defects had significant lower improvement than femoral defects [30]. Moreover, Bentley et al. reported failure of all five patients treated with OAT, possibly due to the difference in thickness of donor and recipient cartilage which can make healing and incorporation difficult [10]. Because of the difficult local topography and the risk of donor-site morbidity, allograft patellar resurfacing is preferred over OAT in patients with severe articular cartilage disease if available. Jamali et al. found a 72 % success rate in 18 such patients (mean age 42) treated with fresh osteochondral allografts after a mean of 8 years [35]. For isolated cartilage defects in the patellofemoral joint, clinical results seem to be improving in recent years, possibly due to the increase in experience with ACI and focus on the biomechanical shearing forces of the extensor mechanism [59]. Pascual-Garrido et al. reported significant short-term improvement in patients receiving ACI for defects (mean size 4.2 cm^2) in the patellofemoral joint [62]. The 50 % of patients who received a concomitant anteromedialization (AMZ) achieved statistically higher clinical scores. However, it remains difficult to compare the treatment effect of each individual procedure and a randomized trial for ACI with or without concomitant AZM is lacking. Nevertheless, a variety of reports have demonstrated success rates of 70–90 % for ACI with or without concomitant correction of the extensor mechanism [20, 24, 27, 31, 52, 77]. Others have shown no significant difference in clinical outcome after ACI compared to other locations supporting its use as primary treatment for defects in the patellofemoral joint [17, 69].

3.7 Early Osteoarthritic Defects and Salvage Repair

Early osteoarthritic defects are increasingly being recognized in younger active patients, creating a new challenging population for the orthopedic surgeon. Compared to OA, early OA is considered more difficult to diagnose as signs and symptoms may still be limited, often becoming manifest after higher strains during sport activities [47]. As standard measures for OA include temporary symptom relief or invasive joint replacement, cartilage repair procedures are increasingly being introduced in this population [26]. Bae et al. evaluated 44 patients with an average lesion size of 3.9 cm^2 with moderate osteoarthritic changes who underwent MF [3]. After a mean of 2.3 years, significant improvement in pain and daily living was seen. In addition, using second-look arthroscopy, defect filling was confirmed. Miller et al. and Steadman et al. evaluated MF for degenerative lesions and high-impact athletics, respectively, with satisfying clinical outcome and return to high-impact sports for more than five seasons [51, 74]. However, these studies were not aimed specifically at (early) OA. Brittberg et al. used drilling and subsequent carbon fiber scaffold implantation for treatment of early osteoarthritic defects in two separate cohorts with a short-term success rate of over 80 % in terms of pain and clinical outcome [11, 17]. Minas et al. reported on a large cohort consisting of 153 patients (mean age 38 years) with early OA treated with ACI and followed for up to 11 years [53]. At 5 years, 92 % of patients were functioning well, delaying the need for joint replacement. At final follow-up, eight percent of joints were considered failures while 50–75 % experienced significant improvement. Although limited clinical data are available, OAT has been implemented in early OA. Hangody et al. used OAT in 82 professional athletes with signs of OA. In this 17-year prospective study, similar success rates were found to that of less athletic patients, although high motivation resulted in better subjective evaluation [30]. Jakob et al. found good results in ten patients with patellofemoral OA treated with OAT [33]. Concomitant procedures for patellofemoral maltracking may be an important confounder. Könst et al. used autologous bone grafting combined with gel-type ACI (GACI) to treat 9 patients with severe osteochondral defects [42]. At 1-year follow-up, statistically significant improvement was demonstrated in eight patients with only one patient needing conversion to total knee arthroplasty (TKA).

3.8 Treatment Algorithm: Summarizing the Findings from the Literature

Although there is no strong evidence supporting a single treatment algorithm, the literature does provide tools for clinical decision making. In short, early diagnostics for cartilage defects and concomitant injuries are required as a disturbed joint homeostasis and treatment delay reduce clinical outcome. Defects smaller than 2.5 cm^2 respond well to MF and OAT, the latter being indicated in deeper osteochondral defects. For larger defects (>2.5 cm^2), ACI is generally the treatment of choice. Depending on availability and experience, (fresh) osteochondral allograft transplantation or the ACI sandwich technique can be used in large osteochondral defects. Cartilage repair procedures for treatment of (early) OA are still in their early phase, and an evidence-based algorithm is difficult to construct. As such, careful treatment selection is warranted, specifically in more advanced OA and younger patients. Current evidence suggests that TKA can be delayed with cartilage repair. Furthermore, the short-term results (up to 5 years) in patients with early osteoarthritic defects are promising [48]. Figure 3.1 provides a summary of the evidence-based treatment algorithm.

3.9 Addendum: Treatment Selection for (Professional) Athletes

The high impact and torsional loads subjected to the knee joint in (professional) athletes are an important cause of cartilage injury and

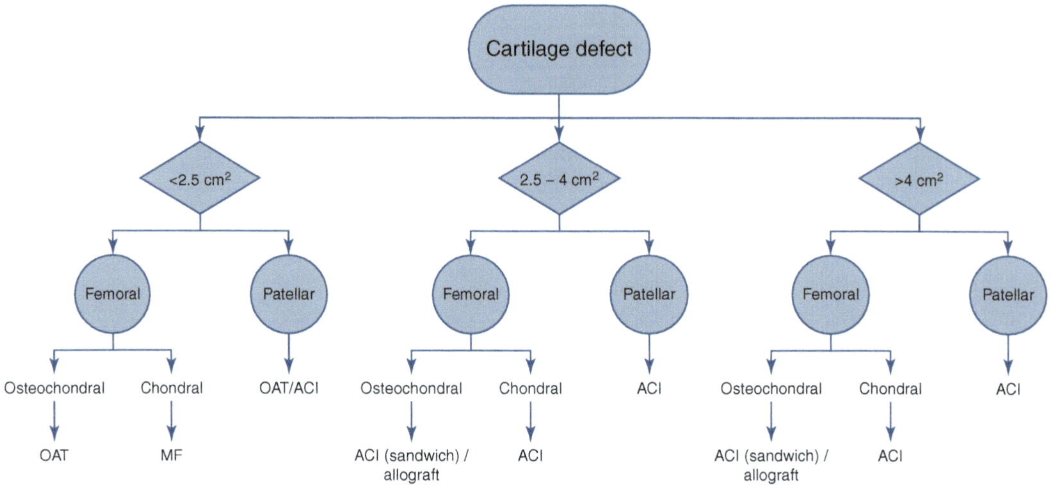

Fig. 3.1 Evidence-based treatment algorithm for articular cartilage repair of the knee

subchondral bone turnover [12]. This in turn may lead to functional disability and (early) OA during and after (professional) sports participation [55]. For professional soccer players and adolescent athletes, ACI resulted in higher functional improvement compared to MF [56, 57]. Indeed Mithoefer et al. showed a decline in sports participation after MF in 47 % of athletes while 87 % of patients treated with ACI remained at the pre-injury level [54]. OAT also showed superior clinical outcome in a randomized study among both professional and recreational athletes [29]. For defects larger than 2 cm^2, both MF and OAT showed significantly worse clinical outcome and a lower return to sports when compared to smaller defects [49, 56]. Although it seems ACI provides a more durable return to sports participation, especially in larger defects, the average time to return to sports is higher (18 months) compared to MF (8 months) and OAT (7 months). Therefore, in reviewing the literature for athletes, Bekkers et al. previously suggested to use OAT or MF as treatment of choice in defects smaller than 2 cm^2. If ACI is the treatment of choice, a surgical debridement of the traumatic defect with additional biopsy during the season and subsequent transplantation during the off-season might optimize professional sports participation [8].

Conclusion

Each patient should be assessed individually based on physical demands and expectations, concomitant injuries, previous treatments, symptom to treatment duration, as well as defect characteristics such as chronicity, location, size, and depth. Although age as such should not limit treatment selection, careful consideration in terms of patient expectations is warranted for patients older than 40 years. According to the available evidence, defect size seems to be a reliable primary indicator for treatment selection. Finally, based on this literature review, an extensive evidence-based treatment algorithm was created (Fig. 3.1).

References

1. Alford JW, Cole BJ (2005) Cartilage restoration, part 2: techniques, outcomes, and future directions. Am J Sports Med 33:443–460
2. Asik M, Ciftci F, Sen C, Erdil M, Atalar A (2008) The microfracture technique for the treatment of full-thickness articular cartilage lesions of the knee: mid-term results. Arthroscopy 24:1214–1220
3. Bae DK, Yoon KH, Song SJ (2006) Cartilage healing after microfracture in osteoarthritic knees. Arthroscopy 22:367–374
4. Bartlett W, Gooding CR, Carrington RW, Skinner JA, Briggs TW, Bentley G (2005) Autologous chondrocyte

implantation at the knee using a bilayer collagen membrane with bone graft. A preliminary report. J Bone Joint Surg Br 87:330–332
5. Beaver RJ, Mahomed M, Backstein D, Davis A, Zukor DJ, Gross AE (1992) Fresh osteochondral allografts for post-traumatic defects in the knee. A survivorship analysis. J Bone Joint Surg Br 74:105–110
6. Bedi A, Feeley BT, Williams RJ III (2010) Management of articular cartilage defects of the knee. J Bone Joint Surg Am 92:994–1009
7. Bekkers JE, Inklaar M, Saris DB (2009) Treatment selection in articular cartilage lesions of the knee: a systematic review. Am J Sports Med 37(Suppl 1): 148S–155S
8. Bekkers JEJ, de Windt T, Brittberg M, Saris DBF (2012) Cartilage repair in football (soccer) athletes. Cartilage 3:43S–49S
9. Benthien JP, Schwaninger M, Behrens P (2011) We do not have evidence based methods for the treatment of cartilage defects in the knee. Knee Surg Sports Traumatol Arthrosc 19:543–552
10. Bentley G, Biant LC, Carrington RW, Akmal M, Goldberg A, Williams AM, Skinner JA, Pringle J (2003) A prospective, randomised comparison of autologous chondrocyte implantation versus mosaicplasty for osteochondral defects in the knee. J Bone Joint Surg Br 85:223–230
11. Brittberg M, Faxen E, Peterson L (1994) Carbon fiber scaffolds in the treatment of early knee osteoarthritis. A prospective 4-year followup of 37 patients. Clin Orthop Relat Res 304:155–164
12. Buckwalter JA, Mankin HJ (1998) Articular cartilage: degeneration and osteoarthritis, repair, regeneration, and transplantation. Instr Course Lect 47:487–504
13. Bugbee WD, Convery FR (1999) Osteochondral allograft transplantation. Clin Sports Med 18:67–75
14. Cole BJ, Pascual-Garrido C, Grumet RC (2010) Surgical management of articular cartilage defects in the knee. Instr Course Lect 59:181–204
15. de Windt TS, Bekkers JE, Tsuchida A, Ouwerkerk J, Saris DB (2011) The technovolution of cartilage repair. Nederlands Tijdschrift voor Fysiotherapie 2:11–17
16. de Windt TS, Bekkers JE, Creemers LB, Dhert WJ, Saris DB (2009) Patient profiling in cartilage regeneration: prognostic factors determining success of treatment for cartilage defects. Am J Sports Med 37(Suppl 1):58S–62S
17. de Windt TS, Concaro S, Lindahl A, Saris DB, Brittberg M (2012) Strategies for patient profiling in articular cartilage repair of the knee: a prospective cohort of patients treated by one experienced cartilage surgeon. Knee Surg Sports Traumatol Arthrosc. doi:10.1007/:s00167-011-1855-8
18. Dozin B, Malpeli M, Cancedda R, Bruzzi P, Calcagno S, Molfetta L, Priano F, Kon E, Marcacci M (2005) Comparative evaluation of autologous chondrocyte implantation and mosaicplasty: a multicentered randomized clinical trial. Clin J Sport Med 15:220–226
19. Engen CN, Engebretsen L, Aroen A (2010) Knee cartilage defect patients enrolled in randomized controlled trials are not representative of patients in orthopedic practice. Cartilage 1:312–319
20. Farr J (2007) Autologous chondrocyte implantation improves patellofemoral cartilage treatment outcomes. Clin Orthop Relat Res 463:187–194
21. Filardo G, Kon E, Di MA, Iacono F, Marcacci M (2011) Arthroscopic second-generation autologous chondrocyte implantation: a prospective 7-year follow-up study. Am J Sports Med 39:2153–2160
22. Fu FH, Zurakowski D, Browne JE, Mandelbaum B, Erggelet C, Moseley JB Jr, Anderson AF, Micheli LJ (2005) Autologous chondrocyte implantation versus debridement for treatment of full-thickness chondral defects of the knee: an observational cohort study with 3-year follow-up. Am J Sports Med 33:1658–1666
23. Gille J, Schuseil E, Wimmer J, Gellissen J, Schulz AP, Behrens P (2010) Mid-term results of Autologous Matrix-Induced Chondrogenesis for treatment of focal cartilage defects in the knee. Knee Surg Sports Traumatol Arthrosc 18:1456–1464
24. Gobbi A, Kon E, Berruto M, Francisco R, Filardo G, Marcacci M (2006) Patellofemoral full-thickness chondral defects treated with Hyalograft-C: a clinical, arthroscopic, and histologic review. Am J Sports Med 34:1763–1773
25. Gomoll AH, Farr J, Gillogly SD, Kercher JS, Minas T (2011) Surgical management of articular cartilage defects of the knee. Instr Course Lect 60:461–483
26. Gomoll AH, Filardo G, de Girolamo L, Esprequeira-Mendes J, Marcacci M, Rodkey WG, Steadman RJ, Zaffagnini S, Kon E (2012) Surgical treatment for early osteoarthritis. Part I: cartilage repair procedures. Knee Surg Sports Traumatol Arthrosc 20:450–466
27. Gomoll AH, Minas T, Farr J, Cole BJ (2006) Treatment of chondral defects in the patellofemoral joint. J Knee Surg 19:285–295
28. Gross AE, Shasha N, Aubin P (2005) Long-term followup of the use of fresh osteochondral allografts for posttraumatic knee defects. Clin Orthop Relat Res 435:79–87
29. Gudas R, Simonaityte R, Cekanauskas E, Tamosiunas R (2009) A prospective, randomized clinical study of osteochondral autologous transplantation versus microfracture for the treatment of osteochondritis dissecans in the knee joint in children. J Pediatr Orthop 29:741–748
30. Hangody L, Dobos J, Balo E, Panics G, Hangody LR, Berkes I (2010) Clinical experiences with autologous osteochondral mosaicplasty in an athletic population: a 17-year prospective multicenter study. Am J Sports Med 38:1125–1133
31. Henderson IJ, Lavigne P (2006) Periosteal autologous chondrocyte implantation for patellar chondral defect in patients with normal and abnormal patellar tracking. Knee 13:274–279
32. Iwasaki N, Kato H, Kamishima T, Suenaga N, Minami A (2007) Donor site evaluation after autologous

osteochondral mosaicplasty for cartilaginous lesions of the elbow joint. Am J Sports Med 35:2096–2100
33. Jakob RP, Franz T, Gautier E, Mainil-Varlet P (2002) Autologous osteochondral grafting in the knee: indication, results, and reflections. Clin Orthop Relat Res 401:170–184
34. Jakobsen RB, Engebretsen L, Slauterbeck JR (2005) An analysis of the quality of cartilage repair studies. J Bone Joint Surg Am 87:2232–2239
35. Jamali AA, Emmerson BC, Chung C, Convery FR, Bugbee WD (2005) Fresh osteochondral allografts: results in the patellofemoral joint. Clin Orthop Relat Res 437:176–185
36. Jungmann PM, Salzmann GM, Schmal H, Pestka JM, Sudkamp NP, Niemeyer P (2012) Autologous chondrocyte implantation for treatment of cartilage defects of the knee: what predicts the need for reintervention? Am J Sports Med 40:58–67
37. Kirkley A, Birmingham TB, Litchfield RB, Giffin JR, Willits KR, Wong CJ, Feagan BG, Donner A, Griffin SH, D'Ascanio LM, Pope JE, Fowler PJ (2008) A randomized trial of arthroscopic surgery for osteoarthritis of the knee. N Engl J Med 359:1097–1107
38. Knutsen G, Drogset JO, Engebretsen L, Grontvedt T, Isaksen V, Ludvigsen TC, Roberts S, Solheim E, Strand T, Johansen O (2007) A randomized trial comparing autologous chondrocyte implantation with microfracture. Findings at five years. J Bone Joint Surg Am 89:2105–2112
39. Knutsen G, Engebretsen L, Ludvigsen TC, Drogset JO, Grontvedt T, Solheim E, Strand T, Roberts S, Isaksen V, Johansen O (2004) Autologous chondrocyte implantation compared with microfracture in the knee. A randomized trial. J Bone Joint Surg Am 86-A:455–464
40. Kon E, Filardo G, Condello V, Collarile M, Di MA, Zorzi C, Marcacci M (2011) Second-generation autologous chondrocyte implantation: results in patients older than 40 years. Am J Sports Med 39:1668–1675
41. Kon E, Gobbi A, Filardo G, Delcogliano M, Zaffagnini S, Marcacci M (2009) Arthroscopic second-generation autologous chondrocyte implantation compared with microfracture for chondral lesions of the knee: prospective nonrandomized study at 5 years. Am J Sports Med 37:33–41
42. Konst YE, Benink RJ, Veldstra R, van der Krieke TJ, Helder MN, van Royen BJ (2012) Treatment of severe osteochondral defects of the knee by combined autologous bone grafting and autologous chondrocyte implantation using fibrin gel. Knee Surg Sports Traumatol Arthrosc. doi:10.1007/:s00167-012-1891-z
43. Kreuz PC, Erggelet C, Steinwachs MR, Krause SJ, Lahm A, Niemeyer P, Ghanem N, Uhl M, Sudkamp N (2006) Is microfracture of chondral defects in the knee associated with different results in patients aged 40 years or younger? Arthroscopy 22:1180–1186
44. Kreuz PC, Steinwachs MR, Erggelet C, Krause SJ, Konrad G, Uhl M, Sudkamp N (2006) Results after microfracture of full-thickness chondral defects in different compartments in the knee. Osteoarthritis Cartilage 14:1119–1125
45. Krishnan SP, Skinner JA, Bartlett W, Carrington RW, Flanagan AM, Briggs TW, Bentley G (2006) Who is the ideal candidate for autologous chondrocyte implantation? J Bone Joint Surg Br 88:61–64
46. Laprade RF, Botker JC (2004) Donor-site morbidity after osteochondral autograft transfer procedures. Arthroscopy 20:e69–e73
47. Luyten FP, Denti M, Filardo G, Kon E, Engebretsen L (2012) Definition and classification of early osteoarthritis of the knee. Knee Surg Sports Traumatol Arthrosc 20:401–406
48. Luyten FP, Vanlauwe J (2012) Tissue engineering approaches for osteoarthritis. Bone 51:289–296
49. Marcacci M, Kon E, Zaffagnini S, Iacono F, Neri MP, Vascellari A, Visani A, Russo A (2005) Multiple osteochondral arthroscopic grafting (mosaicplasty) for cartilage defects of the knee: prospective study results at 2-year follow-up. Arthroscopy 21:462–470
50. Mastbergen SC, Saris DB, Lafeber FP (2013) Nat Rev Rheumatol 9(5):277–290
51. Miller BS, Steadman JR, Briggs KK, Rodrigo JJ, Rodkey WG (2004) Patient satisfaction and outcome after microfracture of the degenerative knee. J Knee Surg 17:13–17
52. Minas T, Bryant T (2005) The role of autologous chondrocyte implantation in the patellofemoral joint. Clin Orthop Relat Res 436:30–39
53. Minas T, Gomoll AH, Solhpour S, Rosenberger R, Probst C, Bryant T (2010) Autologous chondrocyte implantation for joint preservation in patients with early osteoarthritis. Clin Orthop Relat Res 468: 147–157
54. Mithoefer K, Hambly K, Della VS, Silvers H, Mandelbaum BR (2009) Return to sports participation after articular cartilage repair in the knee: scientific evidence. Am J Sports Med 37(Suppl 1):167S–176S
55. Mithoefer K, McAdams TR, Scopp JM, Mandelbaum BR (2009) Emerging options for treatment of articular cartilage injury in the athlete. Clin Sports Med 28: 25–40
56. Mithoefer K, Williams RJ III, Warren RF, Wickiewicz TL, Marx RG (2006) High-impact athletics after knee articular cartilage repair: a prospective evaluation of the microfracture technique. Am J Sports Med 34: 1413–1418
57. Mithofer K, Peterson L, Mandelbaum BR, Minas T (2005) Articular cartilage repair in soccer players with autologous chondrocyte transplantation: functional outcome and return to competition. Am J Sports Med 33:1639–1646
58. Moseley JB, O'Malley K, Petersen NJ, Menke TJ, Brody BA, Kuykendall DH, Hollingsworth JC, Ashton CM, Wray NP (2002) A controlled trial of arthroscopic surgery for osteoarthritis of the knee. N Engl J Med 347:81–88
59. Mouzopoulos G, Borbon C, Siebold R (2011) Patellar chondral defects: a review of a challenging entity. Knee Surg Sports Traumatol Arthrosc 19:1990–2001
60. Niemeyer P, Kostler W, Salzmann GM, Lenz P, Kreuz PC, Sudkamp NP (2010) Autologous chondrocyte

implantation for treatment of focal cartilage defects in patients age 40 years and older: a matched-pair analysis with 2-year follow-up. Am J Sports Med 38:2410–2416
61. Ossendorf C, Steinwachs MR, Kreuz PC, Osterhoff G, Lahm A, Ducommun PP, Erggelet C (2011) Autologous chondrocyte implantation (ACI) for the treatment of large and complex cartilage lesions of the knee. Sports Med Arthrosc Rehabil Ther Technol 3:11
62. Pascual-Garrido C, Slabaugh MA, L'Heureux DR, Friel NA, Cole BJ (2009) Recommendations and treatment outcomes for patellofemoral articular cartilage defects with autologous chondrocyte implantation: prospective evaluation at average 4-year follow-up. Am J Sports Med 37(Suppl 1):33S–41S
63. Paul J, Sagstetter A, Kriner M, Imhoff AB, Spang J, Hinterwimmer S (2009) Donor-site morbidity after osteochondral autologous transplantation for lesions of the talus. J Bone Joint Surg Am 91:1683–1688
64. Peterson L, Minas T, Brittberg M, Lindahl A (2003) Treatment of osteochondritis dissecans of the knee with autologous chondrocyte transplantation: results at two to ten years. J Bone Joint Surg Am 85-A(Suppl 2):17–24
65. Peterson L, Vasiliadis HS, Brittberg M, Lindahl A (2010) Autologous chondrocyte implantation: a long-term follow-up. Am J Sports Med 38:1117–1124
66. Salzmann GM, Niemeyer P, Steinwachs M, Kreuz PC, Sudkamp NP, Mayr HO (2011) Cartilage repair approach and treatment characteristics across the knee joint: a European survey. Arch Orthop Trauma Surg 131:283–291
67. Saris DB, Dhert WJ, Verbout AJ (2003) Joint homeostasis. The discrepancy between old and fresh defects in cartilage repair. J Bone Joint Surg Br 85:1067–1076
68. Saris DB, Vanlauwe J, Victor J, Almqvist KF, Verdonk R, Bellemans J, Luyten FP (2009) Treatment of symptomatic cartilage defects of the knee: characterized chondrocyte implantation results in better clinical outcome at 36 months in a randomized trial compared to microfracture. Am J Sports Med 37(Suppl 1):10S–19S
69. Schneider U, Rackwitz L, Andereya S, Siebenlist S, Fensky F, Reichert J, Loer I, Barthel T, Rudert M, Noth U (2011) A prospective multicenter study on the outcome of type I collagen hydrogel-based autologous chondrocyte implantation (CaReS) for the repair of articular cartilage defects in the knee. Am J Sports Med 39:2558–2565
70. Shasha N, Krywulak S, Backstein D, Pressman A, Gross AE (2003) Long-term follow-up of fresh tibial osteochondral allografts for failed tibial plateau fractures. J Bone Joint Surg Am 85-A(Suppl 2): 33–39
71. Shelbourne KD, Jari S, Gray T (2003) Outcome of untreated traumatic articular cartilage defects of the knee: a natural history study. J Bone Joint Surg Am 85-A(Suppl 2):8–16
72. Steadman JR, Briggs KK, Rodrigo JJ, Kocher MS, Gill TJ, Rodkey WG (2003) Outcomes of microfracture for traumatic chondral defects of the knee: average 11-year follow-up. Arthroscopy 19:477–484
73. Steadman JR, Miller BS, Karas SG, Schlegel TF, Briggs KK, Hawkins RJ (2003) The microfracture technique in the treatment of full-thickness chondral lesions of the knee in National Football League players. J Knee Surg 16:83–86
74. Steadman JR, Ramappa AJ, Maxwell RB, Briggs KK (2007) An arthroscopic treatment regimen for osteoarthritis of the knee. Arthroscopy 23:948–955
75. Strauss EJ, Fonseca LE, Shah MR, Yorum T (2011) Management of focal cartilage defects in the knee – is ACI the answer? Bull NYU Hosp Jt Dis 69:63–72
76. Vanlauwe J, Saris DB, Victor J, Almqvist KF, Bellemans J, Luyten FP (2011) Five-year outcome of characterized chondrocyte implantation versus microfracture for symptomatic cartilage defects of the knee: early treatment matters. Am J Sports Med 39: 2566–2574
77. Vasiliadis HS, Lindahl A, Georgoulis AD, Peterson L (2011) Malalignment and cartilage lesions in the patellofemoral joint treated with autologous chondrocyte implantation. Knee Surg Sports Traumatol Arthrosc 19:452–457

Part II

Marrow Stimulation Techniques

4 Stimulation Techniques: Microfracturing, Drilling

Christoph Erggelet

Contents

C. Erggelet, MD, PhD
University of Freiburg Medical Center
Freiburg/Germany, Center for Biologic Joint Surgery,
Kraftstrasse 29CH-8044, Zurich, Switzerland

Department for Orthopaedic Surgery
and Traumatology, Albert-Ludwigs-University
Medical Center, Freiburg, Germany
e-mail: info@drerggelet.ch

4.1 Introduction

Microfracture has been established as a gold standard for the treatment of articular cartilage defects. The technique and initial results were published in 1994 [28]. It was originally performed in patients with post-traumatic lesions of the knee that progressed to full-thickness chondral defects. Unstable articular cartilage and degenerative changes were also indications for microfracture in the presence of normal leg alignment.

Microfracture follows the principle of bone marrow stimulation. The intrinsic repair mechanisms are activated by perforating the subchondral bone plate. As a result, the medullary bleeding carries proteins and pluripotent cells into the cartilage defect, starting a cascade of physiological cell differentiation. In many cases, with the predominant existence of fibroblasts in those conglomerates, the development of fibrous cartilage is described [30]. Other studies did not support this theory [14]. Various techniques are reported pioneered by the simple perforation of the subchondral bone plate with a drill or a K-wire in 1959 by Pridie [13, 27]. With an intact cartilage surface, a retrograde technique should

A.A. Shetty et al. (eds.), *Techniques in Cartilage Repair Surgery*,
DOI 10.1007/978-3-642-41921-8_4, © ESSKA 2014

be preferred. Motorised shaver systems enable the resection of the superficial sclerosised layer of the subchondral bone plate to expose the healthy spongious tissue – so-called abrasion chondroplasty [8]. The microfracture technique was developed by Steadman using specially designed instruments to open the subchondral bone space without harming the subchondral bone plate.

Multiple clinical trials show good results for microfracture; other studies present a variable outcome. Although the microfracture technique is performed by many orthopaedic surgeons, clinical experience has shown that some patient populations may benefit more from microfracture than others.

4.2 Surgical Technique

For the arthroscopical procedure, three portals are recommended: one for the inflow cannula and one each for the arthroscope and the working instruments. After assessing the full-thickness articular cartilage lesion, the exposed bone is debrided of all remaining unstable cartilage. A full-radius resector and/or a handheld curved curette is used to debride loose or marginally attached cartilage to form a stable perpendicular edge of healthy cartilage around the defect. The crater surrounded by normal cartilage forms a pool that helps to hold the bone marrow clot. The calcified cartilage layer that remains is removed by using a curette (Fig. 4.1). Thorough and complete removal of the calcified cartilage layer is extremely important according to Frisbie et al. [9] (Fig. 4.2). To avoid excessive damage to the subchondral bone, an arthroscopic awl then is used to make multiple perforations, or microfractures, into the exposed subchondral bone plate [33]. The holes should be placed 3–4 mm apart without breaking the subchondral bone plate between them (Fig. 4.3). Fat emerging from the marrow cavity indicates the appropriate depth (2–4 mm of penetration). Thermal damage to the bone does not occur with this technique. When the blood flow from the bone marrow seems to be adequate in all areas of the defect after reducing the irrigation fluid pressure, the procedure is terminated. Intra-articular drains are not recommended (Fig. 4.4).

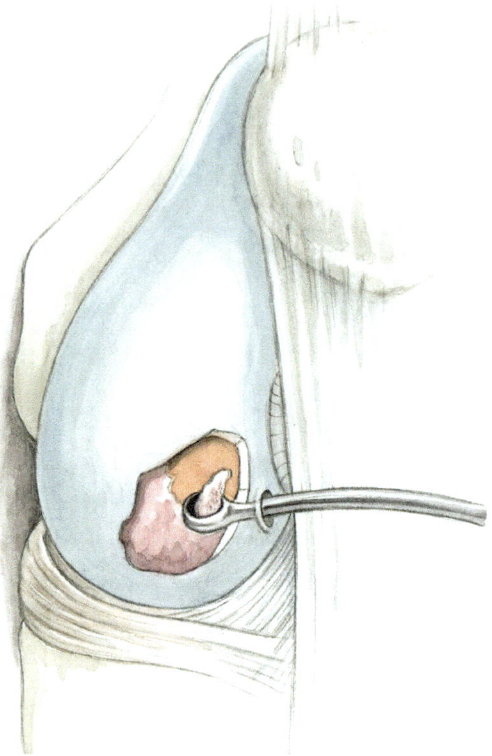

Fig. 4.1 Debridement of cartilage defect with removal of the sclerotic layer of the subchondral bone (Reproduced from Erggelet and Mandelbaum [35])

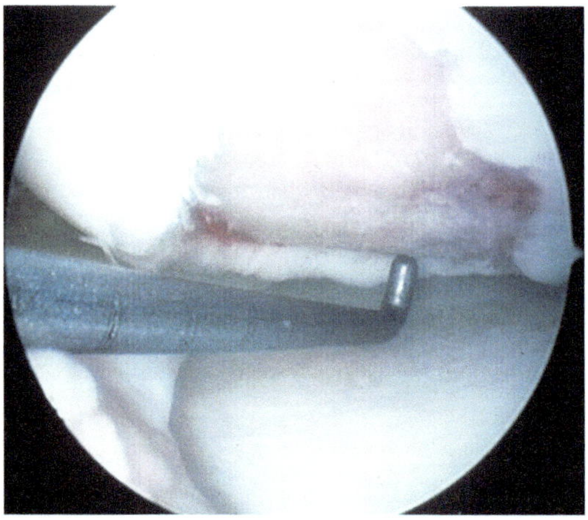

Fig. 4.2 Arthroscopic picture of a debrided cartilage defect

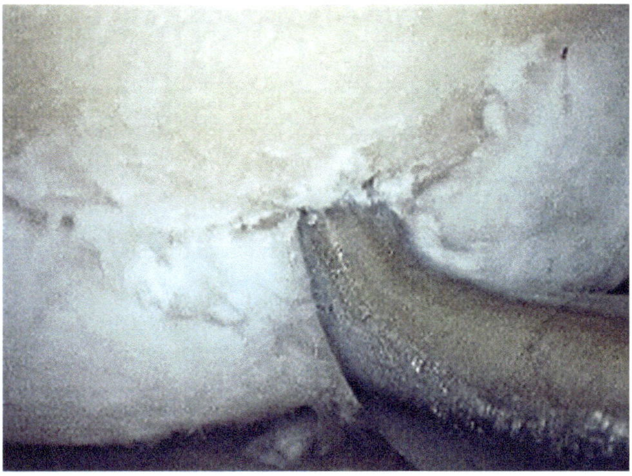

Fig. 4.3 Perforation of the subchondral bone with a round awl

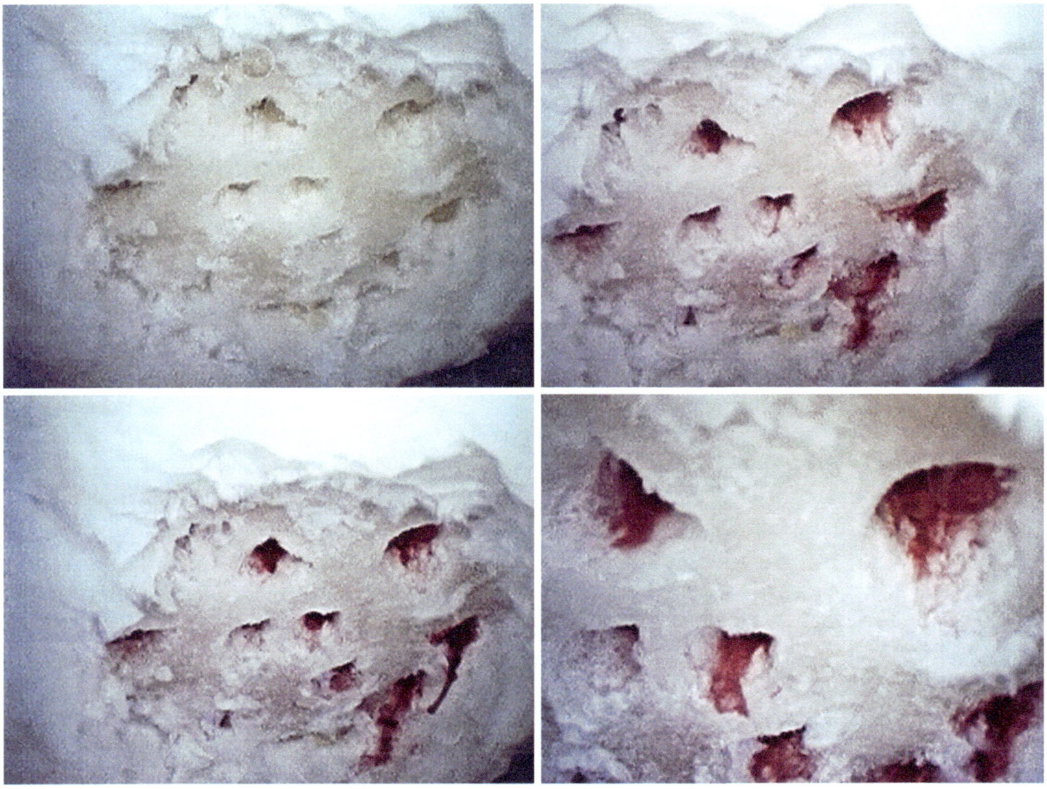

Fig. 4.4 Blood flow from the microfractures after intra-articular pressure release

4.3 Control of Bleeding

Releasing tourniquet pressure will allow moderate bleeding into the defect as well as blood clot formation. If this cannot be observed, perforation/abrasion has to be repeated.

4.4 Pitfalls

- Fracture of subchondral bone plate by overly dense or non-perpendicular perforations
- Incomplete defect filling because of wide gaps between perforations

4.5 Postoperative Treatment

- Unrestricted CPM (exclusion – lesions of the femoropatellar joint; apply flexion restriction of 60° for 2–6 weeks in these cases)
- Unloading of the affected joint for 4–6 weeks
- Gait training with weight-bearing limitation ('soul contact' only) after procedures of knee and ankle joint

It may take up to one year until fibrocartilage formation is completed. Hence, revision surgery is usually not indicated within a postoperative period of at least one year.

4.6 Rehabilitation

The exact rehabilitation protocol is discussed controversely.

Rodrigo emphasised the importance of rehabilitation after microfracture. Rehabilitation should promote the ideal physical environment in which newly recruited mesenchymal stem cells from the marrow can differentiate into appropriate articular cartilage like cell lines. Location of the defect, size and concurrently treated pathologies determine the postoperative protocol. In general, continuous passive motion (CPM) is started in the recovery room with an increasing range of motion at one cycle per minute for 6–8 h per day [33]. Crutch-assisted touch-down weight bearing is allowed for 6–8 weeks, depending on the size of the lesion. Elastic cord exercises and weight training are progressed to full function. The return to more demanding sports should not be earlier than 4–6 months after microfracture.

4.7 Indications

- Full-thickness cartilage defects of all joints.
- Maximum defect size varies with overall body size.
- Stable defect shoulder and intact joint containment are necessary, as early regenerates are usually soft and need protection by healthy surrounding cartilage.

4.8 Advantages

- Arthroscopic technique
- Cost-efficient

4.9 Disadvantages

- Fibrocartilage formation only with chance of deterioration over time
- Injury of the subchondral bone plate

4.10 Drilling

Above recommendations are also applicable for antegrade drilling. K-wires or small drill bits with a diameter of 1.5–2 mm are to be used to perforate the subchondral bone plate (Fig. 4.5).

OD lesions are special cases requiring retrograde drilling. Given an intact cartilage surface but visible demarcation of the fragment (yellowish colour, soft spot), the underlying sclerotic bone has to be perforated with a drill bit. Special guide instruments (e.g. from the ACL reconstruction set) or image intensifiers are used to perform retrograde drilling without injuring overlying cartilage. Refrain from antegrade drilling through the fragment to avoid additional cartilage injury.

Heat-related necrosis and accidental injury of overlying cartilage are remaining problems of this particular technique. However, there seems to be evidence that the quality of the regenerated repair tissue is better after subchondral drilling than microfracture. The use of a 1 mm K-wire in oscillating mode down a min depth of 8 mm does not create overheating and promotes the release of more active pluripotent cells [4].

4.11 Results

- Arthroscopic: Regenerates appear to be soft with fibrillated surface even under ideal circumstances within the first 12 months. In case of a missing stable defect, shoulder regenerates are likely to be torn off, resulting in failure of the procedure.

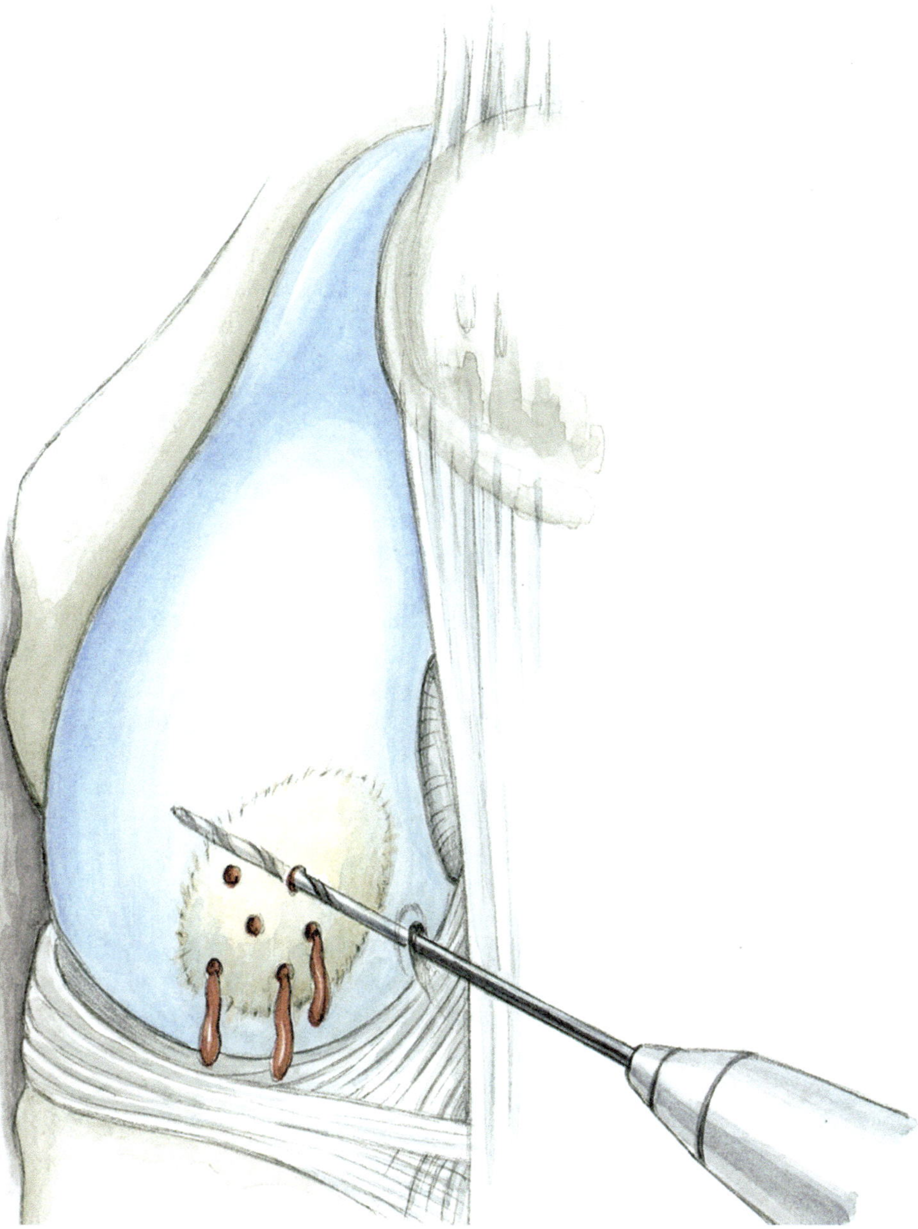

Fig. 4.5 Anterograde defect drilling with deep perforation of the subchondral bone (Reproduced from Erggelet and Mandelbaum [35])

- Macroscopic: Even complete defect filling with stable, smooth fibrocartilage does not necessarily result in success of the procedure. Reasons for this phenomenon are unknown.
- Histological: Histological processing of regenerates shows characteristic fibrocartilaginous structure even under ideal conditions, differing significantly from hyaline cartilage.
- Clinical: Deterioration of initially good results after 3–5 years is more likely with microfracture in patients older than 40 years.

4.12 Amplified Results/Literature

The first study was published by Rodriogo et al. in 1994 [28]. They examined 77 patients after microfracture treatment, all of whom had second-look arthroscopy for various reasons. In a level III retrospective comparative series, they compared one group who were treated with postoperative continuous passive motion (CPM) to a second group without postoperative CPM. After a follow-up time of 64 weeks for group one and 73 weeks for group two, macroscopic rating from 1 (excellent) to 5 (bad) showed an improvement of 2.67 grades for the group treated with CPM in comparison to 1.67 grades for the group treated without CPM. They concluded that CPM should be used after microfracture.

Blevins et al. in 1998 compared the outcomes of 48 professional athletes to 188 recreational athletes after microfracture [3] in a level IV case series. The clinical outcome scores showed significantly better results in both groups from baseline to follow-up at 3.7 and 4.0 years, respectively. Thirty-one of 48 professional athletes responded to the outcome questionnaire of which 23 returned to the same athletic level. Blinded evaluation was performed on 26 arthroscopic videos in the group of professional athletes and 54 of the recreational athletes. The examiner had no information whether the lesion was being reviewed at the time of initial treatment or at second look. The cartilaginous findings were graded on a scale from I to IV adapted from the Outerbridge classification. The average improvement from baseline to follow-up was 1.6 for the professional athletes and 14 for the recreational athletes. Thirty-five per cent of the recreational athletes showed no improvement with exposed subchondral bone compared to 8 % showing no improvement in the professional group.

In 2003 Steadman et al. presented data with an average follow-up of 11 years after microfracture for traumatic chondral defects of the knee [31] as a level IV case series. Sixty-eight patients (71 knees) younger than 45 years of age were questioned regarding their functional outcome with scores from 1 (unable to perform activities) to 10 (no limitation in performing). The rating for Activity in Daily Living was 5.4 preoperatively, 8.3 after 2 years and 8.2 after 7 years. The function for strenuous work showed a scoring of 5 preoperatively and 7.4 after 2 and 7 years. Sports activity was judged with 4.2 preoperatively compared to 7.3 after year 2 and 7.2 after year 7. In another case series with an evidence level of IV, Steadman et al. reported that 19 of 25 national football league players returned to play an average of 56 games after microfracture [32].

In the microfracture arm of his level IV case series, Bachmann included seven patients with a mean age of 33 years (± 6) and found a clinical improvement using the Lysholm score from 45.5 to 74.2 [1]. A complete defect fill on MRI was detected in 2 of 7 patients after 2 years.

Miller et al. presented outcome data 2.6 years (2–5) after microfracture of degenerative cartilage lesions [23] in a level IV case series. All 81 patients were 40 years and older (40–70) and had an average defect size of 2.29 cm^2 (0.25–20). The Tegner score increased from 53.8 (19–85) preoperatively to 83.1 (44–100) at follow-up. Patient's satisfaction was 8.2 (1–10) and it corresponded to an increase in the Tegner activity scale from 2.9 (1–6) to 4.5 (2 7). Five failures were reported (total knee arthroplasty) as well as 13 rearthroscopies were performed due to pain. The authors concluded that arthroscopic microfracture can consistently achieve significant symptomatic and functional improvement in the degenerative knee.

At a mean follow-up time of 72 months (36–120), Gobbi et al. evaluated a cohort of competitive athletes (26 professionals and 27 recreational) after microfracture [10]. A total of 33 males and 20 females with a mean age of 38 (19–55) showed large (mean 4.0 cm^2) grade III and IV cartilage lesions in this level IV case series. The Lysholm, IKDC and Tegner scales all showed a significant increase at follow-up. Clinical examination was also performed with a functional one-leg hop test. Ten per cent were not able to jump more than 50 % of the distance covered using the normal leg whereas 70 % performed normal or nearly normal. Two of three failures were treated with autologous chondrocyte implantation. Ten biopsies after second-look arthroscopy showed areas of fibromyxoid tissue with differentiation and a transition zone with some cartilage tissue in the areas with initial hyaline transformation.

In 2005, Gudas et al. presented a prospective randomised clinical study with an evidence level of I comparing mosaic osteochondral autologous transplantation to microfracture [11]. Thirty patients with comparable demographics were randomly assigned to two groups. CPM was not used in either group postoperatively. Contrary to the ICRS score at a follow-up time of 36 months, the mean HSS score declined after the first year in the microfracture group. Fourteen biopsies were obtained at 12 months postoperatively. Fibrocartilage was present in eight cases, and in six cases fibroelastic tissue was present, or there was no coverage. MRIs on 21 patients, 12 months after surgery, revealed seven cysts with only 18 % of defect coverage.

A prospective cohort study was published in 2005 by Mithoefer et al. on 52 individuals (37 males and 11 females) who underwent microfracture due to persistent pain [24]. In this case series, the patients were a mean of 48 years of age (16–60) with a mean defect size of 4.8 to cm^2 (2.4–20). At an average follow-up of 41 months (24–54), 48 patients completed a subjective questionnaire. Good or excellent results were found in 32 cases, fair results in 12 cases and poor results in 4 cases. Thirty-two patients showed a decrease in the IKDC score 24 months postoperatively. Patients with a BMI greater than 30 seemed to do worse, whereas patients with an age <30 did better after microfracture. MRI revealed a persistent gap between the tissue in the defect and the surrounding articular cartilage on MRI for 22 of 24 patients at 12 months after surgery.

The value of continuous passive motion after microfracture was studied by Marder et al. in a retrospective comparative level III study in 2005 [20]. The study included 25 patients in each group with a cartilage lesion surface area less than 2 cm^2 with a circumferentially stable margin of intact cartilage. Postoperatively 25 patients were treated by continuous passive motion and touchdown weight bearing for 6 week and 25 patients were allowed to weight bearing as tolerated without CPM. After a mean follow-up time of 5.2 years (2–9), the mean Lysholm score increased from 37 to 81 in the CPM group and from 33 to 85 in the group with full weight bearing and no CPM. Correspondingly, the pain was much less in both groups and there was no significant difference between the groups. No failures were reported but five re-arthroscopies were performed due to pain.

Kreuz et al., in a retrospective level IV study [19], concluded that microfracture of lesions on the femoral condyles shows better clinical outcome compared to other locations. Seventy patients with lesions in 4 locations (femoral condyle, patella, trochlear and tibia) were evaluated 36 months after microfracture using the ICRS score. The author concluded that the results of microfracture of the femoral condyles were better when compared to microfracture of lesions in other locations.

Another publication by Kreuz et al. [18] presented data examining the influence of age on the outcome of microfracture in the knee joint [18]. Thirty-two males and 37 females with cartilage defects ICRS grades 3b and c were grouped for age under 40 years and over 40 years (18–55) for a level IV case series. Clinical examination and scoring according to the criteria of the Lysholm, ICRS and SF-36 scores were performed at 6, 18 and 36 months postoperatively. MR imaging was performed preoperatively at 18 and 36 months after surgery. ICRS scores suggested a deterioration between 18 and 36 months in the age group over 40. Patella and trochlear lesions showed more unfavourable results after 18 months.

A challenging group of patients with osteoarthritic knees were treated by Bae et al. with microfracture [2]. Forty-six patients, the majority of whom were female aged 57 years (41–77) with a mean defect size of 3.9 cm^2 (1–6), presented with persistent knee pain. At follow-up of this level IV case series using Baumgaertners knee scale, 36 % of the patients rated excellent, 53 % good and 11 % fair. Second-look arthroscopies, performed at 1 year (10–15 months), demonstrated cartilage healing of greater than 80 % in 36 cases and less than 50 % in 3 cases. Histological analysis including Western Blotting and immunohistochemistry revealed a significantly reduced content of collagen II in the repair tissue with a mean of 44 % compared to a normal control tissue. Eight cases had more than 70 % of type II collagen compared to the normal control group, seven cases had collagen II in the range of 20–70 % of normal and only six cases showed less than 20 % collagen II in the repair tissue.

Mithoefer et al. reported the results of 32 high-impact athletes (3 % professional, 59 % competitive and 38 % recreational) after treatment with microfracture [25] in a level IV case series. Fourteen patients returned to sports and 8 patients returned to sports on the same level. At a minimum follow-up of 2 years, this cohort with an average lesion size of 4.9 to cm^2 (2.4–20) showed significant improvement according to the criteria of the Brittberg rating scale, the Tegner activity score and the Marx activity rating scale. Two failures were reported.

The goal of a study by Domayer et al. was to correlate clinical outcome with MRI T2 mapping after microfracture [6]. Therefore, 24 patients with a mean age of 41 years (± 14) and mean defect size of 2.0 cm^2 (0.825) were included in this level IV case series and examined 29 months (± 14) after microfracture both clinically and with MRI. All patients reported improvement after surgery with the mean Lysholm score of 80.6 (SD 18.5). The mean outcome of the subjective IKDC form was 70.0 (SD 23.8). In the IKDC rating, the knee status was normal in 41.7 %, nearly normal at 45.8 % and abnormal in 12.5 %. MRI showed that the average volume fill grade of the defect with regenerated tissue was above 75 % in 66.7 % of the cases compared to the adjacent native cartilage. In 4.1 % the filling grade was below 25 %. Since the T2 mapping index correlated with the outcome of the Lysholm score ($r=0.641$) and the IKDC subjective knee evaluation form ($r=0.549$), the authors suggested quantitative T2 mapping as a valuable tool to monitor the progress of cartilage repair.

The findings at 5 years after autologous chondrocyte implantation (ACI) and microfracture were presented by Knutsen et al. after conducting a prospective randomised controlled trial with an evidence level of I [16]. Eighty patients with an average defect size of 4.5 cm^2 after debridement (2–10) were randomly assigned to be treated either with ACI or microfracture. The procedures were performed in a standardised fashion with an identical rehabilitation programme. The patients were examined clinically at 12 and 24 months and a second-look arthroscopy was performed at two years. At the time of the 5-year follow-up, there were nine failures in each group. Clinical data on the patients who did not have a failure were collected at 5 years. The mean Lysholm scores and the mean scores on the visual analogue pain scale remain significantly improved in both groups. Compared with the baseline values, 72 % of the patients had less pain, 80 % had improvement in the Lysholm score, and 72 % had improvement in the SF-36 physical component score. No significant difference between the treatment groups was found in the Lysholm score or the visual analogue score at 5 years after treatment. Younger patients less than 30 years old had a significantly better clinical outcome regardless of their treatment group after 5 years. Evaluation of second-look arthroscopies and histological analysis of the same patient population was presented in an earlier publication by Knutsen et al. [17]. The macroscopic findings of 35 patients after microfracture were graded as nearly normal. Thirty-nine per cent of the biopsy specimens had at least some hyaline cartilage present. In contrast, 43 had fibrocartilage throughout most of their depth. Unscheduled second-look arthroscopy was necessary in four cases in the microfracture group.

The only study in this review with a control group was performed by Matsunaga et al. comparing the repair of articular cartilage and clinical outcome after osteotomy with microfracture or abrasion arthroplasty for medial gonarthrosis [21]. In a retrospective comparative level III study, 104 patients were assigned to three different therapeutic groups. Forty-five patients received a closing-wedge high tibial osteotomy with internal fixation combined with abrasion arthroplasty on the femoral condyle. In 25 patients, abrasion arthroplasty was replaced by microfracture in combination with a high tibial osteotomy. No specific cartilage treatment was performed in 34 patients receiving only high tibial osteotomy serving as a control group. From day 2 postoperatively continuous passive motion exercise was performed for about 3 h daily for 4 weeks. Partial and full weight bearing was allowed from 4 to 6 to 8 weeks after surgery respectively. The same postoperative protocol was followed in all three groups. Repeat arthroscopy was done during removal of the hardware about 1 year after HTO. With an overall follow-up rate of 98 % up to 5 years after surgery, the clinical outcome was assessed using the Japanese Orthopaedic Association score (JOA) at 1, 3 and 5 years after surgery. There was a significant improvement in all three groups after surgery and the clinical score did not deteriorate within 5 years. There were no significant differences of the preoperative or postoperative JOA scores between the three groups at any time of assessment. At arthroscopy one year postoperatively, cartilage repair on the medial femoral condyle was more extensive in the abrasion arthroplasty group than in the HTO group alone, while there was no difference between the microfracture group and the HTO group. The authors concluded that abrasion arthroscopy combined with HTO is more successful in producing repair cartilage than microfracture combined with HTO, although neither procedure improved the clinical outcome within 5 years after surgery in comparison to HTO alone. Although it is generally assumed that covering exposed subchondral bone with repair cartilage should be relevant to the management of osteoarthritis, the authors interpret their results in a way that it is inappropriate to combine HTO with marrow stimulation techniques.

Another level I prospective randomised trial comparing microfracture with autologous chondrocyte implantation was published by Saris and co-workers [29]. Sixty-one patients (41 males and 20 females) with a single defect on the femoral condyle with a mean size of 2.4 cm^2 (± 1.2) were treated in the microfracture arm of the study. The postoperative rehabilitation programme was similar in both groups. They were limited to weight bearing for 6 weeks and an unloader brace for 8 weeks. No detailed information was given regarding continuous passive motion. The follow-up time was 18 months for 51 out of 61 patients after microfracture. The KOOS score improved from an average of 59.53 (± 14.95) to 75.04 (± 14.50) postoperatively. Eight adverse events occurred. The KOOS overall score for the autologous chondrocyte implantation group was 56.3 (± 13.61) at baseline compared to 74.73 (± 17.01) postoperatively at 18 months. The adjusted mean overall histology assessment score was statistically significantly higher for the ACI treatment group than for the microfracture group. The authors attribute this histological difference to the use of characterised chondrocytes with the ACI technique. However, there was no difference in clinical outcome at 18 months.

4.13 Discussion

Despite the fact that microfracture is widely accepted as gold standard for the treatment of cartilage defects, the preponderance of articles on the use of microfracture report data from case series (evidence level IV).

Over time a multitude of scoring systems have been used to evaluate the clinical outcome of patients before and after treatment preventing easy comparison of results (Table 4.1). For future studies in the field of cartilage repair, one might refer to the recommendations of the ICRS (International Cartilage Repair Society).

Table 4.1 Clinical scores

Lysholm [1, 6, 10, 16, 18–20, 23, 31, 32]
ICRS [10, 11, 18, 19]
Tegner [10, 18, 20, 23, 32]
VAS [23]
WOMAC [31]
Modified Cincinnati [19]
Functional outcome level [3, 32]
SF 36 [19, 24, 31]
HSS [11]
Patient satisfaction [23]
IKDC [6, 24]
Return to sport [32]
Baumgaertners knee scale [2]
Brittberg rating [25]
Marx activity rating scale [25]
Knee outcome survey [25]
KOOS [29]
Japanese Orthopaedic Association score JOA [19]

Overall the weakness of the literature has to be emphasised, specifically the low methodological quality of most of the studies. Additionally, publications describing combined treatments with microfracture AND e.g. high tibial osteotomy [22, 34] have to be looked at critically. Duplications of previously published studies are rare but occurring [12] as well as reports about an already included cohort at a different time point. [16] Caution should be executed when citing abstracts without the availability of the original publication [5]. Reports about mixed patient cohorts with e.g. knee and ankle treatment seem not to be relevant as well [26].

The use of a specifically designed data extraction form enable a standardized way to evaluate and compare publications. Details regarding data collection regarding exact reference; objective of the study; study design; demographics of the participants; description of the intervention; possible control groups; outcome data and level of evidence according Journal of Bone and Joint Surgery criteria. [15] should not be overseen and noted. That warrants caution when interpreting the results of microfracture for treatment of chondral injuries. However, there might be some indications on the clinical outcome of microfracture in the literature mentioned above.

4.13.1 Durability of Microfracture

The mean length of follow-up ranged from 12 months to 11.3 years (7–17 years). Functional and other clinical parameters significantly improved in patients who had symptomatic cartilage defects 2–5 years after microfracture [16] and in patients with degenerative knee lesions 2.6 years after microfracture [23]. Consistent with these results are the observations of Steadman et al. of decreased pain and improved function over the first two years and of decreased swelling over the first three years, responses that were maintained up to 7 years [31]. In a study of patients with moderate osteoarthritis, 25/47 (53 %) of the cases had good and 36 % had excellent scores after an average follow-up of 2.3 years (24–44 m) [2].

In contrast, some studies with a duration of 18 months or more showed that initial improvements in patient outcomes may decline at later time points. In the two studies by Kreuz et al. [18, 19], clinical outcome deteriorated between the 18- and 36-month time points depending on the age of the patient and/or the lesion location. In a 48-month study [24], Mithoefer and colleagues found that while activities of daily living, the International Knee Documentation Committee (IKDC) score and the SF-36 physical component score improved up to 24 months following microfracture, the IKDC follow-up score significantly worsened from 24 to 36 months and was no longer significantly different than preoperative by 48 months. In another study on athletes, activity scores initially increased but later declined in almost half of the patients [25]. Similar results were reported by Gudas et al. [11]. and Gobbi et al. who demonstrated that in a longer-term study (mean follow-up up to 6 years), knee function improved significantly following microfracture with 70 % of the patients being considered normal or nearly normal. Although, strenuous sports activities improved in 80 % of subjects at a 2-year follow-up, only 55 % of patients were improved at the final follow-up [10].

The conclusions of durability of microfracture are mixed. There are no apparent reasons to be extracted from the literature. One has to be aware of possible unknown factors influencing the outcome of microfracture – not only in terms of durability: compliance of patients, 'genetic footprint', variations in the physiotherapy regime, medications, drug abuse and many more.

4.13.2 Quality of Cartilage Repair Tissue Following Microfracture

MRI is used [1, 6, 18, 19, 24, 29] to determine the degree of defect filling at given time points. The quality of the repair tissue could not be sufficiently evaluated with MRI. Future developments might help to correlate MRI results with histological quality of regenerated tissue. In one study

MRI findings correlated with the clinical outcome [6].

Histology gradings [2, 10, 11, 16, 21, 29] generally show variable results. Histological grading of the repaired tissue was in most cases based on morphological structure and the absent/reduced content of type II collagen. With microfracture, the normal, hyaline cartilage structure cannot be restored. However, the regeneration of a repair tissue with inferior quality within a cartilage defect may reduce pain and improve joint function.

4.13.3 Effect of Age on the Outcome of Microfracture

There is evidence from the described studies that patients under 30–40 years might benefit more from the microfracture technique [18, 19, 28, 32]. A possible explanation for this finding could be the higher biological quality of the emerging stem cell as well as better nutritional support of the regenerating tissue due to the more effective blood supply in younger individuals.

4.13.4 Effect of Lesion Location on the Outcome of Microfracture

Kreuz et al. reported that patients with femoral condyle lesions treated with microfracture had better clinical improvement, quality of cartilage repair and defect filling than patients treated for lesions of the trochlea, tibia and/or patella [19]. In contrast, lesion location was not found to influence Lysholm scores in a study of patients 40 years and over with degenerative knee lesions [23]. When lesions in the medial femoral condyle, lateral femoral condyle and trochlea were compared, defect location did not influence MRI parameters including repair cartilage signal, repair cartilage fill, repaired lesion morphology, peripheral cartilage repair integration and subchondral oedema [24].

No consensus can be found to evaluate the influence of defect location for the outcome of microfracture. Maybe a larger number of included patients would reveal an answer to this question.

4.13.5 Effect of Lesion Size on the Outcome of Microfracture

For the most part, studies show that patients with smaller lesions have better clinical outcomes and quality of cartilage repair tissue following microfracture than patients with larger lesions [2, 10, 16, 23, 25, 28]. The results of Steadman in 2003 [31], indicating that larger lesion size was significantly associated with greater improvement in clinical scores at final follow-up, could be explained with the lower scoring at baseline leaving more room for improvement. Another factor for this inconsistency could be the technique of sizing a cartilage defect. Even the most accurate method with a scaled needle leaves room for errors. Additionally the size of a defect has to be seen in comparison to the overall appearance of the individual treated. A 3 cm^2 cartilage defect has possibly more clinical impact in a female ballet dancer weighing 95 lbs compared to a male janitor with 240 lbs.

4.13.6 How Important Are Postoperative CPM and Weight Bearing for the Outcome of Microfracture

Extensive postoperative CPM and prolonged touchdown weight bearing after microfracture is thought to be essential for a successful clinical outcome by numerous authors. Even so, the literature presents conflicting results. Rodrigo showed better results when CPM was used 6–8 h a day. [28] Most researchers adhered more or less to this regimen with variations regarding duration of CPM and degree of weight bearing from toe touch to partial.

In contrast, a study that examined the difference between patients who were toe-touch weight bearing and receiving CPM postoperatively and those who had no CPM and were allowed weight bearing as tolerated showed that clinical improvement was not affected by postoperative treatment [17].

Again, the results appear to be conflicting. A prospective randomised study might be necessary to evaluate the importance of the postoperative regime after microfracture.

Most of the factors possibly influencing the outcome of microfracture cannot be adequately analysed because of the inconsistencies in the literature. Those inconsistencies are mainly due to comparing results of studies that included patients who have lesions in different locations, different patient populations and, possibly, different surgical techniques. Additionally the results are analysed with a multitude of different outcome instruments. The conclusions regarding the impact of these factors and the results of microfracture must be judged vis-a-vis to the limitations of the literature. Consequently, there is limited support for analysis of the secondary hypothesis. Future directives should include analyzing these gaps of knowledge with prospective randomised trials, which address these deficiencies.

Conclusion

The evidence for the effectiveness of the microfracture procedure is largely derived from case series and few randomised trials. Clinical outcomes improve with microfracture for the most part, but in some studies these effects are not sustained. The quality of cartilage repair following microfracture is variable and inconsistent for unknown reasons. Younger patients have better clinical outcomes and quality of cartilage repair than older patients. When lesion location was shown to affect microfracture outcome, patients with lesions of the femoral condyle seem have the best clinical improvements and quality of cartilage repair compared with patients who had lesions in other areas. Patients with smaller lesions can possibly expect to have better clinical improvement than patients with larger lesions. The necessity of long postoperative CPM and restricted weight bearing is widely accepted but not completely supported by the evidence in the literature.

Maybe new developments like the scaffold augmented microfracture [7] will show even more consistent clinical and biological results as well as faster rehabilitation for the treatment of small- to medium-sized cartilage defects in younger individuals.

References

1. Bachmann G, Basad E, Lommel D, Steinmeyer J (2004) MRI in the follow-up of matrix-supported autologous chondrocyte transplantation (MACI) and microfracture. Radiologe 44:773–782
2. Bae DK, Yoon KH, Song SJ (2006) Cartilage healing after microfracture in osteoarthritic knees. Arthroscopy 22:367–374
3. Blevins FT, Steadman JR, Rodrigo JJ, Silliman J (1998) Treatment of articular cartilage defects in athletes: an analysis of functional outcome and lesion appearance. Orthopedics 21:761–767; discussion 767–8
4. Chen H, Sun J, Hoemann CD, Lascau-Coman V, Ouyang W, McKee MD, Shive MS, Buschmann MD (2009) Drilling and microfracture lead to different bone structure and necrosis during bone-marrow stimulation for cartilage repair. J Orthop Res 27(11):1432–1438
5. Coleman SH, Malizia R, Macgillivray J, Warren RF (2001) Treatment of isolated articular cartilage lesions of the medial femoral condyle. A clinical and MR comparison of autologous chondrocyte implantation vs. microfracture. Ortop Traumatol Rehabil. (2001);3: 224–226
6. Domayer SE, Kutscha-Lissberg F, Welsch G, Dorotka R, Nehrer S, Gabler C, Mamisch TC, Trattnig S (2008) T2 mapping in the knee after microfracture at 3.0T: correlation of global T2 values and clinical outcome – preliminary results. Osteoarthritis Cartilage 16:903–908
7. Erggelet C, Neumann K, Endres M, Haberstroh K, Sittinger M, Kaps C (2007) Regeneration of ovine articular cartilage defects by cell-free polymer-based implants. Biomaterials 28:5570–5580
8. Ficat RP, Ficat C, Gedeon P,Toussaint JB (1979) Spongialization: a new treatment for diseased patellae. Clin Orthop Relat Res:(144):74–83.
9. Frisbie DD, Trotter GW, Powers BE, Rodkey WG, Steadman JR, Howard RD, Park RD, McIlwraith CW (1999) Arthroscopic subchondral bone plate microfracture technique augments healing of large chondral defects in the radial carpal bone and medial femoral condyle of horses. Vet Surg 28:242–255
10. Gobbi A, Nunag P, Malinowski K (2005) Treatment of full thickness chondral lesions of the knee with microfracture in a group of athletes. Knee Surg Sports Traumatol Arthrosc 13:213–221
11. Gudas R, Kalesinskas RJ, Kimtys V, Stankevicius E, Toliusis V, Bernotavicius G, Smailys A (2005) A prospective randomized clinical study of mosaic osteochondral autologous transplantation versus microfracture for the treatment of osteochondral defects in the knee joint in young athletes. Arthroscopy 21:1066–1075

12. Gudas R, Stankevicius E, Monastyreckiene E, Pranys D, Kalesinskas RJ (2006) Osteochondral autologous transplantation versus microfracture for the treatment of articular cartilage defects in the knee joint in athletes. Knee Surg Sports Traumatol Arthrosc 14:834–842
13. Insall J (1974) The Pridie debridement operation for osteoarthritis of the knee. Clin Orthop Relat Res: (101):61–67
14. Johnson LL (1986) Arthroscopic abrasion arthroplasty historical and pathologic perspective: present status. http://jbjs.org/public/instructionsauthors.aspx. Arthroscopy 2:54–69
15. Surgery JoBaJ (2008) Instructions for Authors – Levels of Evidence for primary research question. J Bone Joint Surg Am:90-A number 1, http://jbjs.org/public/instructionsauthors.aspx
16. Knutsen G, Drogset JO, Engebretsen L, Grontvedt T, Isaksen V, Ludvigsen TC, Roberts S, Solheim E, Strand T, Johansen O (2007) A randomized trial comparing autologous chondrocyte implantation with microfracture. Findings at five years. J Bone Joint Surg Am 89:2105–2112
17. Knutsen G, Engebretsen L, Ludvigsen TC, Drogset JO, Grontvedt T, Solheim E, Strand T, Roberts S, Isaksen V, Johansen O (2004) Autologous chondrocyte implantation compared with microfracture in the knee. A randomized trial. J Bone Joint Surg Am 86-A:455–464
18. Kreuz PC, Erggelet C, Steinwachs MR, Krause SJ, Lahm A, Niemeyer P, Ghanem N, Uhl M, Sudkamp N (2006) Is microfracture of chondral defects in the knee associated with different results in patients aged 40 years or younger? Arthroscopy 22:1180–1186
19. Kreuz PC, Steinwachs MR, Erggelet C, Krause SJ, Konrad G, Uhl M, Sudkamp N (2006) Results after microfracture of full-thickness chondral defects in different compartments in the knee. Osteoarthritis Cartilage 14:1119–1125
20. Marder RA, Hopkins GJ, Timmerman LA (2005) Arthroscopic microfracture of chondral defects of the knee: a comparison of two postoperative treatments. Arthroscopy 21:152–158
21. Matsunaga D, Akizuki S, Takizawa T, Yamazaki I, Kuraishi J (2007) Repair of articular cartilage and clinical outcome after osteotomy with microfracture or abrasion arthroplasty for medial gonarthrosis. Knee:14(6):465–471
22. Miller BS, Joseph TA, Barry EM, Rich VJ, Sterett WI (2007) Patient satisfaction after medial opening high tibial osteotomy and microfracture. J Knee Surg 20:129–133
23. Miller BS, Steadman JR, Briggs KK, Rodrigo JJ, Rodkey WG (2004) Patient satisfaction and outcome after microfracture of the degenerative knee. J Knee Surg 17:13–17
24. Mithoefer K, Williams R Jr, Warren RF, Potter HG, Spock CR, Jones EC, Wickiewicz TL, Marx RG (2005) The microfracture technique for the treatment of articular cartilage lesions in the knee. A prospective cohort study. J Bone Joint Surg Am 87:1911–1920
25. Mithoefer K, Williams R Jr, Warren RF, Wickiewicz TL, Marx RG (2006) High-impact athletics after knee articular cartilage repair: a prospective evaluation of the microfracture technique. Am J Sports Med 34:1413–1418
26. Passler HH (2000) Microfracture for treatment of cartilage detects. Zentralbl Chir 125:500–504
27. Pridie KH (1959) A method of resurfacing osteoarthritic knee joints. J Bone Joint Surg Am 41-B: 618–619
28. Rodrigo JJ, Steadman JR, Silliman J, Fulstone HA (1994) Improvement of full thickness chondral defect healing in the human knee after debridement and microfracture using continuous passive motion. Am J Knee Surg 7:109–116
29. Saris DB, Vanlauwe J, Victor J, Haspl M, Bohnsack M, Fortems Y, Vandekerckhove B, Almqvist KF, Claes T, Handelberg F, Lagae K, van der Bauwhede J, Vandenneucker H, Yang KG, Jelic M, Verdonk R, Veulemans N, Bellemans J, Luyten FP (2008) Characterized chondrocyte implantation results in better structural repair when treating symptomatic cartilage defects of the knee in a randomized controlled trial versus microfracture. Am J Sports Med 36:235–246
30. Shapiro F, Koide S, Glimcher MJ (1993) Cell origin and differentiation in the repair of full-thickness defects of articular cartilage. J Bone Joint Surg Am 75:532–553
31. Steadman JR, Briggs KK, Rodrigo JJ, Kocher MS, Gill TJ, Rodkey WG (2003) Outcomes of microfracture for traumatic chondral defects of the knee: average 11-year follow-up. Arthroscopy 19:477–484
32. Steadman JR, Miller BS, Karas SG, Schlegel TF, Briggs KK, Hawkins RJ (2003) The microfracture technique in the treatment of full-thickness chondral lesions of the knee in National Football League players. J Knee Surg 16:83–86
33. Steadman JR, Rodkey WG, Briggs KK (2002) Microfracture to treat full-thickness chondral defects: surgical technique, rehabilitation, and outcomes. J Knee Surg 15:170–176
34. Sterett WI, Steadman JR (2004) Chondral resurfacing and high tibial osteotomy in the varus knee. Am J Sports Med 32:1243–1249
35. Erggelet C, Mandelbaum B (2008) Principles of Cartilage Repair. Steinkopff/Springer, Heidelberg

Part III

Acellular Matrix Based Cartilage Regeneration Techniques

Matrix-Enhanced Microfracture: Autologous Matrix-Induced Chondroneogenesis (AMIC™)

5

Matthias Reinhard Steinwachs,
B. Waibl, and M. Mumme

Contents

M.R. Steinwachs, PD Dr. med. (✉)
Center for Orthobiologics and Cartilage Repair, Schulthess Clinic Zurich, Lengghalde 2, CH-8008 Zurich, Switzerland

Department of Orthopedics and Trauma Surgery, University Hospital Freiburg, Freiburg, Germany
e-mail: matthias.steinwachs@kws.ch

B. Waibl • M. Mumme
Center for Orthobiologics and Cartilage Repair, Schulthess Clinic Zurich, Lengghalde 2, CH-8008 Zurich, Switzerland

5.1 Introduction

Various surgical techniques have been developed over the last 20 years for the treatment of articular cartilage defects. In the past years microfracture, autologous chondrocyte implantation, and osteochondral transplantation have been investigated extensively. Especially for these methods, a sufficient number of validated studies on a good level of evidence are available. Cartilage repair has become a valid, standardized treatment. It is integrated in the daily work of surgeons worldwide and is element of the training of orthopedic surgeons by the specialized societies such as ICRS, AAOS, AGA, and ESSKA. In addition to these proven methods, new methods or modifications are introduced regularly.

Due to the fact that adult cartilage has lost its ability to repair cartilage defects [1–4], these defects have a very limited, age-dependent, self-healing capacity. There are two main reasons for this fact: First, tissue-bound differentiated cartilage cells are not able to replicate. Second, the metabolic activity of tissues nourished solely by diffusion is very limited. Hence, the reparative capacity of cartilage is insufficient to effectively repair defects of the biomechanically burdened cartilage matrix by the means of augmented matrix synthesis. A surgical approach is therefore required in adults with symptomatic ICRS grade III/IV defects of the knee joint.

For biologic tissue regeneration, the "sine qua non" is the presence of specific cells, which possess the ability of tissue regeneration. These cells

A.A. Shetty et al. (eds.), *Techniques in Cartilage Repair Surgery*,
DOI 10.1007/978-3-642-41921-8_5, © ESSKA 2014

are recruited from the bone marrow in marrow-stimulating techniques, released by establishing access to the medullary cavity and subsequent bleeding into the defect area [5–8]. In particular, ingrowing stem cells are intended to transform the resulting blood clot into "fibrous cartilage." Arthroscopically, these techniques have formerly been used as Pridie drillings with moderate success [9, 10]. A modification of this technique, the "microfracturing," has replaced it since the late 1990s [5].

Due to the fact that microfracturing is a minimally invasive method with limited expenses and that it offers the possibility to combine it with other arthroscopic procedures such as ligamentous and meniscus repair, microfracture surgery is the worldwide most often used cartilage repair technique. Microfracturing promotes the formation of fibrous tissue with a histologic range from primitive scar tissue up to mixed fibrous-hyaline cartilage under local biochemical and biomechanical factors [11, 12].

Analyses of more than 3,000 patients with a follow-up of up to 17 years indicate that microfracturing shows an initial clinical improvement in 47–90 % of the patients but, after 18–36 months, a deterioration in function and pain can be observed. The medium-term revision rates reported are up to 31 % [13–16]. Drawbacks of the technique are the inferior mechanical tissue properties and the formation of intralesional osteophytes.

In athletes, return to sport on the pre-injury level after microfracture surgery can be expected in 45–67 % after 8–17 months. Onset of symptoms of less than 12 months prior to surgery is associated with a significantly higher return to sports rate (67 %) compared to a longer history of more than 12 months (14 %) [17]. This technique is still considered in young (<40 years) and active patients with small and isolated defects (<2.5 cm^2), low body-mass index, and a short duration of preoperative symptoms [7, 8].

Besides incomplete defect filling, in particular the histologically inferior tissue quality seems to be the reason for inconsistent clinical results over time [4, 18]. The frequently observed intralesional ossification goes along with poor clinical results as well and represents an important negative predictive factor concerning mid- and long-term outcome together with persistent subchondral bone marrow edema in MRI [11, 12, 14, 16].

In combination with different biomaterials, microfracture techniques have been used to treat large cartilage defects for several years (e.g., chondroplasty, AMIC™, MaioRegen™, CaRes-S™) [8, 19]. As a modification of the abovementioned techniques, antegrade or retrograde drilling with K-wires or fine drills is utilized to stimulate the healing of the often pathologically altered subchondral bone.

5.2 Patient Selection

The AMIC™ technique is suitable for symptomatic chondral and osteochondral defects of the knee joint, ankle joint, and hip joint with a size of about 2–5 cm^2 [22, 23].

In osteochondral defects, reconstruction of the osseous defect area is accomplished during the same intervention via transfer of cancellous bone or a cortico-cancellous plug. This operative technique is applicable also in revision cases and early osteoarthritis where ACI is no longer an option.

The prerequisite for a successful treatment is simultaneous correction of concomitant pathologies as, e.g., joint instability, maltracking, and axis deformities [21]. This technique should not be chosen in hemophilic joints, rheumatoid disorders, severe metabolic arthropathies, toxic cartilage damage, or joint infections. In advanced osteoarthritis (Kellgren & Lawrence grade III/IV), AMIC™ is an option as palliative concept only in exceptional cases. Defect situations of the patella, which cannot be treated alternatively, can be treated in a symptom-modifying fashion if the altered biomechanical environment is addressed simultaneously. All the necessary concomitant interventions shall be accomplished in one operation in order to avoid an unnecessary prolongation of the rehabilitation time.

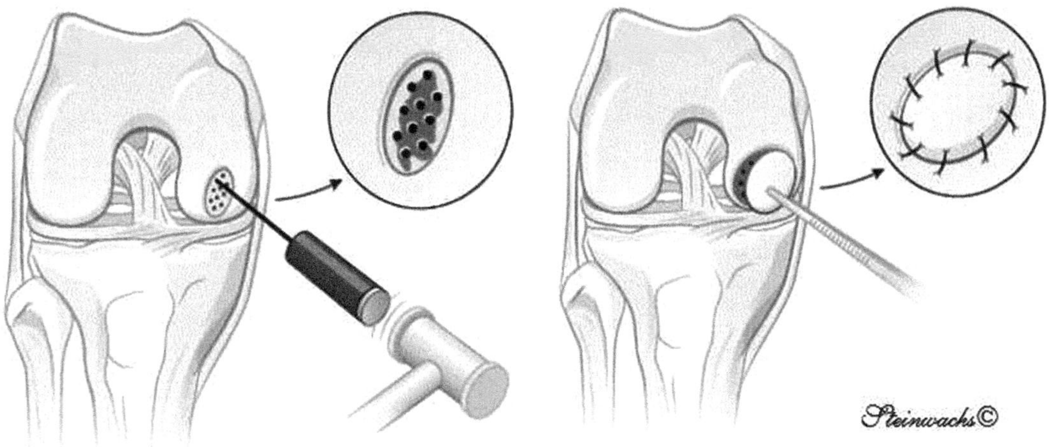

Fig. 5.1 AMIC technique

5.3 Surgical Technique

5.3.1 Chondral Reconstruction

Usually, the patient is placed on the operating table in a supine position with a tourniquet mounted at the thigh. Manipulation of the leg has to be allowed during the intervention. A foot rest to arrest the joint in flexion is optional.

Depending on the defect localization, the joint is opened via a mini-arthrotomy placed directly over the defect. The defect is then circumcised with a blade No. 15 perpendicularly to the surface sparingly in healthy tissue. With the aid of special curettes, the destroyed cartilage is prepared off the subchondral lamina.

Additional damage to the underlying bone plate of the defect ground shall be avoided. Solid sclerotic subchondral bone or hypertrophic areas of bone/intralesional osteophytes have to be equalized with a high-speed burr. Microfracture holes are then tapped in a distance of approximately 3 mm to each other with special microfracture awls (e.g., K. Storz, Arthrex, S&N) (Fig. 5.1).

If the obligatory preoperative MRI scan confirms a deep subchondral bone marrow edema, the perforations shall be accomplished with a K-wire (1.6–2.0 mm) to allow for the deeper bony pathology to be addressed simultaneously in the sense of a stimulation drilling. After microfracture or drilling, the defect ground has to be liberated of tiny bony fragments. With the help of an aluminum template, an imprint of the defect is made, and shape and size are transferred onto a Chondro-Gide™ collagen membrane (Geistlich, Wolhusen, Switzerland). The dry collagen membrane is cut to size 10 % smaller considering some swelling in humid condition.

After sealing of the osseous defect ground with some fibrin glue (e.g., Tissucol™, Baxter), the membrane is inserted with the porous surface facing the defect ground and is humidified with some saline solution. As a next step, the membrane is secured avoiding any overlap at the surface with single sutures (e.g., PDS™ 6-0, Ethicon) in a circular manner. The sutures are sealed with some fibrin glue in a final step. The absorbable biomaterial ensures that the bone marrow blood discharged after releasing the tourniquet is kept in the defect [8, 19]. The formed blood clot and the stromal cells within are able to build up fibrous cartilage and ensure a homogenous defect filling (Fig. 5.2) [20].

The joint is rinsed thoroughly and hemostasis accomplished. The joint is closed layer by layer

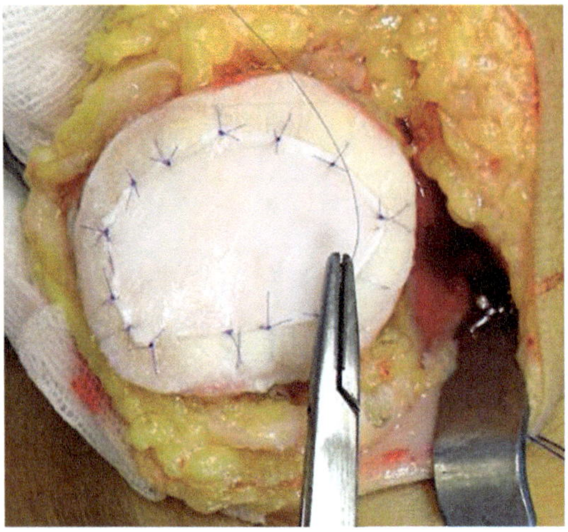

Fig. 5.2 Sutured Chondro-Gide™ Membrane during AMIC™ procedure on the patella

and an intra-articular and a subcutaneous drainage without vacuum are installed. At the end of the operation, an immobilizing initial brace is mounted.

5.3.2 Osteochondral Reconstruction

Patient setting is conducted in analogy to chondral reconstruction. A standard arthrotomy is performed to access the joint. After exposition of the defect, the cartilage borders are prepared with a blade No. 15 perpendicularly to the surface. The destroyed cartilage is abraded with special curettes. Sclerotic areas, cysts, or necrotic bone is removed with a curette or high-speed burr in a radical fashion until healthy cancellous tissue is reached. The defect ground is then drilled (deepness approx. 1 cm) with a 2.0 mm drill to ensure optimal integration of the subsequently inserted cancellous bone.

Harvesting of the cancellous bone can be accomplished at the tibial head, the distal femoral metaphysis, or the anterior or posterior iliac crest. We prefer bone graft harvesting at the distal femoral metaphysis. The periosteum and the synovial tissue layer are incised electrothermically (incision approx. 2 cm) and stripped off the bone with a raspatorium superior to the medial trochlear facet. A large bone cylinder is harvested with an OATS™ or Diamond Bone Cutting System™. Alternatively, access to the femoral medullary cavity is gained via preparation of an osseous lid with a chisel. With the help of a curette, an adequate amount of cancellous bone is then harvested from the medullary cavity. The medullary cavity is sealed by reinserting the cortico-cancellous cylinder or bone lid with some fibrin glue. The periosteum is closed with some sutures to prevent pronounced formation of a hematoma. The harvested cancellous bone is impacted into the defect cavity in several layers stabilized intermittently with the aid of fibrin glue until the bone-cartilage border is reached.

An imprint of the defect is made in analogy to the previously described chondral repair technique, and shape and size are transferred onto a Chondro-Gide™ collagen membrane (Geistlich, Wolhusen, Switzerland). The membrane is cut to size approximately 10 % smaller than the actual defect size in dry condition. After sealing the defect ground with some fibrin glue (e.g., Tissucol™, Baxter), the membrane is fitted into the defect with the porous side facing the osseous surface and moistened with some saline solution. The membrane is then secured with single sutures (e.g., PDS™ 6-0, Ethicon) in a circular manner. The sutures are sealed with some fibrin glue in a final step. The joint is rinsed thoroughly and hemostasis accomplished. The joint is closed layer by layer and an intra-articular and a subcutaneous drainage without vacuum are installed. At the end of the operation, an immobilizing brace is mounted (Figs. 5.3 and 5.4).

5.4 Rehabilitation

The limb is placed in an elevated position until the first postoperative day. The knee joint is cooled and a sufficient pain management is ensured with a regional catheter system and an anti-inflammatory pharmacotherapy.

From the first day on for the first week postoperatively, mobilization with crutches and foot contact (5 kg) is carried out by the physiotherapists,

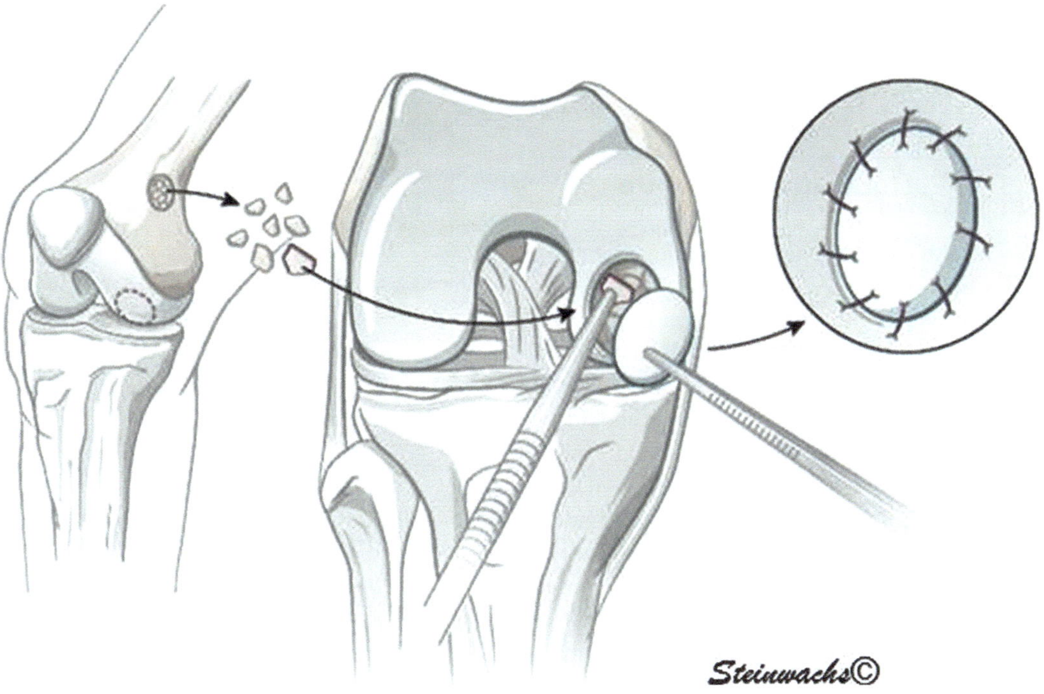

Fig. 5.3 Technique of membrane-covered bone grafting

Fig. 5.4 Clinical application of a membrane-covered bone grafting

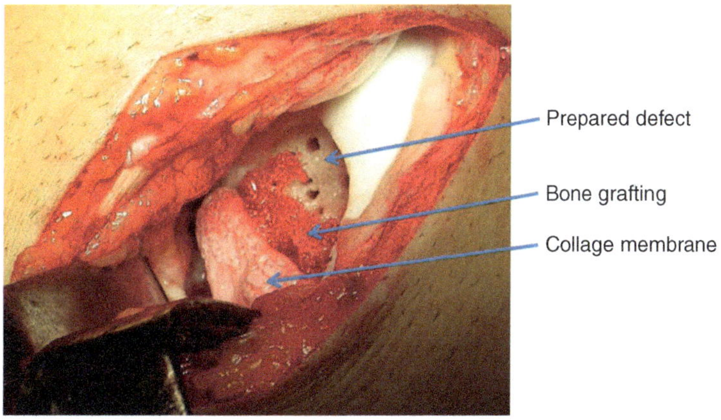

followed by a period of progressive weight bearing for 5 weeks. Physiotherapy is recommended two to three times per week in the initial postoperative phase.

After reconstruction of patellofemoral cartilage defects, flexion is limited to 30° for 2 weeks and 60° and 90°, respectively, for each two subsequent weeks. The use of a CPM device is obligatory for at least 3 h per day for 6 weeks postoperatively.

In defects of the femoral condyles, flexion is restricted to 90° for the first 6 weeks. To support our patients in obeying these limits, we equip them with an adjustable soft brace for the time of restricted motion and weight bearing. We recommend pharmacological thrombosis prophylaxis during the partial weight-bearing period.

After the protection phase (week 0–6) [26], full weight bearing is accomplished over a time period of 1–2 weeks, followed by a physiotherapeutic gait training, coordinative training, and a muscle-strengthening program. Return to sports is allowed not before 6 months after the operation.

5.5 Postoperative Follow-Up

We recommend an outpatient appointment for removal of the stitches after 10–12 days. After termination of the unloading phase 6 weeks postoperatively, a further clinical evaluation is performed. Joint mobility should have reached 90° of flexion and patellar mobility should be sufficient at this date. A further clinical evaluation can be arranged. A reevaluation after 6 months together with an MRI scan is obligatory to be able to evaluate the morphologic result of the intervention. Depending on the clinical result and MRI evaluation, reintegration to sport is arranged. The prerequisite for this step is competence in stabilizing the limb and having reached quadriceps force levels of about 80 % compared to the contralateral lower extremity.

The AMIC™ technique is a relatively new procedure not yet allowing a conclusion in respect to mid- and long-term results to date. The available case–control studies (level of evidence IV) with short follow-up periods are encouraging [22–24].

Nevertheless, we have to expect the same problems as with all marrow stimulation techniques in the future. This expectation already found its confirmation in a comparative study of ACI and AMIC™ of Dorotka and coworkers [25].

References

1. Fuller JA, Ghadially FN (1972) Ultrastructural observations on surgically produced partial-thickness defects in articular cartilage. Clin Orthop 86:193–205
2. Grande DA, Pitman MI, Peterson L, Menche D, Klein M (1989) The repair of experimentally produced defects in rabbit articular cartilage by autologous chondrocyte transplantation. J Orthop Res 7(2): 208–218
3. Mankin HJ (1982) The response of articular cartilage to mechanical injury. J Bone Joint Surg 64A:460–466
4. Shapiro F, Koide S, Glimcher MJ (1993) Cell origin and differentiation in the repair of full-thickness defects of articular cartilage. J Bone Joint Surg (A) 75(4):532–553
5. Steadman JR, Rodkey WG, Briggs KK (2002) Microfracture to treat full-thickness chondral defects: surgical technique, rehabilitation and outcomes. J Knee Surg 15(3):170–176
6. Steadman JR, Briggs KK, Rodrigo JJ, Kocher MS, Gill TJ, Rodkey WG (2003) Outcomes of microfracture for traumatic chondral defects of the knee: average 11-year follow-up. Arthroscopy 19(5):477–484
7. Steinwachs MR, Kreuz PC, Krause S, Lahm A (2003) Klinische Ergebnisse nach Mikrofrakturierung bei der Behandlung von Gelenkknorpeldefekten. Sportortho Sporttrauma 19:291–294
8. Steinwachs MR, Guggi T, Kreuz PC (2008) Marrow stimulation technique. Injury 39S1:26–31
9. Pridie KH (1959) A method of resurfacing osteoarthritic knee joints. J Bone Joint Surg (Br) 41:618–619
10. Tippet JW (1996) Articular cartilage drilling and osteotomy in osteoarthritis of the knee. In: McGinty JB, Caspari RB, Jackson RW, Poehling GG (eds) Operative arthroscopy, 2nd edn. Raven Press, Philadelphia, pp 411–426
11. Saris DB, Vanlauwe J, Victor J, Almqvist KF, Verdonk R, Bellemans J, Luyten FP (2007) Characterized chondrocyte implantation results in better structural repair when treating symptomatic cartilage defects of the knee in a randomized controlled trial versus microfracture. Am J Sports Med 36:235–246
12. Saris DB, Vanlauwe J, Victor J, Almqvist KF, Verdonk R, Bellemans J, Luyten FP (2009) Treatment of symptomatic cartilage defects of the knee: characterized chondrocyte implantation results in better clinical outcome at 36 months in a randomized trial compared to microfracture. Am J Sports Med 37(Suppl 1): 10S–19S
13. Kreuz PC, Erggelet C, Steinwachs MR, Krause SJ, Lahm A, Niemeyer P, Ghanem N, Uhl M, Südkamp N (2006) Is microfracture of chondral defects in the knee associated with different results in patients aged 40 years or younger? Arthroscopy 22(11):1180–1186
14. Kreuz PC, Steinwachs MR, Erggelet C, Krause SJ, Konrad G, Uhl M, Südkamp N (2006) Results after microfracture of full-thickness chondral defects in different compartments in the knee. Osteoarthritis Cartilage 14(11):1119–1125
15. Mithoefer K, Williams RJ, Warren RF, Potter HG, Spock CR, Jones EC, Wickiewicz TL, Marx RG (2005) The microfracture technique for the treatment of articular cartilage lesions in the knee. A prospective cohort study. J Bone Joint Surg Am 87(9): 1911–1920
16. Mithoefer K, McAdams T, Williams RJ, Kreuz PC, Mandelbaum BR (2009) Clinical efficacy of the microfracture technique for articular cartilage repair in the knee: an evidence-based systematic analysis. Am J Sports Med 37(10):2053–2063
17. Steinwachs MR, Engebretsen L, Brophy RH (2012) Scientific evidence base for cartilage injury and repair in the athlete. Cartilage 3:11S–17S

18. Wakitani S, Goto T, Pineda SJ, Young RG, Mansour JM, Caplan AI, Goldberg VM (1994) Mesenchymal cell-based repair of large, full-thickness defects of articular cartilage. J Bone Joint Surg (A) 76(4):579–592
19. Behrens P (2005) Matrixgekoppelte Mikrofrakturierung. Arthroskopie 18:193–197
20. Steinwachs MR, Waibl B, Niemeyer P (2011) Use of human progenitor cells in the treatment of cartilage damage. Bundesgesundheitsblatt Gesundheitsforschung Gesundheitsschutz 54(7):797–802
21. Niemeyer P, Andereya S, Angele P, Ateschrang A, Aurich M, Baumann M, Behrens P, Bosch U, Erggelet C, Fickert S, Fritz J, Gebhard H, Gelse K, Günther D, Hoburg A, Kasten P, Kolombe T, Madry H, Marlovits S, Meenen NM, Müller PE, Nöth U, Petersen JP, Pietschmann M, Richter W, Rolauffs B, Rhunau K, Schewe B, Steinert A, Steinwachs MR, Welsch GH, Zinser W, Albrecht D (2013) Autologous chondrocyte implantation (ACI) for cartilage defects of the knee: a guideline by the working group "Tissue Regeneration" of the German Society of Orthopaedic Surgery and Traumatology (DGOU). Z Orthop Unfall 151(1):38–47
22. Valderrabano V, Miska M, Leumann A, Wiewiorski M (2013) Reconstruction of osteochondral lesions of the talus with autologous spongiosa grafts and autologous matrix-induced chondrogenesis. Am J Sports Med 41(3):519–527
23. Leunig M, Tibor LM, Naal FD, Ganz R, Steinwachs MR (2012) Surgical technique: second-generation bone marrow stimulation via surgical dislocation to treat hip cartilage lesions. Clin Orthop Relat Res 470(12):3421–3431
24. Gille J, Schuseil E, Wimmer J, Gelissen J, Schulz AP, Behrens P (2010) Mid-term results of autologous matrix-induced chondrogenesis for treatment of focal cartilage defects in the knee. Knee Surg Sports Traumatol Arthrosc 18(11):1456–1464
25. Dorotka R, Bindreiter U, Macfelda K, Windberger U, Nehrer S (2005) Marrow stimulation and chondrocyte transplantation using a collagen matrix for cartilage repair. Osteoarthritis Cartilage 13(8):655–664
26. Hambly K, Silvers H, Steinwachs M (2012) Rehabilitation after articular cartilage repair in the football player. Cartilage 3(Suppl 1):505–565

Autologous Collagen-Induced Chondrogenesis (ACIC™)

6

Asode Ananthram Shetty, Seok-Jung Kim, and Vishvas A. Shetty

Contents

A.A. Shetty, MD, PhD, MCh, FRCS Ed., FRCS Eng., FRCS Orth (✉)
Department of Minimally Invasive Surgery, Faculty of Health and Social Sciences, Canterbury Christ Church University, Pembroke Court 30, ME4 4UF Chatham Maritime, Kent, UK

Faculty of Stem Cell Research and Regenerative Medicine, NITTE University, Mangalore, India
e-mail: aashetty@hotmail.com

S.-J. Kim, MD, PhD, FRCS
Department of Orthopedic Surgery, Uijeongbu St. Mary's Hospital, College of Medicine, The Catholic University of Korea, 480-717 Gyeonggi-do, Republic of (South Korea)

Faculty of Stem Cell Research and Regenerative Medicine, NITTE University, Mangalore, India
e-mail: orthopland@naver.com

V.A. Shetty
Department of Minimally Invasive Surgery, Faculty of Health and Social Sciences, Canterbury Christ Church University, Pembroke Court 30, ME4 4UF, Chatham Maritime, Kent, UK

6.1 Introduction

Articular cartilage defects in the knee joint are commonly seen in today's clinical practice [1]. They were recognised early on by the likes of Galen and William Hunter, though we have begun to effectively diagnose and treat them only in the last few decades [2, 3].

In the last three decades, the treatment of chondral defects has steadily evolved across the world, striving towards better quality cartilage and minimally invasive techniques. Since the 1980s, microfracture remains popular despite conclusive evidence that it results in the formation of fibrocartilage [4]. Osteochondral grafting replaces the defect with native hyaline cartilage but is limited by the size and number of lesions [5]. ACI forms hyaline-like cartilage and can be used for large lesions, but two surgical procedures, delamination and morbidity of arthrotomy, prove expensive for all [6, 7].

The use of single-stage arthroscopic procedure has obvious advantages. Apart from being less expensive, it reduces rehabilitation time for the patient and avoids the complications of an arthrotomy [6, 7]. The novel technique described below treats chondral defects arthroscopically, utilising autologous collagen and a fibrin gel preparation which ensures good fixation and growth of hyaline-like cartilage.

The use of autologous collagen and cell-free collagen scaffolds in cartilage repair is well established [8, 9]. They are known to form an effective scaffold for cartilage regeneration and help in forming hyaline-like cartilage. Atelocollagen is

A.A. Shetty et al. (eds.), *Techniques in Cartilage Repair Surgery*,
DOI 10.1007/978-3-642-41921-8_6, © ESSKA 2014

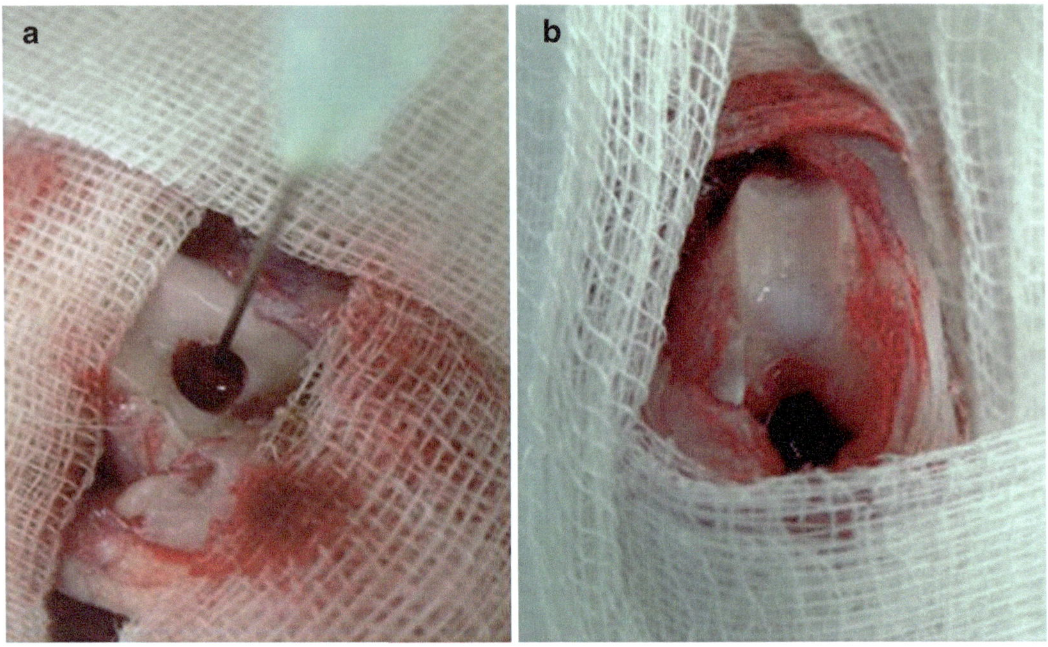

Fig. 6.1 (**a**) Microdrilling and (**b**) injection of atelocollagen gel in rabbit model

known for its biocompatibility and low risk of adverse reactions. [9] (Figs. 6.1, 6.2, 6.3, and 6.4).

Collagen-based scaffolds and gels have been tested to promote better fixation of the graft [10]. Collagen is the connective tissue protein which is important in maintaining the morphology of tissue. The form used in our technique is atelocollagen, which is a highly purified type I collagen obtained following the treatment of pepsin from skin dermis. The removal of telopeptide (A-telocollagen) renders it immunologically neutral [9]. For this reason, atelocollagen has been used for the purposes of wound healing, vessel prosthesis, bone substitute and hemostatic agent.

Fibrin gel is used as it mimics final step of the coagulation and helps control bone bleeding [11]. Fibrin is also useful in cartilage regeneration as it has high biocompatibility and is a suitable carrier for generating neo-cartilage [12, 13]. Due to its gel form, various sized defects can be treated. On combination of thrombin and fibrin, the gel hardens in about 5 min and holds the collagen mixture in place. Kim et al. [14] demonstrated that fibrin can form fibrous and solid wall-like structures, 200–1,000 nm in diameter. Hence, fibrin gels are used as material for a scaffold in cartilage repair and regeneration [15].

The CO_2 in this technique is bolstered by its extensive use in laparoscopic surgery [16]. Animal studies have shown no untoward events on continuous intravenous infusion [17]. Microdrilling to the depth of 6 mm produces greater subchondral haematoma with increased access to marrow stroma; this improves stem cell recruitment [18]. These channels also provide rotational stability for the graft [19]. However, the results of the rabbit study by Chen et al. [18] still have to be confirmed by clinical human studies.

6.2 Autologous Collagen

The autologous collagen filler used is ACIC™. ACIC™ consists of 3 ml of porcine-derived atelocollagen that induces cell conduction and induction. In combination with marrow stimulation techniques (microdrilling, microfracture, etc.) and fibrin gel, it is known to form a stable matrix structure that secures and stimulates marrow cells. ACIC™ should be stored at 1–30 °C.

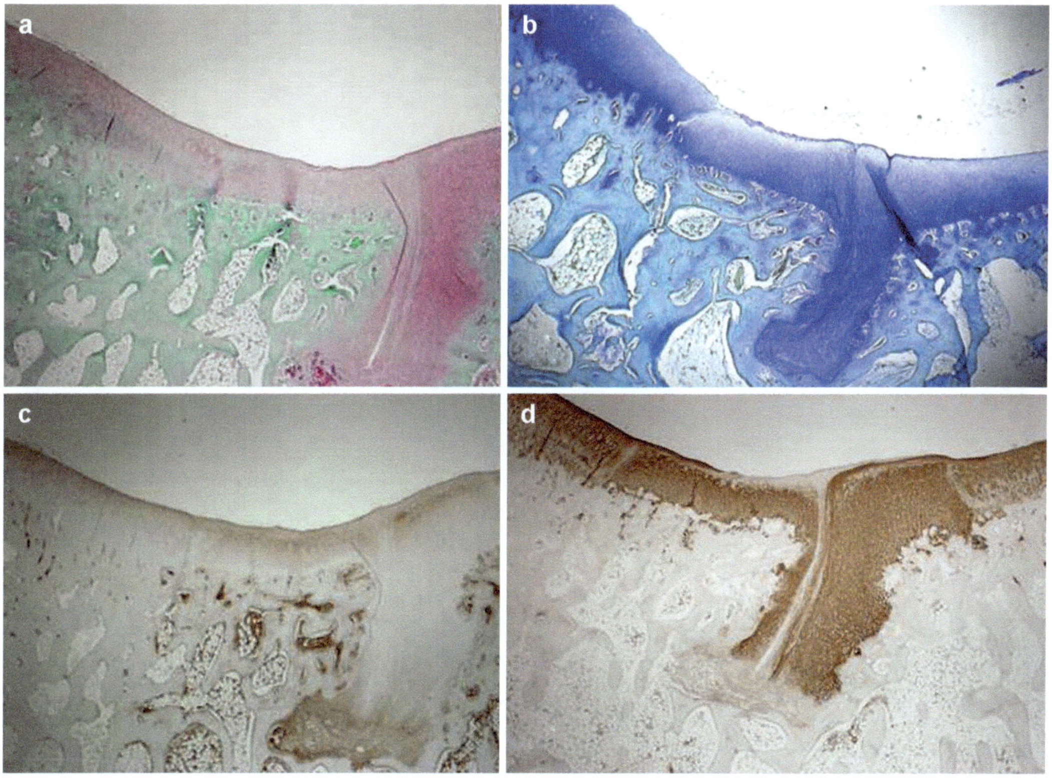

Fig. 6.2 (a) Safranin-O and (b) toluidine blue staining showing smooth cartilage. (c) Immunohistochemical staining with anti-collagen type I antibody and (d) immunohistochemical staining with anti-collagen type II antibody (×40). Immunohistochemistry showing minimal type 1 collagen and mainly type 2 collagen

6.3 Patient Selection

Patient selection is the key to the success of the procedure. This includes associated conditions apart from chondral damage which contribute to the pain and affect the outcome of surgery.

Suitable candidates undergo a thorough clinical examination, including a detailed history. Significant medical comorbidities which may increase perioperative mortality may preclude surgery. Advice regarding weight loss, diet and smoking cessation is given throughout the perioperative period. The stability of the knee, flexed flexion deformity and range of movement is tested at this stage, along with function of the hip and ankle joints.

If found suitable for the procedure, they undergo the cartilage imaging protocol, which consists of the following:

- Weight-bearing long-leg radiograph
- Lateral and skyline radiographic views of affected knee
- MRI (DESS sequencing) of affected knee
- CT patellar tracking of both knees

Alignment is measured on the long-leg radiograph. Corrective osteotomy would be considered for malalignment (varus or valgus) more than 5°. Patellofemoral maltracking is corrected by tibial tubercle transfer. Instability is orrected by suitable ligament reconstruction.

MRI scans have been deemed suitable for detecting and quantifying chondral lesions. With newer sequences, even early lesions can be detected with reasonable accuracy [20]. Associated conditions such as meniscal tears, ligamentous insufficiencies and loose bodies are also noted and are treated simultaneously.

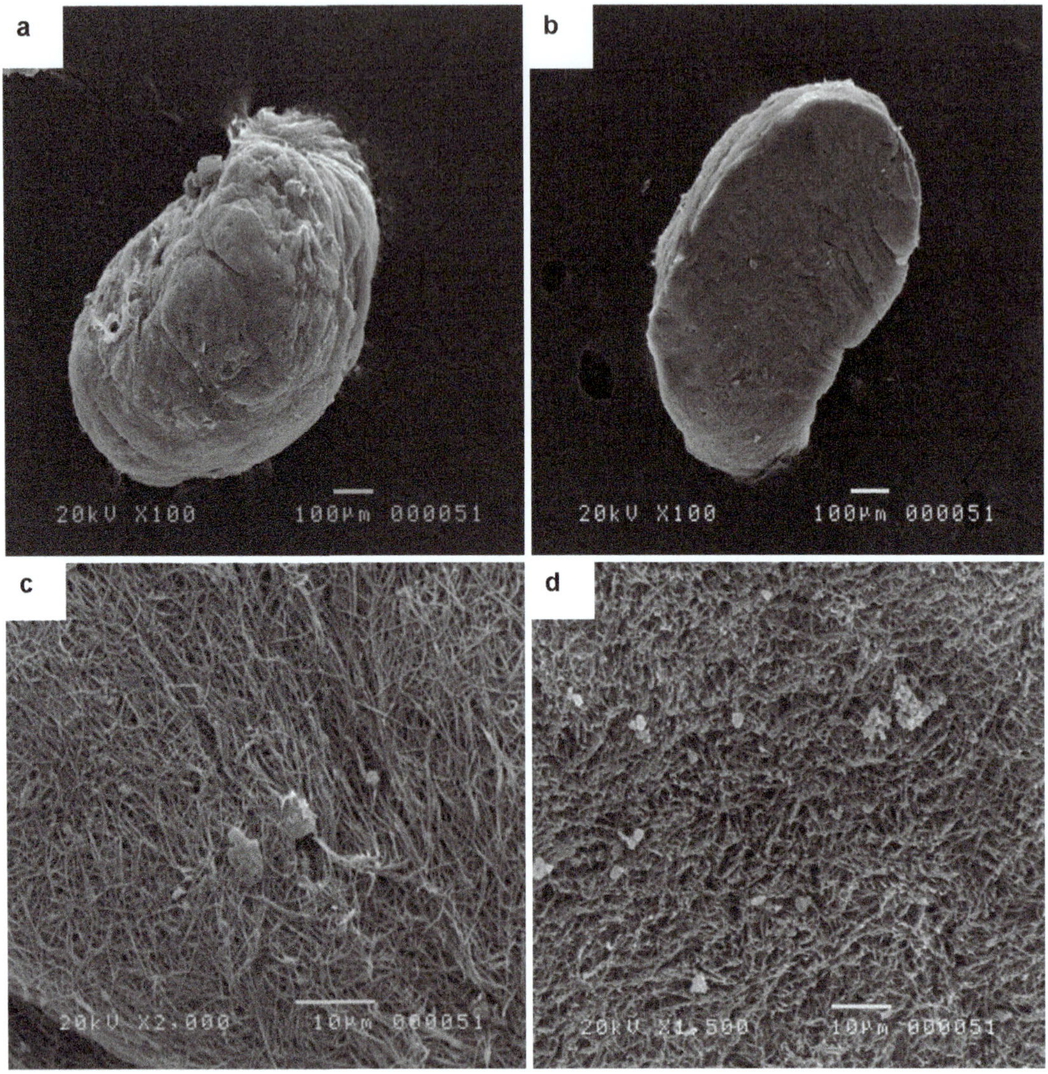

Fig. 6.3 The microstructures of MSC-collagen beads at 21 days (**a–d**) Scanning electron microscopic images of the surfaces (**a**, **b**) and insides (**c**, **d**) of MSC-collagen gel beads culture

6.3.1 Inclusion Criteria

- Patients aged 18–65 years
- Diagnosed with articular cartilage defect in the knee (ICRS/outer bridge grade III/IV cartilage lesions as assessed on MRI scan)
- Less than three lesions, measuring more than 2 cm^2 and less than 9 cm^2
- Symptoms less than 3 years' duration

6.3.2 Exclusion Criteria

- Age below 18 and over 65 years
- Generalised and/or inflammatory arthritis
- Active joint inflammation
- More than three lesions
- Lesions more than 9 cm^2
- Ligament instability

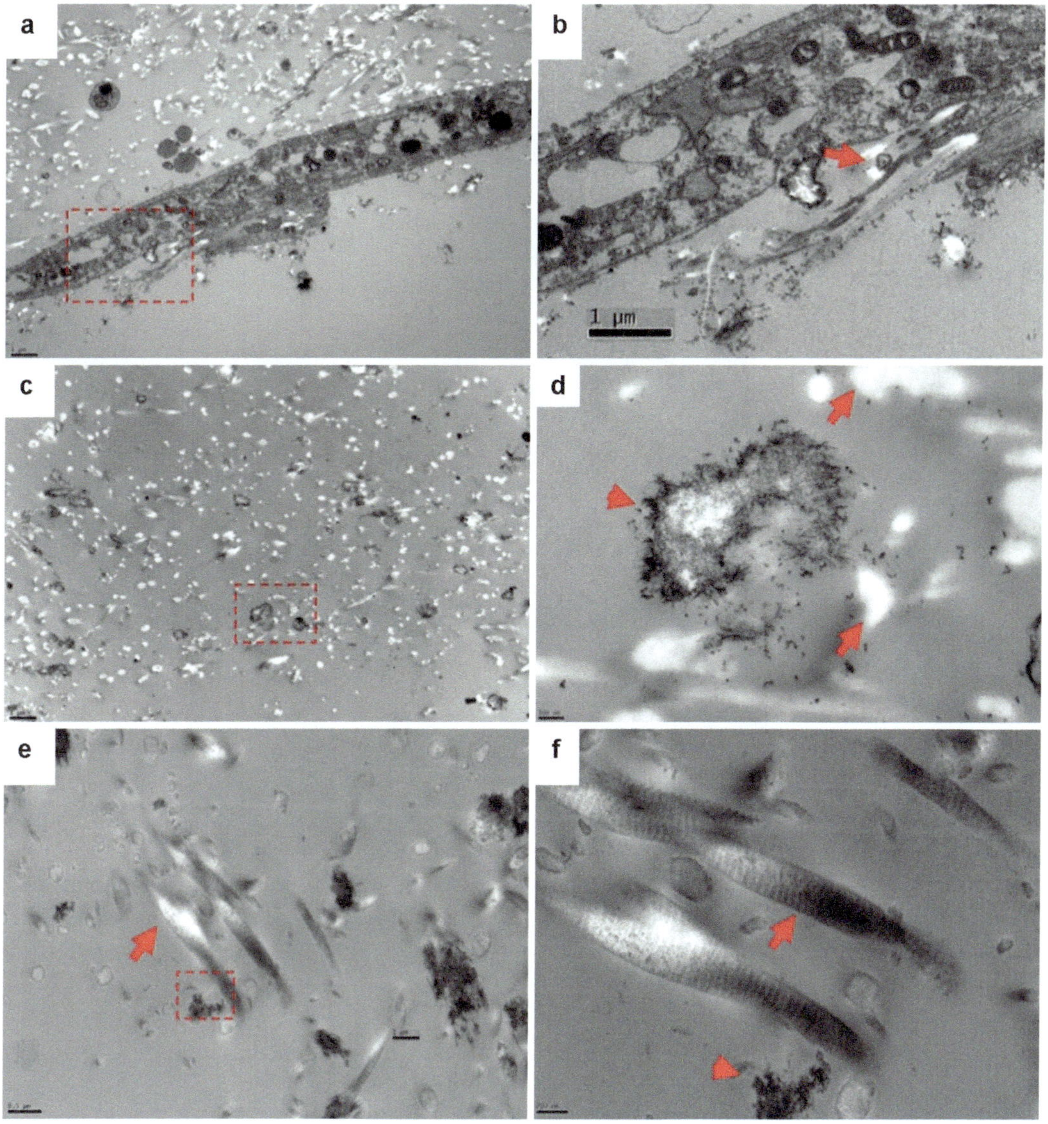

Fig. 6.4 (**a–f**) Scanning electron microscopic images of MSC-collagen gel beads culture. Transmission electron microscopic images revealed newly biosynthesised collagen fibres. Only newly synthesised collagen fibres (*arrows*) and incorporated cells were visible in the TEM pictures of MSC-collagen hydrogel beads. Collagen scaffolds made of atelocollagen were not visualised by TEM (**b**, **d** and **f** are the enlarged versions of the area within the *dotted boxes* in **a**, **c** and **e**)

6.4 Theatre and Patient Setup

Theatre setup is similar to routine arthroscopy. The surgeon is seated on the side being operated and the stack system is placed on the opposite side for comfortable visualisation of the monitor. The CO_2 pump is placed on the stack system trolley with a filter and sterile insufflation tubing (insufflation tubing with Wolf adaptor, Leonhard Lang UK Ltd., Stroud, UK).

Patient is positioned supine with the table horizontal at an appropriate height. Lateral supports are preferable for medial compartment lesions, especially with associated meniscal

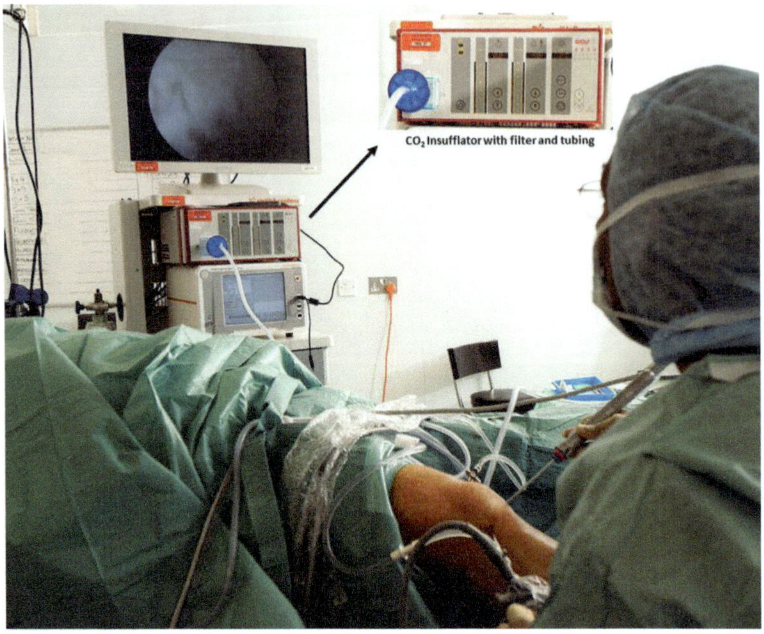

Fig. 6.5 Theatre setup

tears. A tourniquet is applied as high up on the thigh as possible and inflated to 100 mg above systolic blood pressure.

Patient is anesthetised using general or spinal anaesthesia. NSAIDs are withheld as these drugs are known to be chondrotoxic. Appropriate antibiotic is administered intravenously prior to inflation of tourniquet (Fig. 6.5).

6.5 Surgical Technique

6.5.1 Preparation of Atelocollagen Mixture

Unpack contents of atelocollagen (ACIC™, CYP biotech, Seoul, Korea) and fibrin sealant (TISSEEL®, Baxter, Thetford, UK):

- With sterile precautions, transfer 1 ml of the aprotinin solution into the vial containing fibrinogen powder. Completely dissolve the fibrinogen powder by careful stirring without excessive frothing. Transfer 1 ml of this mixture into one of the DUPLOJECT syringes (step 1).
- With sterile precautions, transfer 1 ml of the calcium chloride into the vial containing thrombin powder (human thrombin lyophilised) and stir until the thrombin powder is dissolved. A syringe containing 0.2 ml of the thrombin and the atelocollagen implant syringe are then attached to a connector and mix. Transfer 1 ml of this mixture into one of the DUPLOJECT syringes (steps 1 and 2).
- Both DUPLOJECT syringes (A and B) are placed in the kit.

The mixed contents are ready to be applied onto the cartilage defect (step 3) (Fig. 6.6).

6.6 Preparation of Chondral Defect for Implantation

The standard anterolateral and anteromedial arthroscopic portals were used to approach the knee, and normal saline under pressure was infused. A superomedial portal was used for an outflow cannula. Under arthroscopic vision, the number, size and location of the lesions are confirmed. If considered suitable for surgery, the lesions are then carefully debrided to bare subchondral bone. It is imperative that a stable shoulder of healthy cartilage is maintained at the

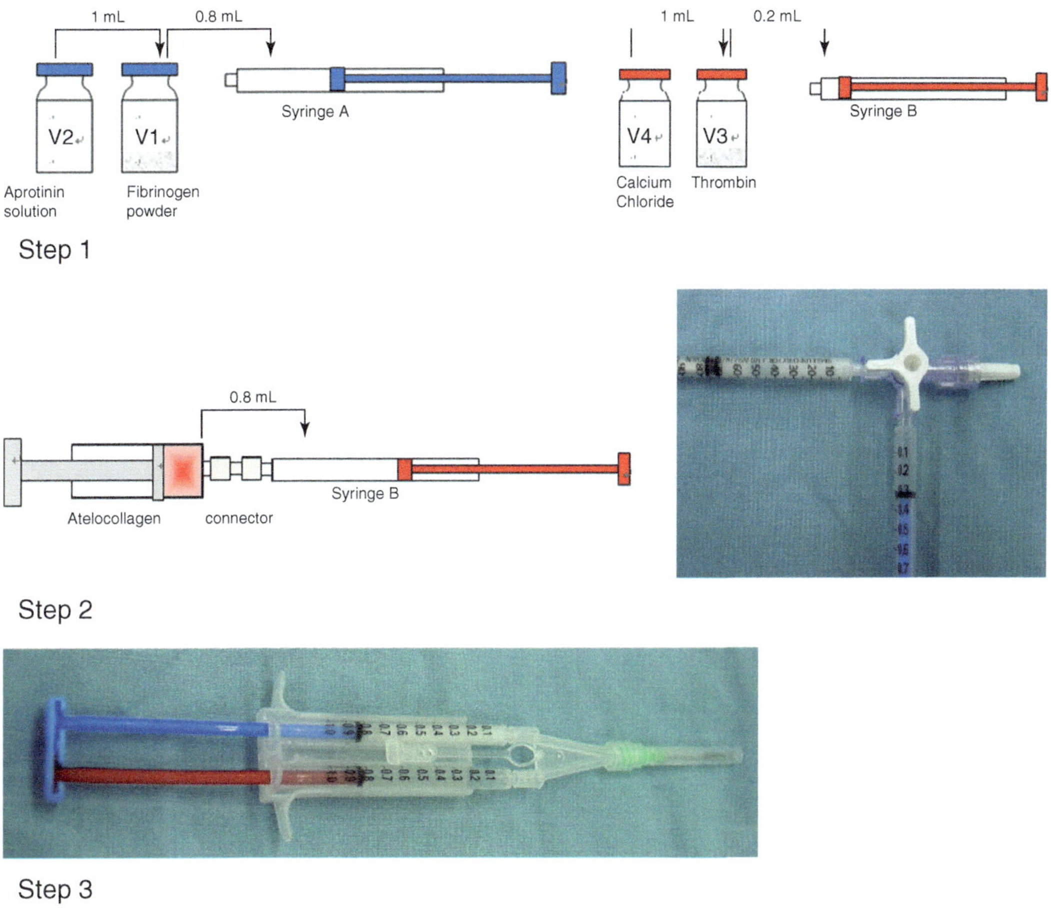

Fig. 6.6 Preparation of autologous collagen and fibrin gel mixture. *Step 1* Syringe A. B preparation. *Step 2* Mix with atelocollagen and syringe B preparation. *Step 3* Ready to use

periphery of the lesions. The subchondral bone was drilled with a 45°-angled drill (PowerPick drill, Arthrex, UK) up to a depth of 6 mm, at 3-mm intervals.

Once ready for implantation, normal saline is switched off and CO_2 is insufflated at 20 mm of Hg, flowing at 20 l/min. The CO_2 is introduced via a Wolf cannula (Karl Storz GmbH, Tuttlingen, Germany) and disposable tubing with a filter (insufflation tubing with Wolf adaptor, Leonhard Lang UK Ltd., Stroud, UK) through the superolateral portal. Any residual saline is aspirated via an angled suction tube (Exmoor, Taunton, UK) and the chondral lesion is dried using cotton buds.

A 20-gauge needle (inner diameter 0.9 mm, length 90 mm) (spinal needle, Becton Dickinson, Madrid, Spain) is inserted into the joint via any suitable portal and connected to the previously prepared DUPLOJECT syringe. Under arthroscopic vision, a layer of gel was applied into the defect. For patellofemoral joint lesions, a patellar clamp (AO or Lewin bone clamp) can be used to lift and stabilise the patella. Once this first layer becomes firm (after about 1–2 min), a second layer can be injected deep to the first layer. A McDonalds dissector (Bolton Surgical, UK) is used to shape the graft in situ, within 5 min, after which the gel hardens. The knee is taken through its range of motion to test the stability of the graft and to mould it further.

Once the stability of the graft was established, all instruments were withdrawn. Hyaluronic acid

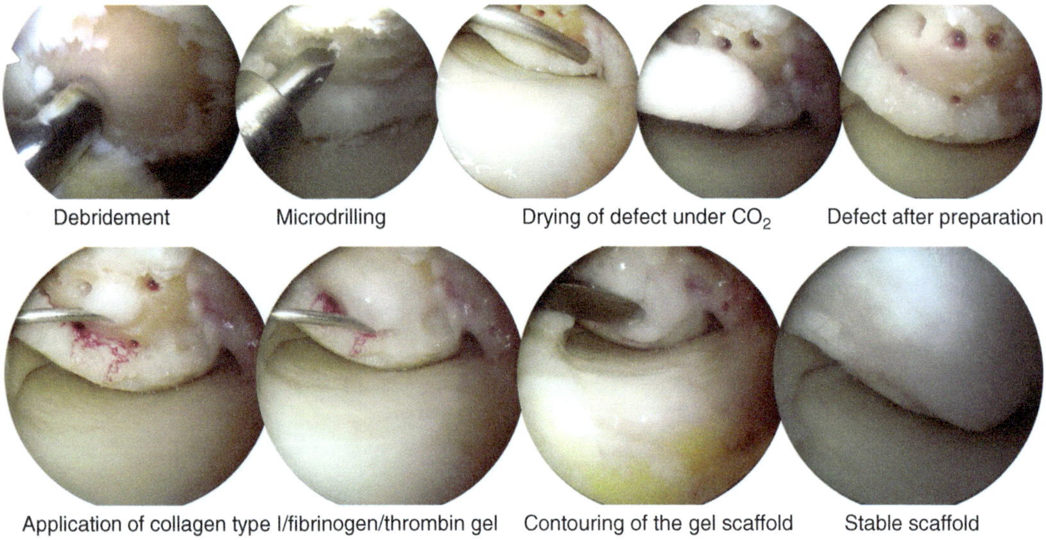

Fig. 6.7 Surgical technique for preparation of lesion and implantation of collagen-fibrin gel

(Highhyal, Huons, Seoul, Korea) was injected into the joint and local anaesthetic was injected around the portals. The skin was closed either by sutures or butterfly stitches (Fig. 6.7).

6.7 Postoperative Rehabilitation

Following surgery, CPM is initiated for 4–6 h while the patient remains in the hospital. Patients with tibiofemoral lesions are instructed to partially weight bearing on the operated leg, starting of 25 % of full weight on day 0 and gradually building up to 100 % of full weight at 6 weeks [21]. Patients with patellofemoral lesions are fitted with a brace on the operated leg and flexion is increased by 20° a week, up to 6 weeks, when the brace is removed [19]. Patients are advised not to return to active sport for at least 9–12 months following the surgery [19]. They are allowed low-resistance, cycling, swimming (avoiding breast stroke) and walking to keep fit.

Patients are advised to avoid NSAIDs for pain control for at least 12 weeks following surgery as these drugs have toxic on cell membranes [22]. Alternate pain medication is prescribed. Any other medication being taken is monitored and coexisting medical conditions are treated effectively.

All patients underwent MRI scans at 12 and 18 months following the surgery. At 12 months, cartilage was imaged using DESS sequencing and T2* mapping. A d-GEMRIC scan was done at 18 months.

6.8 Results

The technique described above has been in use for over 4 years now and encouraging results have been seen, both clinically and radiologically. Patients were asked to complete the Lysholm Score, IKDC score and the KOOS score pre- and postoperatively. They also underwent MRI scans with cartilage specific protocols prior to surgery and at 12 and 18 months following surgery. The Lysholm score improved from 51.7 ± 27.1 (mean ± standard deviation) preoperatively to 81.3 ± 24.6 at 2-year follow-up ($p < 0.05$). The mean MOCART score at 1-year follow-up was 70.4 ± 20.2 ranging from 15 to 95 [9]. The mean MOCART score at 1-year follow-up was 71.7 ± 21.0 ranging from 25 to 95. The mean T2* relaxation times were 30.6 ± 11.3 ms and 28.8 ± 6.8 ms for the repair tissue and surrounding native cartilage, respectively. The T2* ratio between the repair tissue and native cartilage was 105 ± 30 %, indicating repair tissue properties similar to native cartilage [23].

References

1. Elders MJ (2000) The increasing impact of arthritis on public health. J Rheumatol Suppl 60:6–8
2. Hirshorn KC, Cates T, Gillogly S (2010) Magnetic resonance imaging-documented chondral injuries about the knee in college football players: 3-year National Football League Combine data. Arthroscopy 26(9):1237–1240. doi:10.1016/j.arthro.2010.01.025, Epub 2010 Jul 14
3. Hunter W (1743) On the structure and diseases of articulating cartilage. Philos Trans R Soc Lond B Biol Sci 42B:514–521
4. Carey JL (2012) Fibrocartilage following microfracture is not as robust as native articular cartilage: commentary on an article by Aaron J. Krych, MD, et al.: "Activity levels are higher after osteochondral autograft transfer mosaicplasty than after microfracture for articular cartilage defects of the knee. A retrospective comparative study". J Bone Joint Surg Am 94(11):e80. doi:10.2106/JBJS.L.00319
5. Robb CA, El-Sayed C, Matharu GS, Baloch K, Pynsent P (2012) Survival of autologous osteochondral grafts in the knee and factors influencing outcome. Acta Orthop Belg 78(5):643–651
6. Gardner OF, Archer CW, Alini M, Stoddart MJ (2013) Chondrogenesis of mesenchymal stem cells for cartilage tissue engineering. Histol Histopathol 28(1):23–42
7. Ipach I, Schäfer R, Lahrmann J, Kluba T (2011) Stiffness after knee arthrotomy: evaluation of prevalence and results after manipulation under anaesthesia. Orthop Traumatol Surg Res 97(3):292–296. doi:10.1016/j.otsr.2011.01.006, Epub 2011 Apr 11
8. Efe T, Theisen C, Fuchs-Winkelmann S et al (2012) Cell-free collagen type I matrix for repair of cartilage defects-clinical and magnetic resonance imaging results. Knee Surg Sports Traumatol Arthrosc 20(10): 1915–1922
9. Shetty AA, Kim SJ, Bilagi P, Stelzeneder D (2013) Autologous collagen-induced chondrogenesis: single-stage arthroscopic cartilage repair technique. Orthopedics 36(5):e648–e652. doi:10.3928/01477447-20130426-30
10. Efe T, Theisen C, Fuchs-Winkelmann S et al (2011) Cell-free collagen type I matrix for repair of cartilage defects-clinical and magnetic resonance imaging results. Knee Surg Sports Traumatol Arthrosc 20(10):1915–1922
11. Mawatari M, Higo T, Tsutsumi Y et al (2006) Effectiveness of autologous fibrin tissue adhesive in reducing postoperative blood loss during total hip arthroplasty: a prospective randomised study of 100 cases. J Orthop Surg 14:117
12. Keller J, Andreassen TT, Joyce F et al (1985) Fixation of osteochondral fractures, fibrin sealant tested in dogs. Acta Orthop Scand 56:323
13. Peterson L, Brittberg M, Kiviranta I et al (2002) Autologous chondrocyte transplantation: biomechanics and long-term durability. Am J Sports Med 30:2
14. Jang J-D, Moon Y-S, Kim Y-S, Choi N-Y, Mok H-S, Kim Y-J, Shetty AA, Kim S-J (2013) Novel repair technique for articular cartilage defect using a fibrin and hyaluronic acid mixture. Tissue Eng Regen Med 10(1):1–9. doi:10.1007/s13770-013-0361-0
15. Davis H, Binder BY, Schaecher P, Yakoobinsky D, Bhat A, Leach JK (2013) Enhancing osteoconductivity of fibrin gels with apatite-coated polymer microspheres. Tissue Eng Part A 19:1773–1782
16. Hirai F, Beppu T, Nishimura T, Takatsu N, Ashizuka S, Seki T, Hisabe T, Nagahama T, Yao K, Matsui T, Nakashima R, Inada N, Tajiri E, Mitsuru H, Shigematsu H (2011) Carbon dioxide insufflation compared with air insufflation in double-balloon enteroscopy: a prospective, randomized, double-blind trial. Gastrointest Endosc 73(4):743–749, doi:S0016-5107(10)02188-7 [pii]
17. Corson SL, Hoffman JJ, Jackowski J, Chapman GA (1988) Cardiopulmonary effects of direct venous CO2 insufflation in ewes. A model for CO2 hysteroscopy. J Reprod Med 33(5):440–444
18. Chen H, Sun J, Hoemann CD, Lascau-Coman V, Ouyang W, McKee MD, Shive MS, Buschmann MD (2009) Drilling and microfracture lead to different bone structure and necrosis during bone-marrow stimulation for cartilage repair. J Orthop Res 27(11):1432–1438. doi:10.1002/jor.20905
19. Jang J-D, Moon Y-S, Kim Y-S, Choi N-Y, Mok H-S, Kim Y-J, Shetty AA, Kim S-J (2013) Novel repair technique for articular cartilage defect using aFibrin and hyaluronic acid mixture. Tissue Eng Regen Med 10(1):1–9
20. Roemer FW, Crema MD, Trattnig S, Guermazi A (2011) Advances in imaging of osteoarthritis and cartilage. Radiology 260(2):332–354, doi: 260/2/332 [pii]
21. Reinold MM, Wilk KE, Macrina LC, Dugas JR, Cain EL (2006) Current concepts in the rehabilitation following articular cartilage repair procedures in the knee. J Orthop Sports Phys Ther 36:774–794
22. Pereira-Leite C, Nunes C, Reis S (2013) Interaction of nonsteroidal anti-inflammatory drugs with membranes: in vitro assessment and relevance for their biological actions. Prog Lipid Res 52(4):571–584. doi:10.1016/j.plipres.2013.08.003, pii: S0163-7827(13)00048-9
23. Stelzeneder D, Shetty AA, Kim SJ, Trattnig S, Domayer SE, Shetty V, Bilagi P (2013) Repair tissue quality after arthroscopic autologous collagen-induced chondrogenesis (ACIC) Assessed via T2* mapping. Skeletal Radiol 42(12):1657–1664

TruFit®

7

Richard W. Kang, Richard Ma, Delia A. Pais, and Riley J. Williams III

Contents

R.W. Kang, MS, MD (✉) • R. Ma, MD • D.A. Pais, BA
R.J. Williams III, MD
Departments of Sports Medicine and Shoulder Service, Hospital for Special Surgery, 535 East 70th Street, New York, NY 10021, USA
e-mail: kangr@hss.edu; mar@hss.edu; paisd@hss.edu; williamsr@hss.edu

7.1 Technical Details

The TruFit® CB (cartilage/bone) (Smith & Nephew, San Antonio, TX) is a resorbable implant consisting of semiporous 75:25 poly D,L-LACTIDE-CO-glycolide (PLG) copolymer, calcium sulfate, polyglycolide acid (PGA) fibers, and surfactant [1]. The implant is designed to replicate mechanical properties of the superficial (articular cartilage) and deep (bone) aspects of an osteochondral lesion. The superficial phase is softer and functions as a scaffold to facilitate cartilage regeneration. The deep phase contains calcium sulfate, which improves its strength. Incorporation of the PGA fibers has been shown to improve the implant's compressive modulus and yield strength [2].

7.2 Patient Selection

As with any newer technique, the indications and contraindications will become clearer over time. However, our understanding of osteochondral autograft and allograft procedures can help elucidate our indications for TruFit®. Patients with symptomatic unipolar osteochondral or full-thickness cartilage lesions would be indicated for the TruFit® procedure. Patients with smaller lesions may benefit from implantation of a single synthetic plug. For patients with larger lesions, but smaller than 600 mm^2, synthetic scaffold mosaicplasty would be indicated. Absolute contraindications include, but are not limited to, generalized arthritis, inflammatory arthritis, and

A.A. Shetty et al. (eds.), *Techniques in Cartilage Repair Surgery*,
DOI 10.1007/978-3-642-41921-8_7, © ESSKA 2014

joint infection. Relative contraindications for this procedure would include bipolar lesions, malalignment, ligamentous laxity, and significant meniscal deficiency. It is possible to address these comorbid pathologies through performing concomitant or staged procedures.

Obtaining preoperative cartilage-sensitive MRI imaging is an important tool in determining whether patients are indicated for surgery. Moreover, MRI studies can help characterize the size and location of the lesion, which can facilitate surgical planning.

7.3 Patient Setup and Bone Marrow Concentrate (BMC) Preparation

1. Place patient supine on the operating room table and apply a non-sterile thigh tourniquet.
2. Prep a sterile field for the ipsilateral iliac crest bone marrow harvest.
3. Place and mallet in the Jamshidi needle into the ipsilateral iliac crest (Fig. 7.1).
4. Aspirate approximately 50 ml of bone marrow aspirate from the iliac crest (Fig. 7.2).

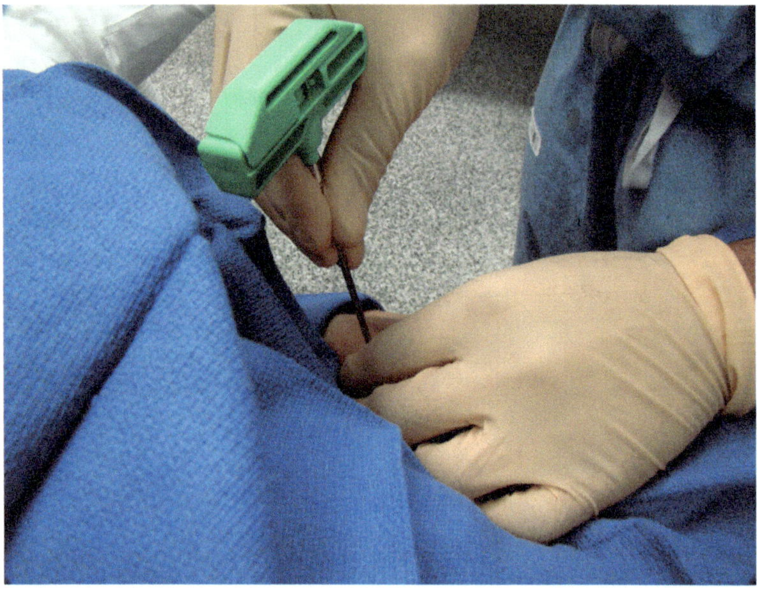

Fig. 7.1 Jamshidi needle placed into ipsilateral iliac crest

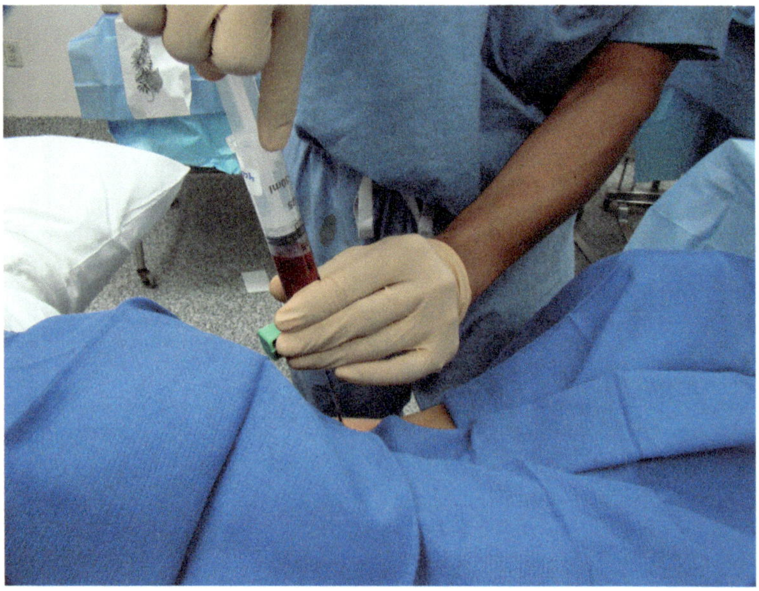

Fig. 7.2 Bone marrow aspiration. 50 cc of aspirate will be obtained

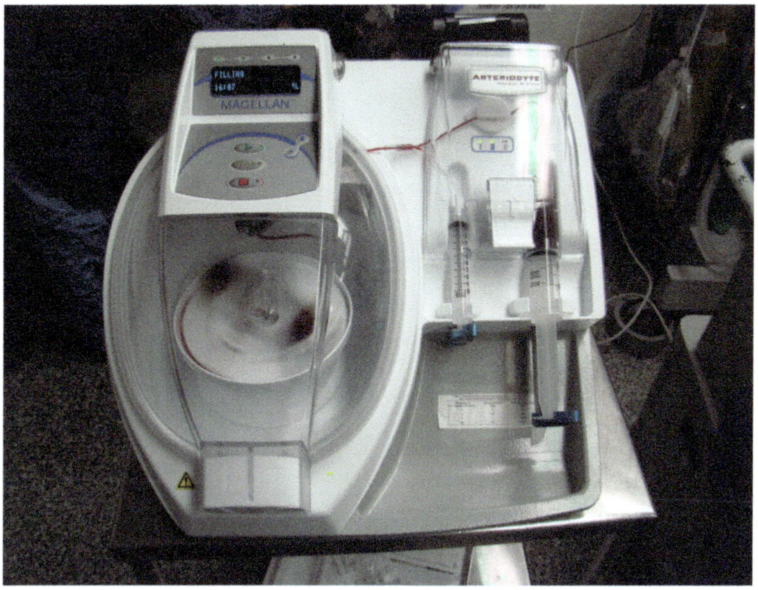

Fig. 7.3 Preparation of bone marrow concentrate using Magellan Autologous Platelet Separator (Arteriocyte Medical Systems, Cleveland, OH). 4 cc of bone marrow concentrate is prepared

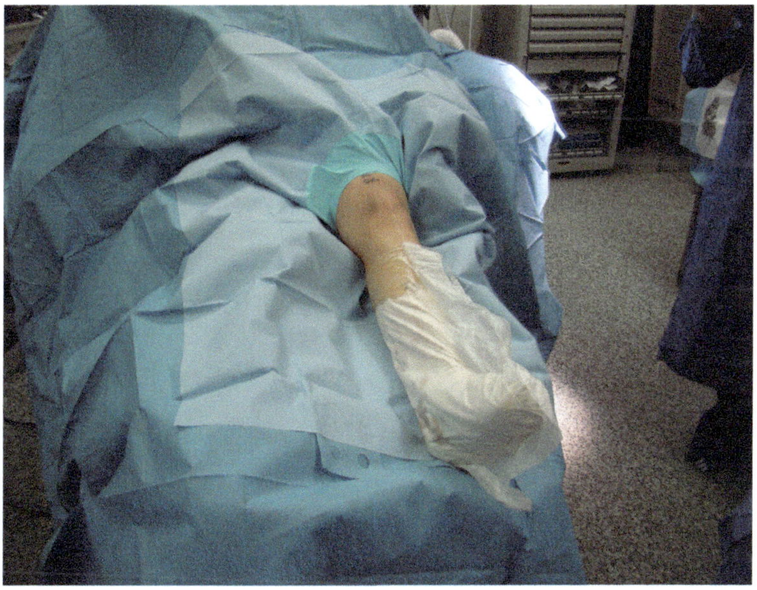

Fig. 7.4 Sterile prep of patient's leg. This step is performed after the bone marrow aspiration is completed

5. Use the bone marrow aspirate (50 ml) to prepare the BMC (4 ml) utilizing any method of choice. Our preferred system is the Magellan Autologous Platelet Separator (Arteriocyte Medical Systems, Cleveland, OH) (Fig. 7.3).
6. Sterile prep and drape of patient's leg can be done after bone marrow aspirate is obtained (Fig. 7.4).
7. The TruFit® plugs are soaked in the BMC for at least 10 min prior to implantation into the defect (Fig. 7.5).

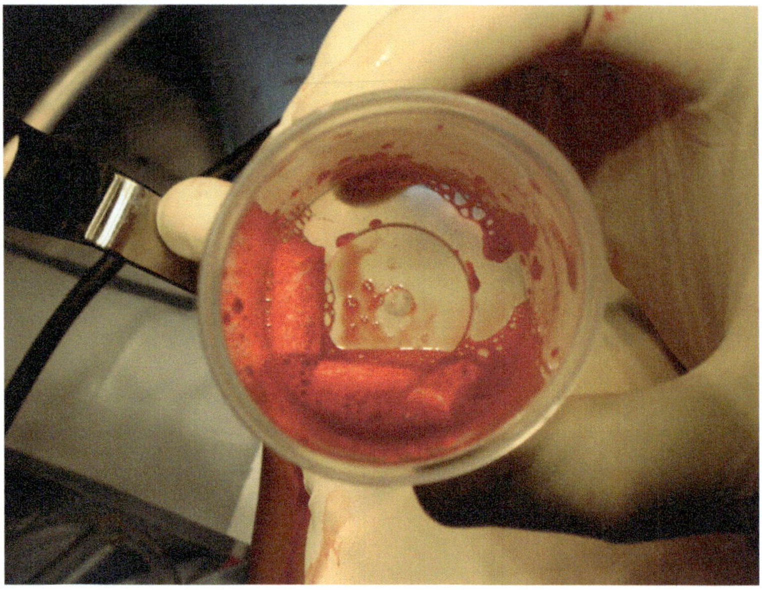

Fig. 7.5 TruFit® plugs bathed in bone marrow concentrate for at least 10 min prior to implantation

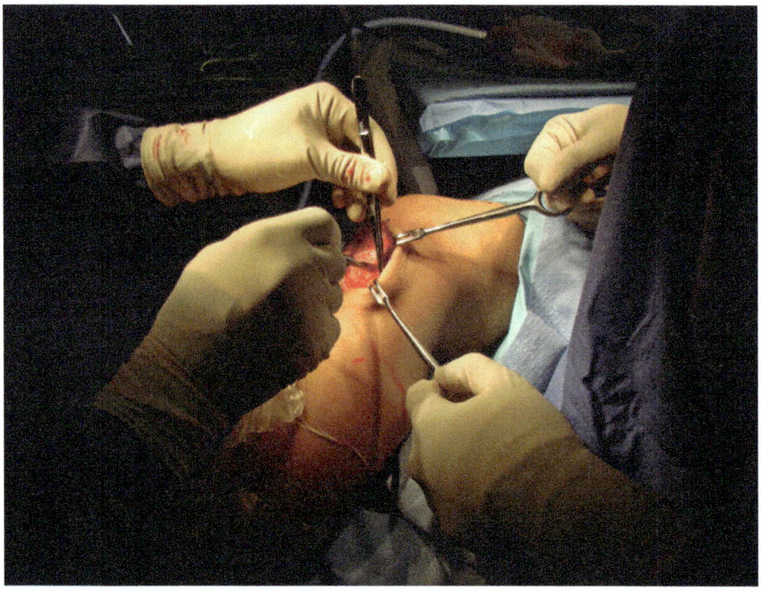

Fig. 7.6 Arthrotomy of knee

7.4 Surgical Approach

1. Conduct standard diagnostic arthroscopy to assess the cartilage lesion and perform any concomitant procedures (i.e., meniscectomy or meniscal repair).
2. After exsanguinating the leg and inflating the tourniquet, create an arthrotomy of the knee and expose the lesion. The arthrotomy can be medial or lateral depending on the location of the lesion (Figs. 7.6 and 7.7).
3. Place an appropriately sized drilling trochar over the lesion and gently mallet into the cartilage until secured (Fig. 7.8).
4. Use drill through the center of the trochar to prepare the recipient hole to a depth of about 8 mm (Figs. 7.9 and 7.10).
5. Load the TruFit® loading device with a TruFit® plug (Fig. 7.11).
6. Place the back end of the loading device into the recipient hole and push the plug in until the plunger behind it bottoms out. This step

sets the depth of the plug needed to fill the recipient hole (Fig. 7.12).

7. Cut the excess plug off using a serrated knife (Fig. 7.13).
8. Fill the recipient hole with the previously prepared BMC prior to implantation of the plug (Fig. 7.14).
9. Insert the TruFit® plug with the loading device and finish with a tamp. Appropriate contouring of the plugs is then confirmed in at least two planes (Figs. 7.15, 7.16, and 7.17).
10. If needed, repeat the steps above to conduct a mosaicplasty (Fig. 7.18).
11. Apply fibrin sealant over final construct. Our preferred sealant is EVICEL® Fibrin Sealant (Ethicon, Somerville, NJ) (Figs. 7.19 and 7.20).

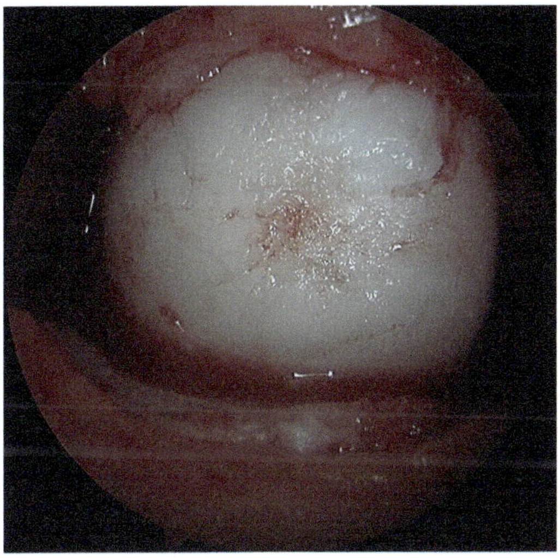

Fig. 7.7 Chondral lesion exposed

7.5 Potential Complications and Troubleshooting

Several complications have been noted with bioabsorbable implants made from poly(h-hydroxy esters) such as persistent effusions, inflammatory reaction [3, 4], early resorption, loosening, and breakage [5]. To date, no device-related complications have been observed in our patient population consisting of more than a 100 patients since 2005 [6]. However, the complication rate with long-term use of this device is unclear.

7.6 Rehabilitation

The advantage of TruFit® over techniques such as microfracture is the ability to accelerate a patient's rehab. This will allow for minimal muscle wasting

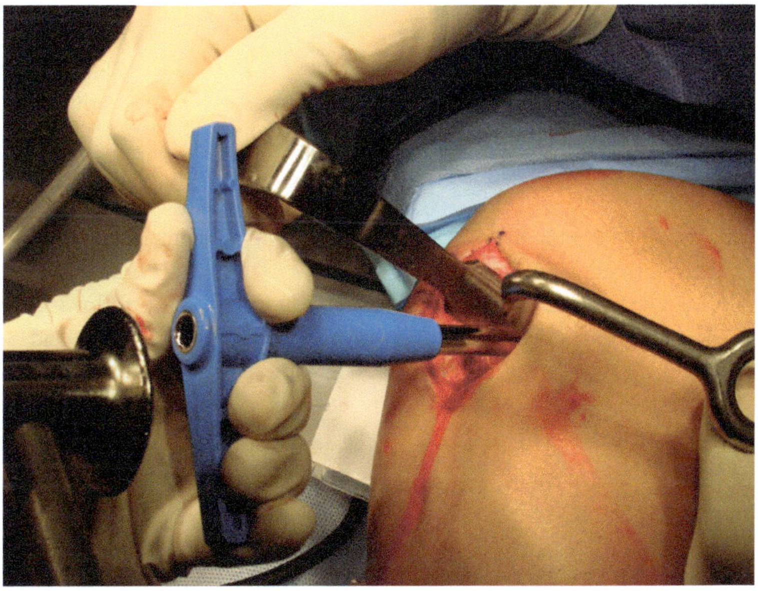

Fig. 7.8 Drilling trochar malleted into chondral lesion

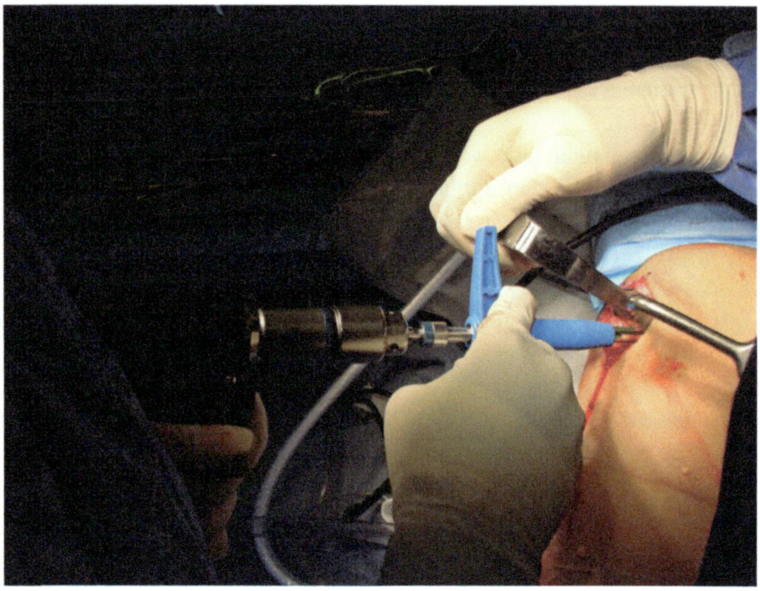

Fig. 7.9 Drill placed through center of trochar to prepare the recipient hole to a depth of 8 mm

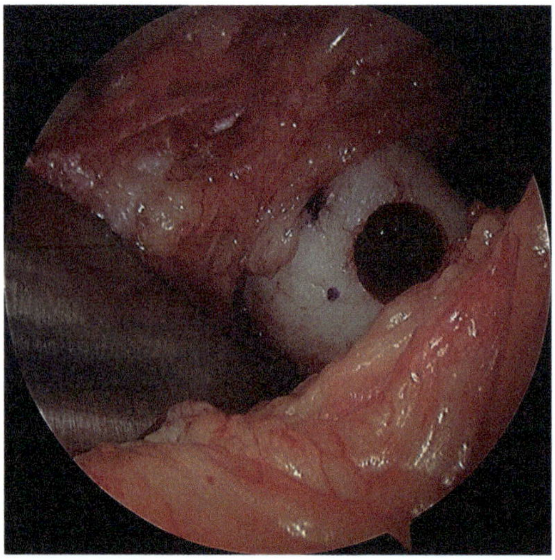

Fig. 7.10 Recipient hole after preparation

and possibly shorten the overall recovery period. The rehabilitation will consist of:

- Week 1: toe-touch weight bearing with a brace
- Week 2: weight bearing as tolerated with brace
- Week 3: weight bearing as tolerated with an open brace
- Week 4: brace is discontinued

7.7 Postoperative Follow-Up

Clinical follow-up begins with a 2 and 6-week visit. Subsequent visits are accompanied by MRI to assess the implant's position and degree of integration. These visits are typically scheduled for 3 months, 1, 2, and 5 years.

7.8 Outcomes

Early experiences following use of TruFit® osteochondral scaffolds are beginning to emerge [7–11]. Dhollander et al. evaluated a small series of 20 consecutive patients who had a focal chondral lesion (patella, trochlea, or medial or lateral femoral condyle) treated with the TruFit® plug. The authors reported modest but significant improvement in patient pain visual analog scale (VAS) (preoperative mean 64.84 ± 24.75 mm versus 1-year follow-up 29.85 ± 27.09 mm, $p=0.006$) and in total and subdomain Knee Injury and Osteoarthritis Outcome Scale (KOOS) scores [9]. The evaluation of cartilage fill by the TruFit® plug using the magnetic resonance observation of

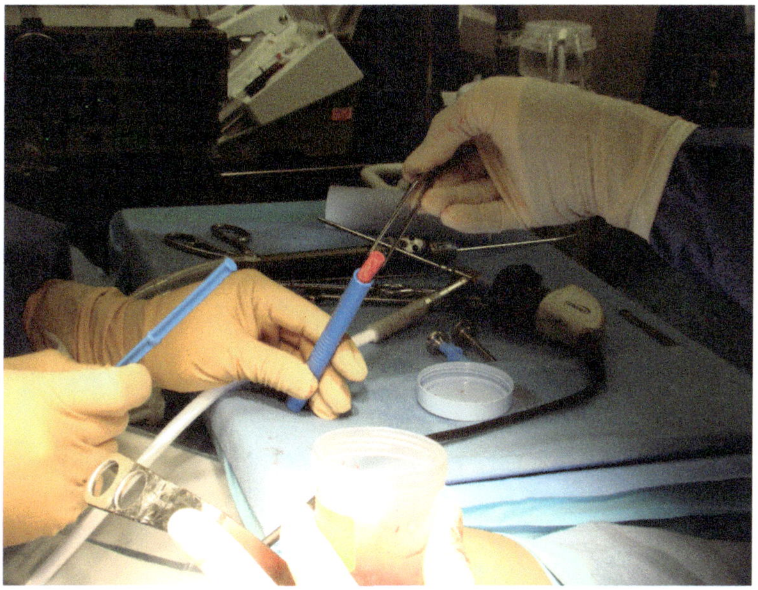

Fig. 7.11 TruFit® plug placed into loading device

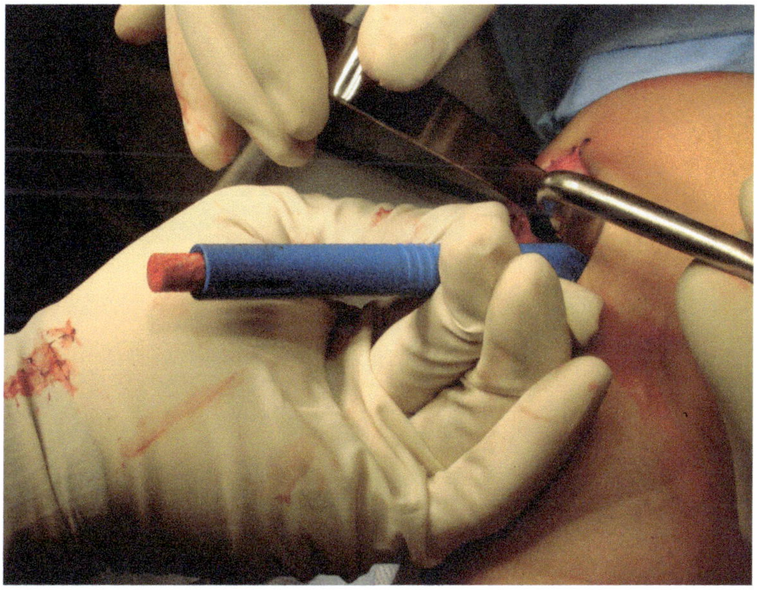

Fig. 7.12 Depth measurement taken with the back end of the loading device. By bottoming out the device into the recipient hole, the amount of the TruFit® plug to be cut is exposed

cartilage repair tissue (MOCART) demonstrated stable cartilage-like repair tissue at 6 and 12 months. One interesting MRI finding was the consistent edema associated with the bony part of all implanted TruFit® plugs, which may suggest the scaffold is incompletely incorporated even at 1 year after surgery. In a separate study evaluating use of TruFit® for patellar osteochondral lesions, results at 2 years have been less promising [10]. Failures of the plugs were attributed to delayed subchondral lamina formation, which may have led to loss of the initial chondral fill.

The issue of delayed integration of TruFit® plugs has been highlighted in the literature [7, 8].

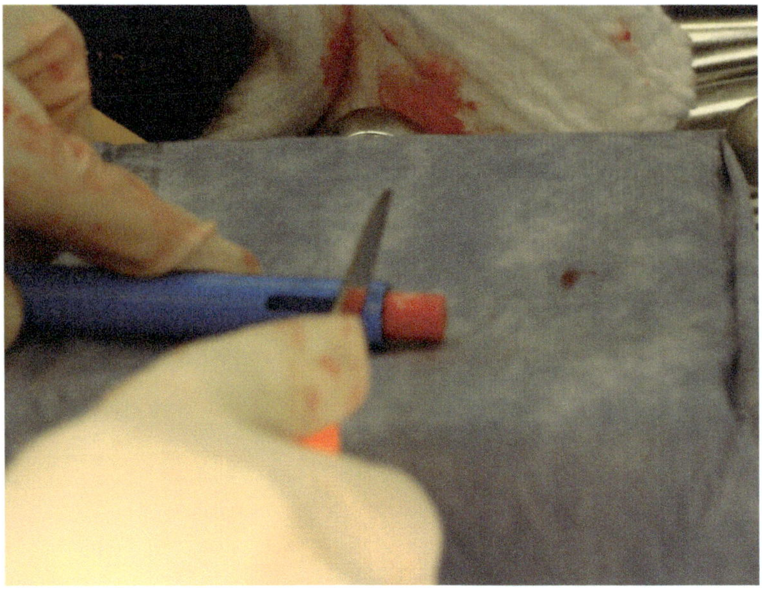

Fig. 7.13 TruFit® plug is cut down with a serrated knife

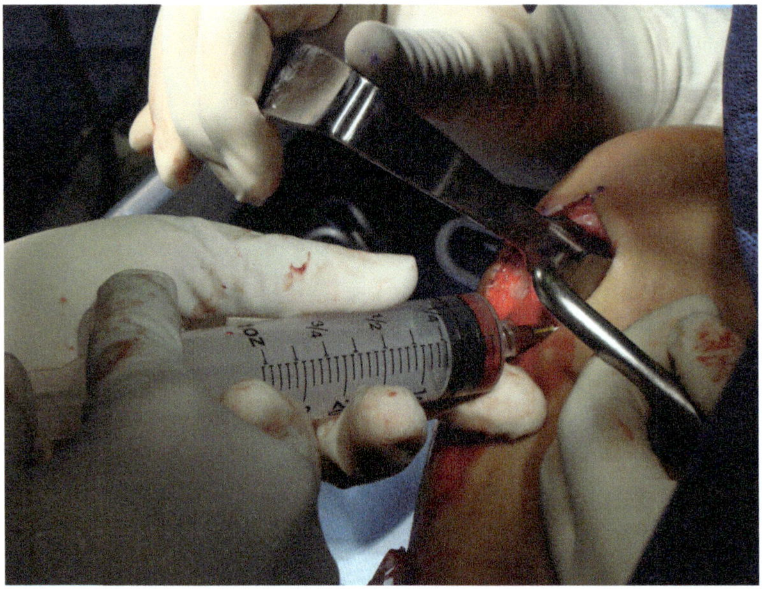

Fig. 7.14 Bone marrow concentrate is injected into the recipient hole prior to insertion of the TruFit® plug

Our institution's experience following the incorporation of TruFit® plugs has demonstrated a similar slow maturation process following implantation [7]. In the early postoperative period (≤6 months), TruFit® plugs demonstrate favorable appearances on MR images with 75 % (33 of 46) and 78 % (36 of 46) demonstrating flushed morphology and exhibiting near-complete or complete fill of the defect, respectively. At 12 months, there is a deterioration in appearance of

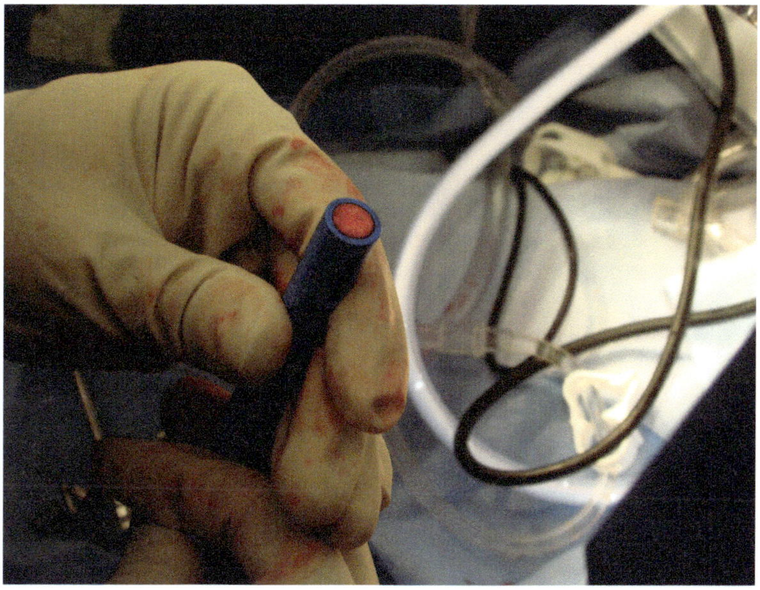

Fig. 7.15 TruFit® plug after being cut down and prepared for insertion into recipient hole

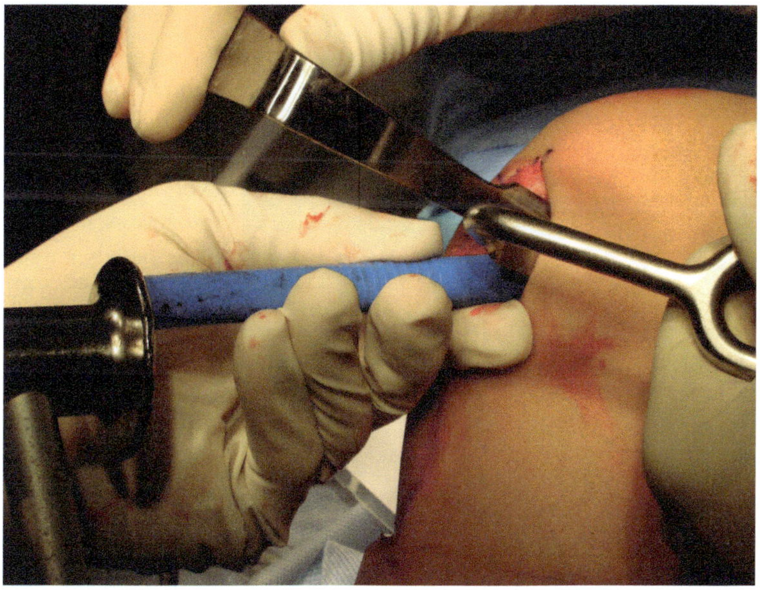

Fig. 7.16 Insertion of TruFit® plug with mallet

the plugs with only 26 % (12 of 46) demonstrating a flush morphology and 52 % (24 of 46) of the plugs exhibiting near-complete or complete fill of the defect. Only 3 % of the plugs demonstrated complete incorporation at 1 year. The MR appearance of TruFit® plugs substantially improved with longer postoperative duration (≥16 months) with 64 and 26 % of the plugs demonstrating complete and progressing partial incorporation, respectively. The MR changes likely

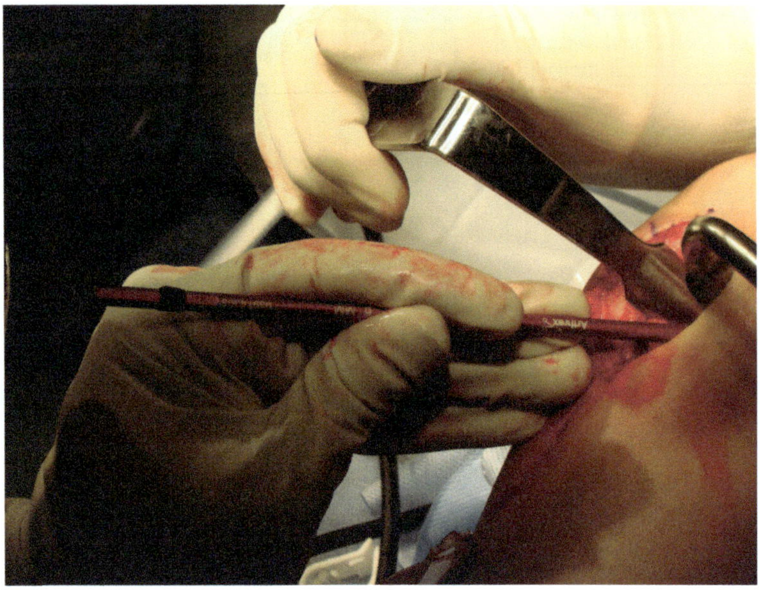

Fig. 7.17 Tamp is used to make TruFit® plug flush with neighboring cartilage

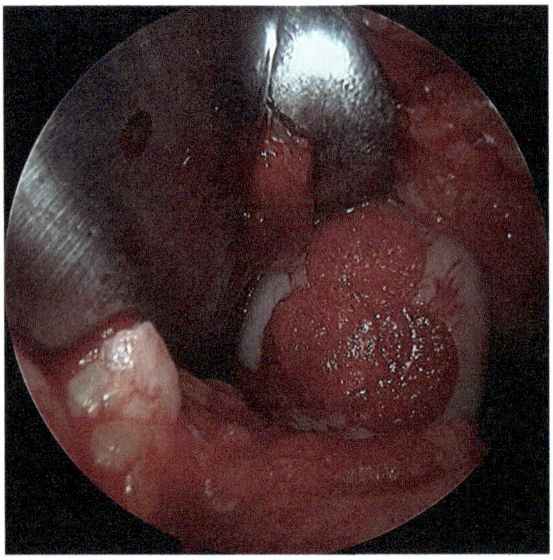

Fig. 7.18 Final construct of TruFit® plug mosaicplasty

parallel the biologic integration of the TruFit® plug. During the first 6 months following implantation, the plug largely retains its mechanical properties; hence, it is able to maintain its flush morphology and good fill. As the scaffold is resorbed (9–12 months), its morphology may become depressed leading to deterioration in its MR appearance. As the incorporation process progresses, however, the plug appearance on MRI substantially improves to demonstrate a high percentage of lesion fill, good incorporation, and restoration of a flush morphology at repair surface. The relatively poor filling characteristics of these synthetic plugs at an intermediate postoperative interval (~12 months) should therefore not be automatically misinterpreted as a failure of the cartilage repair procedure but rather a normal phase in the natural history of incorporation of the scaffold into host bone [7, 8].

In summary, reported outcomes using TruFit® scaffolds have been mainly early experiences. Some series have been promising. Integration and maturation of the plug may still be ongoing out to 2 years following implantation, which may lead to delayed patient symptom alleviation.

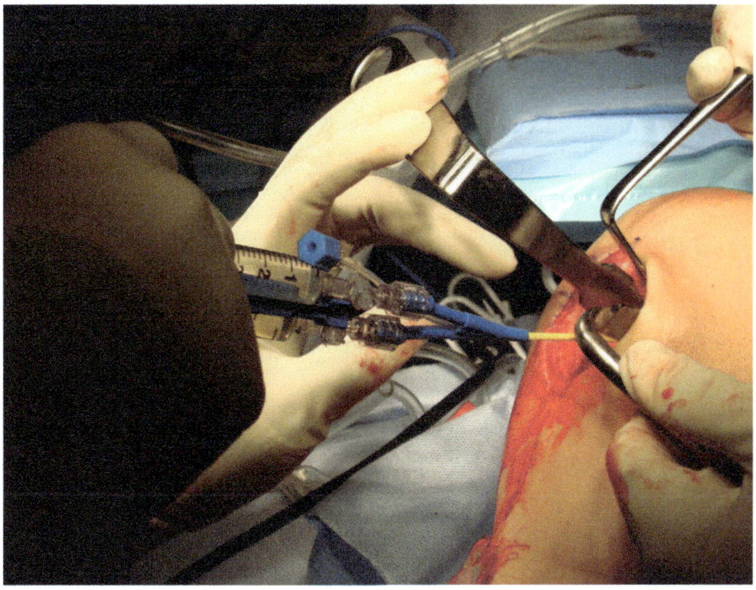

Fig. 7.19 EVICEL® Fibrin Sealant (Ethicon, Somerville, NJ) placed over the repair construct

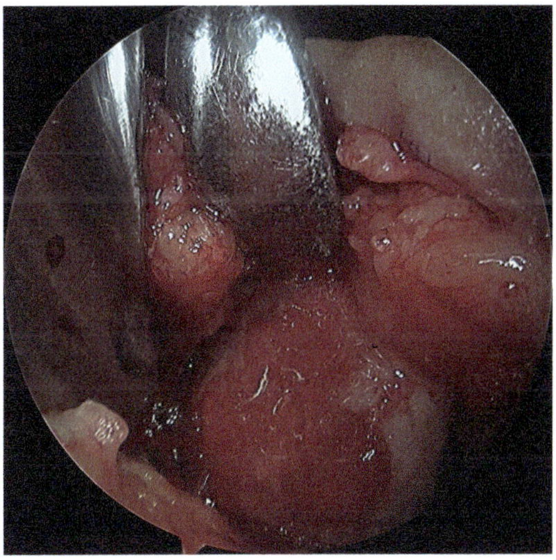

Fig. 7.20 TruFit® plug mosaicplasty covered with fibrin sealant

Ultimately, longer follow-up will be essential to validate not only the early promise that these implants hold but also adaptation of this new technology for widespread use.

References

1. Niederauer GG, Slivka MA, Leather-bury NC et al (2000) Evaluation of multiphase implants for repair of focal osteochondral defects in goats. Biomaterials 21:2561–2574
2. Slivka MA, Leatherbury NC, Kieswetter K, Niederauer GG (2001) Porous, resorbable, fiber-reinforced scaffolds tailored for articular cartilage repair. Tissue Eng 7:767–780
3. Bostman OM, Pihlajamaki HK (1998) Late foreign-body reaction to an intraosseous bioabsorbable polylactic acid screw: a case report. J Bone Joint Surg Am 80:1791–1794
4. Burkart A, Imhoff AB, Roscher E (2000) Foreign-body reaction to the bioabsorbable suretac device. Arthroscopy 16:91–95
5. Sassmannshausen G, Sukay M, Mair SD (2006) Broken or dislodged poly-L-lactic acid bioabsorbable tacks in patients after SLAP lesion surgery. Arthroscopy 22:615–619
6. Williams RJ III, Gamradt S (2008) Articular cartilage repair using a resorbable matrix scaffold. Instr Course Lect 57:563–571
7. Bedi A, Foo LF, Williams RJ III, Potter HG, Group tCS (2010) The maturation of synthetic scaffolds for osteochondral donor sites of the knee. Cartilage 1(1):20–28

8. Carmont MR, Carey-Smith R, Saithna A, Dhillon M, Thompson P, Spalding T (2009) Delayed incorporation of a TruFit plug: perseverance is recommended. Arthroscopy 25(7):810–814
9. Dhollander AA, Liekens K, Almqvist KF et al (2012) A pilot study of the use of an osteochondral scaffold plug for cartilage repair. Arthroscopy 28(2): 225–233
10. Joshi N, Reverte-Vinaixa M, Diaz-Ferreiro EW, Dominguez-Oronoz R (2012) Synthetic resorbable scaffolds for the treatment of isolated patellofemoral. Am J Sports Med 40(6):1289–1295
11. Melton JT, Wilson AJ, Chapman-Sheath P, Cossey AJ (2010) TruFit CB bone plug: chondral repair, scaffold design, surgical technique and early experiences. Expert Rev Med Devices 7(3):333–341

MaioRegen: Our Experience

8

Elizaveta Kon, Francesco Perdisa, Giuseppe Filardo, and Maurilio Marcacci

Contents

E. Kon (✉)
NAno-BIotechnology Laboratory,
II Orthopaedic Clinic, Codivilla-Putti Research Center, Rizzoli Orthopaedic Institute,
Via di Barbiano 1/10, 40136 Bologna, Italy
e-mail: e.kon@biomec.ior.it

F. Perdisa
NAno-BIotechnology Laboratory,
II Orthopaedic Clinic, Rizzoli Orthopaedic Insitute,
Via di Barbiano 1/10, 40136 Bologna, Italy

G. Filardo
Biomechanics Laboratory,
II Orthopaedic Clinic, Rizzoli Orthopaedic Insitute,
Via di Barbiano 1/10, 40136 Bologna, Italy

M. Marcacci
NAno-BIotechnology Laboratory,
II Orthopaedic Clinic, Rizzoli Orthopaedic Insitute,
Via di Barbiano 1/10, 40136 Bologna, Italy

8.1 Introduction

The rationale of using a scaffold is to have a temporary three-dimensional structure of biodegradable polymers for the growth of living cells. The ideal scaffold should mimic biology, architecture, and structural properties of the native tissue, thus facilitating cell infiltration, attachment, proliferation, and differentiation. Other important properties include biocompatibility and biodegradability through safe biochemical pathways at suitable time intervals to support the first phases of tissue formation and gradually be replaced by the regenerating tissue. We think that an ideal graft would be an off-the-shelf product from both a surgical and commercial standpoint.

Actually there is an increasing interest in a new treatment approach for regenerative medicine in clinical practice, which involves the implant of various biomaterials for "in situ" cartilage repair exploiting bone marrow stem cell differentiation induced by the scaffold properties. In fact, some scaffolds may have a potential themselves

A.A. Shetty et al. (eds.), *Techniques in Cartilage Repair Surgery*,
DOI 10.1007/978-3-642-41921-8_8, © ESSKA 2014

to promote chondral or osteochondral regeneration favoring the self-regenerative potential of the body. The possibility to produce a cell-free implant that is "smart" enough to provide the joint with the appropriate stimuli to induce orderly and durable tissue regeneration is really attractive, and different new biomaterials are recently proposed to induce "in situ" cartilage regeneration after direct transplantation onto the defect site both in research and in clinical practice.

The awareness on the importance of the subchondral bone for its role in the etiopathogenic processes of articular surface damage has recently increased also. In fact, the subchondral bone may be involved in the pathological process not only primarily, such as in osteochondritis dissecans (OCD), osteonecrosis, and severe trauma, but also secondarily in large degenerative cartilage lesions and even focal chondral defects, if left untreated, may increase in size over time and present with concomitant changes of the underlying subchondral bone plate [13]. There's evidence that even small and focal chondral defects of the knee represent a risk to more extensive joint damage, mainly due to the higher mechanical stress on the lesion's edge.

Most of the available surgical options aimed at reconstructing a functional joint surface focus on the cartilage layer and offer good results if applied to small traumatic lesions on otherwise healthy joints, whereas they lack indication in more compromised knees [17, 31].

For this kind of osteochondral articular defects, different specific scaffolds have been developed. In fact, the treatment is biologically challenging since two different tissues are involved (bone and articular cartilage) with a distinctly different intrinsic healing capacity.

Several groups thus focused on using tissue engineering to generate osteochondral composite materials with various approaches [2, 8, 29, 32, 48]. Heterogeneous scaffolds, combining distinct but integrated layers corresponding to the cartilage and bone regions, appeared to be one of the most promising approaches. These devices aim at supplying the different requirements to regenerate cartilage and bone of an osteochondral defect, preventing the risk of delamination of different components. Initially, integrated bilayered osteochondral scaffolds have been proposed using a-hydroxy acid polymers (i.e., polylactic acid, poly lactic-co-glycolic acid) combined with a ceramic component (i.e., hydroxyapatite, tricalcium phosphate) in the region corresponding to the subchondral bone [37, 39]. Then biphasic but monolithic materials were formed by freeze-drying and chemical cross-linking collagen-based materials (i.e., mineralized or coupled with hyaluronic acid), as well as by ionotropic gelation of alginate-based materials (i.e., containing or not hydroxyapatite ceramic particles), allowing to achieve specific mechanical properties (i.e., elasticity or compression strength) [12, 13].

This chapter is focused on resuming our preclinical and clinical experience on a newly developed three-layered nanostructured scaffold for osteochondral regeneration.

8.2 Technical Details

Tampieri et al. [42] applied bioengineering criteria to design a biomimetic osteochondral composite scaffold resembling the composition of the extracellular matrices of cartilage and bone tissue, respectively, using nucleation of hydroxyapatite (HA) nanocrystals onto self-assembled collagen fibers [14, 41], to generate a chemically and morphologically graded hybrid biomaterial by stacking a lower mineralized layer, an intermediate layer with reduced amount of mineral (tidemark-like) and an upper layer formed by collagen and hyaluronic acid (reproducing some cartilaginous cues).

Equine type I collagen (Coll) was chosen as organic component, working as matrix for the mineralization process, due to its good physicochemical stability and processability and high safety and biocompatibility profile, related to the removal of all potentially immunogenic telopeptides.

Three different layers where prepared in order to generate a scaffold with morphological and mineralization gradient:

- Cartilaginous upper layer: Type I collagen. Thickness: 2.0 mm

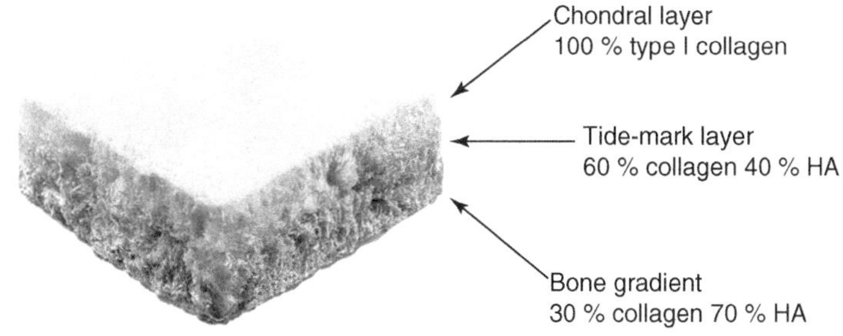

Fig. 8.1 The MaioRegen scaffold. The three different layers are visible

- Intermediate bony layer (tidemark): HA/Coll (40/60 %). Thickness: 1.5 mm
- Lower bony layer (subchondral bone): HA/Coll (70/30 %). Thickness: 2.5 mm

The thicknesses of the different layers were selected on the basis of the technological limitations (to prepare layers thinner than 1.5 mm is challenging) and the dimension of native articular cartilage of the animal model (sheep) selected for the in vivo extensive trials.

8.2.1 Scaffold Preparation

The osteochondral (OC) biomimetic scaffold (*MaioRegen®* Fin-Ceramica Faenza S.p.A., Faenza, Italy) has a porous 3D composite tri-layered structure, mimicking the whole osteochondral anatomy. The mineral phase, represented by magnesium–hydroxyapatite (Mg–HA), was directly nucleated onto collagen fibers during their self-assembling. Magnesium ions were introduced to increase the physicochemical, structural, and morphological affinities of the composite with newly formed natural bone [38]. The cartilaginous layer, consisting of type I collagen, has a smooth surface. The intermediate layer (tidemark-like) consists of a combination of type I collagen (60 % of weight) and Mg–HA (40 % of weight), whereas the lower layer consists of a mineralized blend of type I collagen (30 % of weight) and Mg–HA (70 % of weight), reproducing the subchondral bone layer (Fig. 8.1). Each layer is separately synthesized, starting from an atelocollagen aqueous solution (1 % w/w) in acetic acid, isolated from equine tendon; the upper nonmineralized chondral layer is obtained by dissolving 200 g of acetic solution of type I collagen (Opocrin S.p.A., Corlo di Formigine, Modena, Italy) in 200 mL of bi-distilled water, after setting the pH at 5.5. By adding 0.1 NaOH, the precipitate obtained is homogenized by moderate stirring and rinsed in distilled water. The assembled collagen fibers are subsequently cross-linked with 42 mL of 0.5 g/L 1,4-butanediol diglycidyl ether (BDDE) solution (Fluka, Sigma-Aldrich Group, St. Louis, MO) and stored at 4 °C for 48 h. The intermediate and the lower layers are obtained by nucleating bone-like nanostructured non-stoichiometric HA into self-assembling collagen fibers, as occurs in the natural biological neo-ossification process. The mineralized intermediate layer is obtained starting from two reagents prepared as follows: reagent A, prepared by diluting 300 g of type I collagen acetic solution with H_3PO_4 40 mM, to reach a final pH of 3.0; reagent B, prepared by mixing 480 mL of a 42 mM $Ca(OH)_2$ solution with 20 mL of 48 mM MgC12 $6H_2O$ solution and 24 mL of SBF (simulated body fluid). Under gentle stirring conditions, reagent A is dripped into reagent B until HA nanoparticles are nucleated into the auto-assembled collagen fibers, reaching a final pH of 6.0. The obtained precipitate, composed of 60 % collagen and 40 % of HA, is rinsed in distilled water, cross-linked with 63 mL of BDDE cross-linking solution, and stored at 48 °C for 48 h. The lower layer is also prepared starting from two reagents: reagent C, obtained by adding 200 g of type I collagen acetic solution with 40 mM of H_3PO_4, achieving a pH of 3.0; reagent D, obtained by mixing 1,100 mL of 42 mM $Ca(OH)_2$ solution with 50 mL of 48 mM $MgCl_2$ $6H_2O$ solution and 55 mL of SBF (simulated body fluid). Under stirring conditions, reagent C is dripped into reagent D until precipitation of HA occurs into auto-assembled collagen fibers, with a final pH of close to 7.0. The composite precipitate is 70 % HA and 30 % collagen, respectively. Subsequently, after thoroughly rinsing in bi-distilled water, self-assembled collagen–HA fibers are cross-linked with 63 mL of BDDE solution and then stored at 48 °C for 48 h. The final construct is obtained by physically combining the layers on top of a Mylar sheet and finally freeze-dried and gamma-sterilized at 25 kg ray.

8.2.2 Composite Characterization and Biological Validation

Composite samples were characterized by analyzing the ion content of the mineral phase, such as Mg^{2+}, Ca^{2+}, and $PO4^{3-}$, using an inductive coupled plasma–atomic emission spectrometer (ICP–AES) and examined by environmental scanning electron microscopy (ESEM) and infrared spectroscopy.

Enzymatic tests were performed for each material to study the kinetics of degradation using a UV-visible spectrophotometer to observe the different absorbance in function of time. Mechanical tests on three mineralized specimens for each different final porosity in the range 45–65 vol% were performed measuring Young's modulus. The scaffold was chemically cross-linked through a biocompatible organic reticulation agent [49] to provide stability, thus increasing in situ hydrophilic properties and good handling properties, including flexibility.

Human expanded chondrocytes and sheep bone marrow stromal cells were processed as previously described [37, 39] and used, as they can differentiate towards the chondrogenic and osteogenic lineages, respectively. Either expanded human chondrocytes suspension (concentration of 2×10^8 cells/mL) or expanded sheep BMSCs resuspended at 2.0×10^7 cells/mL were statically loaded onto the composites (8-mm-diameter and 6-mm-height disks) either in the cartilaginous or subchondral bone layer. The scaffolds seeded with expanded chondrocytes were then cultured for 2 weeks in a chondrogenic medium, with medium changes twice a week. BMSCs/scaffold composites were subcutaneously implanted on the back of immunodeficient mice of 1 month of age, which then were sacrificed. Three constructs were implanted in three different mice.

Histological characterization demonstrated that the cartilaginous layer of the composite scaffold is permissive to human articular chondrocyte differentiation and cartilaginous matrix deposition, whereas only a fibrous tissue could develop in the subchondral bone layer. Conversely, bone tissue formation was supported within the subchondral layer of the composite, but not in the cartilaginous region. Also mechanical pulling tests on dry and wet samples proved the good adhesion between the mineralized layers and the cartilaginous one.

This first in vitro study [42], testing the nanostructured collagen-HA scaffold, loaded with differentiated cells (e.g., articular chondrocytes) or BMSCs, showed to support cartilage and bone tissue formation selectively in ectopic models.

8.3 Animal Studies

8.3.1 Horses

After the promising results obtained in vitro, the newly developed scaffold was preliminary tested in vivo in horses, comparing two different configurations: either bi- or tri-layered to reproduce, respectively, chondral and osteochondral anatomy [21]. Articular cartilage repair should be accompanied by an adequate restoration of the underlying subchondral bony structure, enhancing the effective union with surrounding host tissues [39]. Since the bone-to-bone interface integrates faster than the cartilage-to-cartilage interface, this multilayered osteochondral construct appeared promising also in order to obtain a firm anchorage for a cartilage substitute to natural surrounding tissues [29]. The horse was chosen as an animal model because its cartilage thickness is similar to that of the human knee and thus ideal to test implant surgical feasibility and mechanical stability.

The three-layered scaffold was the same as previously described, the bi-layered one was instead constituted of only cartilage (type I collagen) and an underlying layer comprised of type I collagen (60 %) and HA (40 %), separately synthetized and assembled as reported above for the three-layered one. Two adult horses were selected and chondral defects (lateral condyle) and deep osteochondral defects (medial condyle) were made in the distal epiphysis of the third metacarpal bone of both forelimbs, for a total of four implants for each animal. Defect dimensions and preliminary graft stability were defined in a previous cadaver study. A 10-mm-diameter defect was created in the weight-bearing area of both condyles. Lateral condyles were treated with superficial debridement and abrasion of the subchondral bone to induce the bleeding; a 8–10-mm-deep osteochondral defect was instead created into the medial condyle, where bleeding was inducted by deep perforation of the subchondral bone. Both grafts were implanted using press-fit fixation and the procedures were simultaneously performed. A second-look arthroscopy was performed at 2 months of follow-up, showing good filling of chondral and osteochondral defects, with fibrocartilage appearance of grafted tissue. In the medial condyle residual osteochondral scaffold was still visible while, at contrary, no traces of residual biomaterial were observed in the chondral side. No inflammatory reaction but a light fibrosis was observed.

Macroscopic and gross appearance evaluation using a modified scoring system from Fortier et al. [11] and a score proposed by Niederaurer et al. [33] did not show any inflammation in all eight implant sites nor significant differences on the macroscopic scores of the two animals. In the osteochondral lesions, fibrous tissue was found covering the osteochondral defect with a cartilage-like regeneration tissue, smooth, stiff, and with regular borders, firmly fixed to the healthy cartilage. No fibrous tissue was present on the lateral condyles and the regenerating tissue was cartilage-like, without any gap between the newly formed tissue and the surrounding healthy cartilage and with a firm fixation of the graft. No significant differences were found between the two animals for both chondral and osteochondral lesions at histological evaluation on either undecalcified (fast green, toluidine blue, and acid fuchsin) or decalcified (toluidine blue) sections. Osteochondral lesions that were stained had evident growth of trabecular bone in the osteochondral lesion, well integrated with the surrounding bone. Only in one case fibrocartilaginous tissue filled the whole thickness of the lesion. The formation of a tidemark line was evident between the newly formed bone and the regenerated cartilage. In chondral lesions a newly formed cartilage-like tissue was present which completely filled the lesions, and on the other hand, the underlying trabecular bone was not distinguishable from the healthy bone, with no bone infiltrating into the cartilage surface. Collagen fibers though had immature morphology, with initial longitudinal alignment recognizable at polarized light. Decalcified specimens showed in all cases a demarcation line between the regenerative cartilage and the native one.

In conclusion the scaffold demonstrated perfect ability to adhere and fit both the chondral and osteochondral defects, despite the intrinsic high motility of the experimental model (metacarpophalangeal joint of the horse, without any postoperative cast) and the use of press-fit fixation only. While a significant regrowth of good-quality subchondral bone was noticed in the deepest areas, some other areas still showed distinguishable osteoid tissue, and fibrocartilaginous tissue was mostly detected in the cartilaginous layer. However, it is known that the kinetics of the cartilaginous and bony regrowth certainly exceed 6 months time; therefore, the regenerative processes were still in evolution at the evaluation point. These results allowed us to test this osteochondral scaffold in larger experimental studies. It was finally guessable that adding autologous chondrocytes or growth factors could improve the regenerated cartilage tissue quality.

After the promising results of the first study on horses, confirming the good stability of the osteochondral scaffold and feasibility of the procedure, our group decided to apply this composite scaffold to a sheep animal model, in order to test extensively in vivo its regenerative and integrative properties after implantation inside osteochondral defects [18].

8.3.2 Sheep

Twelve skeletally mature female adult sheep were used for this study, divided in three different groups: (1) biomimetic scaffold alone

(S-group), possibly exploiting bone marrow stem cells recruitment from underlying subchondral bone; (2) biomimetic scaffold combined with in vitro cultured autologous chondrocytes (S-ACI group); and (3) spontaneous cartilage and bone control repair (C-group). Sheep model was chosen due to the relevant loading that their limbs bear more similarity to humans than, for example, the rabbit model [6].

A total of 24 osteochondral lesions were performed on the right medial and lateral femoral condyles, with eight lesions assigned to each of the three experimental groups. The left stifle joints were used as comparison. In the group treated with autologous chondrocytes, cells were isolated starting from cartilage biopsies collected from the left stifle joint, then culture-expanded and seeded drop by drop onto the 1 cm^2 of the scaffold surface, which was then gently and repeatedly pressed for a few times to help penetration and dispersion of the cells within the matrix meshes. After adding thrombin to induce fibrinogen polymerization, and a medium, the cell/material constructs were cultured in a cell incubator at 37 °C, 5 % CO_2 for 5 days. Surgery included a medial arthrotomy and a parapatellar approach to the lateral and medial condyles. Then, an osteochondral lesion was induced on each femoral condyle. A specifically designed drill was used to create a 7-mm-diameter and 9-mm-deep defect in the weight-bearing area of both condyles. Following implantation by press-fit, grafts were flush to the cartilage surface. A total of 16 osteochondral grafts were implanted, while 8 lesions were left untreated and used as a control.

Macroscopic evaluation after 6 months' sacrifice showed all grafts still in their original site, with no signs of inflammation, except for slightly hyperemic synovium. Small osteophytes were detected in medial condyles of all groups. The healthy chondral surface and newly formed hyaline-like tissue were well integrated except for the control group and scaffold alone, and scaffold with autologous chondrocytes had better bone regeneration. No difference in cartilage and bone reconstruction and in the filling of the defect was noted between cell-seeded and cell-free groups. These results were confirmed also by the macroscopic evaluation with the modified Fortier [11] and Niederaurer [33] scores. Microradiographic evaluation showed the appearance of newly formed bone in the deepest area of the osteochondral implant: with better improvement in subchondral bone healing for the experimental groups, compared to the control one, which showed lytic holes that were filled by fibrous tissue as proved by histological staining. No bone growth in the chondral layer was observed in any of the groups.

Histological evaluation confirmed the macroscopic results with complete reabsorption of the implanted biomaterial, without any inflammatory reactions or giant cells in the grafted area, on the other hand. The newly formed repair tissue was associated with good integration of the scaffolds with host cartilage for both scaffold groups, containing a hyaline-like tissue, with a strong proteoglycan staining and columnar rearrangement of chondrocytes, and an underlying well-structured subchondral trabecular bone, which was distinguishable from the healthy adjacent bone. Moreover, both the experimental groups had better bone regeneration, with no difference between S and S-ACI groups, while in the control group, the defect was filled with amorphous fibrous tissue. This findings were generally confirmed by immunohistochemical staining for collagen types I and II: the experimental groups displayed a rather orderly pattern of tissue repair, with positivity for type II collagen in the cartilaginous layer down to the interface with subchondral bone, and type I collagen uniformly positive in the subchondral tissue or in association with single cells in the chondral region. Instead, in the C-group, type II collagen was either negative or positive in scattered areas, whereas positive staining for type I collagen in the extracellular matrix was extended throughout the repair tissue up to the joint space. The reconstruction of both hyaline-like cartilage and structured bone tissue anchored to the interface of adjacent healthy tissues was observed at 6 months, and even without addition of other bioactive agents, the healing of the defect was evident and confirmed by histology. However, it is well known that the kinetics of cartilaginous and bone regrowth occurs over a period longer than 6 months of follow-up, and therefore the processes observed were still ongoing; in fact, the marked regrowth of good-quality subchondral bone observed at 6 months was characterized by well-defined cortex in most of the areas, while in some other osteoid tissue was still distinguishable, confirming that physiological processes of bone regeneration end within 10–12 months.

Finally, the presence into the subchondral compartment of areas positively stained for type II collagen and of cells with hypertrophic chondrocyte morphology suggested that the scaffold-mediated regeneration of subchondral bone followed an endochondral ossification process. Considering the result obtained also by the cell-free scaffold, it was likely that the process was mediated by mesenchymal precursor cells resident in the subchondral bone and recruited within the material. This finding would thus be consistent with a previously proposed concept [5] as well as the results from another study that advocated the contribution of mesenchymal stem cells attracted from the bone marrow towards autologous matrix-induced chondrogenesis [23].

Our group then reported a second study on sheep model to investigate the possible enhancement of the good regenerative potential shown by this new scaffold, implanting it in association with platelet-rich plasma (PRP), which is an inexpensive minimally invasive source of growth factors (GFs) and cytokines that govern and regulate the tissue healing processes of most tissues [20].

In vitro studies showed that PRP could enhance both chondral and osseous tissues in the osteochondral regeneration induced by the scaffold [1, 9, 47]. Platelet concentrates stimulate the initial recruitment of bone marrow cells for migration [34], mitogenesis, differentiation into osteoblasts, and angiogenesis [45]. Also on chondral regeneration it has been shown that PRP enhances proliferation of chondrocytes and biosynthesis of the cartilage matrix proteins [1, 9], but just a few clinical studies were reported at the time on PRP for osteochondral regeneration [3, 40, 47].

Twelve animals, randomly divided in 3 groups of 4 sheep each, underwent a total of 24 osteochondral lesions, performed on the right medial and lateral femoral condyles. Each animal received the same treatment on both condyles. The groups were (1) biomimetic scaffold alone (S-group), (2) biomimetic scaffold combined with PRP (S-PRP group), and (3) a control group of spontaneous cartilage and bone repair (C-group).

The scaffold was the same previously used, while the PRP was prepared according to Weibrich et al. [46]: within 1 h before the operation, 20 mL of peripheral venous blood was drawn from the radial vein into siliconized tubes containing 3.8 % sodium citrate (blood/citrate ratio: 9/1), then the blood was centrifugated at 1,000 rpm for 5 min to obtain PRP. Two milliliters of PRP were activated using a 10 % solution of $CaCl_2$ in 50 μL/mL proportion and soaked into the scaffold immediately after use. Surgical procedure for scaffold implantation, animal sacrifice, and explant of the samples at 6 months after surgery were performed as described above [18].

Gross evaluation showed no bone and cartilage defect healing in the control group. Good integration of the healthy chondral surface, newly formed hyaline-like tissue, and better bone regeneration were observed in the group implanted with the scaffold alone (S-group), whereas incomplete bone defect filling and irregularity of the bone–cartilage surface were detected in the S-PRP group. Evaluation of the macroscopic appearance using modified Fortier and Niederaurer scores [11, 33] showed better results in both experimental groups compared with the control group. However, the S-group appeared significantly better than the others in both scores. Microradiographic evaluation showed newly formed bone in the deepest area of the implant for both study groups, with better bone regeneration for the scaffold alone than in addition to PRP. Bone growth into the chondral layer was not observed in any of the groups. Histology confirmed significant superior results for both study groups and, between them, worse results were for the S-PRP group.

The reabsorption of the implant was complete, without any inflammatory reaction or giant cells present. S-group presented a repair tissue well integrated with the host cartilage and with strong proteoglycan staining; underlying subchondral trabecular bone appeared to be well structured and distinguishable from the adjacent bone. Also better bone regeneration was observed for this group compared to the S-PRP group. Immunohistochemical staining for collagen types I and II generally confirmed that for S-group type II collagen stained positive in the cartilaginous layer down to the interface with the subchondral bone, where type I collagen was uniformly positive. Into the subchondral tissue discrete areas were positive for type II collagen; the hypertrophic chondrocyte morphology suggested ongoing remodeling towards a bone matrix, whereas in S-PRP and C-groups type II collagen resulted either negative or positive in scattered areas, whereas a positive staining for type I collagen in the extracellular matrix was extended throughout the repair tissue up to the joint space.

The conclusion of this study is that, despite in vitro premises and theoretical assumptions, the addition of multiple bioactive factors contained in PLT concentrate had a negative influence on bone and cartilage regeneration demonstrated by this kind of scaffold, leading to a highly amorphous cartilaginous repair tissue and poorly spatially organized underlying bone tissue, thus we decided to implant scaffold alone in our first pilot clinical study.

8.4 Clinical Application

8.4.1 Indications

- Symptomatic chondral defect: ICRS grade III–IV
- Etiology: traumatic, degenerative, and osteochondritis dissecans (OCD)
- Defect size: about 2–8 cm^2
- Age: less than 60 years (even if there is still lack of a precise cutoff for this scaffold, it is known that, as for bone marrow stimulating techniques, a high regenerative potential is needed) [15]
- Body mass index (BMI): less or equal to 30

8.4.2 Contraindications

- Medium to severe osteoarthritis
- Untreated comorbidities such as malalignment or ligament stability deficiency
- Rheumatic and autoimmune diseases, infections

8.4.3 Surgical Technique [19]

Mini-arthrotomic (medial or lateral) approach is necessary.

- Identification and debridement of the osteochondral lesion
- Preparation of the defect in order to remove:
  - Damaged surface
  - Sclerotic subchondral bone (depth: 8 mm)
- Cut of the scaffold to the right size and shape
- Press-fit fixation and tourniquet release (the scaffold swells with getting wet after tourniquet release)
- Stability tests (cyclic bending and extension of the knee)

8.4.4 Postoperative Rehabilitation

Management of postoperative pain allows for early mobilization that, in turn, contributes to faster resolution of swelling, promotes defect healing and joint nutrition, and prevents the development of adhesions. On the second postoperative day, self-assisted mobilization of the knee or continuous passive motion (CPM) for 6 h daily with one cycle per minute is recommended until 90° of flexion is reached. Early isometric and isotonic exercises and controlled mechanical compression are performed. Muscular voluntary contraction and neuromuscular electrical stimulation (NMES) are indicated and can be started at patient discharge. In the third or fourth week, weight touchdown with crutches is allowed and the patient can then move progressively towards full weight bearing.

8.5 Clinical Results

The ability of the scaffold to induce orderly osteochondral tissue repair without necessarily including autologous cells made it attractive (1) from a practical and commercial standpoint, because it could be used as an off-the-shelf graft in a one-step surgical procedure; (2) from a surgical standpoint, it could be inserted under minimally invasive conditions due to its flexibility; and (3) from a biological standpoint, because the problems related to the cell culture would be eliminated. Moreover, the possibility of treating complex defects is very attractive for cases wherein tissue damage extends to the subchondral bone, involving 2 tissues characterized by different intrinsic healing capacities. Thus, we decided to introduce to the clinical practice the use of this scaffold in a pilot experimental trial on 30 patients to evaluate the safety and feasibility of the procedure and analyze the clinical results. Considering the previous in vitro and animal studies [18, 20, 21], we decided to implant the scaffold alone, without any biological augmentation.

Preliminary results were reported on 13 patients (15 defects), focusing on the surgical technique and the intrinsic mechanical stability of the implants without any other fixation technique [19]. Since MRI had become the method of choice for noninvasive follow-up of patients undergoing cartilage repair, and it has been demonstrated that MRI allows for evaluation of both the biochemical and biomechanical status of cartilage, in addition to its morphology we thought it represents a well-accepted powerful tool for postoperative monitoring of osteochondral lesions and tissue repair [26–28, 43]. High-resolution MRI technique was used for the evaluation of the graft adherence at 5–8 weeks after implantation and for evaluation of further graft stability and maturation at 6 months. At 1 month, with a simple evaluation system, we scored the transplant as completely attached, partially attached, or detached. To reduce evaluation bias, all MRI scans were read by two independent experienced radiologists.

Fifteen lesions in 13 patients were prospectively analyzed. At the earliest evaluation time (5–8 weeks), complete attachment and adherence was found in 13 of the implantation sites. Partial attachment was found in two patients. The possible reason for the early detachment of the implanted biomaterials could be weak mechanical fixation due to inadequate surgical technique with insufficient shoulder coverage of the prepared implantation site. Further analysis at 6 months revealed partial reabsorption of the graft in one case with an incomplete cartilage layer and a complete subchondral structure, while in the other case an inhomogeneous tissue filled in the entire treated area, probably due to the development of fibrous tissue. The MRI evaluation at 6 months showed good filling of the lesion and integration of the graft, and the mean MOCART score presented a satisfying value considering the ongoing evolutionary process. In fact, the estimation of scaffold maturation in bone and cartilage tissues showed normal osteochondral structure in only nine (60 %) of the cases and a not-differentiated inhomogeneous signal in the implanted area in the rest of the patients, as predicted at early follow-up. The histological analysis, although only performed in two cases, revealed the presence of a perfectly formed subchondral bone and complete biomaterial reabsorption. The cartilage repair tissue analyzed 6 months after treatment appeared to be in different degrees of remodeling, but the presence of two partially differentiated tissues in an ongoing healing process without any presence of "bone step-in" is very promising. The clinical outcome at 6 months follow-up was also analyzed. Such an early clinical evaluation is not useful for determining the success rate of the procedure; however, the objective and subjective IKDC scores obtained documented the return to normal daily activities with a marked improvement relative to the preoperative level. More intensive activities are not advisable at an early stage and, consequently, were not performed. A correlation between clinical outcome and total MOCART score could not be identified, probably due to the low number of cases evaluated. However, in analyzing the single parameters, a correlation was shown between the patient's age and effusion that might be related to the slower healing process and recovery of older patients after surgical trauma. This short observation period provided promising preliminary results for the attachment rate and healing process obtainable using this new technique.

We reported also the case of a 46-year-old athletic patient [16] who, treated with ACL reconstruction at the same knee 10 years before, complained of anteromedial left knee pain after playing tennis for the last 6 months. The pain had progressed to the point where he could no longer engage in athletic activity. On physical examination there was a mild effusion. The patient's active range of motion was 0–110°, and he was tender on palpation along the medial joint line. There was no anteroposterior nor varus–valgus instability. Plain radiographs showed a 10° varus deformity and moderate medial joint space narrowing. At MRI there was evidence of deep and extended osteochondral lesions, involving the medial femoral condyle, the trochlea, and the patella. The chondral lesions were inspected arthroscopically and were graded as four according to the ICRS classification. A closing-wedge high tibial osteotomy was performed to restore the lower limb's normal axis and unload the medial compartment. Next, the biomimetic osteochondral scaffold was implanted through a medial parapatellar approach to regenerate the damaged articular surface using the technique previously described.

At 1-year follow-up the patient was pain-free, had full range of motion, and returned to his preoperation level of tennis. MRI performed 6 and 12 months after surgery showed stable implants and a hyaline-like signal with good restoration of the articular surface at 6 months. Subchondral edema then progressively decreased over time and at 12 months it was barely evident. The principal finding of the present study was the promising outcome obtained also in a patient affected by degenerative cartilage lesions on the medial femoral condyle, trochlea, and patella treated with a closing-wedge high tibial osteotomy and the new osteochondral scaffold.

Currently we are prospectively following a group of 30 patients (9 F, 21 M, mean age 29 years) affected by either chondral or osteochondral lesions of the knee who underwent the scaffold implantation at 36-month follow-up, whose results have previously been reported at 24 months of follow-up [22]. The inclusion criteria of the study were patients with clinical symptoms such as knee pain or swelling affected by grade III–IV chondral and osteochondral lesions of the knee (International Cartilage Repair Society Evaluation Package) [44]. The exclusion criteria were non-corrected axial deviation and knee instability, as evaluated clinically and via radiographic examination. As reported above, patients with an ACL lesion at the time of surgery underwent the associated surgical procedure of ACL reconstruction in the same surgical session as the osteochondral grafting. Patients with infectious, neoplastic, metabolic, and inflammatory pathologic changes were excluded from the study. All patients gave informed consent, and treatment was approved by the local ethics board. Twenty-eight out of 30 patients were analyzed prospectively at 6, 12, 24, and 36 months using the Cartilage Standard Evaluation Form, as proposed by the ICRS, and a high-resolution MRI; 2 patients were lost to follow-up. Twenty-two patients presented a single lesion, while multiple lesions were detected in 6 cases (34 lesions in total). The sites of the defects were the following: 8 medial femoral condyles, 5 lateral femoral condyles, 12 patellae, 7 trochlea, and 2 lateral tibial plateaux. The average size of the defects was 2.9 ± 1.3 cm^2 (range: 1.5–6.0 cm^2). Etiology was traumatic in 5 cases, microtraumatic/degenerative in 16 cases, and 7 patients were affected by OCD. Seventeen patients were athletically active, being well trained or practicing sports at a competitive level, whereas 11 patients were less active, practicing sports at only an amateur level or not

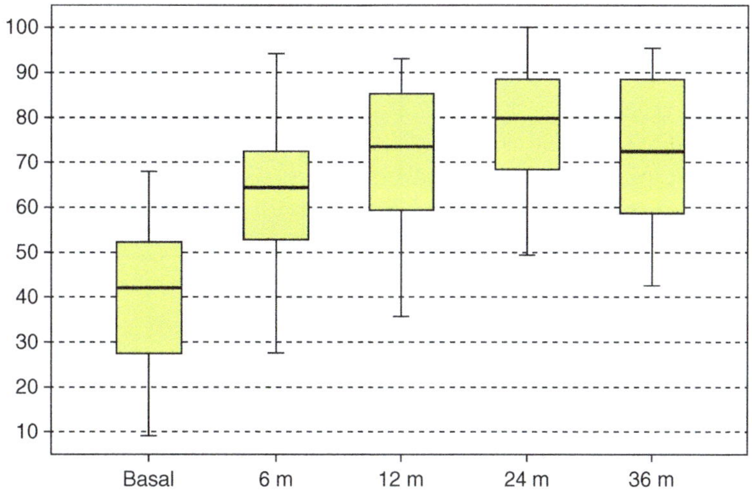

Graphic 8.1 IKDC subjective score at 36 months

practicing any sport at all. Nine patients were operated on for the first time, whereas 19 patients had undergone previous surgery (11 patients had previous cartilage treatment). In 15 patients, other associated procedures were performed during the same operation: 4 osteotomies, 3 patellar realignments, 2 lateral releases, 1 patellar tendon suturing, 1 ACL reconstruction with arthroscopic meniscectomy, 1 meniscal allograft, 1 patellar lateral facet removal, 1 lateral tibial plateau elevation with external fixator implantation, and 1 hardware removal. The evaluation of these 28 patients was performed using the subjective and objective scores of the International Knee Documentation Committee (IKDC); the Tegner score was used to assess the level of regular physical activity of the patient. A high-resolution MRI of each patient was also analyzed using the MOCART (Magnetic Resonance Observation of Cartilage Repair Tissue) score [4, 13, 14, 24, 25, 27, 29].

During the follow-up period, 10 patients suffered minor adverse events like articular swelling, bleeding, or temperature: in all cases resolution was observed within 1 month, with the exception of two patients whose articular stiffness required arthroscopic treatment. In one case, we performed a second-look arthroscopy in a patient treated with multiple scaffolds implantation and complaining for persistent articular pain: we observed loosening of one of the scaffolds, which was subsequently debrided. The mean preoperative subjective score of the 28 patients was 40.4 (±14.6); 12 months after surgery the average score raised to 71.9 (±14.3), at 24 months of follow-up a further increase was registered (76.7 ± 14) whereas at 36 months follow-up we reported a little, not significant decrease at mean score of 72.8: however, the results at 3 years of follow-up showed a statistically significant ($p<0.005$) improvement from basal evaluation (Graphic 8.1). This improvement has been confirmed even at objective IKDC evaluation: from basal to 36-month follow-up, we reported an increase from 50 to 89.3 % of "normal" (objective IKDC=A) or "nearly normal" (objective IKDC=B) knees. Mean pre-injury Tegner score was 5.2 (±2.5), whereas at pretreatment evaluation it was 1.6 (±1.1). A significant increase was registered at 12 months of follow-up with a mean value of 4.0 (±1.6), which was confirmed at 24 months. The 36-month follow-up evaluation revealed a further rise up to 4.5 (±1.9). These results show a statistically significant improvement ($p<0.0005$) from presurgery to 3 years of follow-up, even if the final sport activity level is lower than the pre-injury one (Graphic 8.2). The lesion site comes out to be clinically relevant at 6 and 12 months follow-up: there is a lower improvement in patients with patellar lesions ($p=0.037$ at 6 months and $p=0.05$ at 12 months), probably due to the difficulty in restoring patellar articular surface and its tracking. However, no significant differences were observed at longer follow-ups. Another influencing factor was the sport activity level: in fact

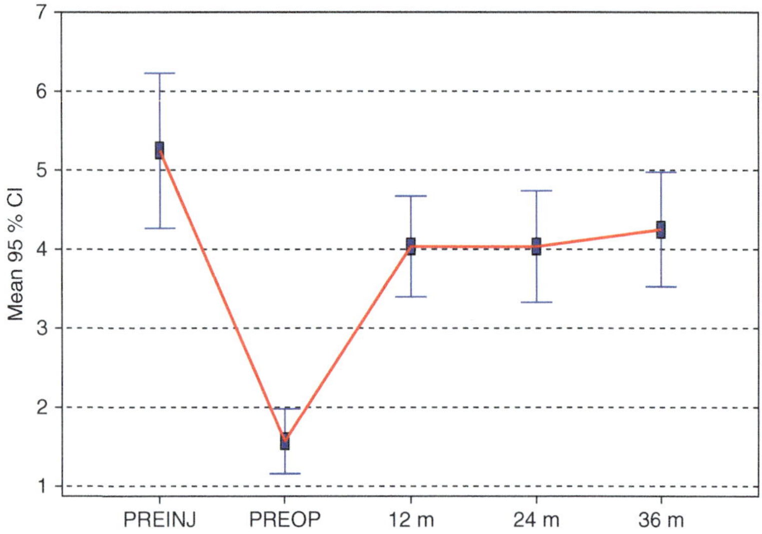

Graphic 8.2 Tegner score at 36 months

active patients had statistically better results than non-active ones. Furthermore we noticed that age, gender, lesion dimension, and previous surgery do not correlate with clinical outcome. We performed 17 MRI evaluations (21 lesions in total) at 36 months after surgery and we analyzed them using the MOCART score. The analysis revealed a complete degree of repair and filling of the defect in 66.7 % of cases and complete integration of the scaffold with the adjacent cartilage in 66.7 % of cases, even if the surface of the repair tissue appeared perfectly intact in just 38.1 % of cases (average MOCART score=74). Anyway our data at 36 months revealed no significant difference when compared to MOCART score analysis performed on 29 patients at 24 months of follow-up. A statistically relevant improvement was nonetheless observed comparing the final MOCART score with the first one performed 6 months after surgery. We performed 3 arthroscopic biopsies: one was made during a concurrent meniscectomy 8 months after the scaffold implantation; another was done during a concurrent hardware removal at 11 months of follow-up; the last one was performed during an arthroscopic second-look made to address the recurrence of articular pain at 18 months after scaffold implantation. These biopsies showed regeneration of the subchondral bone associated with complete biomaterial reabsorption and presence of hyaline-like cartilage rich in proteoglycans and type II collagen.

8.6 Discussion and Conclusion

When approaching lesions of the articular surface, regenerative techniques, like second-generation ACI, have already shown good results at short- and medium-term follow-up [10, 17, 36], but with some limitations: the need for a two-step surgery and the possibility to treat only cartilage damages [13]. The subchondral bone is also involved in big chondral lesions and it needs to be treated in order to have a correct restoration of the most superficial layers of the joint [35]. This is the reason why different osteochondral scaffolds have been created, even if only for two of them clinical results have already been reported [7, 16, 19, 22, 30]. In particular, after extensive in vitro and in vivo preclinical evaluation, we decided to implant MaioRegen® scaffold in our pilot clinical trial on 30 patients affected by either chondral or osteochondral lesions to evaluate the efficacy of this new synthetic, biomimetic, and multilayered scaffold. Statistical analysis made on the 28 patients' results at 3 years of follow-up showed significant improvement of the scores compared to the basal control. IKDC subjective showed over time stability of the good outcomes already achieved 12 months after surgery. The IKDC objective evaluation score increased from 50 % at basal control to 89.3 % at the final follow-up of "normal" (objective IKDC=A) or "nearly normal" (objective IKDC=B) knees. Tegner score

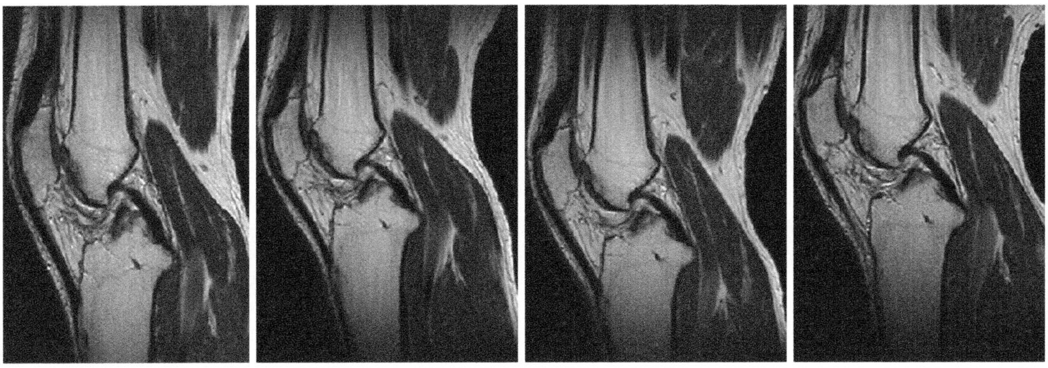

Fig. 8.2 MaioRegen implant on trochlea: MRI follow-ups at 6, 12, 24, and 36 months

showed a statistically significant improvement from preoperative time (mean score of 1.6 ± 1.1) to 3 years of follow-up (mean score of 4.5 ± 1.9), with stable trend, even if the final sport activity level was lower than the pre-injury one. MRI evaluation through MOCART analysis revealed a complete degree of repair and filling of the defect in 66.7 % of cases, showing with the same percentage a complete integration of the scaffold with the adjacent cartilage (Fig. 8.2). These encouraging data, both clinical and radiological, suggest that this particular one-step surgical approach, based on a cell-free biomimetic scaffold, could be successfully performed in knee chondral or osteochondral lesions. From a technical point of view, the plasticity of the graft allows large osteochondral lesions to be treated through minor incisions. Since one of the major concerns with the use of biomaterials for cartilage and osteochondral defects repair with no surgical graft fixation is graft detachment, which can lead to graft failure, also this aspect has been examined in our early studies, showing the safety and feasibility of the procedure.

Concluding, this scaffold-based one-step repair is in our opinion a new interesting approach for the treatment of deep chondral and osteochondral lesions. The advantage of these techniques is the possibility of a one-step procedure, on-the-shelf availability of the material, more simple and fast surgical technique, and lower costs. By the way, even if promising preliminary results have been already reported, these materials are new and require further clinical investigation with longer-term follow-ups and a higher number of patients to attest the efficacy and durability over time, as showed by the preliminary results.

References

1. Akeda K, An HS, Okuma M et al (2006) Platelet-rich plasma stimulates porcine articular chondrocyte proliferation and matrix biosynthesis. Osteoarthritis Cartilage 14:1272–1280
2. Bernhardt A, Lode A, Boxberger S et al (2008) Mineralised collagen–an artificial, extracellular bone matrix–improves osteogenic differentiation of bone marrow stromal cells. J Mater Sci Mater Med 19:269–275
3. Brehm W, Aklin B, Yamashita T et al (2006) Repair of superficial osteochondral defects with an autologous scaffold-free cartilage construct in a caprine model: implantation method and short-term results. Osteoarthritis Cartilage 14:1214–1226
4. Brittberg M (2008) Autologous chondrocyte implantation–technique and long-term follow-up. Injury 39(Suppl 1):S40–S49
5. Buma P, Pieper JS, Van Tienen T et al (2003) Cross-linked type I and type II collagenous matrices for the repair of full-thickness articular cartilage defects–a study in rabbits. Biomaterials 24:3255–3263
6. Buma P, Schreurs W, Verdonschot N (2004) Skeletal tissue engineering-from in vitro studies to large animal models. Biomaterials 25:1487–1495
7. Carmont MR, Carey-Smith R, Saithna A et al (2009) Delayed incorporation of a TruFit plug: perseverance is recommended. Arthroscopy 25:810–814
8. Domaschke H, Gelinsky M, Burmeister B et al (2006) In vitro ossification and remodeling of mineralized collagen I scaffolds. Tissue Eng 12:949–958
9. Drengk A, Zapf A, Sturmer EK et al (2009) Influence of platelet-rich plasma on chondrogenic differentiation and proliferation of chondrocytes and mesenchymal stem cells. Cells Tissues Organs 189:317–326
10. Filardo G, Kon E, Di Martino A et al (2011) Arthroscopic second-generation autologous chondrocyte

implantation: a prospective 7-year follow-up study. Am J Sports Med 39:2153–2160
11. Fortier LA, Mohammed HO, Lust G et al (2002) Insulin-like growth factor-I enhances cell-based repair of articular cartilage. J Bone Joint Surg Br 84: 276–288
12. Gelinsky M, Welzel P, Simon P, Bernhardt A, Konig U (2008) Porous threedimensional scaffolds made of mineralized collagen: preparation and properties of a biomimetic nanocomposite material for tissue engineering of bone. Chem Eng J 137:84–96
13. Gomoll AH, Madry H, Knutsen G et al (2010) The subchondral bone in articular cartilage repair: current problems in the surgical management. Knee Surg Sports Traumatol Arthrosc 18:434–447
14. Jiang CC, Chiang H, Liao CJ et al (2007) Repair of porcine articular cartilage defect with a biphasic osteochondral composite. J Orthop Res 25:1277–1290
15. Kai Mithoefer K, Saris D, Farr J, Kon E, Zaslav K, Cole BJ, Ranstam J, Yao J, Shive M, Levine D, Dalemans W, Brittberg M (2011) Guidelines for the design and conduct of clinical studies in knee articular cartilage repair: international cartilage repair society recommendations based on current scientific evidence and standards of clinical care. Cartilage 2:100–121
16. Kon E, Delcogliano M, Filardo G et al (2009) Novel nano-composite multi-layered biomaterial for the treatment of multifocal degenerative cartilage lesions. Knee Surg Sports Traumatol Arthrosc 17:1312–1315
17. Kon E, Verdonk P, Condello V et al (2009) Matrix-assisted autologous chondrocyte transplantation for the repair of cartilage defects of the knee: systematic clinical data review and study quality analysis. Am J Sports Med 37(Suppl 1):156S–166S
18. Kon E, Delcogliano M, Filardo G et al (2010) Orderly osteochondral regeneration in a sheep model using a novel nano-composite multilayered biomaterial. J Orthop Res 28:116–124
19. Kon E, Delcogliano M, Filardo G et al (2010) A novel nano-composite multi-layered biomaterial for treatment of osteochondral lesions: technique note and an early stability pilot clinical trial. Injury 41:693–701
20. Kon E, Filardo G, Delcogliano M et al (2010) Platelet autologous growth factors decrease the osteochondral regeneration capability of a collagen-hydroxyapatite scaffold in a sheep model. BMC Musculoskelet Disord 11:220
21. Kon E, Mutini A, Arcangeli E et al (2010) Novel nanostructured scaffold for osteochondral regeneration: pilot study in horses. J Tissue Eng Regen Med 4:300–308
22. Kon E, Delcogliano M, Filardo G et al (2011) Novel nano-composite multilayered biomaterial for osteochondral regeneration: a pilot clinical trial. Am J Sports Med 39:1180–1190
23. Kramer J, Bohrnsen F, Lindner U et al (2006) In vivo matrix-guided human mesenchymal stem cells. Cell Mol Life Sci 63:616–626
24. Marcacci M, Berruto M, Brocchetta D et al (2005) Articular cartilage engineering with Hyalograft C: 3-year clinical results. Clin Orthop Relat Res 435:96–105
25. Marlovits S, Singer P, Zeller P et al (2006) Magnetic resonance observation of cartilage repair tissue (MOCART) for the evaluation of autologous chondrocyte transplantation: determination of interobserver variability and correlation to clinical outcome after 2 years. Eur J Radiol 57:16–23
26. Marlovits S, Striessnig G, Kutscha-Lissberg F et al (2005) Early postoperative adherence of matrix-induced autologous chondrocyte implantation for the treatment of full-thickness cartilage defects of the femoral condyle. Knee Surg Sports Traumatol Arthrosc 13:451–457
27. Marlovits S, Striessnig G, Resinger CT et al (2004) Definition of pertinent parameters for the evaluation of articular cartilage repair tissue with high-resolution magnetic resonance imaging. Eur J Radiol 52:310–319
28. Marlovits S, Daniels VG, Resinger C et al (2007) Clinical and radiological outcome of matrix induced autologous chondrocyte implantation (MACI) after 24 months. Osteoarthritis Cartilage 15(suppl B, P68):105
29. Martin I, Miot S, Barbero A et al (2007) Osteochondral tissue engineering. J Biomech 40:750–765
30. Melton JT, Wilson AJ, Chapman-Sheath P et al (2010) TruFit CB bone plug: chondral repair, scaffold design, surgical technique and early experiences. Expert Rev Med Devices 7:333–341
31. Mithoefer K, Mcadams T, Williams RJ et al (2009) Clinical efficacy of the microfracture technique for articular cartilage repair in the knee: an evidence-based systematic analysis. Am J Sports Med 37: 2053–2063
32. Newman AP (1998) Articular cartilage repair. Am J Sports Med 26:309–324
33. Niederauer GG, Slivka MA, Leatherbury NC et al (2000) Evaluation of multiphase implants for repair of focal osteochondral defects in goats. Biomaterials 21:2561–2574
34. Oprea WE, Karp JM, Hosseini MM et al (2003) Effect of platelet releasate on bone cell migration and recruitment in vitro. J Craniofac Surg 14:292–300
35. Pape D, Filardo G, Kon E et al (2010) Disease-specific clinical problems associated with the subchondral bone. Knee Surg Sports Traumatol Arthrosc 18:448–462
36. Peterson L, Brittberg M, Kiviranta I et al (2002) Autologous chondrocyte transplantation. Biomechanics and long-term durability. Am J Sports Med 30:2–12
37. Scheck RM, Taboas JM, Segvich SJ, Hollister SJ, Krebsbach PH (2004) Engineered osteochondral grafts using biphasic composite solid free-form fabricated scaffolds. Tissue Eng 10:1376–1385
38. Serre CM, Papillard M, Chavassieux P et al (1998) Influence of magnesium substitution on a collagen-

apatite biomaterial on the production of a calcifying matrix by human osteoblasts. J Biomed Mater Res 42:626–633
39. Sherwood JK, Riley SL, Palazzolo R et al (2002) A three-dimensional osteochondral composite scaffold for articular cartilage repair. Biomaterials 23:4739–4751
40. Sun Y, Feng Y, Zhang CQ et al (2010) The regenerative effect of platelet-rich plasma on healing in large osteochondral defects. Int Orthop 34:589–597
41. Tampieri A, Celotti G, Landi E et al (2003) Biologically inspired synthesis of bone-like composite: self-assembled collagen fibers/hydroxyapatite nanocrystals. J Biomed Mater Res A 67:618–625
42. Tampieri A, Sandri M, Landi E et al (2008) Design of graded biomimetic osteochondral composite scaffolds. Biomaterials 29:3539–3546
43. Trattnig S, Mamisch TC, Pinker K et al (2008) Differentiating normal hyaline cartilage from post-surgical repair tissue using fast gradient echo imaging in delayed gadolinium-enhanced MRI (dGEMRIC) at 3 Tesla. Eur Radiol 18:1251–1259
44. Van Den Borne MP, Raijmakers NJ, Vanlauwe J et al (2007) International Cartilage Repair Society (ICRS) and Oswestry macroscopic cartilage evaluation scores validated for use in Autologous Chondrocyte Implantation (ACI) and microfracture. Osteoarthritis Cartilage 15:1397–1402
45. Van Den Dolder J, Mooren R, Vloon AP et al (2006) Platelet-rich plasma: quantification of growth factor levels and the effect on growth and differentiation of rat bone marrow cells. Tissue Eng 12: 3067–3073
46. Weibrich G, Hansen T, Kleis W et al (2004) Effect of platelet concentration in platelet-rich plasma on peri-implant bone regeneration. Bone 34:665–671
47. Wu W, Zhang J, Dong Q et al (2009) Platelet-rich plasma – a promising cell carrier for micro-invasive articular cartilage repair. Med Hypotheses 72: 455–457
48. Yokoyama A, Gelinsky M, Kawasaki T et al (2005) Biomimetic porous scaffolds with high elasticity made from mineralized collagen–an animal study. J Biomed Mater Res B Appl Biomater 75:464–472
49. Zeeman R, Dijkstra PJ, Van Wachem PB et al (2000) The kinetics of 1,4-butanediol diglycidyl ether cross-linking of dermal sheep collagen. J Biomed Mater Res 51:541–548

BST-CarGel®: An Enhanced Bone Marrow Stimulation Treatment

9

Alberto Restrepo, Stéphane Méthot, William D. Stanish, and Matthew S. Shive

Contents

A. Restrepo, MD (✉) • S. Méthot, PhD
M.S. Shive, PhD
Piramal Life Sciences, Bio-Orthopaedic Division,
475 Armand Frappier Boulevard,
Laval (QC) H7V 4B3, Canada
e-mail: alberto.restrepo@piramal.com

W.D. Stanish, MD
Department of Surgery, Dalhousie University,
5595 Fenwick Street, Suite 311,
Halifax (NS) B3H 4M2, Canada

9.1 Introduction

Bone marrow stimulation techniques such as abrasion arthroplasty [1], Pridie drilling [2], and microfracture [3] attempt to use the natural wound repair response elicited by a blood clot originating from the bone marrow. Channels surgically made in the subchondral bone below the cartilage lesion permit access to marrow blood and blood components including stem cells intended to provide an environment for wound healing that ultimately leads to cartilage regeneration. Microfracture, which has been frequently used as a first-line treatment for small cartilage lesions, has the advantage of being simple and safe, cost-effective, and minimally invasive with a low morbidity rate [4, 5]. On the other hand, the procedure results in a mixed repair tissue with mainly fibrous or fibrocartilaginous properties [6–10], limited collagen type II and glycosaminoglycan (GAG) levels, and poor mechanical properties compared to native hyaline cartilage. Indeed, the long-term durability of this repair tissue has been questioned with many reports showing a failure of repair tissue and a return of associated clinical symptoms starting as early as 24 months post-treatment [8, 11, 12].

In an effort to guide or enhance the regeneration of more hyaline-like cartilage tissue following bone marrow stimulation, these procedures have been combined with scaffolds and/or growth factors or other biological materials [13]. These so-called enhanced bone marrow stimulation

A.A. Shetty et al. (eds.), *Techniques in Cartilage Repair Surgery*,
DOI 10.1007/978-3-642-41921-8_9, © ESSKA 2014

techniques may have the potential to overcome the main drawback of poor repair tissue quality and durability while still being safe and cost-effective, requiring a single-step, minimally invasive surgery.

9.2 BST-CarGel® Background

9.2.1 The Product

BST-CarGel® (Piramal Healthcare (Canada) Ltd.) is a new liquid scaffold that was developed to physically stabilize the blood clot in the cartilage lesion following a one-step bone marrow stimulation procedure, in order to promote hyaline cartilage formation. BST-CarGel® is based on a patented thermogel platform technology [14]. BST-CarGel® is a physiological solution (in terms of pH and osmolarity) comprised of chitosan, a buffer called β-glycerophosphate (β-GP), and hydrochloric acid (HCI). The natural biopolymer chitosan is a linear, cationic polysaccharide composed of D-glucosamine and *N*-acetyl-D-glucosamine and has been extensively studied for regenerative medicine and other biotechnological applications [15–18] due to its desirable biodegradability, biocompatibility, and mucoadhesivity.

BST-CarGel® is an implantable medical device designed to be a liquid at room temperature, mixed with fresh autologous whole blood (BST-CarGel®/blood mixture ratio of 1:3), and delivered to a cartilage lesion surgically prepared by debridement and bone marrow stimulation. BST-CarGel® is packaged as a 2-component system made up of the *Mixing Vial* (red cap) and the *Additive Vial* (blue cap) (Fig. 9.1). The *Mixing Vial* contains the chitosan solution and stainless steel beads to facilitate mixing with whole blood, while the *Additive Vial* contains the β-GP solution. The final BST-CarGel® product is obtained by combining the two solutions just prior to the addition of fresh autologous whole blood. Once the whole blood is added, BST-CarGel® is ready to be applied to the cartilage lesion where BST-CarGel® permits natural blood clotting and the in situ formation of a hybrid clot that provides a three-dimensional scaffold supporting the blood components over the marrow holes and guiding the repair process.

9.2.2 Primary Mode of Action

Many intrinsic (lesion type, location, size, and depth) and extrinsic factors (surgical technique, postoperative rehabilitation) are important in the success of a bone marrow stimulation procedure

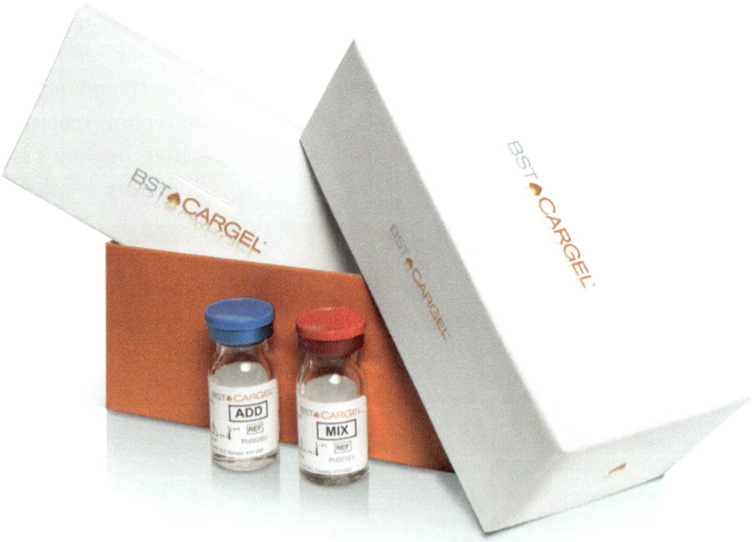

Fig. 9.1 BST-CarGel® product packaging. BST-CarGel® is a 2-component system comprised of the *Mixing Vial* (MIX; *red cap*) and the *Additive Vial* (ADD; *blue cap*). The *Mixing Vial* contains the chitosan solution and stainless steel beads to facilitate mixing with the whole blood, while the *Additive Vial* contains the β-glycerophosphate buffer solution

for cartilage repair. The properties of the bone marrow-derived blood clot (volume, adhesiveness, and stability) and its residency in the cartilage lesion should be maximized to maintain critical blood components over the marrow channel and drive repair. Following bone marrow stimulation techniques, the loss in volume of a blood clot due to retraction can be as much as 50 % [19], resulting in a deficient healing response including a poorly filled lesion, poor tissue quality, and lack of integration of the regenerated tissue with native cartilage.

On the other hand, the mixture of BST-CarGel® with fresh autologous whole blood permits natural clot formation [20] but inhibits retraction of the fibrin scaffolding [19], thus providing a more space-filling provisional matrix for repair (Fig. 9.2). Since hyaline cartilage is

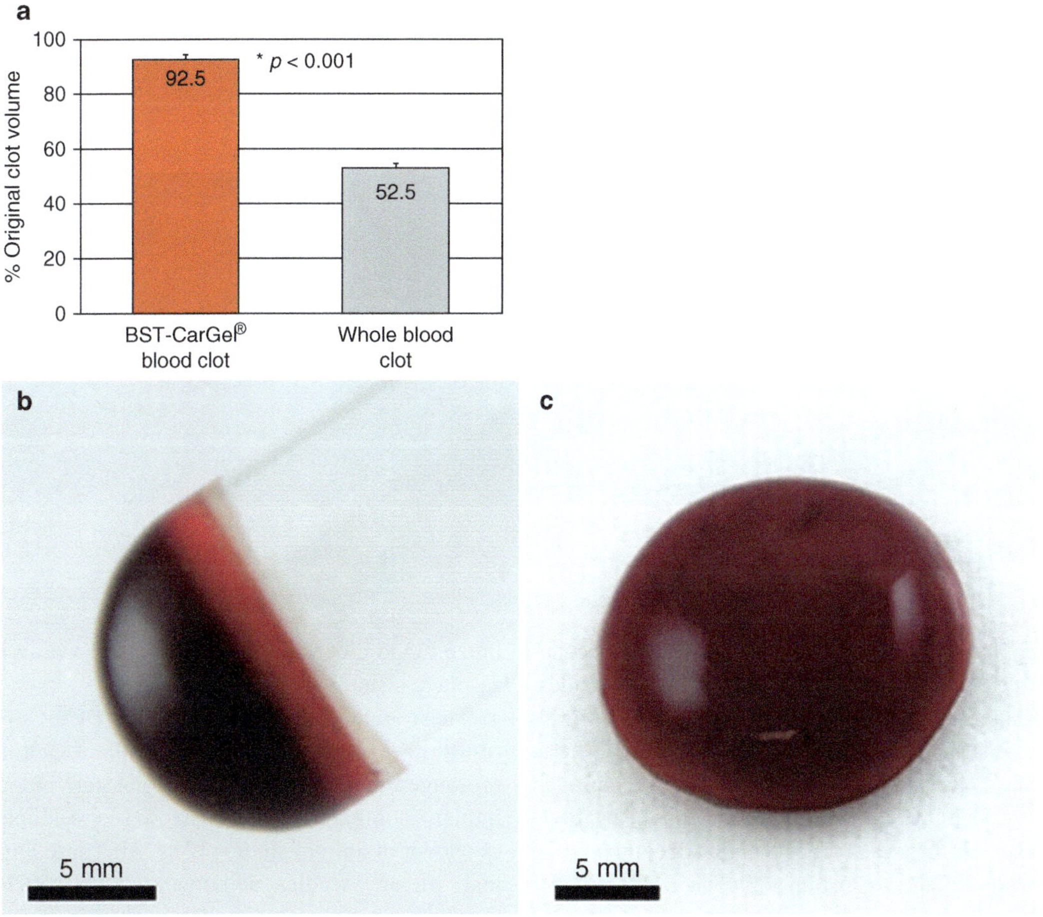

Fig. 9.2 Blood clot retraction and histology. (**a**) Clot retraction after 60 min at 37 °C was calculated from clot weights obtained before and after removal of exudated plasma ($n=25$). BST-CarGel® significantly inhibits clot retraction (92.5 % of original volume maintained) compared to whole blood only (52.5 %). (**b**) BST-CarGel®/blood clot in a glass tube and (**c**) petri dish exhibiting a bright red color, relatively little plasma exudation, and minimal retraction. (**d**) Whole blood clot in a glass tube and (**e**) petri dish exhibiting a darker red color (due to densely packed erythrocytes), plasma exudation, and significant retraction. (**f**) Histology of a BST-CarGel®/blood clot (toluidine blue staining). The chitosan (*light blue*; *empty arrowheads*) is homogenously dispersed throughout the erythrocytes (*green; black arrowheads*), and white blood cells (*dark blue*) are observed to co-localize with chitosan. The BST-CarGel®/blood clot appears less dense (less retraction) compared to the whole blood clot and does not suffer from cracking artifacts resulting from histological processing (more stable). (**g**) Histology of a whole blood clot (toluidine blue staining) demonstrating densely packed erythrocytes (significant retraction) and cracking artifacts (fragile clot)

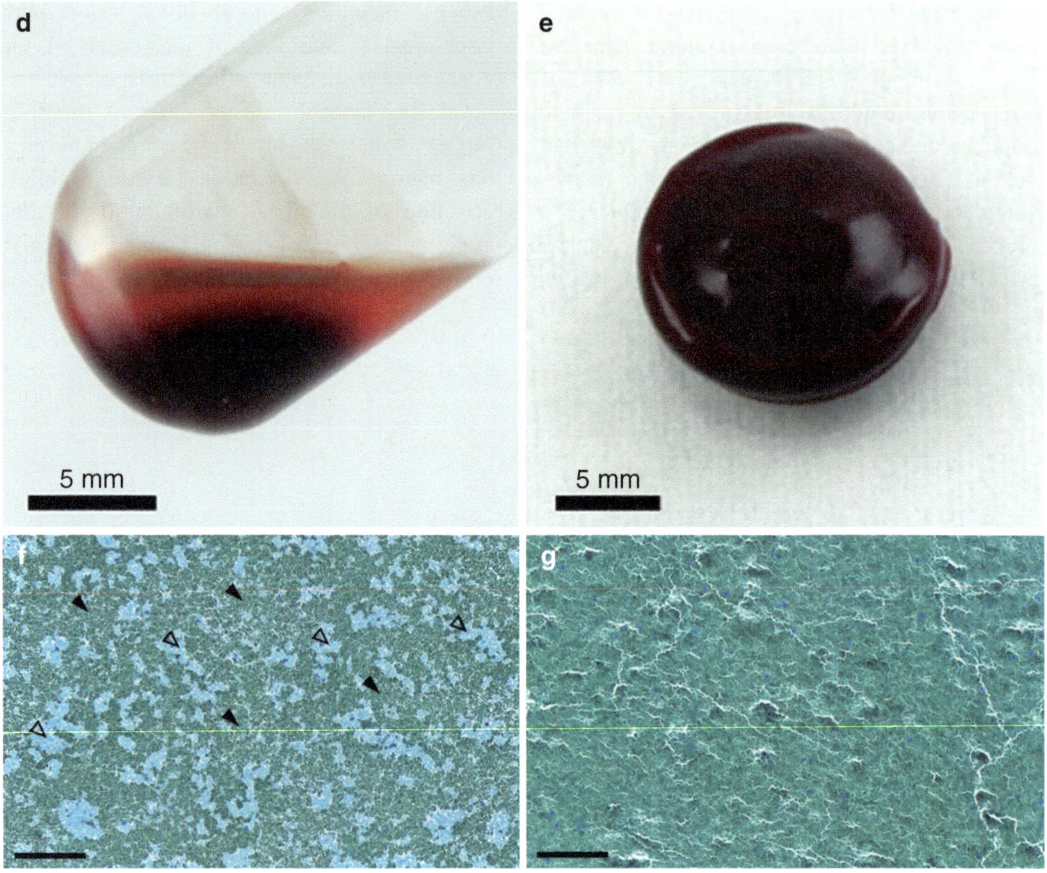

Fig. 9.2 (continued)

comprised of the negatively charged, disaccharide glycosaminoglycan (GAG) macromolecules, chitosan, the primary component of this scaffold, offers superior adhesion to the lesion surfaces due to its cationic charge [21–24]. The improved clot stabilization and adhesion brought by BST-CarGel® can easily be visualized compared to whole blood, as in Fig. 9.3. The BST-CarGel®/blood mixture provides a structurally stable and effective scaffolding with improved residency for cartilage regeneration driven by pluripotent bone marrow-derived stem cells [19–21, 23, 25]. Moreover, chitosan is biodegradable through endogenous chitosan-degrading enzymes and cells, which results in complete resorption from the implant site [14, 21, 23, 26–28].

Table 9.1 summarizes the mechanical contributions that BST-CarGel® brings in order to maximize blood clot volume and residency within a cartilage lesion.

These unique properties of BST-CarGel® result in a more voluminous implant and a prolonged residency of the BST-CarGel®/blood implant compared to the marrow blood alone, as shown in animal studies [21, 23]. These animal efficacy studies demonstrated that BST-CarGel® treatment led to (1) a greater lesion filling with a better integrated repair tissue, (2) a more cellular repair tissue with cells having a more chondrogenic phenotype, (3) an increase in glycosaminoglycan content in repair tissue (via Safranin-O staining), (4) a higher concentration of collagen type II in repair tissue (via immunohistochemistry), and (5) a more porous and vascularized subchondral bone plate [19, 21, 23].

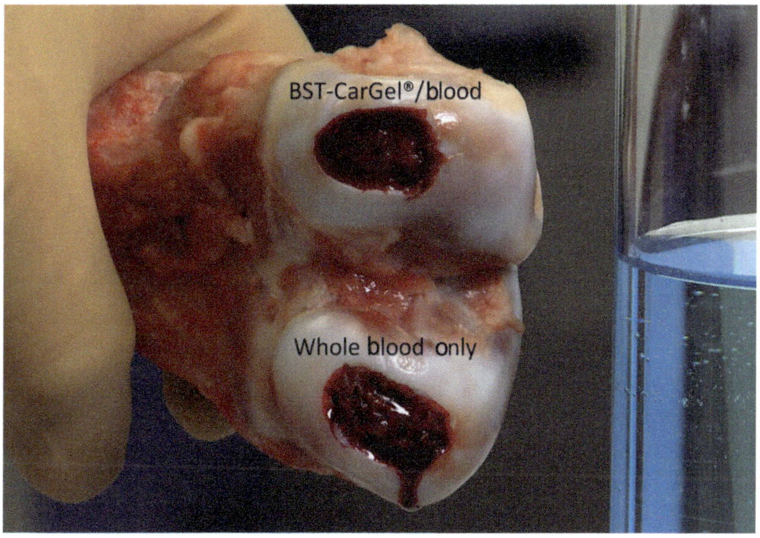

Fig. 9.3 Blood clot stabilization and increased adhesion by BST-CarGel®. BST-CarGel®/blood mixtures and whole blood were applied to microfractured lesions created on warmed pig femurs and left to clot for 15 min at 37 °C. When the femurs were then rotated to 90°, the superior adhesion of the BST-CarGel®/blood clot is observed, a result of the cationic chitosan's unique mucoadhesivity

Table 9.1 BST-CarGel®: primary mode of action

Acts as a scaffold to physically stabilize the blood clot in the cartilage lesion
Resists blood clot retraction while permitting normal clotting, thus providing a space-filling provisional matrix for repair
Adheres to the cartilage lesion surfaces

The repair processes by which the quantity and quality of repair tissue are improved by BST-CarGel® have been shown to differ significantly from those of bone marrow stimulation techniques in three enhanced healing events at early stages: (1) increased inflammatory and marrow-derived stromal cell recruitment; (2) increased vascularization of the provisional repair tissue; and (3) increased intramembranous bone formation and subchondral bone remodeling. These unique characteristics support a dynamic cartilage repair environment where resolution of the chitosan-induced wound healing leads to improved hyaline cartilage formation [21]. The development of this hyaline tissue appears to be modulated by BST-CarGel® in the timing, maturation, and position relative to articular surface of chondrogenic foci found in subchondral holes and which resemble natural cartilage growth processes [29].

The ability of BST-CarGel® to improve upon the morphology and biology of subchondral bone and the entire osteochondral unit and not just the articular surface [21, 30–32] is a critical finding as recent reviews have emphasized the important role of the osteochondral unit [33, 34]. Moreover, controversy exists regarding the potential influence of subchondral bone changes following marrow stimulation, where some reports show higher failure rates on subsequent revision surgery [35, 36] while others do not [37, 38]. The beneficial effects of BST-CarGel® on subchondral bone could potentially alleviate this issue.

9.3 BST-CarGel® Use

9.3.1 Indications/Contraindications

Correct patient profiling is an essential aspect of any cartilage repair technique. Multiple variables, as opposed to a single demographic or surgical factor, contribute to the success or failure of a given procedure. The best surgical technique, even with a proven product, can still fail if critical variables such as limb malalignment, joint instability, and obesity are not adequately assessed. If present, these contraindications for cartilage repair should be corrected, either before or concomitant with the procedure. Furthermore, lesion chronicity should also be considered since clinical outcomes, regardless of treatment, have

Table 9.2 BST-CarGel®: indications/contraindications

Indications	Contraindications
Grade 3 or 4 focal chondral or osteochondral lesions	Kissing lesions
Femoral condyles	Knee malalignment of more than 5°
Lesion area up to 7 cm^2	Meniscal insufficiencies
Traumatic or degenerative etiology	Ligamentous instability Shellfish allergy

been shown to be negatively correlated with chronicity [12].

Patient expectations must also be managed. Although factors such as age, activity level, comorbidities, and previous cartilage repair surgeries may have an impact on the outcome of the procedure (notwithstanding those listed above), the relative success or failure of a procedure will ultimately be judged from the patient's perspective. Consequently, it is critical for clinicians to establish the expectations of what a patient can reasonably expect for a given cartilage repair procedure based on the combination of these factors. The approach for BST-CarGel® should not differ from this.

From the current understanding of BST-CarGel® derived from the animal and clinical experience, the potential indications for BST-CarGel® are currently limited to localized or focal cartilage damage. Determining the suitability for BST-CarGel® treatment should take into account lesion grade (depth), location, and size as well as the status of the opposing chondral surface. Both traumatic cartilage damage and focal damage resulting from degenerative processes are considered indications for BST-CarGel®, the latter representing a large symptomatic patient population who are considered too young for total knee replacement. Furthermore, as already described, the mechanistic evidence from animal data has shown that BST-CarGel® has a reproducible and positive effect on subchondral bone remodeling [21, 31, 32], suggesting that cartilage loss emanating from subchondral bone pathologies, such as osteochondritis dissecans or cysts, may be addressed through BST-CarGel® treatment. A summary of indications is shown in Table 9.2 and supported by the randomized clinical trial described in Sect. 9.5.2. The presence of coexisting pathology that may adversely affect BST-CarGel®-mediated repair must be addressed before or concomitantly with the application of BST-CarGel®, including ligamentous instability, tibiofemoral malalignment, bone deficiency, patellofemoral malalignment, and meniscal pathology. The future use of scaffold-guided regenerative medicine (SGRM) using BST-CarGel® for in situ chondroinduction (ICI) can be envisioned in other joints in which chondral and osteochondral lesions are extensively found. Lesions in the ankle and hip joints might additionally be suitable for BST-CarGel® therapy because of the pathological similarities and their arthroscopic accessibility.

The approved indication for use of BST-CarGel®, according to the current labeling, is for the repair of single, symptomatic grade 3 or 4 focal cartilage lesions on the femoral condyles of the knee with an area up to 7 cm^2 in patients between 18 and 55 years old.

9.3.2 Concomitant Medications

The BST-CarGel® approach relies on the intrinsic properties of the human blood clot derived from the bone marrow, which upon clotting naturally initiates a cascade of signaling and biological events leading to wound healing through inflammatory pathways. Thus, anticoagulants and aspirin or heparin, as well as anti-inflammatory medications as tolerated, should ideally be discontinued at least 7 days prior to BST-CarGel® treatment and should not be resumed for 24 h posttreatment unless otherwise prescribed. Patients taking routine anticoagulation therapy, or when indicated, can resume their therapy 6 h after the end of the surgical procedure.

9.3.3 Surgical Technique

No unique tools or requirements in terms of facilities are needed to treat a patient with BST-CarGel® outside of a standard operating room equipped for arthroscopic surgery. A standard set of surgical instruments and retractors for open knee surgery is helpful if a mini-arthrotomy approach is used.

BST-CarGel® is applied as a viscous mixture of the product mixed on-site with fresh whole peripheral blood to a lesion which has already been debrided and treated with bone marrow stimulation (e.g., microfracture). The surgical technique for BST-CarGel® consists of three steps:

1. Preparation of the lesion through careful debridement and bone marrow stimulation
2. Preparation of the BST-CarGel®/blood mixture
3. Delivery of the BST-CarGel®/blood mixture to the lesion

Lesion Preparation

An arthroscopic probe is used to assess the targeted lesion, its limits, and the stability of its margins as well as the rest of the joint. Rough articular cartilage, flaps, and loose debris are meticulously debrided using a shaver and a curette to entirely remove the calcified cartilage layer without impinging on the subchondral bone. A contained lesion with stable vertical margins is thus created and necessary to hold the BST-CarGel® mixture adequately. Bone marrow stimulation (e.g., microfracture) is then performed as originally described [3, 4, 39]. Strict adherence to the bone marrow stimulation procedure is crucial particularly with regard to debridement and removal of the calcified cartilage considering that both noncalcified and calcified cartilage act as barriers to marrow-derived repair [40].

BST-CarGel® Preparation

BST-CarGel® should be prepared by a trained, non-sterile assistant, normally while the lesion is being surgically prepared. First, exactly 0.3 mL of the β-GP solution is removed from the *Additive Vial* using a 1 cc syringe and added slowly (at least 5 s) to the chitosan solution in the *Mixing Vial*. The mixture is then allowed to stand undisturbed for at least 10 min.

Lesion preparation and leg positioning should be performed before adding the fresh autologous whole blood to the prepared BST-CarGel®. First, 5 mL of peripheral whole blood is drawn from the patient into a plastic 5 mL syringe. Larger syringes are not recommended as they lack necessary volume gradations. Then, exactly 4.5 mL of blood is immediately added to the *Mixing Vial* using a disposable sterile hematological dispensing pin and shaken vigorously by hand for 10 s by the non-sterile assistant. A second pin is used by a sterile assistant to slowly withdraw an amount of 4–5 mL of the BST-CarGel®/blood mixture into a sterile 5 cc syringe, before handing this syringe to the treating surgeon for the delivery of the mixture into the already prepared lesion (Fig. 9.4).

Lesion Positioning and BST-CarGel® Delivery

Following bone marrow stimulation, the lesion can be accessed via an arthroscopically assisted mini-arthrotomy. The length of the incision will vary with the lesion size, but 3–4 cm usually allows sufficient visualization of the lesion to permit accurate application of the BST-CarGel®/blood mixture to the prepared lesion. Alternatively, an all arthroscopic approach is feasible if the lesion size and location allows for full visualization of the lesion and an accurate delivery of the BST-CarGel®/blood mixture. With either approach, the joint must be fully suctioned of perfusion liquid and blood, and the lesion swabbed with gauze in an attempt to create a "dry field" before applying the BST-CarGel®/blood mixture. As BST-CarGel® is implanted as a viscous mixture, the knee must be positioned such that the prepared lesion is horizontal. This position is achieved by flexing the hip and knee by approximately 90° each (Fig. 9.5) and can be maintained with the use of a Mayo table or leg holder.

The mixture is then applied to the prepared lesion in a dropwise manner using an 18G needle. The amount applied varies according to the size of the lesion. The lesion must be filled until it is almost full (Fig. 9.6). Overfilling should be avoided. The hybrid clot is allowed to solidify in place for 15 min prior to incision closure. After the 15-min solidification period, minimal manipulation of the knee and leg is essential during closing, cleaning, and wrapping. The leg should be straightened in only one motion, ensuring optimal conditions for residency of the BST-CarGel®/blood clot. A standard knee dressing is applied followed by an extension soft brace which should not be removed for 24 h after surgery.

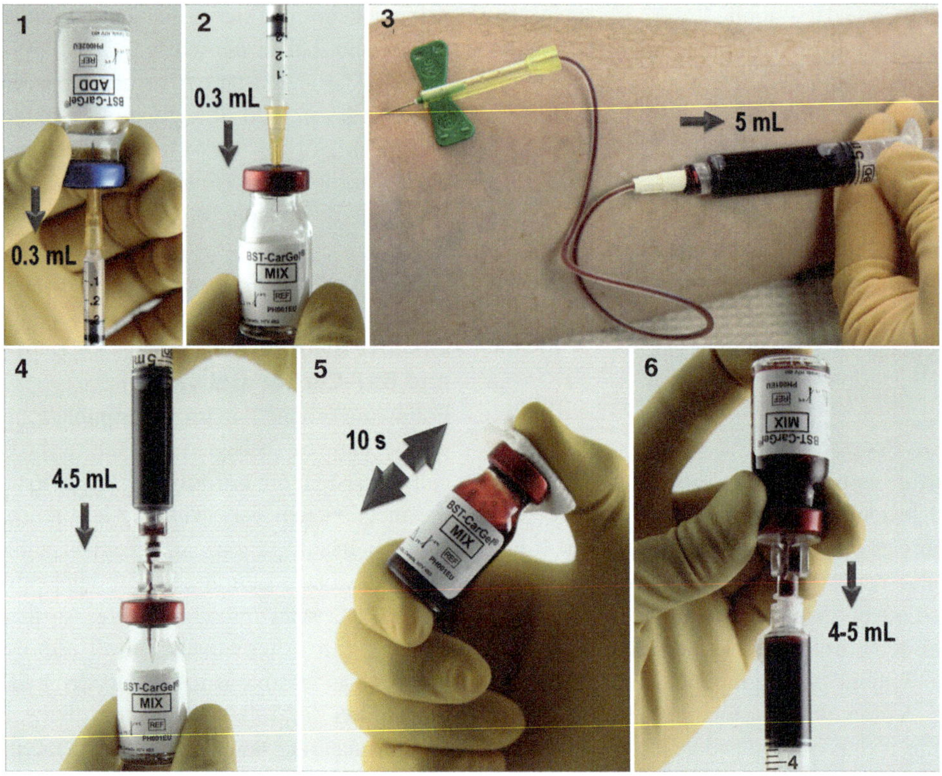

Fig. 9.4 BST-CarGel® product preparation. (*1*) The *Additive Vial* (ADD) is inverted and exactly 0.3 mL of solution (without bubbles) is removed using a sterile 1 mL syringe mounted with a sterile needle. (*2*) Taking at least 5 s, the *Additive Vial* solution is injected dropwise into the *Mixing Vial* (MIX). The *Mixing Vial* is not shaken and left upright and undisturbed for a minimum of 10 min. (*3*) When the lesion has been prepared with bone marrow stimulation, 5 mL of fresh, untreated, peripheral whole blood is collected from the patient via a peripheral vein using a 5 mL syringe. (*4*) The *Mixing Vial* septum is then wiped with alcohol before inserting a dispensing pin into the vial septum with a twisting motion. The blood-filled syringe is attached to the dispensing pin, and exactly 4.5 mL of blood is slowly injected into the *Mixing Vial*. The pin is removed and discarded. (*5*) The *Mixing Vial* is immediately and vigorously shaken for 10 s. (*6*) A second dispensing pin is inserted into the shaken BST-CarGel®/blood-filled vial and attached to a 5 mL sterile syringe. The vial is inverted and any bubbles present in the mixture are allowed to rise for 3 s. An amount of 4–5 mL of the BST-CarGel®/blood mixture is slowly drawn, being careful not to allow bubbles into the syringe. The BST-CarGel®/blood mixture is ready to be applied to the prepared cartilage lesion

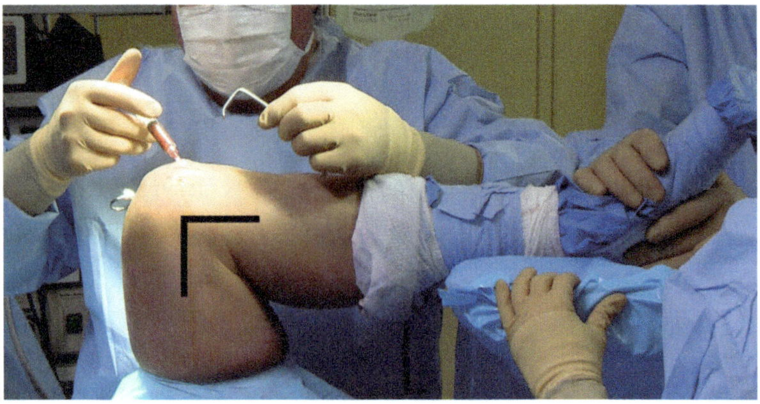

Fig. 9.5 Patient knee positioning for the delivery of BST-CarGel®. BST-CarGel® is implanted as a viscous solution, and thus the knee must be positioned such that the prepared lesion is horizontal. This position is achieved by flexing the hip and knee by approximately 90° each and can be maintained with the use of a Mayo table or a leg holder

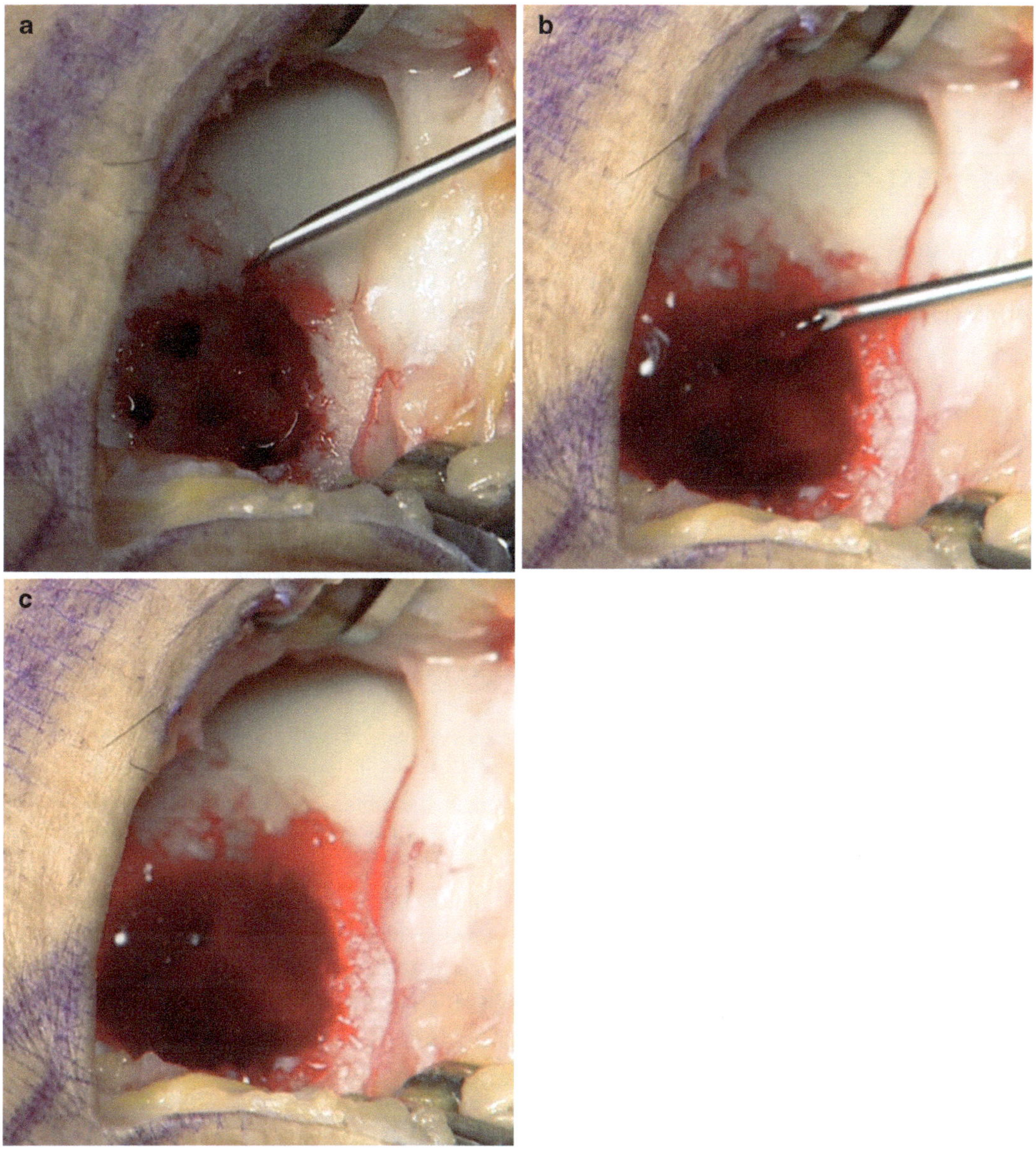

Fig. 9.6 BST-CarGel® delivery to the surgically prepared cartilage lesion. (**a**) The BST-CarGel®/blood mixture is applied to the prepared lesion (**b**) in a dropwise manner using an 18G sterile needle. (**c**) The amount applied varies according to the size of the lesion, but the lesion must be filled until it is almost full. Overfilling should be avoided. The BST-CarGel®/blood mixture is allowed to clot in place for 15 min prior to incision closure. After the 15-min clotting period, minimal manipulation of the knee and leg is essential during closing, cleaning, and wrapping. The leg should be straightened in one single motion, ensuring optimal conditions for residency of the BST-CarGel®/blood clot

9.3.4 Potential Complications and Troubleshooting

Additional points to consider with BST-CarGel® use:

- Due to the viscous liquid nature of the BST-CarGel®/blood mixture, treatment of uncontained lesions should be avoided.
- Lesions with close proximity to the notch or the origin of the posterior cruciate ligament (PCL) without sufficient containment should be avoided since rough mechanical conditions could compromise its residency.
- A second kit of BST-CarGel® should be readily available as backup in the case of overleakage of the mixture from the lesion before

clotting, dislodgement of the implant before the straightening of the leg, or other unforeseen event or delay.

9.4 BST-CarGel® Rehabilitation

The postsurgical rehabilitation program for BST-CarGel® aims at obtaining functional recovery while protecting the developing cartilage tissue from detrimental mechanical overload. Strategically, such a program should look longer term since the maturation process during cartilage repair can last for 18–24 months or more [41, 42].

Only general guidelines are provided as the basis for the rehabilitation program, as there are other demographic and physical factors which need to be considered during rehabilitation. Such factors include patient age, weight, previous activity level, and expectations, as well as surgical factors such as lesion size and location. The basic program should then be adapted to each patient by the treating physiotherapist.

The rehabilitation program following BST-CarGel® treatment is divided into two phases: Phase 1, which generally covers week 1–8 postoperative, and phase 2, which is intended for a full weight-bearing longer-term follow-up for weeks 9–26 postoperative. Table 9.3 lists the rationale and suggestions for modalities to be used.

For phase 1, immediately following surgery, the joint is completely immobilized for the first 24 h with a soft brace in extension which is then used for 14 days during all movement and at night. Frequent sessions with an experienced therapist are desired in phase 1, up to five times for the first week and three times per week for the remaining weeks. Assisted passive motion exercises are used to maintain mobility, increase range of motion, and ensure overall knee health while initiating the mechanical signaling which will modulate the tissue development. Once 110° of flexion is obtained, stationery cycling is permitted. Weight bearing is not allowed for the first 6 weeks, and from week 6–8 the goal is to reach full weight bearing as pain allows. Other standard modalities can be implemented as per therapist preference as shown in Table 9.3. Once the objectives of the phase 1 are attained, the patient can move to phase 2.

Phase 2 implies a normal use of the involved knee joint for activities of daily living, excluding sports-related activities. Strengthening with closed chain kinetic exercises can be implemented to obtain the goals shown in Table 9.3. At the end of this phase, patients are encouraged to begin light sport activities like cycling or swimming. Higher impact or contact sports which involve pivoting are not permitted to resume before 1 year postsurgery, as the maturing tissue is still vulnerable to mechanical loading.

Table 9.3 BST-CarGel® rehabilitation program

Rationale		Modality
Phase 1: 1–8 weeks	Protect and maintain implant residency	6 weeks non-weight bearing
	Control knee pain and swelling	Day 2–7: passive ROM, <35° flexion
	Regain normal range of motion	Day 8–28: passive ROM as tolerated
	Stimulate the new cartilage tissue	Neuromuscular stimulation
		Isometric quad/hamstring contraction
		Hip strengthening
		TheraBand®
Phase 2: 9–26 weeks	Obtain full range of motion	Proprioception exercises with pain-free full weight bearing
	Stimulate maturation of new cartilage tissue	Progressive closed kinetic chain exercises
	Ensure a normal gait pattern	Balance board
	Strengthen muscles and normalize proprioception	Calf raise with progression to unipodal calf raise
	Reinitiate light sport activities (no impact)	Cardiovascular exercise (cycling, walking, swimming, StairMaster) at least 20 min/day

9.5 BST-CarGel® Clinical Experience

9.5.1 Pilot Use

Pilot clinical use of BST-CarGel® occurred from August 2003 to December 2004 under Health Canada's Special Access Program for medical devices intended for compassionate use. Thirty-three patients were treated with BST-CarGel® and encompassed the spectrum of indications, with both traumatic and degenerative lesions, where lesions ranged in size from 0.5 to 12 cm^2 (mean area 4.3 cm^2) for both men and women. One case of osteochondritis dissecans and one exposed subchondral cyst were also treated. Concomitant anterior cruciate ligament replacement preceded treatment with BST-CarGel® in two patients. BST-CarGel® was delivered by arthroscopy for 22 patients and by mini-arthrotomy for 11 patients. This clinical experience is recognized as observational and uncontrolled, but it still yielded an initial assessment of safety as no uncharacteristic observations were made during physical examinations or blood analyses for all patients. At 12 months postoperatively, Western Ontario McMaster (WOMAC) Osteoarthritis Index questionnaires for pain, stiffness, and function improved compared with preoperative baseline scores, and the uniformity of the WOMAC data indicated a clear clinical benefit arising from BST-CarGel® treatment. In addition, surgical experience gained with BST-CarGel® was used to support the development of the clinical protocol for the international multicenter randomized clinical trial described in the following section.

9.5.2 BST-CarGel® Randomized Clinical Trial

A regulated international multicenter trial was performed in accordance with the International Conference on Harmonisation Guidelines for Good Clinical Practice (GCP) to evaluate BST-CarGel® efficacy at 12 months in repairing cartilage lesions and improving patient clinical symptoms, compared to microfracture, the current standard of care. The trial was conducted in 26 clinical centers in Canada, Spain, and South Korea. Eligible male and female patients were 18–55 years of age with an isolated grade 3 or 4 cartilage lesion on the medial or lateral femoral condyle and moderate knee pain (>4 VAS). Patients had stable knees with intact menisci, BMI $\leq$ 30 kg/m^2, and had not undergone previous cartilage or ligament treatments in the study knee within 1 and 2 years of baseline, respectively. The trial enrolled 80 patients, who were randomized (1:1) at the time of surgery to BST-CarGel® or microfracture alone treatment groups, and followed standardized 12-week rehabilitation. This trial represents the first of its kind in cartilage repair using a novel, three-dimensional quantitative MRI to compare repair cartilage structure through standardized data acquisition and blinded analyses for the co-primary endpoints of quantity and quality of new cartilage tissue. The degree of cartilage lesion filling (lesion % fill) was calculated volumetrically at 12 months as a percentage of the 1 month postoperative lesion baseline and a collagen-based quality parameter was measured at 12 months using the transverse (or T2) relaxation time of the entire volume of new tissue. Secondary endpoints at 12 months included clinical benefit, determined with WOMAC questionnaires, and safety. Supportive data from 38 elective biopsies retrieved at 13 months included International Cartilage Repair Society (ICRS) macroscopic scoring (during retrieval), blinded ICRS I and II histological assessments, and polarization light microscopy (PLM) score for collagen architecture.

BST-CarGel® treatment met both co-primary trial endpoints by achieving statistical superiority over microfracture in both the degree of filling of treated lesions and the quality of the new tissue. The data revealed that compared to the microfracture group, the BST-CarGel®-treated lesions contained a significantly greater volume of repair cartilage which exhibited a more ordered collagen structure by T2 than that of microfracture, with characteristics approaching that of native hyaline cartilage. WOMAC assessments for pain, stiffness, and function yielded equivalent and statistically significant improvements from baseline for both groups. Safety was comparable for both groups. Compared to microfracture, BST-CarGel® showed improved ICRS macroscopic grading, superior collagen organization by PLM, and improvements in most ICRS I and II histological parameters.

Overall, BST-CarGel® treatment resulted in greater lesion filling and superior repair tissue quality at 12 months as shown by multiple, independent indicators. Such striking structural improvement should be predictive of longer-term durability of repair and sustained clinical benefit compared to microfracture.

BST-CarGel® has only been approved for sale in Europe at this time.

Acknowledgements BST-CarGel® has been developed by Piramal Healthcare Bio-Orthopedics (formerly BioSyntech Canada Inc.). We are indebted to Professors Michael Buschmann and Caroline Hoemann, the inventors of BST-CarGel®, along with the Biomaterials and Cartilage Laboratory at Ecole Polytechnique of Montreal, who established the basic scientific foundation for BST-CarGel®. We are grateful to Dr. Jun Sun and Dr. Mark Hurtig for their animal surgery expertise. We thank Drs. Nicolas Duval and Pierre Ranger for their contributions with the pilot clinical use of BST-CarGel®. The critical efforts of the BST-CarGel® Clinical Study Group, including the investigators, sub-investigators, research coordinators, and physiotherapists who tirelessly contributed to the success of the clinical trial are warmly acknowledged. Other clinical trial activities carried out by Cato Canada (Montreal), MRI activities by VirtualScopics (Rochester, NY) and Qmetrics (Rochester, NY), and statistical expertise by Dr. Alex Yaroshinsky (San Andreas, CA) are appreciated.

References

1. Johnson LL (1986) Arthroscopic abrasion arthroplasty historical and pathologic perspective: present status. Arthroscopy 2(1):54–69
2. Insall JN (1967) Intra-articular surgery for degenerative arthritis of the knee. A report of the work of the late K. H. Pridie. J Bone Joint Surg Br 49(2): 211–228
3. Steadman JR, Rodkey WG, Singleton SB, Briggs KK (1997) Microfracture technique for full-thickness chondral defects: technique and clinical results. Oper Tech Orthop 7(4):300–304
4. Mithoefer K, Williams RJ 3rd, Warren RF, Potter HG, Spock CR, Jones EC, Wickiewicz TL, Marx RG (2006) Chondral resurfacing of articular cartilage defects in the knee with the microfracture technique. Surgical technique. J Bone Joint Surg Am 88(Suppl 1 Pt 2):294–304
5. Steadman JR, Briggs KK, Rodrigo JJ, Kocher MS, Gill TJ, Rodkey WG (2003) Outcomes of microfracture for traumatic chondral defects of the knee: average 11-year follow-up. Arthroscopy 19(5): 477–484
6. Frisbie DD, Trotter GW, Powers BE, Rodkey WG, Steadman JR, Howard RD, Park RD, McIlwraith CW (1999) Arthroscopic subchondral bone plate microfracture technique augments healing of large chondral defects in the radial carpal bone and medial femoral condyle of horses. Vet Surg 28(4):242–255
7. Knutsen G, Drogset JO, Engebretsen L, Grontvedt T, Isaksen V, Ludvigsen TC, Roberts S, Solheim E, Strand T, Johansen O (2007) A randomized trial comparing autologous chondrocyte implantation with microfracture. Findings at five years. J Bone Joint Surg Am 89(10):2105–2112
8. Mithoefer K, Williams R Jr, Warren RF, Potter HG, Spock CR, Jones EC, Wickiewicz TL, Marx RG (2005) The microfracture technique for the treatment of articular cartilage lesions in the knee. A prospective cohort study. J Bone Joint Surg Am 87(9): 1911–1920
9. Saris DB, Vanlauwe J, Victor J, Haspl M, Bohnsack M, Fortems Y, Vandekerckhove B, Almqvist KF, Claes T, Handelberg F, Lagae K, van der Bauwhede J, Vandenneucker H, Yang KG, Jelic M, Verdonk R, Veulemans N, Bellemans J, Luyten FP (2008) Characterized chondrocyte implantation results in better structural repair when treating symptomatic cartilage defects of the knee in a randomized controlled trial versus microfracture. Am J Sports Med 36(2):235–246
10. Steadman JR, Rodkey WG, Rodrigo JJ (2001) Microfracture: surgical technique and rehabilitation to treat chondral defects. Clin Orthop 391(Suppl): S362–S369
11. Kreuz PC, Steinwachs MR, Erggelet C, Krause SJ, Konrad G, Uhl M, Sudkamp N (2006) Results after microfracture of full-thickness chondral defects in different compartments in the knee. Osteoarthritis Cartilage 14(11):1119–1125
12. Vanlauwe J, Saris DB, Victor J, Almqvist KF, Bellemans J, Luyten FP (2011) Five-year outcome of characterized chondrocyte implantation versus microfracture for symptomatic cartilage defects of the knee: early treatment matters. Am J Sports Med 39(12):2566–2574
13. Gomoll AH (2012) Microfracture and augments. J Knee Surg 25(1):9–15
14. Chenite A, Chaput C, Wang D, Combes C, Buschmann MD, Hoemann CD, Leroux JC, Binette F, Selmani A (2000) Novel injectable neutral solutions of chitosan form biodegradable gels *in-situ*. Biomaterials 21:2155–2161
15. Di Martino A, Sittinger M, Risbud MV (2005) Chitosan: a versatile biopolymer for orthopaedic tissue-engineering. Biomaterials 26(30):5983–5990

16. Kumar MN, Muzzarelli RA, Muzzarelli C, Sashiwa H, Domb AJ (2004) Chitosan chemistry and pharmaceutical perspectives. Chem Rev 104(12):6017–6084
17. Kurita K (2006) Chitin and chitosan: functional biopolymers from marine crustaceans. Mar Biotechnol (NY) 8(3):203–226
18. Shi C, Zhu Y, Ran X, Wang M, Su Y, Cheng T (2006) Therapeutic potential of chitosan and its derivatives in regenerative medicine. J Surg Res 133(2):185–192
19. Hoemann CD, Sun J, McKee MD, Chevrier A, Rossomacha E, Rivard GE, Hurtig M, Buschmann MD (2007) Chitosan-glycerol phosphate/blood implants elicit hyaline cartilage repair integrated with porous subchondral bone in microdrilled rabbit defects. Osteoarthritis Cartilage 15(1):78–89
20. Marchand C, Rivard GE, Sun J, Hoemann CD (2009) Solidification mechanisms of chitosan-glycerol phosphate/blood implant for articular cartilage repair. Osteoarthritis Cartilage 17(7):953–960
21. Chevrier A, Hoemann CD, Sun J, Buschmann MD (2007) Chitosan-glycerol phosphate/blood implants increase cell recruitment, transient vascularization and subchondral bone remodeling in drilled cartilage defects. Osteoarthritis Cartilage 15(3):316–327
22. Henriksen I, Green KL, Smart JD, Smistad G, Karlsen J (1996) Bioadhesion of hydrated chitosans: an in vitro and in vivo study. Int J Pharm 145:231–240
23. Hoemann CD, Hurtig M, Rossomacha E, Sun J, Chevrier A, Shive MS, Buschmann MD (2005) Chitosan-glycerol phosphate/blood implants improve hyaline cartilage repair in ovine microfracture defects. J Bone Joint Surg Am 87(12):2671–2686
24. van den Berg WB, van Lent PL, van de Putte LB, Zwarts WA (1986) Electrical charge of hyaline articular cartilage: its role in the retention of anionic and cationic proteins. Clin Immunol Immunopathol 39(2):187–197
25. Iliescu M, Hoemann CD, Shive MS, Chenite A, Buschmann MD (2008) Ultrastructure of hybrid chitosan-glycerol phosphate blood clots by environmental scanning electron microscopy. Microsc Res Tech 71(3):236–247
26. Chen H, Chevrier A, Hoemann CD, Sun J, Ouyang W, Buschmann MD (2011) Characterization of subchondral bone repair for marrow-stimulated chondral defects and its relationship to articular cartilage resurfacing. Am J Sports Med 39(8):1731–1740
27. Muzzarelli RA (1997) Human enzymatic activities related to the therapeutic administration of chitin derivatives. Cell Mol Life Sci 53(2):131–140
28. Varum KM, Myhr MM, Hjerde RJ, Smidsrod O (1997) In vitro degradation rates of partially N-acetylated chitosans in human serum. Carbohydr Res 299(1–2):99–101
29. Chevrier A, Hoemann CD, Sun J, Buschmann MD (2011) Temporal and spatial modulation of chondrogenic foci in subchondral microdrill holes by chitosan-glycerol phosphate/blood implants. Osteoarthritis Cartilage 19(1):136–144
30. Chen G, Sun J, Lascau-Coman V, Chevrier A, Marchand C, Hoemann CD (2011) Acute osteoclast activity following subchondral drilling is promoted by chitosan and associated with improved cartilage repair tissue integration. Cartilage 2(2):173–185
31. Hoemann CD, Chen G, Marchand C, Tran-Khanh N, Thibault M, Chevrier A, Sun J, Shive MS, Fernandes MJ, Poubelle PE, Centola M, El-Gabalawy H (2010) Scaffold-guided subchondral bone repair: implication of neutrophils and alternatively activated arginase-1+ macrophages. Am J Sports Med 38(9):1845–1856
32. Marchand C, Chen G, Tran-Khanh N, Sun J, Chen H, Buschmann MD, Hoemann CD (2012) Microdrilled cartilage defects treated with thrombin-solidified chitosan/blood implant regenerate a more hyaline, stable, and structurally integrated osteochondral unit compared to drilled controls. Tissue Eng Part A 18(5–6): 508–519
33. Goldring MB, Goldring SR (2010) Articular cartilage and subchondral bone in the pathogenesis of osteoarthritis. Ann N Y Acad Sci 1192:230–237
34. Gomoll AH, Madry H, Knutsen G, van Dijk N, Seil R, Brittberg M, Kon E (2010) The subchondral bone in articular cartilage repair: current problems in the surgical management. Knee Surg Sports Traumatol Arthrosc 18(4):434–447
35. Minas T, Gomoll AH, Rosenberger R, Royce RO, Bryant T (2009) Increased failure rate of autologous chondrocyte implantation after previous treatment with marrow stimulation techniques. Am J Sports Med 37(5):902–908
36. Pestka JM, Bode G, Salzmann G, Sudkamp NP, Niemeyer P (2012) Clinical outcome of autologous chondrocyte implantation for failed microfracture treatment of full-thickness cartilage defects of the knee joint. Am J Sports Med 40(2):325–331
37. McNickle AG, L'Heureux DR, Yanke AB, Cole BJ (2009) Outcomes of autologous chondrocyte implantation in a diverse patient population. Am J Sports Med 37(7):1344–1350
38. Zaslav K, Cole B, Brewster R, DeBerardino T, Farr J, Fowler P, Nissen C (2009) A prospective study of autologous chondrocyte implantation in patients with failed prior treatment for articular cartilage defect of the knee: results of the Study of the Treatment of Articular Repair (STAR) clinical trial. Am J Sports Med 37(1):42–55
39. Chen H, Hoemann CD, Sun J, Chevrier A, McKee MD, Shive MS, Hurtig M, Buschmann MD (2011) Depth of subchondral perforation influences the outcome of bone marrow stimulation cartilage repair. J Orthop Res 29(8):1178–1184
40. Frisbie DD, Morisset S, Ho CP, Rodkey WG, Steadman JR, McIlwraith CW (2006) Effects of calcified cartilage on healing of chondral defects treated with microfracture in horses. Am J Sports Med 34(11):1824–1831
41. Brun P, Dickinson SC, Zavan B, Cortivo R, Hollander AP, Abatangelo G (2008) Characteristics of repair

tissue in second-look and third-look biopsies from patients treated with engineered cartilage: relationship to symptomatology and time after implantation. Arthritis Res Ther 10(6):R132
42. Welsch GH, Mamisch TC, Zak L, Blanke M, Olk A, Marlovits S, Trattnig S (2010) Evaluation of cartilage repair tissue after matrix-associated autologous chondrocyte transplantation using a hyaluronic-based or a collagen-based scaffold with morphological MOCART scoring and biochemical T2 mapping: preliminary results. Am J Sports Med 38(5):934–942

Part IV

Concentrated Cell Based Chondrogenesis

Mesenchymal Stem Cell Induced Chondrogenesis (MCIC™)

10

Asode Ananthram Shetty, Seok-Jung Kim, and Vishvas A. Shetty

Contents

The original version of this chapter was revised. An erratum to this chapter can be found at DOI 10.1007/978-3-642-41921-8_32

A.A. Shetty, MD, PhD, MCh, FRCS Ed., FRCS Eng., FRCS Orth (✉)
Department of Minimally Invasive Surgery, Faculty of Health and Social Sciences, Canterbury Christ Church University, Pembroke Court 30, ME4 4UF Chatham Maritime, Kent, UK

Faculty of Stem Cell Research and Regenerative Medicine, NITTE University, Mangalore, India
e-mail: aashetty@hotmail.com

S.-J. Kim, MD, PhD, FRCS
Department of Orthopedic Surgery, Uijeongbu St. Mary's Hospital, College of Medicine, The Catholic University of Korea, 480-717 Gyeonggi-do, Republic of (South Korea)

Faculty of Stem Cell Research and Regenerative Medicine, NITTE University, Mangalore, India
e-mail: orthopland@naver.com

V.A. Shetty
Department of Minimally Invasive Surgery, Faculty of Health and Social Sciences, Canterbury Christ Church University, Pembroke Court 30, ME4 4UF, Chatham Maritime, Kent, UK

10.1 Introduction

In 1743 William Hunter [1] stated, 'an ulcerated cartilage is a troublesome problem and once destroyed, it never repairs'. This statement holds true even today, in spite of new advances in the field of tissue engineering. Cartilage injuries are common in the knee joint and if untreated can become symptomatic and progressively lead to premature arthritis [2]. Galen observed and wrote about premature arthritis in athletes.

Since the 1980s, cartilage repair strategies have improved rapidly and extensively across the world. Our understanding of the disease itself has evolved and so have our tools to treat it. Microfracture is still in practice in some centres despite proof that it leads to the formation of fibrocartilage [3]. Osteochondral grafting relocates healthy hyaline cartilage from non

A.A. Shetty et al. (eds.), *Techniques in Cartilage Repair Surgery*,
DOI 10.1007/978-3-642-41921-8_10, © ESSKA 2014

weight-bearing areas to area of chondral loss. Unfortunately this technique is limited by the size of the lesion and donor site morbidity [4]. Autologous cartilage implantation is known to produce hyaline-like cartilage; unfortunately it is expensive and requires two stages. It also has the added complications of delamination and arthrotomy [5, 6].

The technique described in this chapter is a single-staged arthroscopic technique to regenerate articular cartilage using BMAC, HA and fibrin gel implanted under CO_2 insufflation. It is economical as it is done as a day case and also avoids an arthrotomy. It also reduces rehabilitation time for patient due to the single stage [5, 6]. Using this technique, we achieved encouraging clinical and radiological outcomes at two years.

Recently, there has been a surge in the use of bone marrow aspirate concentrate cells (BMAC), which contains pluripotent mesenchymal stem cells (MSC) and growth factors. These have garnered interest and have proven to be equal to current techniques [7, 8]. Bone marrow is a good source of MSC and mononuclear cell (MNC). A good bone marrow aspirate has the cellularity of marrow, 15–30 million MNC/ml. The average Colony-Forming Unit-f (CFU-f) content of healthy young human bone marrow is about 100 CFU-f/million MNC. We can obtain 1,500–3,000 CFU-f/ml of healthy human bone marrow aspirate [9]. BMAC contains MSC which have proliferatory potential and the ability to differentiate into a multitude of cell types. These cells also have trophic activity and a paracrine effect. Hence, even a limited number of cells can initiate cartilage regeneration [10]. In addition, fibrin gels and collagen-based scaffolds are being used to ensure better fixation of grafts [11].

The fibrin gel used contains activated thrombin and fibrinogen, which when combined form fibrin and mimic the final stage of the coagulation cascade. Its uses in the surgery are manifold. The fibrin gel helps control bone bleeding, and its gel form helps treat lesions of various sizes and depths [12]. Specifically for cartilage regeneration, fibrin has excellent biocompatibility and has proven to be a suitable carrier for generating neo-cartilage [13, 14]. The gel hardens about five minutes after injection, and this makes for a suitable scaffold to hold the graft in place. Kim et al. [15] demonstrated that fibrin can form fibrous and solid wall-like structures, 200–1,000 nm in diameter. Hence, fibrin gels are a good choice as scaffold material in cartilage repair surgery [16].

The subchondral bone is microfractured up to a depth of 3 mm, at intervals of 3 mm. These microfractured channels provide rotational stability for the graft and also provide larger surface area of raw bone [15].

CO_2 provides a dry internal environment and prevents dispersion of the fibrin gel-BMAC mixture after implantation. It also creates a tamponade effect which allows the grafting of lesions against gravity, including patellar lesions. CO_2 has proven to be safe in animal studies and is extensively used in laparoscopic surgery [17, 18].

10.2 Preclinical Study

The preclinical study involved 14 white New Zealand rabbits divided into two equal groups; all rabbits were kept under the same conditions throughout the study. One group was to be treated by microfracture alone (M group), and the other group was to be treated with a bone marrow concentrate and fibrin gel mixture (MB group).

10.2.1 Surgical Technique

After adequate anesthetizing with a mixture of 35 mg/kg of ketamine hydrochloride and 5 mg/kg of xylazine, a lesion was created in the trochlear region (4 mm in diameter) of all the rabbits. For the MB group, 3 ml of bone marrow was drawn from the proximal tibia. The bone marrow aspirate was combined an equal volume of Dulbecco's phosphate-buffered saline (DPBS; Gibco, NY, USA) and then resuspended and gently layered onto Ficoll-Paque Premium (density 1.077 g/ml; GE Healthcare Bio- Sciences AB,

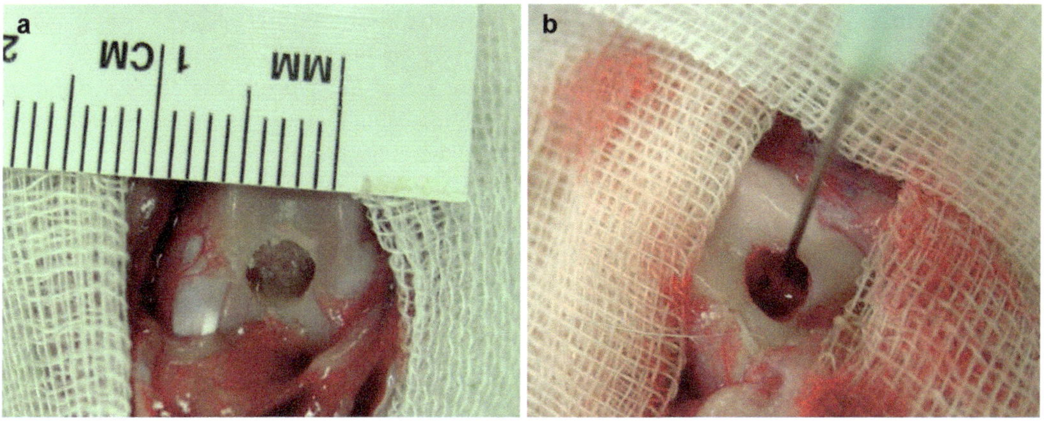

Fig. 10.1 (**a**) A round hole with a diameter of 4 mm down to the subchondral bone was made in the trochlear region. (**b**) Microfracture was performed using a 23-gauge needle

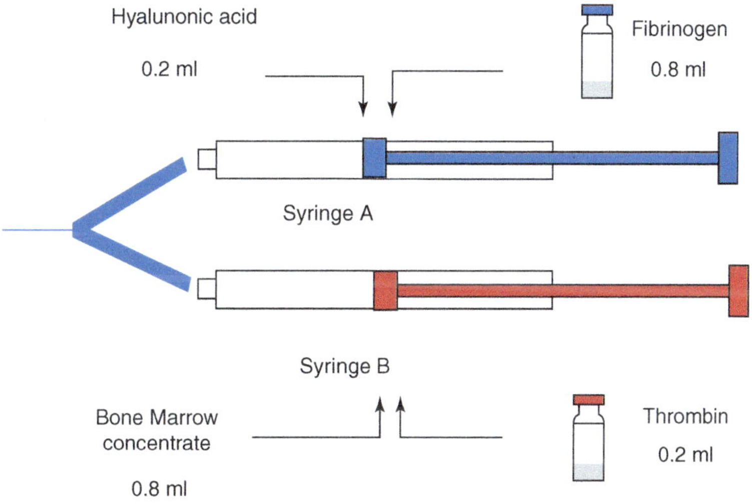

Fig. 10.2 Mixing procedure for hyaluronic acid, fibrin and bone marrow concentrate for the MB group

Uppsala, Sweden). This mixture was then centrifuged at 1,153 g for 20 min at 4oC, and nucleated cells were harvested.

Microfracture was performed in both groups with a 23-gauge needle at intervals of 3 mm. For the MB group, application of BM concentrate was done with two 1-ml syringes connected to a Y-shaped mixing catheter. One syringe contains 0.8 ml of fibrinogen and 0.2 ml of hyaluronic acid. The other syringe contains 0.8 ml of bone marrow concentrate and 0.2 ml of thrombin. Under vision, the defect area in the MB group was slowly filled with the mixture. After waiting 5 min for the gel to dry, the wound was closed (Figs. 10.1 and 10.2).

10.2.2 Assessment

At 12 weeks, the rabbits were sacrificed and the repaired area of cartilage was harvested along with a sample of normal cartilage for comparison. The neo-cartilage was compared with normal cartilage by examining gross appearance; histochemical staining with hematoxylin-eosin for tissue morphology, toluidine blue for collagen and Safranin O for GAG content; immunohistochemistry with antibodies IH11 and CIIC1 for collagen type I and II, respectively; and scanning electron microscopy (SEM) and transmission electron microscopy (TEM) to analyse the microstructural morphologies.

10.2.3 Results

Gross Appearance

On gross examination, in both groups there was a lack of synovitis and tissue or adhesion constrictions. In the MB group, the defect was completely filled with neo-cartilage which had a uniform surface and colour and also had good continuity with the surrounding cartilage. In the M group, the defect fill was irregular with white, fibrous and irregularly shaped cartilage (Fig. 10.3).

Histochemical Staining

A total of five factors were studied (cell morphology, thickness of neo-cartilage, matrix staining, surface regularity and integration of graft with the host), with a total score from 0 to 14 points, as described by Pineda et al. Both groups are compared with the Mann-Whitney test; the MB group had good scores on all counts in comparison to the M group which showed incomplete cartilage growth and multiple defects. The MB group showed cartilage thickness and hematoxylin-eosin staining similar to native cartilage, whereas the M group had a thin layer of cartilage with minimal staining.

Immunohistochemistry

As seen in Fig. 10.4, collagen type I was not expressed at all; type II was expressed though with less staining intensity on the newly formed cartilage (Fig. 10.5).

Electron Microscopy

SEM images show that the bone marrow cells have attached well to the porous structure of the mixture (Fig. 10.6). A fibrous polymer structure 200–1,000 nm in diameter was observed inside the pore. TEM images revealed newly synthesized collagen molecules and cells in the structure, along with micro-movement of the cells which indicated active collagen formation (Fig. 10.7).

10.3 Patient Selection

10.3.1 Clinical

Patient selection is the key to the success of the procedure. Potential candidates undergo a thorough clinical examination, including a detailed history. Axial alignment, stability of the knee and patellar tracking are assessed at this stage.

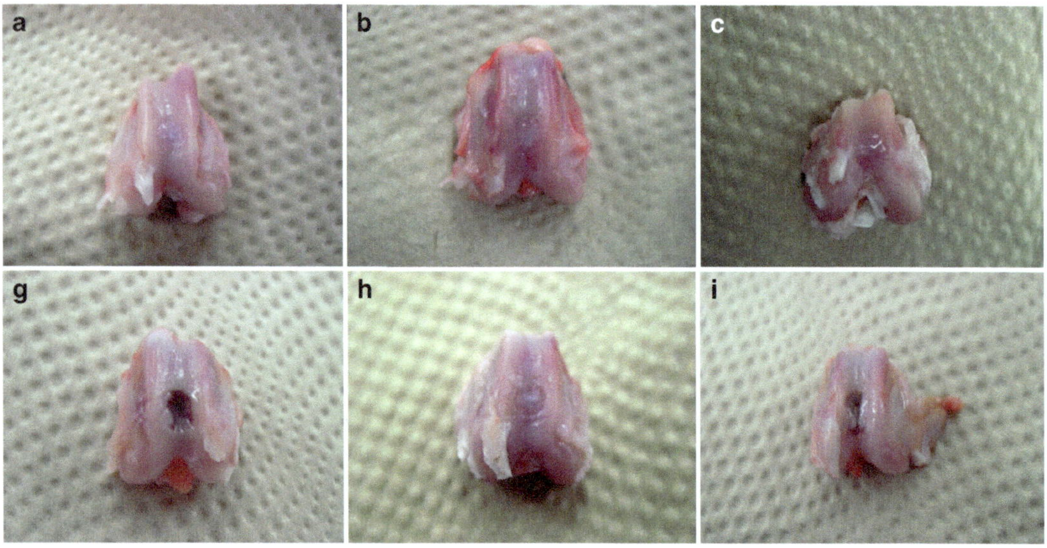

Fig. 10.3 Photographs of the MB (**a**–**c**) and M (**g**–**i**) groups

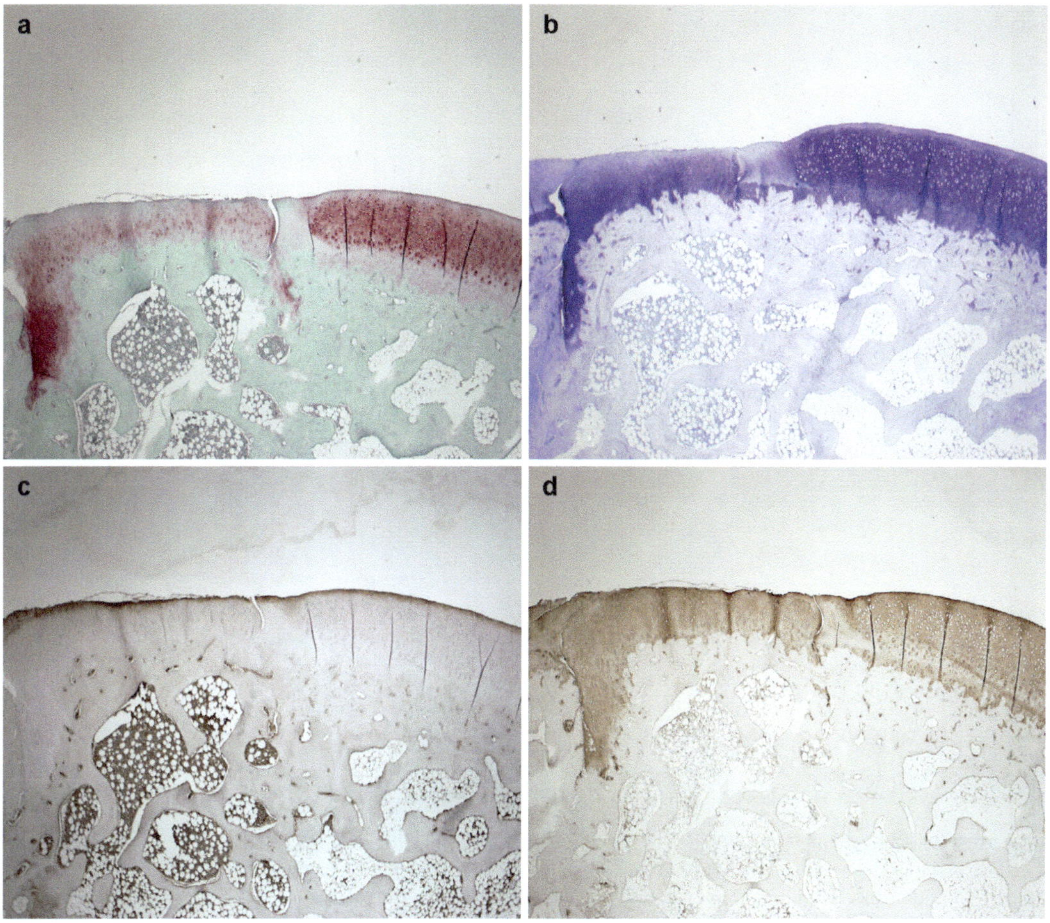

Fig. 10.4 Photomicrograph of the section of regenerated cartilage of the MB group with (**a**) Safranin O staining, (**b**) toluidine blue staining, (**c**) immunohistochemical staining with anti-collagen type I antibody and (**d**) immunohistochemical staining with anti-collagen type II antibody(×40)

Significant medical comorbidities which may increase perioperative mortality may preclude surgery. Advice regarding weight loss, diet and smoking cessation are given throughout the perioperative period.

10.3.2 Radiographic

If found suitable for the procedure, they undergo the cartilage imaging protocol, which consists of the following:

- Weight-bearing long leg radiograph
- Lateral and skyline radiographic views of affected knee
- MRI (DESS sequencing) of affected knee
- CT patellar tracking of both knees

Alignment is measured on the long leg radiograph. Corrective osteotomy would be considered for mal-alignment (varus or valgus) more than five degrees. Patellofemoral mal-tracking is corrected by tibial tubercle transfer. Instability is corrected by suitable ligament reconstruction.

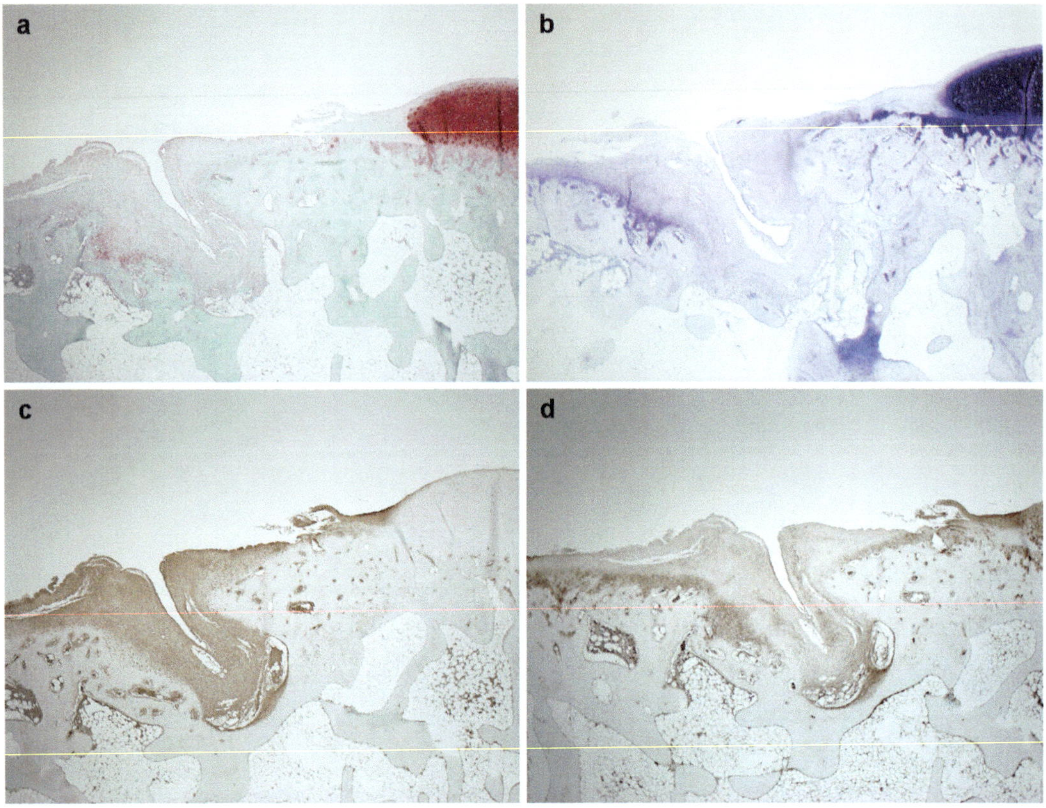

Fig. 10.5 Photomicrograph of the section of the regenerated cartilage of the M group with (**a**) Safranin O staining, (**b**) toluidine blue staining, (**c**) immunohistochemical staining with anti-collagen type I antibody and (**d**) immunohistochemical staining with anti-collagen type II antibody (×40)

MRI scans have been deemed suitable for detecting and quantifying chondral lesions (REF and accuracy). With newer sequences, even early lesions can be detecting with reasonable accuracy [19]. Associated conditions such as meniscal tears, ligamentous insufficiencies, loose bodies etc. are also noted and are treated simultaneously.

Inclusion Criteria

- Patients aged 18–65 years
- Diagnosed with articular cartilage defect in the knee (ICRS/Outerbridge grade III/IV cartilage lesions as assessed on MRI scan)
- Less than three lesions, measuring more than 2 cm^2 and less than 9 cm^2
- Symptoms less than three years' duration

Exclusion Criteria

- Age below 18 and over 65 years
- Generalized and/or inflammatory arthritis
- Active joint inflammation
- More than three lesions
- Lesions more than 9 cm^2
- Ligament instability

10.4 Theatre and Patient Setup

Theatre setup is similar to routine arthroscopy. The surgeon is seated on the side being operated, and the stack system was placed on the opposite side for comfortable visualization of the monitor. The CO_2 pump was placed on the stack system trolley with a filter and sterile insufflation tubing

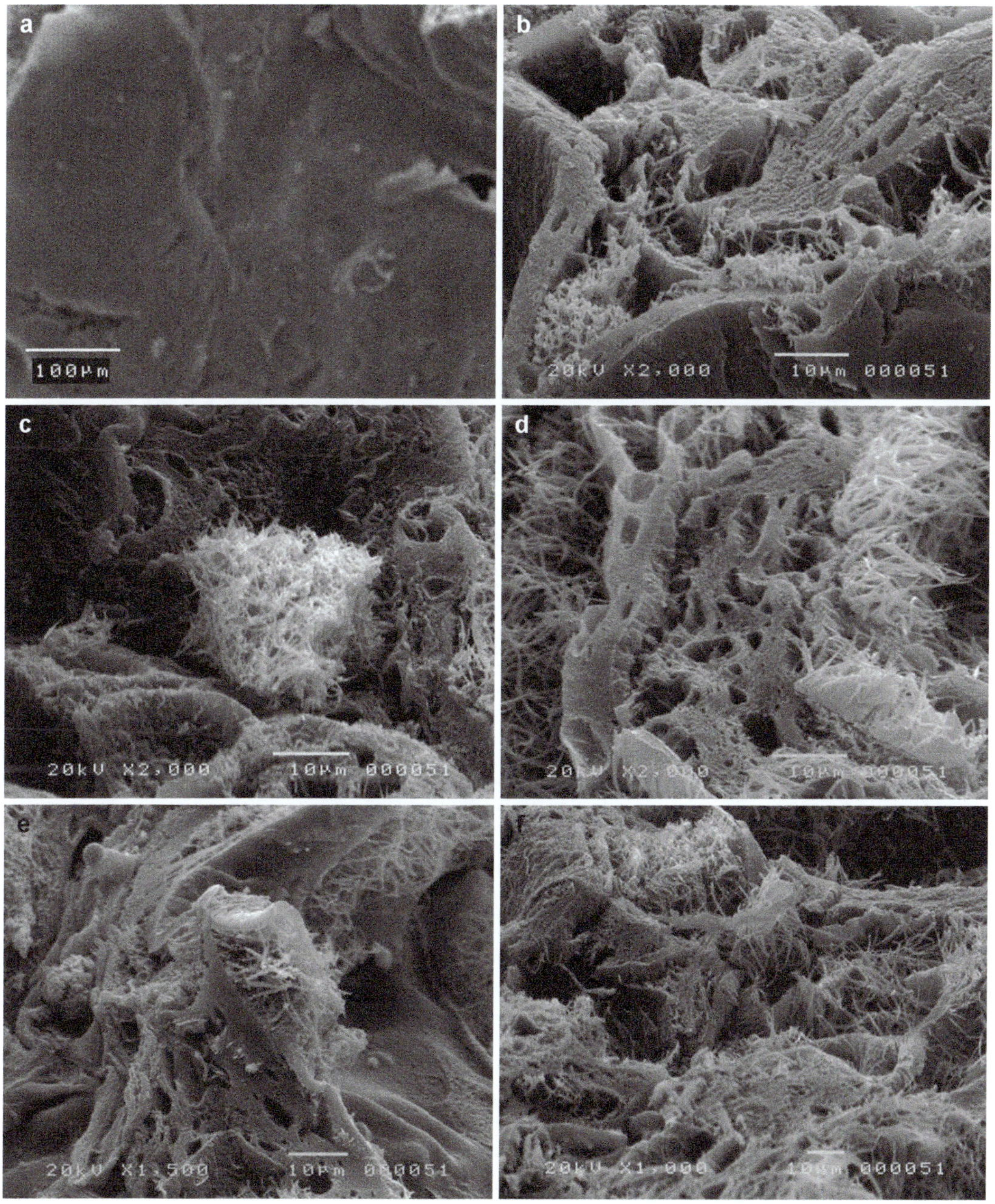

Fig. 10.6 Scanning electron microscopy images of hyaluronic acid/fibrin composites mixed with bone marrow cells revealed that mixing with hyaluronic acid allowed fibrin to show diverse polymerization features ranging from solid, wall-like to fibrous structure. Images of the outside (**a**) and inside (**b**–**f**) of the composite revealed its porous structure. Cells were shown to be attached to the surface of the structure. A fibrous structure with a diameter ranging from 200 to 1,000 nm was observed in the wall-like structure

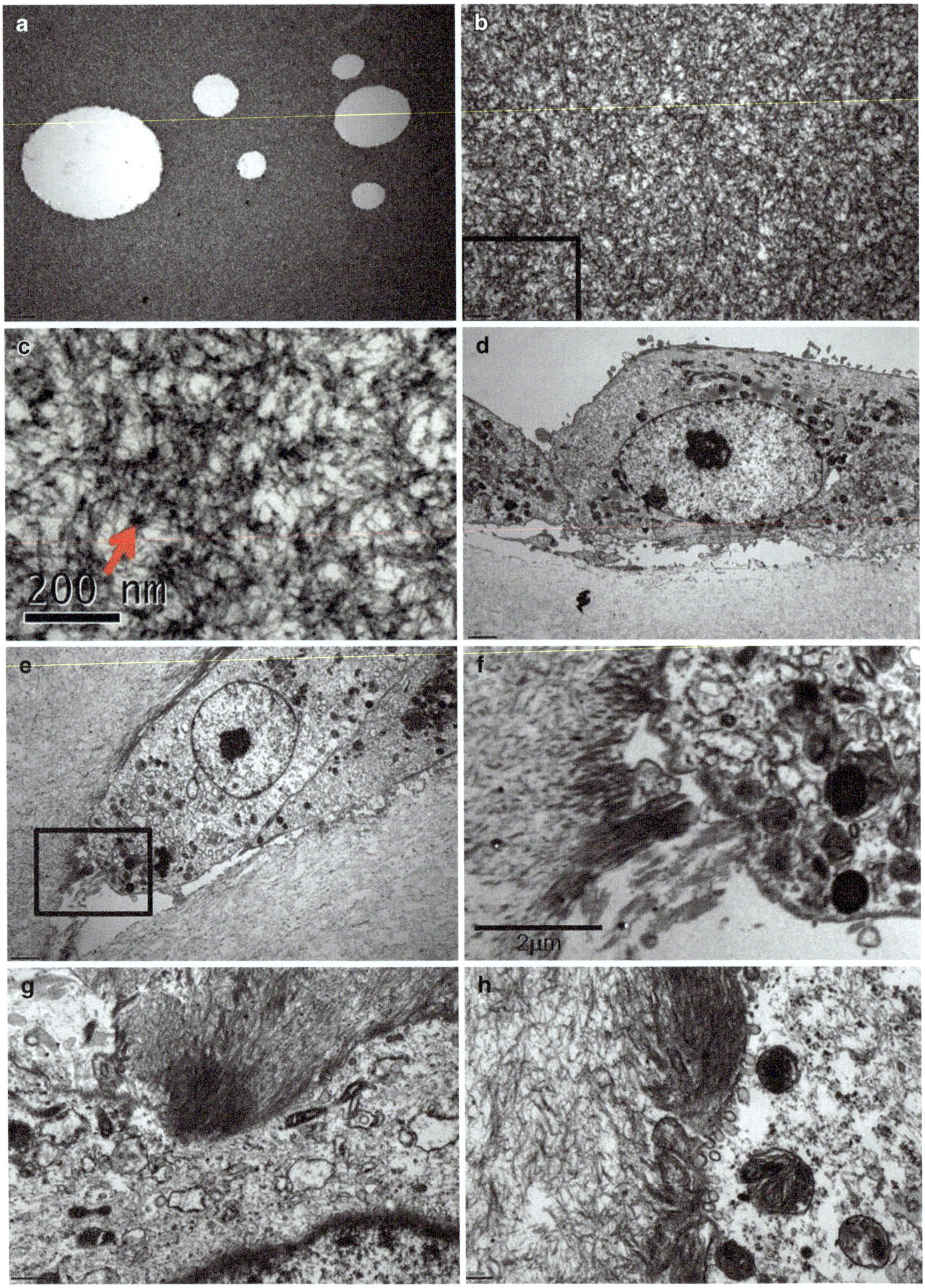

Fig. 10.7 Transmission electron microscopy images of the hyaluronic acid/fibrin composite (**a**–**c**) and the composite mixed with bone marrow cells (**d**–**f**). Low-magnification (**a**) and high-magnification (**b**) images of the composite revealed its porous property. A magnified image (**c**) of a *boxed area* in '**b**' revealed dense areas, thus suggesting a spherical form of the hyaluronic, acid-free chain (*arrow* in **c**). Cells were thoroughly incorporated within the composite and, in some cases, showed directional movement (**e**, **f**) (**f** is the enlarged version of the area within the *black box* in **e**). Newly biosynthesized collagen molecules appeared as distinctive, thin fibres which were not yet formed into striped collagen fibres (**g**, **h**)

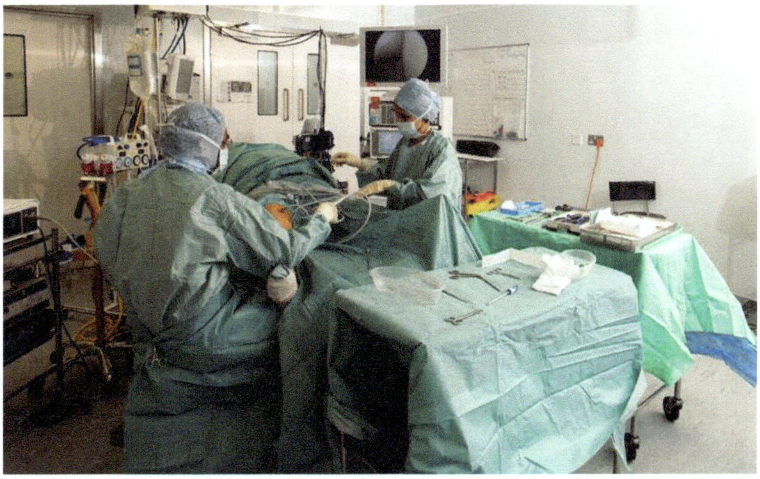

Fig. 10.8 Theatre setup

(Insufflation tubing with Wolf adaptor, Leonhard Lang UK Ltd., Stroud, UK).

Patient is positioned supine with the table horizontal at an appropriate height. Lateral supports are preferable for medial compartment lesions, especially with associated meniscal tears. A tourniquet is applied as high up on the thigh as possible and inflated to 100 mg above systolic blood pressure (Fig. 10.8).

Patient is anesthetised using general or spinal anaesthesia. NSAIDs are withheld as these drugs are known to be chondrotoxic. Appropriate antibiotic is administered intravenously prior to inflation of tourniquet.

10.5 Surgical Technique

10.5.1 Bone Marrow Harvest and Concentration

After suitable anaesthesia, the patient's anterior superior iliac spine (ASIS) is marked, cleaned and draped. If ASIS is not feasible, aspirate can be obtained from the posterior superior iliac spine. Bone marrow aspiration needle (T-Lok™, Angiotech, Gainesville, Florida, USA) and syringes preloaded with 2 ml Anticoagulant Citrate Dextrose solution A (ACD-A, Biomet, Massachusetts, USA) are used to aspirate 42 ml of bone marrow from the iliac crest. The aspiration site is injected with local anaesthetic and covered with a sterile plaster. The bone marrow aspirate is then centrifuged twice in a TriCell bone marrow separation device (CCR kit – CYP Biotech, South Korea) to obtain the required amount of concentrated bone marrow. First cycle is for 6 min at 3,500 rpm, followed by a second cycle for 5 min at 3,600 rpm to obtain BMAC (Fig. 10.9).

10.5.2 Preparation of BMAC and Fibrin Gel (Tissell®, Baxter, Thetford, UK) Mixture (Fig. 10.10)

With sterile precautions, transfer 1 ml of the aprotinin solution into the vial containing fibrinogen powder. Completely dissolve the fibrinogen powder by careful stirring without excessive frothing. Add 0.2 ml of low-molecular-weight hyaluronic acid (Highhyal, Huons, Seoul, Korea) to this vial and, after mixing, transfer the entire contents of this mixture into one of the DUPLOJECT syringes.

- With sterile precautions, transfer 1 ml of the calcium chloride solution into the vial containing thrombin powder (human thrombin lyophilized) and stir until the thrombin powder is dissolved without excessive frothing. Add 0.7 ml of concentrated BMAC to this mixture and, after mixing, transfer the entire contents of this mixture into the other DUPLOJECT syringes.
- A Fibrinotherm (Baxter) can be used to facilitate the mixing of the fibrinogen and thrombin vials (Fig. 10.11).

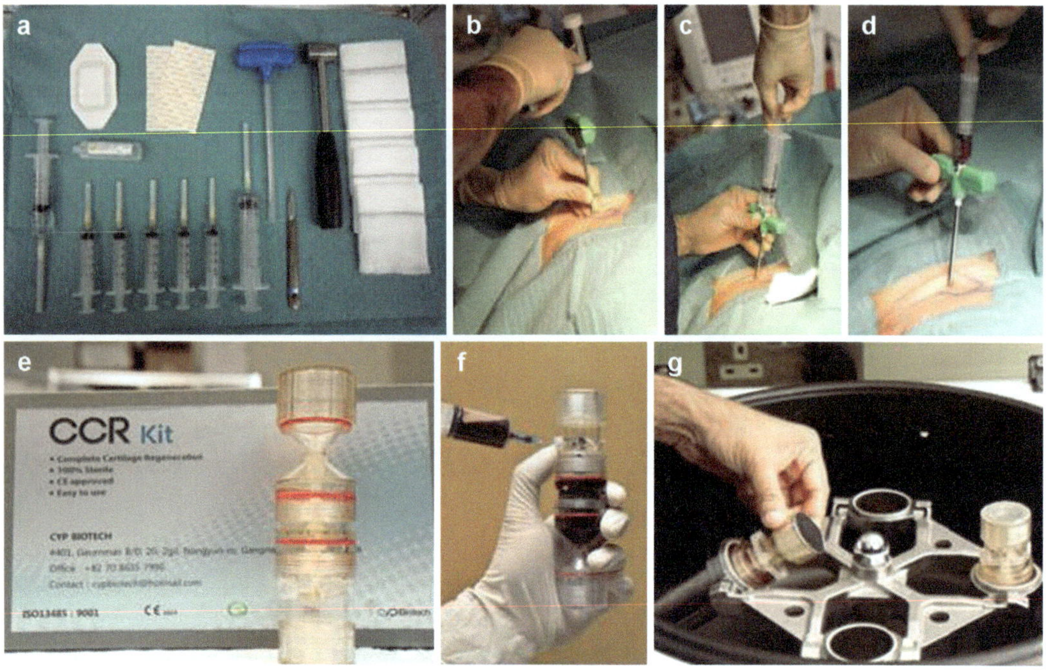

Fig. 10.9 (**a**) Bone marrow aspiration needle and ACD-A preloaded syringes. (**b**) Anchor the bone marrow needle on the iliac crest and gently hammer it in. (**c**) Attach 10-ml syringe and, with constant suction, slowly rotate and withdraw the bone marrow aspiration needle till bone marrow enters the syringe. (**d**) Aspirate 42 ml of bone marrow. (**e, f**) Transfer bone marrow aspirate to CCR™ kit (CYP Biotech, South Korea). (**g**) Place loaded kit into centrifuge with appropriate counterbalance

- Both DUPLOJECT syringes (A and B) are placed in the two syringe clip (C) with the syringe plunger (D) attached to the DUPLOJECT plunger (E) to ensure smooth forward motion. Connect the nozzles of the two syringes to the joining piece (F). Secure the joining piece by fastening the tether strap to the clip (G). Fit an application needle (H) onto the joining piece (F). Do not expel the air remaining inside the joining piece or application needle until you start actual application as the aperture of the needle may clog (Figs. 10.12 and 10.13).

The mixed contents are ready to be applied onto the cartilage defect.

10.5.3 Preparation of Chondral Defect for Implantation

The standard antero-lateral and antero-medial arthroscopic portals were used to approach the knee, and normal saline under pressure was infused. A supero-medial portal was used for an outflow cannula. Under arthroscopic vision, the number, size and location of the lesions are confirmed. If considered suitable for surgery, the lesions are then carefully debrided to bare subchondral bone. It is imperative that a stable shoulder of healthy cartilage is maintained at the periphery of the lesions. The subchondral bone was drilled with a 45°-angled drill (Powerpick drill, Arthrex, UK) up to a depth of 6 mm, at 3 mm intervals.

10.5.4 Implantation of Graft

Once ready for implantation, CO_2 is insufflated at 20 mm of Hg, flowing at 20 l/min. The CO_2 is introduced via a Wolf cannula (Karl Storz GmbH, Tuttlingen, Germany) and disposable tubing with a filter (Insufflation tubing with Wolf adaptor, Leonhard Lang UK Ltd., Stroud, UK) through the supero-lateral portal. Any residual saline is aspirated via an angled suction tube (Exmoor, Taunton, UK), and the chondral lesion is dried using cotton buds (Figs. 10.14 and 10.15).

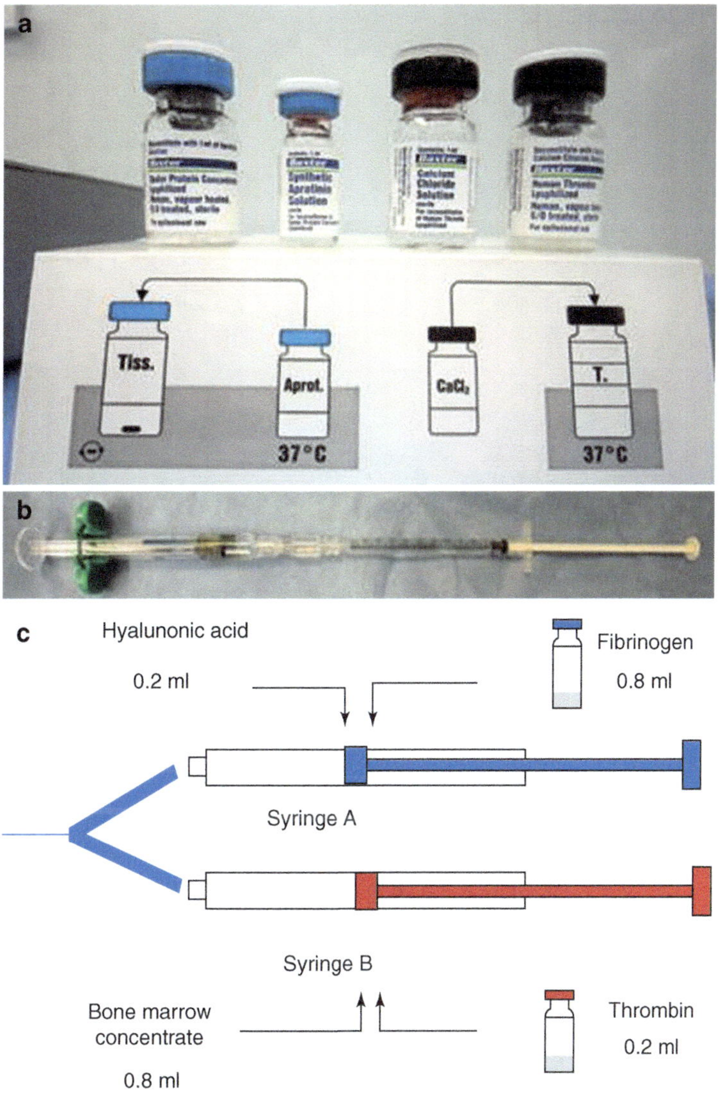

Fig. 10.10 (**a**) Preparation of fibrinogen and thrombin. (**b**) Hyaluronic acid. (**c**) Schematic of final mixing into double syringe

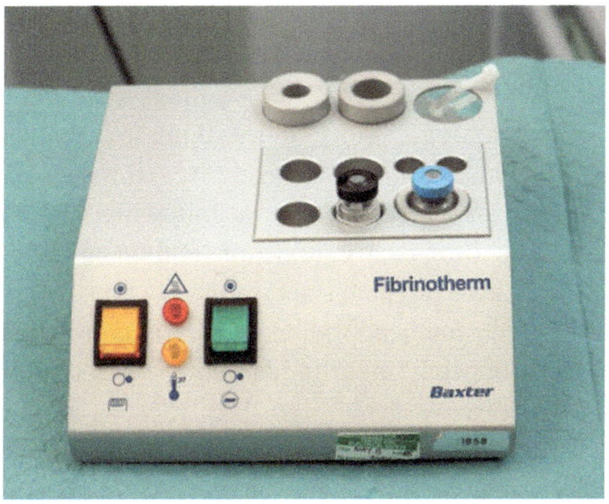

Fig. 10.11 Fibrinotherm facilitates mixing of fibrinogen and thrombin vials

A 20-gauge needle (inner diameter 0.9 mm, length 90 mm) (Spinal needle, Becton Dickinson, Madrid, Spain) is inserted into the joint via any suitable portal and connected to the previously prepared DUPLOJECT syringe. Under arthroscopic vision a layer of gel was applied into the defect. Once this first layer becomes firm (after about 1–2 min), a second layer can be injected deep to the first layer. A McDonald dissector (Bolton Surgical, UK) is used to shape the graft in situ, within five minutes, after which the gel hardens. The knee is taken through its range of motion to test the stability of the graft and to mould it further.

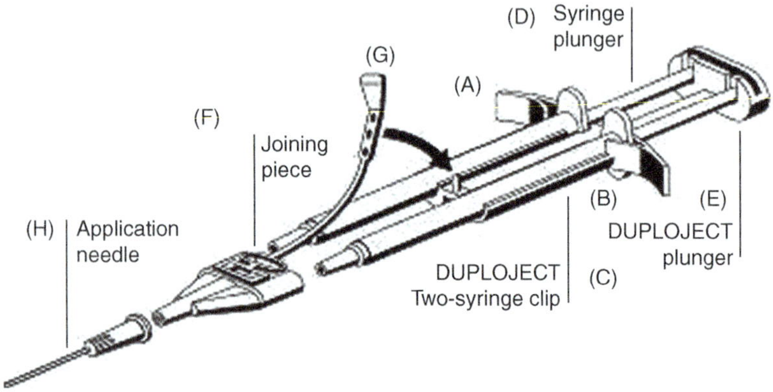

Fig. 10.12 DUPLOJECT assembly

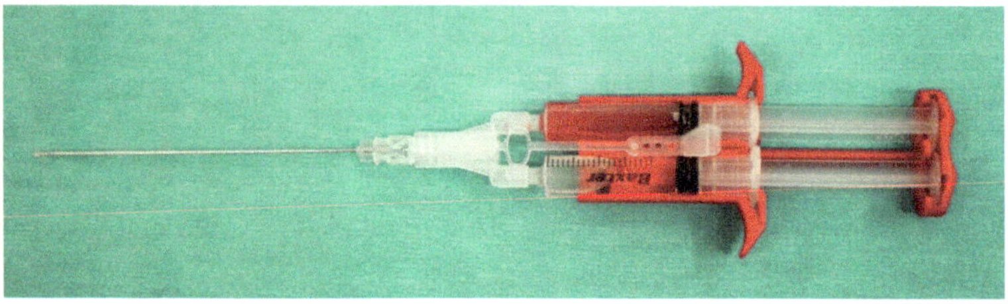

Fig. 10.13 DUPLOJECT syringe ready for application

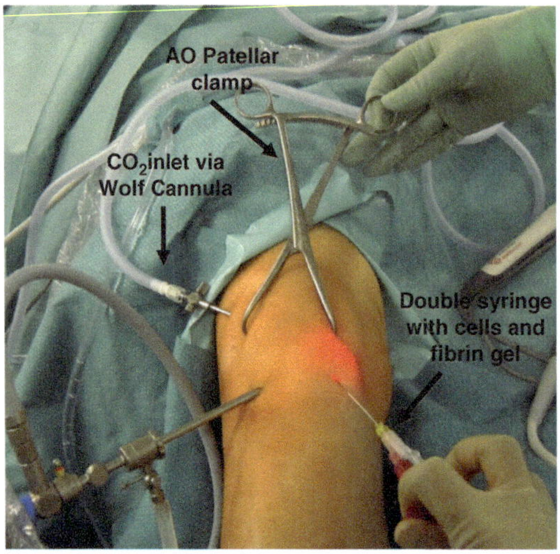

Fig. 10.14 Implantation of graft under CO_2 insufflation

Once the stability of the graft was established, all instruments were withdrawn. Hyaluronic acid (Highhyal, Huons, Seoul, Korea) was injected into the joint, and local anaesthetic was injected around the portals. The skin was closed either by sutures or butterfly stitches.

10.6 Postoperative Rehabilitation

Following surgery, CPM is initiated for 4–6 h while the patient remains in the hospital. Patients with tibio-femoral lesions are instructed to partially weight bearing on the operated leg, starting of 25 % of full weight on day 0 and gradually building up to 100 % of full weight at 6 weeks [20]. Patients with patella-femoral lesions are fitted with a brace on the operated leg, and flexion is increased by 20° a week, up to 6 weeks, when the brace is removed [18]. Patients are advised not to return to active sport for at least 9–12 months following the surgery [18]. They are allowed low-resistance cycling, swimming (avoiding breast stroke) and walking to keep fit.

Patients are advised to avoid NSAIDs for pain control for at least 12 weeks following surgery as these drugs have toxic on cell membranes [21]. Alternate pain medication is prescribed. Any other medication being taken is monitored, and coexisting medical conditions are treated effectively.

All patients underwent MRI scans at 12 and 18 months following the surgery. At 12 months

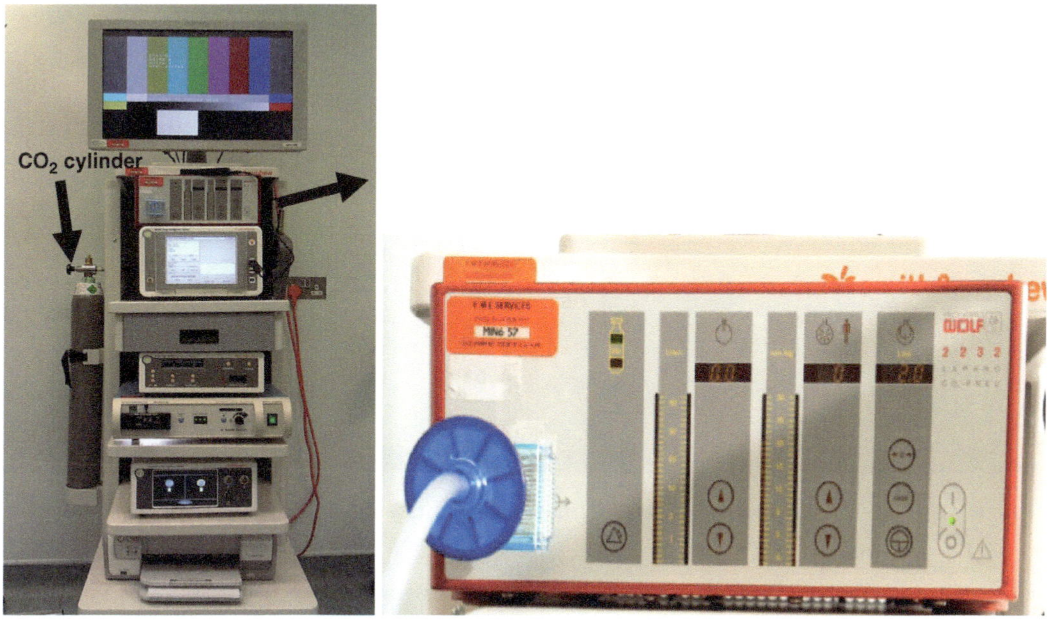

Fig. 10.15 Stack system with carbon dioxide insufflator with filter, tubing and cyclinder

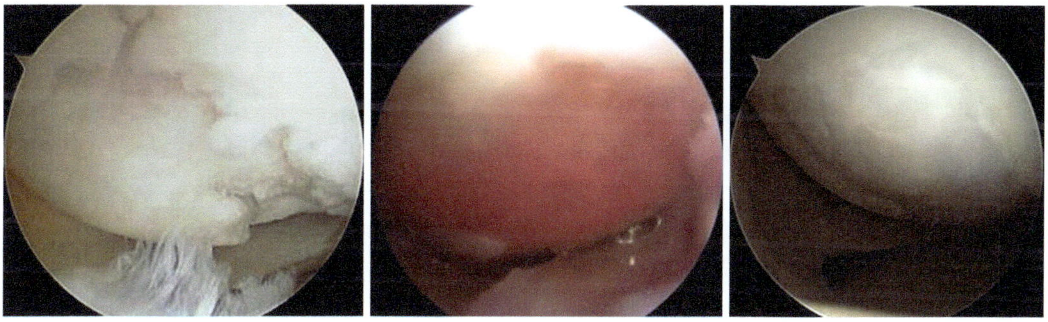

Fig. 10.16 Medial femoral condylar lesion – from left to right – preoperatively, after implantation of cells, at 18 months postoperatively

cartilage was imaged using DESS sequencing and T2* mapping. A d-GEMRIC scan was done at 18 months.

Conclusion

The technique described above has been in use for over 4 years now, and encouraging results have been seen, both clinically and radiologically. Patients were asked to complete the Lysholm score, IKDC score and the KOOS score pre- and postoperatively. They also underwent MRI scans with cartilage-specific protocols prior to surgery and at 12 and 18 months following surgery. At 2-year follow-up, Lysholm score was 80.1, as compared to 50.8 preoperatively ($p<0.05$). KOOS (symptomatic) was 92.1, as compared to 65.7 preoperatively. IKDC (subjective) was 83, up from 39 preoperatively. The mean T2* relaxation times for the repair tissue and native cartilage were 29.1 and 29.9, respectively. This is suggestive of hyaline-like cartilage. Average MOCART score for all lesions was 72 (Figs. 10.16–10.18).

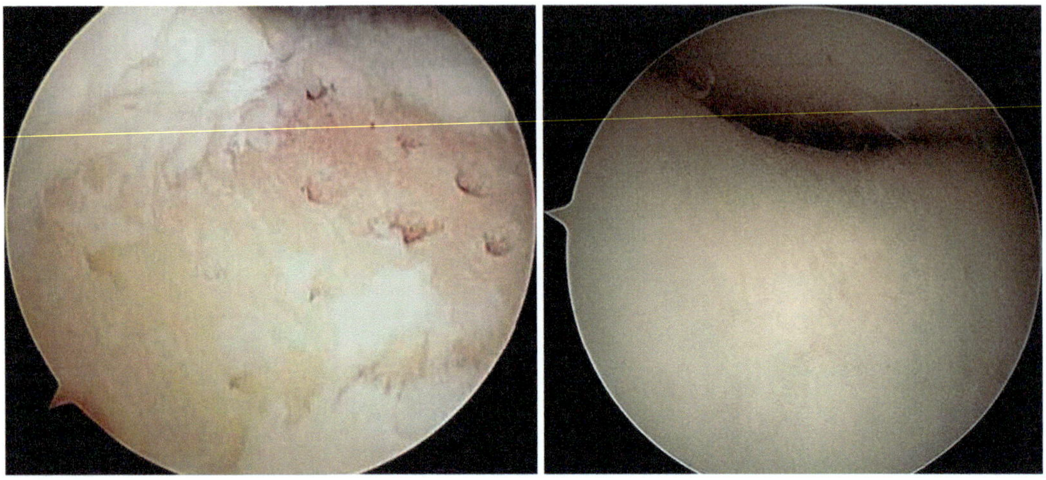

Fig. 10.17 Preoperative (*left*) trochlear lesion and (*right*) postoperatively at 18 months

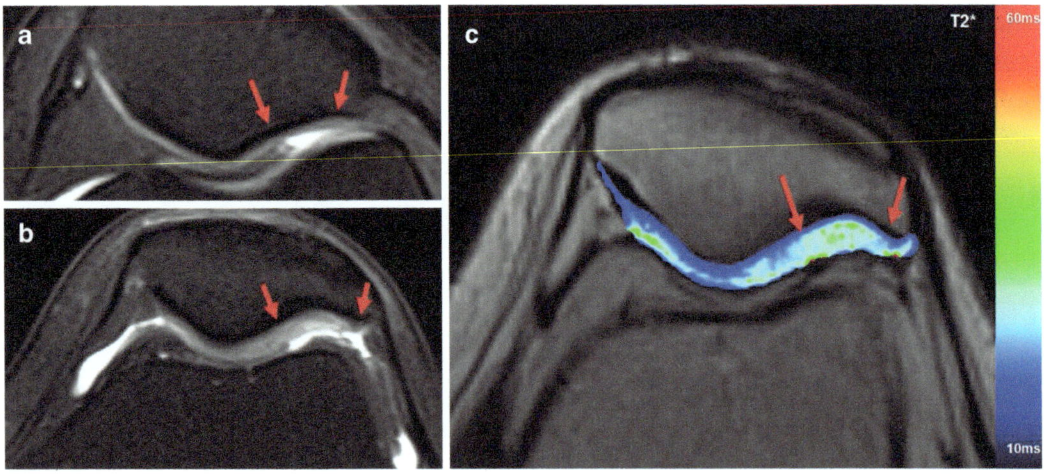

Fig. 10.18 MRI images for patellar femoral joint lesions. The area between the two red arrows indicate area of repaired cartilage lesions. (**a**) Morphological MRI scan pre-operatively. (**b**) Morphological MRI scan post-operatively. (**c**) MRI T2* mapping post-operatively

References

1. Hunter W (1743) On the structure and diseases of articulating cartilage. Phil Trans Roy Soc 42B: 514–521
2. Elders MJ (2000) The increasing impact of arthritis on public health. J Rheumatol Suppl 60:6–8
3. Carey JL (2012) Fibrocartilage following microfracture is not as robust as native articular cartilage: commentary on an article by Aaron J. Krych, MD, et al.: "activity levels are higher after osteochondral autograft transfer mosaicplasty than after microfracture for articular cartilage defects of the knee. A retrospective comparative study". J Bone Joint Surg Am 94(11):e80. doi:10.2106/JBJS.L.00319
4. Robb CA, El-Sayed C, Matharu GS, Baloch K, Pynsent P (2012) Survival of autologous osteochondral grafts in the knee and factors influencing outcome. Acta Orthop Belg 78(5):643–651
5. Gardner OF, Archer CW, Alini M, Stoddart MJ (2013) Chondrogenesis of mesenchymal stem cells for cartilage tissue engineering. Histol Histopathol 28(1):23–42
6. Ipach I, Schäfer R, Lahrmann J, Kluba T (2011) Stiffness after knee arthrotomy: evaluation of prevalence

and results after manipulation under anaesthesia. Orthop Traumatol Surg Res 97(3):292–296. doi:10.1016/j.otsr.2011.01.006, Epub 2011 Apr 11
7. Hui JH, Chen F, Thambyah A, Lee EH (2004) Treatment of chondral lesions in advanced osteochondritis dissecans: a comparative study of the efficacy of chondrocytes, mesenchymal stem cells, periosteal graft, and mosaicplasty (osteochondral autograft) in animal models. J Pediatr Orthop 24(4):427–433
8. Chiang H, Hsieh CH, Lin YH, Lin S, Tsai-Wu JJ, Jiang CC (2011) Differences between chondrocytes and bone marrow-derived chondrogenic cells. Tissue Eng Part A 17(23–24):2919–2929. doi:10.1089/ten.tea.2010.0732, Epub 2011 Sep 6
9. Galotto M, Berisso G, Delfino L et al (1999) Stromal damage as consequence of high-dose chemo/radiotherapy in bone marrow transplant recipients. Exp Hematol 27(9):1460–1466
10. Cantaluppi V, Biancone L, Quercia A, Deregibus MC, Segoloni G, Camussi G (2013) Rationale of mesenchymal stem cell therapy in kidney injury. Am J Kidney Dis 61(2):300–309. doi:10.1053/j.ajkd.2012.05.027, Epub 2012 Aug 30
11. Efe T, Theisen C, Fuchs-Winkelmann S et al (2011) Cell-free collagen type I matrix for repair of cartilage defects-clinical and magnetic resonance imaging results. Knee Surg Sports Traumatol Arthrosc 20:1915–1922
12. Mawatari M, Higo T, Tsutsumi Y et al (2006) Effectiveness of autologous fibrin tissue adhesive in reducing postoperative blood loss during total hip arthroplasty: a prospective randomised study of 100 cases. J Orthop Surg 14:117
13. Keller J, Andreassen TT, Joyce F et al (1985) Fixation of osteochondral fractures, fibrin sealant tested in dogs. Acta Orthop Scand 56:323
14. Peterson L, Brittberg M, Kiviranta I et al (2002) Autologous chondrocyte transplantation: biomechanics and long-term durability. Am J Sports Med 30:2
15. Jang JD, Moon YS, Kim YS, Choi NY, Mok HS, Kim YJ, Shetty AA, Kim SJ (2013) Novel repair technique for articular cartilage defect using a fibrin and hyaluronic acid mixture. Tissue Eng Regen Med 10(1):1–9. doi:10.1007/s13770-013-0361-0
16. Davis H, Binder BY, Schaecher P, Yakoobinsky D, Bhat A, Leach JK (2013) Enhancing osteoconductivity of fibrin gels with apatite-coated polymer microspheres. Tissue Eng Part A 19:1773–1782
17. Hirai F, Beppu T, Nishimura T, Takatsu N, Ashizuka S, Seki T, Hisabe T, Nagahama T, Yao K, Matsui T, Nakashima R, Inada N, Tajiri E, Mitsuru H, Shigematsu H (2011) Carbon dioxide insufflation compared with air insufflation in double-balloon enteroscopy: a prospective, randomized, double-blind trial. Gastrointest Endosc 73(4):743–749, doi:S0016-5107(10)02188-7 [pii]
18. Corson SL, Hoffman JJ, Jackowski J, Chapman GA (1988) Cardiopulmonary effects of direct venous CO_2 insufflation in ewes. A model for CO_2 hysteroscopy. J Reprod Med 33(5):440–444
19. Roemer FW, Crema MD, Trattnig S, Guermazi A (2011) Advances in imaging of osteoarthritis and cartilage. Radiology 260(2):332–354, doi:260/2/332 [pii]
20. Reinold MM, Wilk KE, Macrina LC, Dugas JR, Cain EL (2006) Current concepts in the rehabilitation following articular cartilage repair procedures in the knee. J Orthop Sports Phys Ther 36:774–794
21. Pereira-Leite C, Nunes C, Reis S (2013) Interaction of nonsteroidal anti-inflammatory drugs with membranes: in vitro assessment and relevance for their biological actions. Prog Lipid Res 52:571–584. doi:10.1016/j.plipres.2013.08.003, pii: S0163-7827(13)00048-9

Part V

Repair Techniques

Surgical Techniques in Cartilage Repair Surgery: Osteochondral Autograft Transfer (OATS, Mosaicplasty)

11

László Hangody and Ágnes Berta

Contents

L. Hangody, MD, PhD, DSc (✉)
Á. Berta, MD, MSc, M Res
Department of Orthopaedics and Traumatology, Uzsoki Hospital, Semmelweis University, 1145 Budapest, Uzsoki u. 29, Hungary
e-mail: hangody@t-online.hu; bertaagnes@hotmail.com

11.1 Introduction

Various surgical methods exist for the treatment of focal chondral and osteochondral defects of weight-bearing articular surfaces. Traditional resurfacing techniques provide reparative fibrocartilage coverage of the lesion with poor biomechanical properties and suboptimal clinical outcome. Recent advances in treatment options including osteochondral allografts aim to provide hyaline or hyaline-like repair for articular defects. Although previous publications on autogenous osteochondral transplantation reported long-term hyaline cartilage survival on the transplanted osteochondral block [3, 6, 23, 26], clinical use of single-block osteochondral transfer had been restricted by limited donor-site availability. Also, use of large grafts can cause incongruity at the recipient site, which permanently alters the biomechanics of the joint [5, 7, 9–12]. Our preclinical animal studies performed between 1991 and 1992 showed that the use of small-sized multiple cylindrical grafts, rather than a single large block graft, allows more tissue to be transplanted while preserving donor-site integrity and the mosaic-like implanting fashion permits progressive contouring of the new surface [13, 15].

The basic idea behind autogenous osteochondral transplantation is that mosaic-like transplantation of multiple, small-sized, cylindrical osteochondral grafts can provide a congruent resurfaced area. The grafts are harvested from the relatively less weight-bearing periphery of the patellofemoral joint [8]. The transplanted hyaline

A.A. Shetty et al. (eds.), *Techniques in Cartilage Repair Surgery*,
DOI 10.1007/978-3-642-41921-8_11, © ESSKA 2014

cartilage is capable of surviving and produces a more durable surface than the fibrous repair tissue [3, 6, 23, 26]. Donor-site repair occurs via natural healing processes; the tunnels become filled with cancellous bone and the surface covered by reparative fibrocartilage built by marrow-derived cells [9, 10].

Development of the mosaicplasty resurfacing technique started at the beginning of the early 1990s. The cadaver studies helped to develop an instrumentation which can provide optimal technical conditions for harvesting and mosaic-like transplantation of small-sized cylindrical osteochondral grafts. Since 1991 several series of animal experiments were performed to evaluate the mosaicplasty concept and to identify the ideal donor site, graft dimension, optimal filling rate and congruity [1, 10]. German Shepherd Dogs and horses were subjects of this experimental work, and later veterinary clinical experiences of mosaicplasties on horses were also used in the improvement of technical details and rehabilitation aspects.

The most important findings of these experiments are the following:

- Consistent survival of the transplanted hyaline cartilage could be observed.
- The transplanted grafts integrated to the host tissue.
- There was fibrocartilage formation between the transplanted grafts, which could be promoted by abrasion arthroplasty or sharp curettage of the bony base of the defect.
- Deep matrix integration occurred between the hyaline cap of the grafts and the host cartilage as well as between the graft and host cartilage and the intermediate fibrocartilage, which was present due to defect site preparation.
- Donor tunnels eventually became filled with cancellous bone and covered with fibrocartilage which provided an acceptable gliding surface for these reduced weight-bearing areas.

Biomechanical assessment of press-fit fixation of the implanted grafts was also implemented by our research group and by independent studies. Determination of the pullout forces helped to find the ideal technique of press-fit fixation, which is an important factor in the accelerated rehabilitation process.

Table 11.1 Indications for mosaicplasty procedure

Focal chondral and osteochondral defects of weight-bearing articular surfaces of the knee
Extended indications: articular surfaces of the talus, femoral head and humeral capitulum
The ideal diameter of the defect is between 1 and 3 cm^2, extended indication: 3–4 cm^2
Patient less than 50 years of age, extended indication: 50–55 years
Patient compliance is critical (i.e. weight-bearing limitations)

The first series of instruments were introduced in 1992. Further research in the following years led to the extension of application of the mosaicplasty technique for arthroscopic approach and the development of a second generation of instrumentarium. Driven by the reproducible experimental proof of the mosaicplasty concept, clinical application started on the February 6, 1992. During the subsequent years clinical data reported by various authors confirmed the results seen in animal experiments, and since 1995 the procedure has been used with similar success in numerous institutions throughout the world.

11.2 Indications and Contraindications for Surgery

Small-sized, single focal lesions of femoral condyles are the main indication for mosaicplasty procedures; however, defects on the tibial, patellar and trochlear surfaces can also be treated by osteochondral grafting. Mosaicplasty offers less favourable outcome in multiple defects, especially in kissing lesions. Besides osteochondral defects of the knee, lesions of the talus is a frequent indication, and in exceptional cases capitulum humeri and femoral head lesions can also be treated by mosaicplasty.

The indications for mosaicplasty are summarised in Table 11.1.

Donor-site availability and certain technical considerations limit the optimal extent of defect coverage to 1–4 cm^2. Usually, each patellofemoral peripheries allow graft harvest for 3–4-cm^2-sized defects. When all possible donor sites are

Table 11.2 Contraindications for mosaicplasty procedure

Absolute	Generalised arthritis, rheumatoid and/or degenerative in type
	Infectious or tumour defects
	Lack of appropriate donor area
	Age greater than 55 years
	Defect larger than 8 cm^2
	Osteochondral defect deeper than 10 mm
	Noncompliant patient
Relative	Age between 50 and 55 years
	Defects between 4 and 8 cm^2
	Mild osteoarthritic changes

utilised, defects up to 8–9 cm^2 in size can be resurfaced by mosaicplasty, but such extension of resurfacing can result in a higher rate of donor-site morbidity [13, 16].

Due to decreased repair capacity, 50 years of age constitutes the recommended upper limit for mosaicplasty; this limitation is based on clinical experiences with single-block osteochondral transfer [24, 25].

Contraindications for mosaicplasty include generalised or rheumatoid arthritis and lesions caused by infection or tumours, where the survival of the transplanted hyaline cartilage on the recipient site is hindered by the suboptimal intraarticular biochemical conditions (Table 11.2.).

Although osteoarthritis generally is a contraindication for mosaicplasty, in certain motivated patient groups mosaicplasty can be considered as a salvage intervention for small-sized focal defects. Matching the contour of the defective articular surface to the donor plug can present a technical difficulty; further disadvantages can be donor-site morbidity and the risk of cartilage or bone collapse.

Similar to other resurfacing techniques, mosaicplasty is only one step in the treatment of full-thickness chondral and osteochondral defects; it is also necessary to attend to any accompanying joint abnormalities. Treatment of meniscal and ligamental tears, join instabilities and misalignments must be incorporated in the operative and postoperative rehabilitation algorithms, otherwise early wear of transplanted cartilage or even more progressed degeneration may develop [2, 8, 17, 19]. The most common concomitant surgical interventions are ACL reconstruction, meniscus surgery and femorotibial realignment procedures, and occasionally patellofemoral realignment or lateral release may also be required.

11.3 Operative Technique

11.3.1 Recommendations for Preoperative Preparation

The patient should be positioned supine with the knee capable of 120° flexion, and the contralateral extremity should be placed in a stirrup. General or regional anaesthesia and the use of tourniquet and fluid management system are recommended. Preoperative preparations should include antibiotic prophylaxis. Standard arthroscopic instrumentation and MosaicPlasty Complete System (Smith & Nephew, Inc., Endoscopy Division, Andover, Massachusetts) are required. Besides these reusable instruments, disposable chisels, drill bits and tamps are also available to provide optimal conditions for precise graft harvesting and tunnel preparation. (Dispoposplasty System - Smith & Nephew, Inc., Endoscopy Division, Andover, Massachusetts).

11.3.2 Mosaicplasty Technique

11.3.2.1 Surgical Approach

Surgical approach for mosaicplasty can be arthroscopic (Fig. 11.1) or through miniarthrotomy (Fig. 11.2). The type, size and location of the lesion may require a miniarthrotomy or an open procedure; however, the priority should be an arthroscopic approach.

Portal Selection for Arthroscopic Approach

The majority of femoral condylar defects can be managed arthroscopically, and for most of these lesions, central anterior medial and central anterior lateral working portals allow proper perpendicular access. A 1.2-mm K-wire or an 18-gauge spinal needle can help in the localisation of the portal sites. It should be noted that these portals tend to be more central than the standard portals due to the inward curve of the condyles.

Lesions caused by osteochondritis dissecans on the medial femoral condyle might require an approach from the lateral side.

Occasionally the standard lateral portal proves to be exceedingly oblique; in these cases a central patellar tendon portal can provide a good access to the inner areas of both medial and lateral femoral condyles.

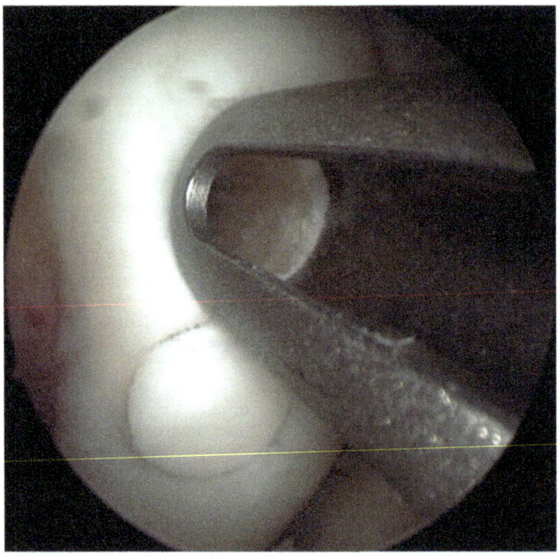

Fig. 11.1 Arthroscopic mosaicplasty on the medial femur condyle of the left knee for the treatment of grade III–IV chondropathy – the first graft is already inserted; dilation of the second recipient tunnel is just performed

Open Mosaicplasty

An open procedure might be chosen during the learning curve or when an arthroscopic approach is not suitable due to the size or location of the lesion. Although certain trochlear defects can be resurfaced arthroscopically, patellotrochlear and tibial lesions always require an open procedure.

The incision can be medial, lateral–anterior–sagittal or an oblique incision; the most suitable can be selected via arthroscopy. Patellotrochlear and tibial implantations may require an extended anteromedial approach.

Further steps and technique of the implantation are identical with the arthroscopic procedure.

11.3.2.2 Defect Preparation

Sharp curette and/or shaver blades should be used to bring the edges of the defect back to intact hyaline cartilage at a correct angle. The bony base of the lesion can be cleaned by an arthroscopic burr (Abrader, Acromionizer) or a half-round rasp to eliminate subchondral sequester layer and refresh subchondral bone. Abrasion arthroplasty of the lesion promotes fibrocartilage grouting from the bony base. The drill guide should be used instead to determine the required

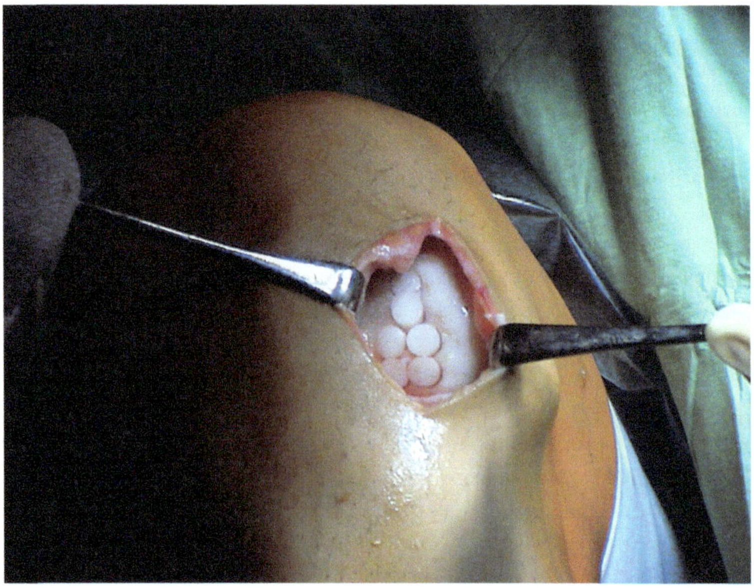

Fig. 11.2 Mosaicplasty from a miniarthrotomy approach on the medial femur condyle of the right knee for the treatment of osteochondritis dissecans; six grafts (8.5 mm diameter) were used

number and size (2.7, 3.5, 4.5, 6.5 and 8.5 mm in diameter) of the grafts, because tapping the cutting edge of the guide into the bony base and removing it can leave a mark on the defect site. Finally, depth of the defect should be measured with the laser marks of the dilator.

Filling the defect with uniform-sized contacting cylindrical grafts allows a filling rate of about 70–80 %; additional smaller graft sizes and cutting the grafts into each other can improve the coverage up to 90–100 %.

11.3.2.3 Graft Harvest

The recommended harvest sites are the area on the medial femoral condyle peripheral of the patellofemoral joint and above the line of the notch. Surface of the lateral femoral condyle above the sulcus terminalis and, in exceptional cases, the notch area can serve as additional donor sites. Grafts harvested from the notch area are less favourable, as they have concave cartilage caps and less elastic underlying bone. Recent publications also suggest the proximal tibiofibular articulation as an exceptional donor site.

The minimal length of the graft should be at least two times of its diameter, but as a rule of thumb, 15-mm long grafts can be taken to resurface chondral lesions and 25-mm long plugs for osteochondral defects.

The optimal viewing angle for graft harvest from the patellofemoral peripheries can be obtained by introducing the scope through the standard contralateral portal. Extending the knee and using the standard ipsilateral portal allows checking whether the access is perpendicular to the donor site. The extended position should provide a perpendicular access to the most superior donor hole. Gradual flexion of the knee allows the harvest of additional grafts from the lower areas of the patellofemoral periphery. The level of graft harvesting should not exceed the top of the intercondylar notch (sulcus terminalis). In case of arthroscopic approach, the medial patellofemoral periphery is more accessible than the lateral one as fluid distension usually moves the patella laterally making perpendicular positioning of the harvesting chisel easier. If the standard portals do not allow a perpendicular access, a spinal needle or a K-wire can be used to determine the location of any additional harvesting portals.

Once location of the portal is determined, the proper-sized tube chisel filled with the matching harvesting tamp should be introduced. Introduction of the harvester along with the tamp can help to eliminate fluid leakage and avoid chondral injuries caused by the sharp cutting edge of the harvester. When the donor site is clearly identified, the chisel should be placed perpendicular to the articular surface. The harvesting tamp is then removed, and the harvester is driven by a hammer to the appropriate depth. The chisel must be hold firmly to avoid shifting at the cartilage–bone interface, producing a crooked graft.

The next step is to insert the appropriate harvesting tamp into the cross-hole in the tubular chisel and to use it as a lever. The chisel should be toggled, not rotated, so the graft can break free at the chisel tip. The grafts should be ejected from the chisel by sliding the appropriately sized chisel guard over the cutting end. The harvesting tamp can be used to push out the graft onto a gauze in a saline-wetted basin.

Donor-site holes will be filled up in a couple of hours with initial repair tissue produced by bleeding mediated mesenchymal stem cells. Adequate rehabilitation can support transformation of this primary repair tissue into cancellous bone with fibrocartilage coverage.

Grafts can also be obtained through a miniarthrotomy (15–20 mm) during the learning curve; determine the site of the incision with the aid of a spinal needle under arthroscopic control.

11.3.2.4 Implantation of the Grafts: "Drill–Dilate–Deliver"

Drill

Bending the knee helps to gain access to the recipient site. Fluid management system can promote proper distension and good visualisation. The first step is to reintroduce the drill guide using the dilator as an obturator and place them perpendicularly to the defected surface. Rotating the arthroscope makes the drill guide and perpendicular position of the laser mark visible from different angles, ensuring proper orientation. Next step is to tap the cutting edge of the guide into the subchondral bone. The appropriately sized drill bit is then inserted and drilled to the desired depth. Generally, a recipient hole a few millimetres deeper than the length of the graft is preferable to minimise high intraosseal pressure and avoid prominent graft positioning. Reducing the inflow helps to minimise leakage. Finally, the drill bit is removed, and bone debris is eliminated by irrigation.

Dilate

First the conical-shaped dilator is reinserted into the drill guide and tapped to the required depth. Depth of dilation depends on the actual stiffness and elasticity of the recipient bone; stiff bone needs more dilation than normal or soft bone. The drill guide must be held firmly while removing the dilator from the hole.

Deliver

The specially designed delivery tamp should be used for graft insertion; depth of insertion can be set by turning the handle. Initially the graft should sit slightly higher than the depth of the defect; it helps to minimise the likelihood of over-penetrating the graft. It is recommended to stop inflow at this step, because fluid flow can force the graft out of the tube. The graft should be delivered under direct visualisation through the drill guide and with the delivery tamp into the recipient hole. The graft can be inserted deeper by turning the handle of the delivery tamp counterclockwise. The graft must be flush with the original articular surface. Removing the drill guide allows inspecting the graft. If the graft is protruded, the drill guide should be reinserted and the graft tapped down gently with the dilator of the appropriate size. Subsequent grafts are inserted with a similar technique by placing the drill guide immediately adjacent to the previously placed grafts. The shoulder of the drill guide must be kept off the previously inserted grafts to avoid inadvertent recessing of the grafts.

It is recommended to start with the most posterior graft and implant further grafts in less bended knee positions. Dilation of the actual recipient hole allows an easy graft insertion (low insertion force on the hyaline cap), and as a main advantage of this step-by-step implantation technique, dilation of the next hole wedges surrounding bone around the previously implanted grafts resulting in a very safe press-fit fixation.

When all grafts are in place, the knee should be moved throughout its range of motion, and depending on the side of the resurfaced area, varus or valgus stress should also be provoked. Suction drainage should be introduced through a superior portal, and after closing the portals, elastic bandage should be applied over the dressing.

11.3.3 Recommendations for Postoperative Care

Postoperative application of ice packs and elastic bandage can help to control extreme bleeding from the donor tunnels. The drain should be removed at 24 h. Appropriate pain control, cold therapy as well as nonsteroidal anti-inflammatory drugs can reduce postoperative complaints. Postoperative thrombosis prophylaxis is also recommended.

11.4 Rehabilitation

Autologous osteochondral mosaicplasty permits immediate full range of motion (ROM) but requires 2 weeks non-weight bearing and further 2–3 weeks partial weight bearing (30–40 kg) period after surgery. The initial non-weight bearing phase is recommended to prevent graft subsidence during osseous integration.

Patients can return to normal daily activity after 8–10 weeks. High-demand sport activity should be delayed till after 5–6 months. The recommended rehabilitation protocol should be modified if concurrent procedures, such as ACL reconstruction, high tibial osteotomy, meniscus reinsertion and meniscus resection, were performed (Table 11.3.).

11.5 Complications

Technical difficulties are frequent during mosaicplasty procedure and can be avoided by following the main principles of the surgical protocol.

Table 11.3 Recommended rehabilitation protocol following mosaicplasty procedure

General guidelines	
Immobilisation	
No immobilisation![a]	
Ambulation[b]	
Two-crutch ambulation, non-weight bearing	Immediate
Two-crutch ambulation, partial loading (30–40 kg)	2–4 weeks
Discontinue crutches, full weight bearing	4–5 weeks
Functional exercises	
Form walking, gait evaluation	4–5 weeks
Step-up	4–5 weeks
Step-down	5–6 weeks
Range of motion (ROM)	
Early ROM is encouraged	
CPM for extended, 2–4 cm^2 lesions (in painless range)	Immediate (first week)
Full extension, flexion as tolerated	Immediate
Stationary bicycle	3 weeks
Strength	
Quadriceps	
Open chain exercises, leg raises	Immediate
Concentric contraction to full extension	1 week (or earlier if tolerated)
Concentric contraction against resistance	2 weeks
Isometric exercises at different angles	Immediate
Eccentric exercises against resistance	3–4 weeks
Hamstrings	
Isometric exercises at different angles	Immediate
Concentric and eccentric strengthening	1–2 weeks
- Against resistance	3–4 weeks
Closed chain exercises[c]	
Pushing soft rubber-ball with foot	Immediate
Closed chain exercises with half weight bearing	2–3 weeks
Closed chain exercises with full weight bearing	5–6 weeks
Stationary bicycle with resistance (if 90° knee flexion achieved)	2–4 weeks
Stairmaster	6–8 weeks
Proprioception	
Balance exercises standing on both feet	5–6 weeks
Balance exercises standing on one foot (hard ground)	6–8 weeks
Balance exercises standing on one foot (trampoline or aerostep)	8–10 weeks
Return to activity	
Jogging	10 weeks
Straight line running	3 months
Directional changes	4–5 months
Shear forces	5 months[d]
Sport-specific adaptations	5 months
Sport activity	5–6 months[e]
Special considerations	
Weight-bearing recommendations based on the location, size and type of the defect	
Femoral or tibial condyle, chondral defect, diameter <15 mm	
Non-weight bearing	1 week
Partial weight bearing	1–3 weeks
Femoral or tibial condyle, chondral defect, diameter ≥15 mm	
Non-weight bearing	2 weeks
Partial weight bearing	2–4 weeks
Femoral or tibial condyle, osteochondral defect	
Non-weight bearing	3 weeks
Partial weight bearing	3–5 weeks
Patellar defect, diameter <15 mm	
Partial weight bearing	2 weeks
Patellar defect, diameter ≥15 mm	
Partial weight bearing	3 weeks
Quadriceps strengthening and patellar mobilisation for patellar defects	
Vastus medialis strengthening!	
Isometric exercises in extension	Immediate
Patellar mobilisation	Immediate!
Isometric exercises at different angles	1 week
Open chain exercises	2 weeks
- Against resistance	3–4 weeks
Eccentric exercises against resistance	4–5 weeks
Closed chain exercises	2–3 weeks
Considerations due to concomitant surgery	
The most frequent combinations are the following:	
LCA reconstruction combined with mosaicplasty	
2–4 weeks non-weight bearing (due to mosaicplasty)	
2 more weeks partial weight bearing	
5°–90° ROM for 4 weeks	
Mainly closed chain exercises for quadriceps strengthening	
Hamstring strengthening in open and closed chain	
Proprioceptive training!	

(continued)

Table 11.3 (continued)

Meniscus reinsertion combined with mosaicplasty
4 weeks non-weight bearing
2 more weeks partial weight bearing
5°–45° ROM for 4 weeks
Retinaculum patellae reconstruction combined with mosaicplasty
2–4 weeks non-weight bearing (due to mosaicplasty)
2 more weeks partial weight bearing
0°–45° ROM for 4 weeks
HTO combined with mosaicplasty
Weight-bearing recommendations (4 weeks with crutches and in extension only) are based on mosaicplasty, pain and degree of correction (undercorrection, non-weight bearing; overcorrection, early weight bearing)

Uzsoki Hospital and Sanitas Private Clinic, Budapest, Hungary

[a]The main goal of rehabilitation is to ensure early motion of the operated joint to promote adequate nutrition of the transplanted cartilage. Cold therapy during the first week can help to avoid postoperative bleeding and decrease postoperative pain. If due to a concomitant procedure external fixation is required (e.g. meniscus reinsertion), limitation of ROM by bracing is permitted for a short period

[b]Extent, type (chondral or osteochondral) and location of the defect can modify weight-bearing recommendations (see special considerations)

[c]Partial loading helps to transform reparative tissue between transplanted plugs into fibrocartilage, especially in the half-weight-bearing period. Certain closed chain exercises (e.g. cycling) can ensure cyclic loading which makes fluid and nutrition transport more efficient between synovial fluid and hyaline cartilage

[d]It takes approximately 4–5 months to form a composite hyaline-like surface over the transplanted area which is able to tolerate shear forces

[e]Depends on the depth and extent of the defect. If strength, power, endurance, balance and flexibility are not satisfying, sport activity should be postponed

Perpendicular harvest and implantation of the grafts are crucial for a successful transplantation, oblique harvest and insertion result in uneven articular surface. Thorough visual control at different angles with the arthroscope can eliminate such complications.

Further technical pitfall might be the extensive implantation of the grafts, which can be avoided by the appropriate use of the delivery tamp. If the grafts are implanted deeper than the desired level, the following steps are recommended:

- Insert the drill guide next to the inadequately implanted graft and drill the applicable recipient hole.
- Remove the guide and use the arthroscopic probe to lift the graft to the required level.
- Continue with the recommended protocol for the rest of the insertions; dilation of the adjacent tunnel provides proper press-fit fixation for the previously implanted graft.

Donor-site morbidity, such as patellofemoral complaints, pain or swelling following strenuous physical activity, is not a frequent complication. Our 17 years of follow-up showed long-term donor-site morbidity in less than 3 % of all operated cases. However, extensive graft harvesting or graft harvesting without considering already existing patellofemoral degeneration can result in higher rate of donor-site morbidity.

Excessive postoperative bleeding from the donor tunnels is also a potential postoperative complication, and according to previous reports, it can occur in 7–8 % of the cases. Postoperative drainage, application of ice packs and elastic bandages can decrease the frequency of this complication.

Septic or thromboembolic complications can be prevented by strict aseptic conditions, single-shot antibiotics and thrombosis prophylaxis.

11.6 Results

Between February 6, 1992, and December 31, 2008, 1,179 mosaicplasties were performed at the authors' institution: 849 implantations on femoral condyles, 171 in the patellofemoral joint, 36 on the tibia condyles, 101 on talar domes, 8 on the capitulum humeri, 3 on humeral heads and 11 on femoral heads. Two thirds of the cases were operated on because of a localised grade III or grade IV cartilage lesion, whereas the rest of the patients underwent surgery due to osteochondral defects. In 81 % of the patients, concomitant surgical interventions were also carried out, which influenced the clinical results of the mosaicplasty procedures. The majority of these concomitant procedures were ACL reconstructions, realignment osteotomies, meniscus surgery and patellofemoral realignment procedures.

Femoral, tibial and patellar implantations were evaluated by the modified Hospital for Special Surgery (HSS), modified Cincinnati, Lysholm and International Cartilage Repair Society (ICRS) scoring systems, while possible donor-site disturbances and morbidity were evaluated by the Bandi scoring system. Patients with talar lesions were subjected to Hannover ankle evaluations. Analysis of clinical scores has shown good to excellent results in 92 % of patients with femoral condylar implantations, 87 % of tibial resurfacings, 74 % of patellar and/or trochlear mosaicplasties and 93 % of talar procedures. Moderate and severe donor-site disturbances were present in 3 % of patients according to the Bandi score (evaluations were done in a 1–10-year interval). Postoperative complications were four deep infections and 56 painful haemarthroses. Arthroscopic or open debridement resolved all deep infections, and 12 cases of haemorrhage also required arthroscopic or open debridement. The remaining patients with haemarthroses were treated by aspiration and cryotherapy. Four patients had minor thromboembolic complications [9, 10, 12–17].

During the recent years several independent centre published retrospective or comparative studies about the clinical outcome of autologous osteochondral mosaicplasty technique. Marcacci et al., in a 2-year follow-up publication, Chow et al. as well as Gudas et al. and Solheim et al. reported the same clinical efficacy [4, 8, 20]. Horas et al. reported outstanding clinical results of mosaicplasty in a comparative, prospective study of mosaicplasty versus autologous chondrocyte transplantation [18]. Nakagawa et al. published trochlear results; Matsusue et al. reported successful tibial outcomes [21, 22]. Duchow et al. and Kordás et al. discuss important details of press-fit implantation in their papers [5, 19].

References

1. Bodó G, Hangody L, Módis L (2004) Autologous osteochondral grafting (mosaic arthroplasty) for the treatment of subchondral cystic lesions in the equine stifle and fetlock. Vet Surg 33:588–596
2. Buckwalter JA, Mankin HJ (1998) Articular cartilage restoration. Arthritis Rheum 41:1331–1342
3. Campanacci M, Cervellati C, Donati U (1985) Autogenous patella as replacement for a resected femoral or tibial condyle. A report of 19 cases. J Bone Joint Surg Br 67:557–563
4. Chow JCY, Hantes ME, Houle JB, Zalavras CG (2004) Arthroscopic autogenous osteochondral transplantation for treating knee cartilage defects: a 2- to 5-year follow-up study. Arthroscopy 20:681–690
5. Duchow J, Hess T, Kohn D (2000) Primary stability of press fit-implanted osteochondral grafts: influence of graft size, repeated insertion and harvesting technique. Am J Sports Med 28:24–27
6. Fabbricciani C, Schiavone Panni A, Delcogliano A (1994) Osteochondral autograft in the treatment of osteochondritis dissecans of the knee. In: American Orthopedic Society for Sports Medicine Annual Meeting, Orlando, pp 78–79
7. Feczkó P, Hangody L, Varga J (2003) Experimental results of donor site filling for autologous osteochondral mosaicplasty. Arthroscopy 19(7):755–761
8. Gudas R, Kalesinskas RJ, Kimtys V (2005) A prospective randomized clinical study of mosaic osteochondral autologous transplantation versus microfracture for the treatment of osteochondral defects in the knee joint in young athletes. Arthroscopy 21:1066–1075
9. Hangody L, Kish G, Kárpáti Z, Eberhart R (1997) Osteochondral plugs – autogenous osteochondral mosaicplasty for the treatment of focal chondral and osteochondral articular defects. Oper Tech Orthop 7(4):312–322
10. Hangody L, Kish G, Kárpáti Z et al (1997) Arthroscopic autogenous osteochondral mosaicplasty for the treatment of femoral condylar articular defects. Knee Surg Sports Traumatol Arthrosc 5:262–267
11. Hangody L, Kish G, Kárpáti Z et al (1997) Treatment of osteochondritis dissecans of talus: the use of the mosaicplasty technique. Foot Ankle Int 18(10):628–634
12. Hangody L, Miniaci A, Kish G (1997) MosaicPlasty* osteochondral grafting – technique guide. Smith and Nephew Inc, Andover
13. Hangody L, Feczkó P, Bartha L et al (2001) Mosaicplasty for the treatment of articular defects of the knee and ankle. Clin Orthop 391(Suppl):328–336
14. Hangody L, Duska ZS, Kárpáti Z (2002) Autologous osteochondral mosaicplasty. Tech Knee Surg 1(1):1–10
15. Hangody L, Füles P (2003) Autologous osteochondral mosaicplasty for the treatment of full thickness defects of weight bearing joints – 10 years experimental and clinical experiences. J Bone Joint Surg 85-A(Supplement 2):25–32
16. Hangody L, Duska ZS, Kárpáti Z (2003) Osteochondral plug transplantation. In: Jackson D (ed) Master techniques in orthopaedics; the knee, 2nd edn. Lippincott-Williams-Wilkins, Philadelphia/Baltimore/New York/London/Buenos Aires/Hong Kong/Sydney/Tokyo, pp 337–352
17. Hangody L, Ráthonyi G, Duska ZS et al (2004) Autologous osteochondral mosaicplasty – surgical technique. J Bone Joint Surg 86-A(suppl I):65–72

18. Horas U et al (2003) Autologous chondrocyte implantation and osteochondral cylinder transplantation in cartilage repair of the knee joint. J Bone Joint Surg 85-A:185–192
19. Kordás G, Szabó JS, Hangody L (2005) The effect of drill-hole length on the primary stability of osteochondral grafts in mosaicplasty. Orthopedics 28: 401–404
20. Marcacci M, Kon E, Zaffagnini S, Iacono F, Neri MP, Vascellari A, Visani A, Russo A (2005) Multiple osteochondral arthroscopic grafting (mosaicplasty) for cartilage defects of the knee: prospective study results at 2-year follow-up. Arthroscopy 21: 462–470
21. Matsusue Y, Kotake T, Nakagawa Y et al (2001) Arthroscopic osteochondral autograft transplantation for chondral lesion of the tibial plateau of the knee. Arthroscopy 17(6):653–659
22. Nakagawa Y, Matsusue Y, Suzuki T, Kuroki H, Nakamura T (2004) Osteochondral grafting for cartilage defects in the patellar grooves of bilateral knee joints. Arthroscopy 20:32–38
23. Outerbridge HK, Outerbridge AR, Outerbridge RE (1995) The use of a lateral patellar autologous graft for the repair of a large osteochondral defect in the knee. J Bone Joint Surg Am 77:65–72
24. Pap K, Krompecher I (1961) Arthroplasty of the knee – experimental and clinical experiences. J Bone Joint Surg 43-A:523–537
25. Solheim E (1999) Mosaicplasty in articular cartilage injuries of the knee. Tidsskr Nor Laegeforen 119:4022–4025 (Norwegian)
26. Yamashita F, Sakakida K, Suzu F, Takai S (1985) The transplantation of an auto-generic osteochondral fragment for osteochondritis dissecans of the knee. Clin Orthop 201:43–50

12 Osteochondral Allograft Transplantation For: "Surgical Techniques in Cartilage Repair Surgery"

William Bugbee

Contents

W. Bugbee, MD
Division of Orthopaedic Surgery, Scripps Clinic, 10666 North Torrey Pines Rd, La Jolla, CA 92037, USA

Department of Orthopaedic Surgery, University of California, San Diego, CA, USA
e-mail: bugbee.william@scrippshealth.org

12.1 Principles of the Osteochondral Allografting Technique

The fundamental concept governing fresh osteochondral allografting is the transplantation of architecturally mature hyaline cartilage with living chondrocytes that survive transplantation and are thus capable of supporting the cartilage matrix [1]. Hyaline cartilage possesses characteristics that make it attractive for transplantation. It is an avascular tissue and therefore does not require a blood supply, meeting its metabolic needs through diffusion from synovial fluid. It is an aneural structure and does not require innervation for function. Thirdly, articular cartilage is relatively immunoprivileged, as the chondrocytes are imbedded within a matrix and are relatively protected from host immune surveillance. The second component of the osteochondral allograft is the osseous portion. This functions generally as a support for the articular cartilage, as well as a vehicle to allow attachment and fixation of the graft to the host. The osseous portion of the graft is quite different from the hyaline portion, as it is a vascularized tissue and cells are not thought to survive transplantation; rather, the osseous structure functions as a scaffold for healing to the host by creeping substitution (similar to other types of bone graft). Generally, the osseous portion of the graft is limited to a few millimeters. It is helpful to consider a fresh osteochondral allograft as a composite graft of both bone and cartilage, with a living mature hyaline cartilage portion and a

A.A. Shetty et al. (eds.), *Techniques in Cartilage Repair Surgery*,
DOI 10.1007/978-3-642-41921-8_12, © ESSKA 2014

nonliving subchondral bone portion. It is also helpful to understand the allografting procedure in the context of a tissue or organ transplantation, as the graft essentially is transplanted as an intact structural and functional unit replacing a diseased or absent component in the recipient joint. The transplantation of mature hyaline cartilage obviates the need to rely on techniques that induce cells to form cartilage tissue, which are central to other restorative procedures.

The cornerstone of an allografting procedure is the availability of fresh osteochondral tissue. Currently, small-fragment osteochondral allografts are not HLA or blood-type matched and are utilized fresh rather than frozen or processed. The rationale for fresh tissue is predicated on the concept of maximizing the quality of the articular cartilage in the graft. It has been demonstrated primarily through retrieval studies that viable chondrocytes and relatively preserved cartilage matrix are present many years after transplantation. These experiences have generally supported the use of fresh versus frozen tissue for small osteochondral allografts in the setting of reconstruction of chondral and osteochondral defects. Understanding the process of tissue procurement, testing, and storage is critically important in the allografting procedure. Historically, the obstacles presented have led to the development of fresh allograft programs only at specialized centers that have a close association with an experienced tissue bank and have put significant investment of resources into setting up protocols specific for safe and effective transplantation of fresh osteochondral tissue. Recently, fresh osteochondral grafts have become commercially available in North America and thus more accessible to the orthopaedic surgical community. The age criterion for the donor pool for fresh grafts is generally between 15 and 35 years of age. The joint surface must also pass a visual inspection for cartilage quality. These criteria ensure, but do not guarantee, acceptable tissue for transplantation. It is extremely important to acknowledge that fresh human tissue is unique and no two donors have the same characteristics. Adherence to tissue-banking standards and to protocols and processes in quality control is critical for both safety and efficacy of fresh allografts. Storage of fresh osteochondral allografts prior to transplantation is an important consideration. Historically, fresh grafts were transplanted within 7 days of donor death, obviating the need for prolonged tissue storage. Current tissue bank protocols call for prolonged storage of fresh osteochondral allografts (for up to 60 days) while processing and testing is completed. Recent studies on allograft storage have shown significant deterioration in cell viability, cell density, and metabolic activity with prolonged storage of fresh osteochondral allografts. Small but statistically significant changes are first detected after storage for 7 days; these changes are pronounced after storage for 28 days. The clinical consequences of these storage-induced graft changes have yet to be determined but have been studied in animal models.

12.2 Indications for Osteochondral Allografts

Fresh osteochondral allografts possess the ability to restore a wide spectrum of chondral and osteochondral pathology. As a result, the clinical indications cover a broad range of pathology. In our experience, allografts can be considered as a primary treatment option for osteochondral lesions >2 cm. in diameter, as is typically seen in osteochondritis dissecans and osteonecrosis. Allografts are useful as a revision cartilage restoration procedure when other cartilage treatments, such as microfracture, osteochondral autologous transfer, or autologous chondrocyte implantation, have been unsuccessful. Allografts are also indicated for salvage reconstruction of posttraumatic defects of the tibial plateau, patella, or the femoral condyle. In selected cases, allografts can be used to treat more severe disease situations such as unicompartmental arthrosis.

12.3 Preoperative Preparation: Graft Sizing

The surgical technique for fresh osteochondral allografting depends on the joint and surface to be grafted. Common to all fresh allografting procedures is matching the donor with recipient. This is done on the basis of size. In the knee, an AP radiograph with a magnification marker is used, and a measurement of the medial-lateral dimension of the tibia is made and corrected for magnification. Some surgeons may prefer to use measurements based on MR or CT images, but we have not found this to be more useful than plain radiographs. The tissue bank makes a direct measurement on the donor tibial plateau. Alternatively, a measurement of the affected femoral condyle can be performed. A match is considered acceptable at ± 2–3 mm; however, it should be noted that there is a significant variability in anatomy, which is not reflected in size measurements. In particular, in treating osteochondritis dissecans, the pathologic condyle typically is larger, wider, and flatter; therefore, a larger donor generally should be used.

12.4 Decision Making for Dowel or Shell Technique

The two commonly used techniques for the preparation and implantation of osteochondral allografts include the press-fit plug technique and the shell graft technique. Each technique has advantages and disadvantages. The press-fit plug technique is similar in principle to autologous osteochondral transfer (OAT). A number of commercially available instruments are available (Fig. 12.1). This technique is optimal for contained condylar lesions

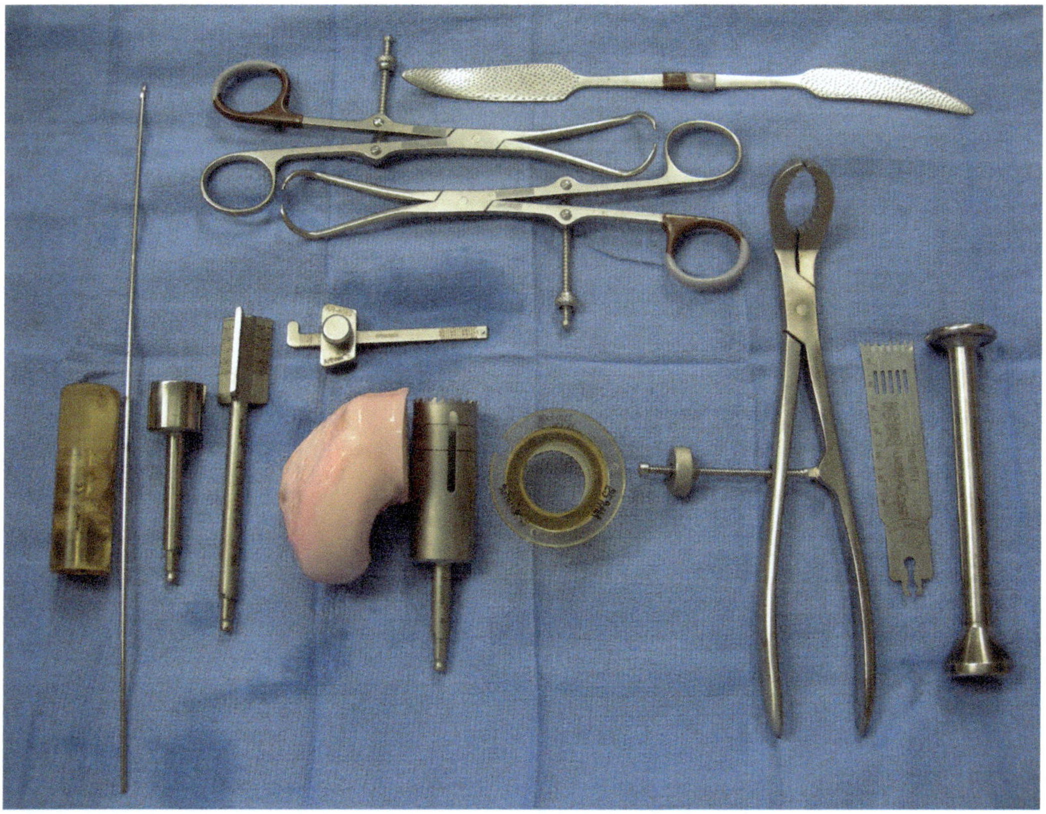

Fig. 12.1 Instruments for preparing dowel graft

between 15 and 35 mm in diameter. Fixation is generally not required due to the stability achieved with the press fit. Disadvantages include the fact that very posterior femoral condyle and tibial plateau lesions are not conducive to the use of a circular coring system and may be more amenable to shell allografts. Additionally, the more ovoid or elongated a lesion is in shape, the more normal cartilage needs to be sacrificed at the recipient site in order to accommodate the circular donor plug. Shell grafts are technically more difficult to perform and typically require fixation. However, depending on the technique employed, less normal cartilage may need to be sacrificed.

12.5 Surgical Approach

The surgical approach for osteochondral allografting involves an arthrotomy of variable size (depending on the position and dimension of the lesion). Usually patients have been previously operated or are at least fully imaged, and the size and location of the lesion(s) are known; otherwise, a diagnostic arthroscopy can be performed prior to the allografting procedure to confirm adequacy of the available graft or to treat coexisting pathology. It is the responsibility of the surgeon to inspect the graft and to confirm the adequacy of the size match and quality of the allograft tissue prior to surgery.

The patient is positioned supine with a proximal thigh tourniquet. A leg or foot holder is extremely helpful to position and maintain the knee in between 70° and 120° of flexion. For most femoral condyle lesions eversion of the patella is not necessary. A standard midline incision is made and elevated subcutaneously, depending on the location of the lesion (either medial or lateral) and the joint entered by incising the fat pad and retinaculum without disrupting the anterior horn of the meniscus or damaging the articular surface. In some cases where the lesion is posterior or very large, the meniscus must be detached and reflected, and, generally, this can be done safely, leaving a small cuff of tissue adjacent to the anterior attachment of the meniscus. Once the joint capsule and synovium have been incised and retractors carefully placed, the knee is brought to a degree of flexion that presents the lesion into the arthrotomy site (Fig. 12.2). Extending the arthrotomy proximal or distal may be necessary to mobilize the extensor mechanism. Once the joint capsule and synovium have been incised and the joint has been entered, retractors are placed medially and laterally to expose the condyle. Care is taken for the positioning of the retractor within the notch, to protect the cruciate ligaments and articular cartilage. The knee is then flexed and/or extended until the proper degree of flexion is noted that presents the lesion into the arthrotomy site.

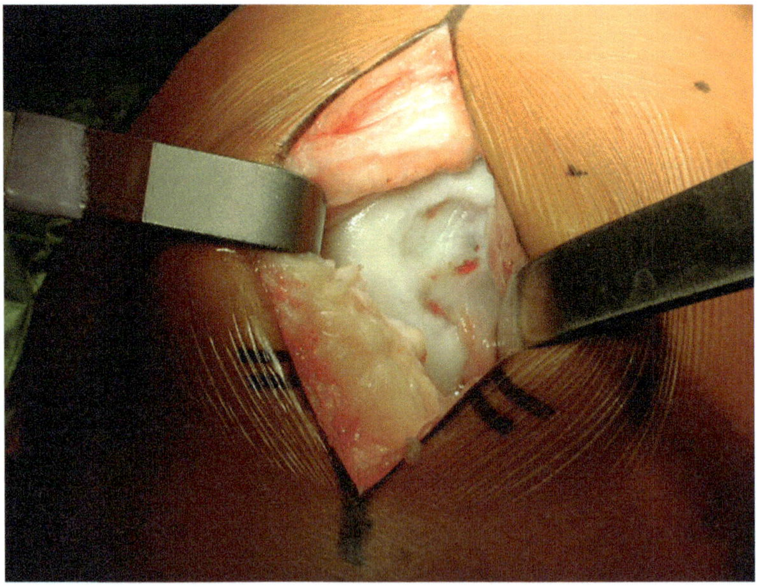

Fig. 12.2 Intraoperative view of the exposed lesion of medial femoral condyle. Note retractor within the femoral notch

12.6 Lesion Inspection and Preparation

The lesion then is inspected and palpated with a probe to determine the extent, margins, and maximum size. The size of the proposed graft then is determined, utilizing sizing dowels. If the lesion falls between two sizes, it is generally preferred to start with the smaller size. At this point the surgeon should also determine if the allograft tissue is adequate in dimension (usually diameter) to harvest the proposed allograft plug (this becomes critical in grafts 25 mm or greater). A guide wire is driven through the sizing dowel into the center of the lesion, perpendicular to the curvature of the articular surface (Fig. 12.3). The cartilage surface is scored, and a special reamer is used to remove the remaining articular cartilage and 3–4 mm of subchondral bone (Fig. 12.4). In deeper lesions, the pathologic bone is removed until there is healthy, bleeding bone. Generally, the preparation depth does not exceed 5–8 mm (Fig. 12.5). It is critical for the surgeon to take care not to inadvertently ream too deep as the

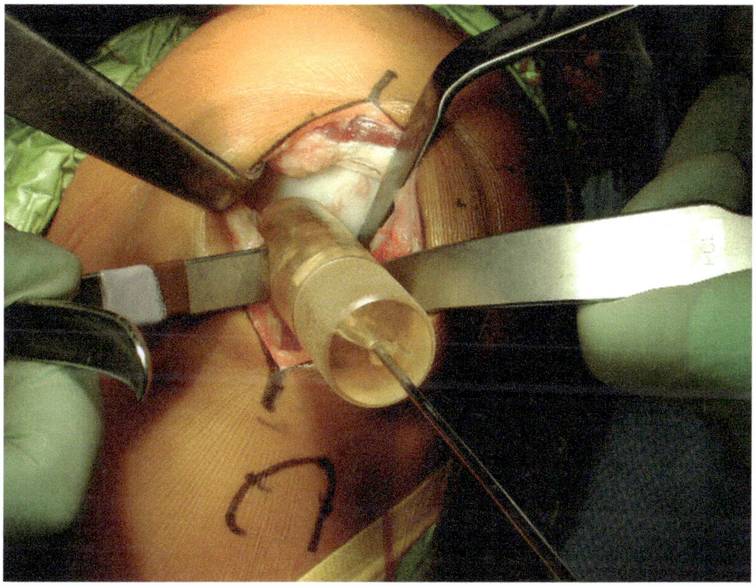

Fig. 12.3 Sizing of lesion and guide pin placement

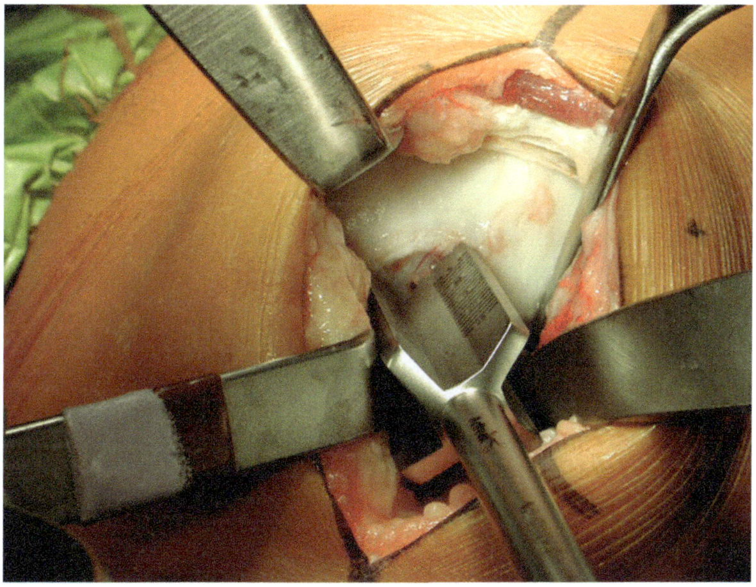

Fig. 12.4 Reaming is performed carefully to desired depth of 5–8 mm. Reaming speed is preferred over drilling for better control and less heat generation

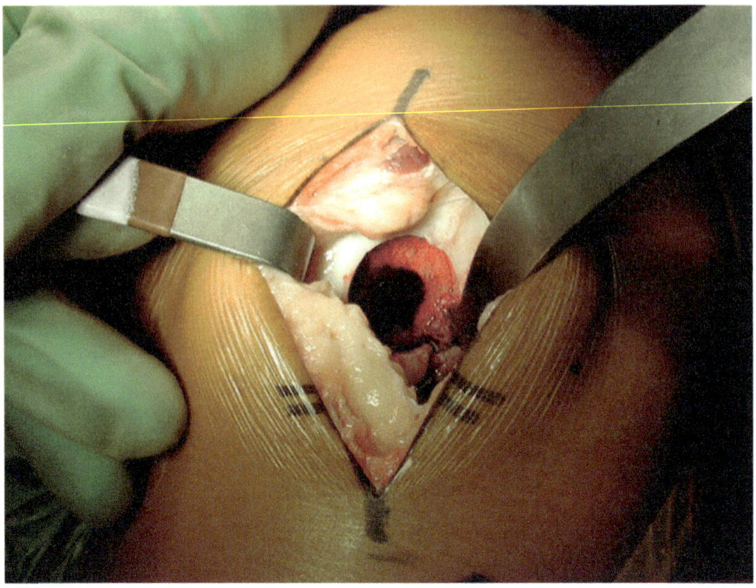

Fig. 12.5 Prepared recipient site. Note bleeding subchondral bone. Depth measurements are made after removal of guide wire

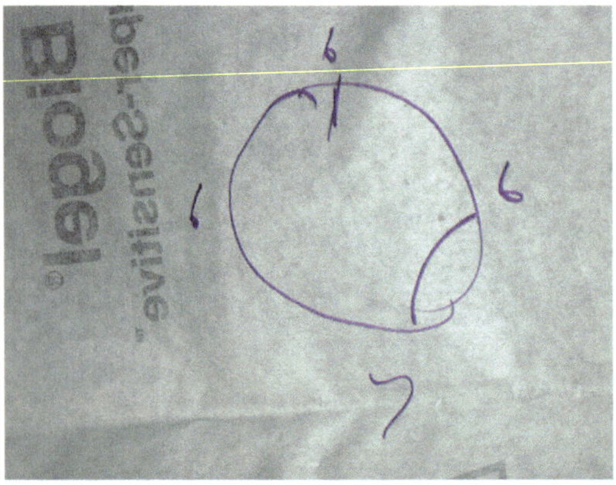

Fig. 12.6 Depth and location map of allograft recipient site to be used in preparation of the donor allograft. The 6 and 7 refer to the measured depths (mm) in each quadrant of the prepared recipient site

bone becomes much softer once the subchondral plate is removed and cancellous bone is encountered. The reamings should be retained for use as bone graft if needed. Bone grafting is performed to fill any deeper or more extensive osseous defects or to modify the fit of the graft if there is a depth mismatch between the recipient socket and allograft plug. At this point the guide pin can be removed and depth measurements are made and recorded in the four quadrants of the prepared recipient site (Fig. 12.6).

12.7 Graft Preparation

The corresponding anatomic location of the recipient site then is identified on the graft. The graft is placed into a graft holder (or alternately, held with bone-holding forceps). A saw guide then is placed in the appropriate position, again perpendicular to the articular surface, exactly matching the orientation used to create the recipient site. The appropriate size matched coring saw is used to core out the graft (Fig. 12.7). The graft can be cut from the donor condyle and removed as a long plug (Fig. 12.8). The allograft plug thickness now must be adjusted. Depth measurements, which were taken from the recipient, are transferred to the graft (Fig. 12.9). The graft is mounted on the graft holder, which serves as a cutting guide and cut with an oscillating saw. Often, this must be done multiple times to ensure precise thickness, matching the prepared defect in the patient (Fig. 12.10). It is also helpful at this time to bevel the edge of the osseous portion of the graft with a small rongeur or rasp to facilitate initial fitting into the recipient socket. The graft should be irrigated copiously with a high-pressure lavage to remove all marrow elements.

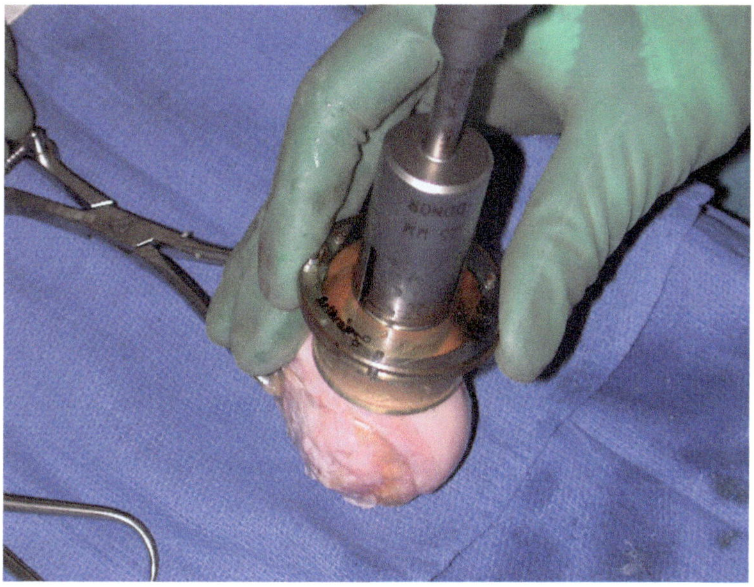

Fig. 12.7 Donor coring saw, saw guide, and medial condyle allograft. Saw guide is placed on the allograft perpendicular to the articular surface at the desired site of graft harvest, and coring saw is used to harvest the graft

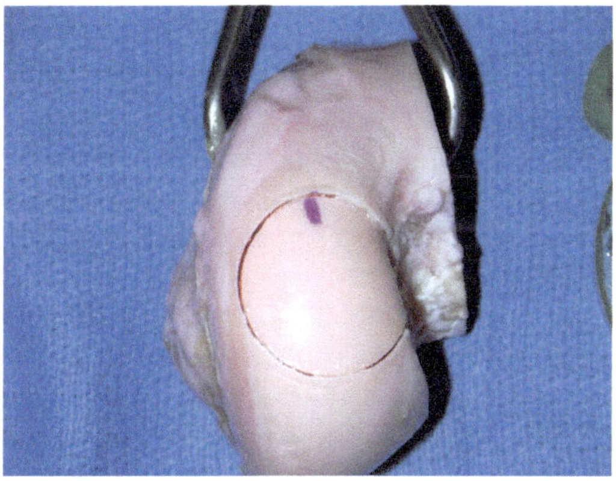

Fig. 12.8 Donor condyle after use of coring saw. Note anatomic location corresponds to lesion site

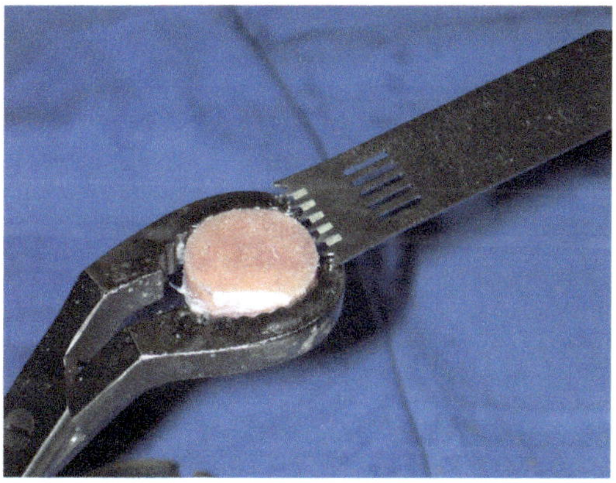

Fig. 12.10 The graft is placed on a graft holder and excess bone is removed with oscillating saw

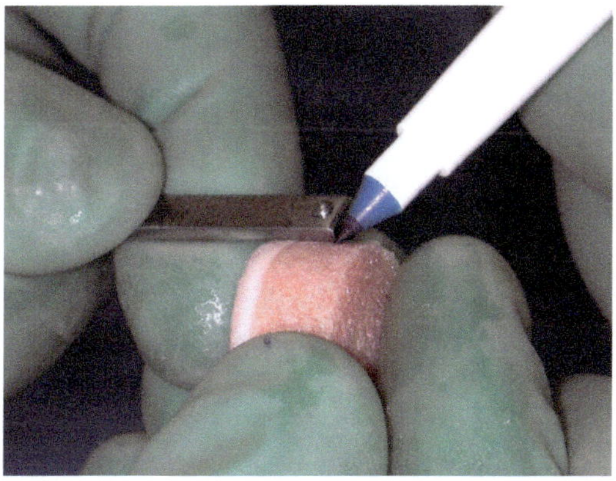

Fig. 12.9 After graft is removed from hemicondyle with oscillating saw, the recipient site measurements are transferred to allograft plug

12.8 Graft Insertion

The graft is then inserted by hand in the appropriate rotation and is gently pressed into place manually (Fig. 12.11). To fully seat the graft, the joint can be carefully brought through a range of motion, allowing the opposing articular surface to seat the graft. Finally, very gentle tamping can be performed to fully seat the graft. Excessive and forceful striking of the graft should be avoided as this leads to chondrocyte necrosis [2]. If the graft does not fit easily, the recipient site can be dilated or reamed again. The graft itself can be further trimmed or beveled. Occasionally,

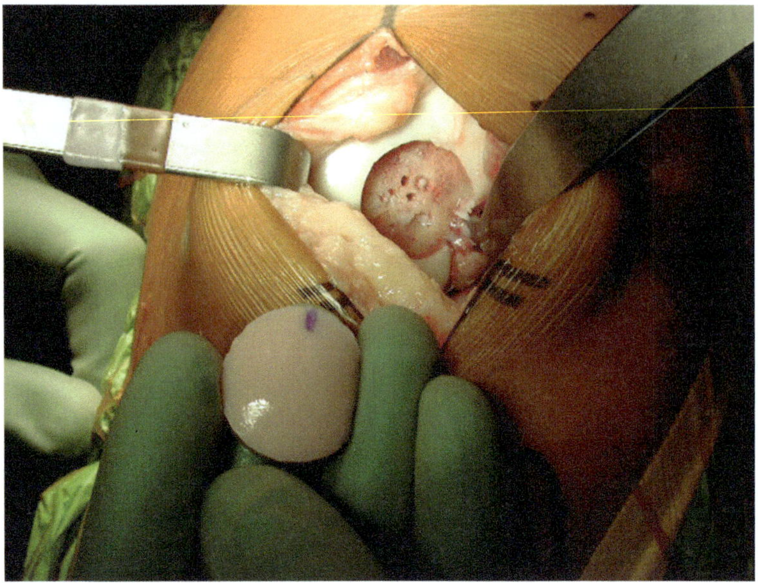

Fig. 12.11 The allograft is ready to be inserted after the graft dimensions and orientation are rechecked, bony edges slightly rounded to facilitate insertion, and the graft lavaged

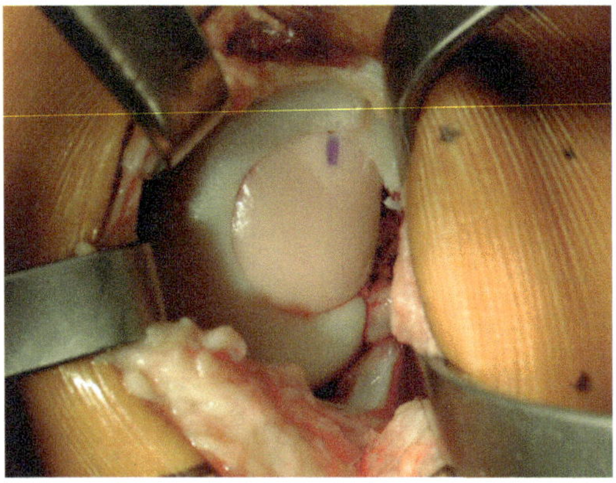

Fig. 12.12 The graft after insertion. Joint compression and range of motion is used to initially seat graft. Gentle tamping can be used for final seating

overhanging cartilage on the margins of the recipient socket or in the graft itself prevents seating, and this can be trimmed with a #15 scalpel blade. Once the graft is seated (Fig. 12.12), a determination is made whether additional fixation is required. Absorbable pins or chondral darts can be utilized. The knee is then brought through a complete range of motion, in order to confirm that the graft is stable and there is no catching or soft-tissue obstruction noted.

12.9 Shell Allograft Technique

Although the dowel or plug allograft method is generally preferred for most lesions, the surgeon should be prepared to perform a shell graft if the lesion size or location does not allow for proper placement of the dowel graft instruments. For the shell graft technique, the defect is identified through the previously described arthrotomy, and the dimensions of the lesion are marked with a surgical pen. Minimizing the sacrifice of normal cartilage, a geometric shape, such as a rectangle or trapezoid, is created that is amenable to hand crafting a shell graft. A #15 scalpel blade is used to demarcate the lesion, and sharp ring curettes are used to remove all tissue inside this mark. Using motorized burrs, sharp curettes, and osteotomes, the subchondral bone is removed down to a depth of 4–5 mm. The shape is transferred to the graft using length, width, and depth measurements or a foil template. A saw is used to cut the basic graft shape from the donor condyle, initially slightly oversizing the graft by a few millimeters. Excess bone and cartilage is removed as necessary through multiple trial fittings. The graft and host bed are then copiously irrigated and the graft placed flush with the articular surface. The need for fixation is based on the degree of inherent stability. Bioabsorbable pins are typically used when fixation is required, but countersunk compression screws may be used as an alternative. After cycling the knee through a full range of motion to ensure graft stability, standard closure is performed.

12.10 Postoperative Management

Initial postoperative management includes attention to control of pain and swelling and restoration of limb control and range of motion. Patients generally are maintained on touchdown weight bearing for 4–6 weeks, depending on the size of the graft and stability of fixation. Patients with patellofemoral grafts are allowed weight bearing as tolerated in extension and generally are limited to 45° of flexion for the first 4 weeks, utilizing an immobilizer or range-of-motion brace. Closed chain exercise such as cycling is introduced between weeks 2 and 4. Weight bearing is progressed slowly between the second and fourth month, with full weight bearing utilizing a cane or crutch. Full weight bearing and normal gait pattern are generally tolerated between the third and fourth month. Recreation and sports are not reintroduced until joint rehabilitation is complete and radiographic healing has been demonstrated, which generally occurs no earlier than 6 months postoperatively

12.11 Potential Complications

Early complications unique to the allografting procedure are few. There does not appear to be any increased risk of surgical site infection with the use of allografts as compared with other procedures. The use of a mini-arthrotomy in the knee decreases the risk of postoperative stiffness. Occasionally, one sees a persistent effusion, which is typically a sign of overuse but which may indicate an immune-mediated synovitis. Delayed union or nonunion of the fresh allograft is the most common early finding. This is evidenced by persistent discomfort and/or visible graft-host interface on serial radiographic evaluation. Delayed union or nonunion is more common in larger grafts, such as those used in the tibial plateau or in the setting of compromised bone, such as in the treatment of osteonecrosis. In this setting, patience is essential and complete healing or recovery may take an extended period. Decreasing activities, the institution of weight-bearing precautions, or use of braces may be helpful in the early management of delayed healing. In this setting, careful evaluation of serial radiographs can provide insight into the healing process, and MRI scans are rarely diagnostic, particularly prior to 6 months postoperatively, as they typically show extensive signal abnormality that is difficult to interpret. The natural history of the graft that fails to osseointegrate is unpredictable. Clinical symptoms may be minimal, or there may be progressive clinical deterioration and radiographic evidence of fragmentation, fracture, or collapse.

Treatment options for failed allografts include observation, if the patient is minimally symptomatic and the joint is thought to be at low risk for further progression of disease. Arthroscopic evaluation and debridement also may be utilized in many cases; revision allografting is performed and generally has led to a success rate equivalent to primary allografting. This appears to be one of the particular advantages to fresh osteochondral allografting, in that fresh allografting does not preclude a revision allograft as a salvage procedure for failure of the initial allograft. In cases of more extensive joint disease, particularly in older individuals, conversion to prosthetic arthroplasty is appropriate.

12.12 Results

Garrett [3] first reported on 17 patients treated with fresh osteochondral allografts for OCD of the lateral femoral condyle utilizing a dowel technique. All patients had failed previous surgery, and in a 2-to-9-year follow-up period, 16 out of 17 patients were reported as asymptomatic. Emmerson et al. [4] reported our experience in the treatment of osteochondritis dissecans of the medial and lateral femoral condyle. Sixty-nine knees in 66 patients were evaluated at a mean of 5.2 years postoperatively. All allografts were implanted within 5 days of procurement. Forty-nine males and 17 females, with a mean age of 28 years (range 15–54), underwent allografting using either the dowel or shell technique. Forty lesions involved the medial femoral condyle and 29 the lateral femoral condyle. An average of 1.6 surgeries had been performed on the knee prior to the allograft procedure. Allograft size was highly variable, with a range from 1 to 13 cm^2. The average allograft size was 7.4 cm^2. Overall, 53/67 (79 %) knees were rated good or excellent, 10/67 (15 %) were rated fair; and 6/67 (6 %) were rated poor. Six patients had reoperations on the allograft: one was converted to total knee arthroplasty, and five underwent revision allografting at 1, 2, 5, 7, and 8 years after the initial allograft. Forty-nine out of 66 patients completed questionnaires: 96 % reported satisfaction with their treatment; 86 % reported less pain. Subjective knee function improved from a mean of 3.5–7.9 on a ten-point scale.

Chu et al. [5] reported on 55 consecutive knees undergoing osteochondral allografting. This group included patients with diagnoses such as traumatic chondral injury, avascular necrosis, osteochondritis dissecans, and patellofemoral disease. The mean age of this group was 35.6 years, with follow-up averaging 75 months (range 11–147 months). Of the 55 knees, 43 were unipolar replacements and 12 were bipolar resurfacing replacements. In this mixed patient population, 42/55 (76 %) of these knees were rated good to excellent, and 3/55 were rated fair, for an overall success rate of 82 %. It is important to note that 84 % of the knees that underwent unipolar femoral grafts were rated good to excellent, and only 50 % of the knees with bipolar grafts achieved good or excellent status.

Aubin et al. [6] reported on the Toronto experience with fresh osteochondral allografts of the femoral condyle. Sixty knees were reviewed with a mean follow-up of 10 years (range 58–259 months). The etiology of the osteochondral lesion was trauma in 36, osteochondritis in 17, osteonecrosis in 6, and arthrosis in one. Realignment osteotomy was performed in 41 patients and meniscal transplantation in 17. Twelve knees required graft removal or conversion to total knee arthroplasty. The remaining 48 patients averaged a Hospital for Special Surgery Score of 83 points. The authors reported 85 % graft survivorship at 10 years.

Williams et al. [7] reported on the outcome of 19 fresh, hypothermically stored allografts, with a mean time to implantation from graft recovery of 30 days. At minimum 2-year follow-up, all patients showed functional improvement, and magnetic resonance imaging demonstrated normal cartilage signal in 18 of 19 grafts and complete or partial osseous incorporation in 14 grafts.

McCulloch et al. [8] reported on a series of 25 fresh, stored osteochondral allografts of the femoral condyle. Statistically significant improvements were seen in all outcome measures, and 22 of 25 were radiographically incorporated into host bone. LaPrade et al. [9] reported on 23 patients treated with osteochondral allografts for focal femoral condyle lesions. At a mean follow-up of 3 years, 22 of 23 grafts were stable and incorporated. Cincinnati and IKDC scores demonstrated significant improvement in this cohort. Most recently Levy reported survivorship of 82 % at 10 years and 74 % at 15 years in a series of 129 femoral condyle allografts performed at our institution.

12.13 Summary

Osteochondral allografting is an extremely useful and versatile technique for managing difficult or complex chondral or osteochondral lesions. The surgical technique relies on common and straightforward principles. Great care should be taken in handling and preparation of the graft. The advantage of allografting lies in its ability to restore both osseous and chondral components of a defect. Reported clinical outcomes are favorable in short and intermediate term.

References

1. Czitrom AA, Keating S, Gross AE (1990) The viability of articular cartilage in fresh osteochondral allografts after clinical transplantation. J Bone Joint Surg Am 72(4):574–581
2. Borazjani BH, Chen AC, Bae WC, Patil S, Sah RL, Firestein GS, Bugbee WD (2006) Effect of Impact on Chondrocyte Viability During the Insertion of Human Osteochondral Grafts. J Bone Joint Surg Am 88A(9):1934–1943
3. Garrett JC (1994) Fresh osteochondral allografts for treatment of articular defects in osteochondritis dissecans of the lateral femoral condyle in adults. Clin Orthop Relat Res 303:33–37
4. Emmerson BC, Gortz S, Jamali AA, Chung C, Amiel D, Bugbee WD (2007) Fresh osteochondral allografting in the treatment of osteochondritis dissecans of the femoral condyle. Am J Sports Med 35(6):907–914
5. Chu CR, Convery FR, Akeson WH, Meyers M, Amiel D (1999) Articular cartilage transplantation. Clinical results in the knee. Clin Orthop Relat Res 360:159–168
6. Aubin PP, Cheah HK, Davis AM, Gross AE (2001) Long-term followup of fresh femoral osteochondral allografts for posttraumatic knee defects. Clin Orthop Relat Res (391 Suppl):S318–327
7. Williams RJ 3rd, Ranawat AS, Potter HG, Carter T, Warren RF (2007) Fresh stored allografts for the treatment of osteochondral defects of the knee. J Bone Joint Surg Am 89(4):718–726
8. McCulloch PC, Kang RW, Sobhy MH, Hayden JK, Cole BJ (2007) Prospective evaluation of prolonged fresh osteochondral allograft transplantation of the femoral condyle: minimum 2-year follow-up. Am J Sports Med 35(3):411–420
9. LaPrade RF, Botker J, Herzog M, Agel J (2009) Refrigerated osteoarticular allografts to treat articular cartilage defects of the femoral condyles. A prospective outcomes study. J Bone Joint Surg Am 91(4):805–811

Suggested Reading

Bonner KF, Bugbee WD (2004) Osteochondral allografting in the knee. In: Mark M, Cole B (eds) Textbook of arthroscopy. Saunders, St. Louis, pp 611–623

Bugbee WD (2004) Osteochondral allograft transplantation. In: Cole B, Mike Malek M (eds) Articular cartilage lesions: a practical guide toward assessment and treatment. Springer, New York, pp 82–94

Bugbee W (2008) Allograft osteochondral plugs. In: Jackson DW (ed) Reconstructive knee surgery, 3rd edn. Lippincott Williams & Wilkins, Philadelphia, pp 475–483

Görtz S, Bugbee WD (2006) Allografts in articular cartilage repair. J Bone Joint Surg Am 88(6):1374–1384

ESSKA Book Series – Techniques in Cartilage Repair Surgery Minced Cartilage: DeNovo and CAIS

13

Jaskarndip Chahal and Brian J. Cole

Contents

J. Chahal, MD, MSc, FRCSC (✉)
University of Toronto Orthopaedic Sports Medicine (UTOSM), Toronto Western Hospital and Women's College Hospital, 399 Bathurst Street–1 East 447, Toronto, ON M5T 2S8, Canada
e-mail: jchahal@utosm.com

B.J. Cole, MD, MBA
Division of Sports Medicine, Rush University Medical Center, 1611 W. Harrison St., Suite 300, Chicago, IL 60612, USA

13.1 Introduction

The burden of illness related to articular cartilage injury of the knee is significant as the prevalence of isolated cartilage injuries has been reported to be approximately 5 % in the general population [14]. A prospective study demonstrated chondral or osteochondral lesions in 61 % of patients, whereas focal defects were found in 19 %. The prevalence of work- and sports-related osteochondral injuries has been estimated to be even higher at 22–50 % [14, 19]. Such injuries can be an important cause of pain, swelling, decreased quality of life, and disability in patients of all ages and represent a significant economic burden on the health-care system [20].

The natural history of focal full-thickness chondral lesions is at best nonprogressive and more likely to continue to enlarge by circumferential expansion. This results in the exposure of increasing amounts of subchondral bone, potentially predisposing the knee to accelerated arthritis [3, 4, 19]. As a result this progression, there has been an emphasis in determining the most favorable surgical technique for the management of such injuries. The ideal surgical approach will generate hyaline cartilage in the defect; recreate normal articular congruity; improve overall functioning, disability, and health; and ultimately prevent the onset of osteoarthritis [3, 4, 7, 19]. At the present time, there are no surgical repair techniques that have satisfied all of these requisite conditions.

A.A. Shetty et al. (eds.), *Techniques in Cartilage Repair Surgery*,
DOI 10.1007/978-3-642-41921-8_13, © ESSKA 2014

Current surgical treatment options for symptomatic cartilage lesions include debridement, marrow-stimulation techniques (e.g. microfracture), osteochondral autograft transplantation system (OATS), fresh osteochondral allograft (OCA), and autologous chondrocyte implantation (ACI) [9]. The concept of using particulated articular cartilage, either as an autograft or allograft, is an emerging concept wherein a few years ago, the idea that chondral grafts alone could be transplanted without an underlying bony component and heal to the recipient site was not widely accepted [9]. This preconceived notion was related to the idea that the ability of chondrocytes to migrate in vivo from their native lacunae site is limited due to the rigidity of the extracellular matrix as well as due to the paucity of cells in articular cartilage, absence of a vascular supply, and exceptional mechanical demands [7, 15].

In 1983, Albrecht and colleagues were the first to demonstrate in a rabbit model that cartilage autograft implantation without bone can lead to defect healing if the cartilage is cut into small pieces [2]. Over two decades later, Lu et al. demonstrated that minced cartilage without cell culture served as an effective intraoperative cell source for cartilage repair [15]. The authors demonstrated that (1) there is an inverse relationship between cartilage fragment size and amount of cartilage outgrowth, (2) the highest level of cellular activity was localized at the minced cartilage edge, and (3) the amount of tissue required approximated one tenth of the area of the entire defect to be treated [15]. It was hypothesized that chondrocytes in the cartilage pieces were able to "escape" from the ECM, migrate, multiply, and form the observed hyaline-like cartilage tissue matrix that integrated with the surrounding host tissue [9, 15]. Unlike cultured chondrocytes that have a spindle-shaped morphology, chondrocytes from the minced cartilage displayed the standard chondrocyte spheroid phenotype [15]. Frisbie et al. also suggested that by reimplanting cartilage fragments immediately into the joint, the fragments are subjected to the normal joint environment which in turn may theoretically serve as the ideal in vivo bioreactor [12].

There are several practical advantages that arise from the use of particulated cartilage when compared with other cartilage repair procedures. Unlike microfracture, there is no violation of the subchondral bone plate [9]. The OATS procedure can only be used for defects smaller than 1–2 cm.[27] Furthermore, there is no need for the creation of a subchondral defect as required with OATS or OCA which in turn obviates the requirement for bony incorporation and may avoid complications such as necrosis or collapse [9]. Finally, compared with ACI, there is no requirement for an exogenous cell culture which in turn helps reduce the cost associated with surgery as well as the need for a second downstream procedure [9, 16, 17].

Currently available products which utilize particulated articular cartilage include the Cartilage Autograft Implantation System (CAIS: DePuy/Mitek, Raynham, MA) and DeNovo Natural Tissue (NT: ISTO, St. Louis, MO). Both CAIS and DeNovo products are small cartilage fragments which serve as a source of viable chondrocytes that can migrate into the surrounding matrix and collagen [17]. In regard to CAIS, autogenous cartilage tissue is processed intraoperatively and loaded onto a scaffold and the resultant construct is fixed into place with bio-absorbable staples [7, 9]. With DeNovo NT, allogeneic juvenile cartilage tissue is processed in advance, is available "on the shelf," and is fixed in place using fibrin glue [6, 11]. With DeNovo, the use of allograft tissue allows for the treatment of very large defects, and the juvenile source of the chondrocytes has the potential for more robust cellular activity than older cartilage tissue [1, 18]. Within the context of tissue engineering, both technologies utilize two requisite features – (1) a bioactive component (i.e., cells or chondrocytes) which drives the biological process and (2) a biomaterial that serves as a carrier or scaffold which in turn provides architectural support and facilitates integration of repaired tissue with contiguous tissue [7]. In essence, the particulate nature of both grafts allows for an optimization of graft surface area for cartilage expansion, and the use of cells and scaffolds creates the potential for a chondro-inductive and chondro-conductive milieu, respectively [16].

13.2 Technical Details

13.2.1 DeNovo NT (NT:ISTO, St. Louis, MO)

DeNovo NT is considered a "minimally manipulated" human tissue allograft, regulated in the United States as a 361 HCT/P product similar to fresh osteochondral allograft, allograft meniscus transplants, and bone-tendon-bone allografts [8, 9]. It is available for clinical application without investigational device exemption [9]. The graft is prepared by removing live cartilage tissue from fresh cadaveric juvenile femoral condyles (up to age 13) and particulating them manually into cubes of approximately 1 cm^3 [11]. The tissue pieces are then packaged into sealed blister packs which contain a proprietary storage medium developed by ISTO Technologies, Inc. (St. Louis, Mo., United States) and are shipped in an aseptic temperature controlling package.

13.2.2 CAIS (DePuy/Mitek, Raynham, MA)

The CAIS involves an instrument which harvests cartilage from an autogenous donor site and distributes the cartilage fragments homogeneously onto an absorbable 3-dimensional (3D) scaffold which consists of 35 % polycaprolactone and 65 % polyglycolic acid and is further reinforced with a polydioxanone (PDO) mesh (Advanced Technologies and Regenerative Medicine, Raynham, MA) [7, 9]. This scaffold is a foam-like material that serves to keep the tissue fragments in place and provides a 3D environment for cartilage matrix generation. The cartilage-scaffold construct is secured to the recipient site using PDO staples [9, 17]. At the present time, CAIS is in the midst of a phase III comparative trial versus microfracture as part of the FDA regulatory process to gain clearance in the United States. It is not currently available for clinical use outside of the multicenter study sites.

13.3 Patient Selection

Patients with symptomatic isolated International Cartilage Repair Society (ICRS) grade III or IV lesions in the femoral or tibial condyles or in the patellofemoral joint are eligible for treatment with DeNovo NT or CAIS. Although no size limitations have been formally recommended, previous reports have suggested that chondral lesions should range in size from 1 to 5 cm^2 [9]. Coexisting malalignment as well as meniscal or ligamentous deficiency is treated concomitantly as required. Patients who undergo patellofemoral procedures will also be treated with an anteromedialization of the tibial tuberosity [5, 10]. Associated patellar instability can be addressed with a medial patellofemoral ligament repair or reconstruction.

Relative contraindications for CAIS and DeNovo NT include bipolar lesions > ICRS grade II, significant underlying bony edema, or osteochondral defects with more than 6 mm of subchondral bone loss [9]. In the latter two situations, our preferred treatment is to use a fresh osteochondral allograft.

13.4 Preoperative Planning

All patients will undergo routine radiographs (anteroposterior, 45° flexion posteroanterior, lateral, skyline) and 1.5 T magnetic resonance imaging (MRI) of the knee to facilitate the preoperative planning process. In cases where there is a clinical concern for malalignment in the coronal or transverse plane, 3'foot standing anteroposterior x-rays (to evaluate the mechanical axis) and computed tomography of the knee (to assess the tibial tuberosity-trochlear groove distance) are ordered, respectively. When patients have had previous surgical procedures, operative reports and arthroscopy photographs are requested to evaluate the status of the cruciate ligaments, articular cartilage, and possible extent of prior meniscal resection.

13.5 Patient Setup

When a concomitant cruciate ligament reconstruction or meniscus allograft transplant is performed, the ipsilateral leg is secured in a leg holder and the contralateral extremity is positioned in a holder with the hip flexed, abducted, and externally rotated. The bed is "reflexed," the end of the operating table is lowered, and the operative extremity is allowed to flex with manual assistance up to 120°. In all other situations, the patient is positioned in the supine position with a lateral post. A tourniquet is applied to the proximal thigh. The knee is prepped and draped in a sterile fashion, and the tourniquet is then inflated.

13.6 Surgical Approach

13.6.1 Diagnostic Arthroscopy

Standard inferomedial and inferolateral arthroscopic portals are established to perform a diagnostic arthroscopy which involves a detailed examination of the patellofemoral, medial, and lateral compartments. Focal cartilage defects are identified and debrided with an arthroscopic shaver in order to allow for defect measurement with an arthroscopic probe. After peripheral cartilage debridement, lesion size should range from 1 to 5 cm^2. For the CAIS procedure, autologous cartilage is harvested at this point in the operation using a specialized instrument (see below).

13.6.2 Exposure

Patellofemoral Joint

A limited anterior midline incision is made from the superior aspect of the patella to a point 2–4 cm below proximal aspect of the tibial tubercle. This is extended as necessary to improve access. Medial and lateral subcutaneous flaps are developed (Fig. 13.1). This is followed by a lateral parapatellar arthrotomy which is commenced just distal to the insertion of the vastus lateralis. Care is taken to avoid iatrogenic injury to anterior horn on the lateral meniscus during exposure. This lateral release is extended distally into the anterolateral compartment – as the exposure is taken distal, an incision is made just lateral to the patellar tendon and subsequently 5 mm lateral to the tibial crest. Once the anterolateral compartment fascia in incised, we then elevate the anterolateral compartment musculature off the tibia using blunt dissection with a Cobb elevator. The posterolateral edge of the tibia is identified, and a Chandler retractor is placed posterolaterally to protect the neurovascular structures.

Next, the T3® *AMZ* System (Arthrex, Naples, FL) with the guide at 60° of inclination is utilized, and a tibial tubercle osteotomy is performed in the standard fashion (Fig. 13.1) [10]. The tibial tubercle wafer of bone, which measures 8–10 cm in length, is moved anteromedially by approximately 10 mm. Fixation is performed with two countersunk 4.5-mm cortical screws in compression (lag) mode (Fig. 13.1). Local bone graft is obtained from the anteromedial aspect of the tibial tuberosity and placed anterolaterally in the defect that remains following translation of the tibial tubercle.

Tibiofemoral Joint

An incision along the medial or lateral border of the patella is made depending on the location of the chondral defect. The incision commences at the equator of the patella and is extended to the level of the joint line with the knee in 90° of flexion. A mini-arthrotomy is performed, and care is taken not to violate the anterior horn of the medial and/or lateral meniscus. In addition, on the medial side a vastus sparing approach is utilized to minimize impairment postoperatively.

13.6.3 Defect Preparation

For both the CAIS and DeNovo techniques, a 15-blade scalpel is used to create a contained chondral defect with clean vertical walls – the ideal construct will have 90° margins around the

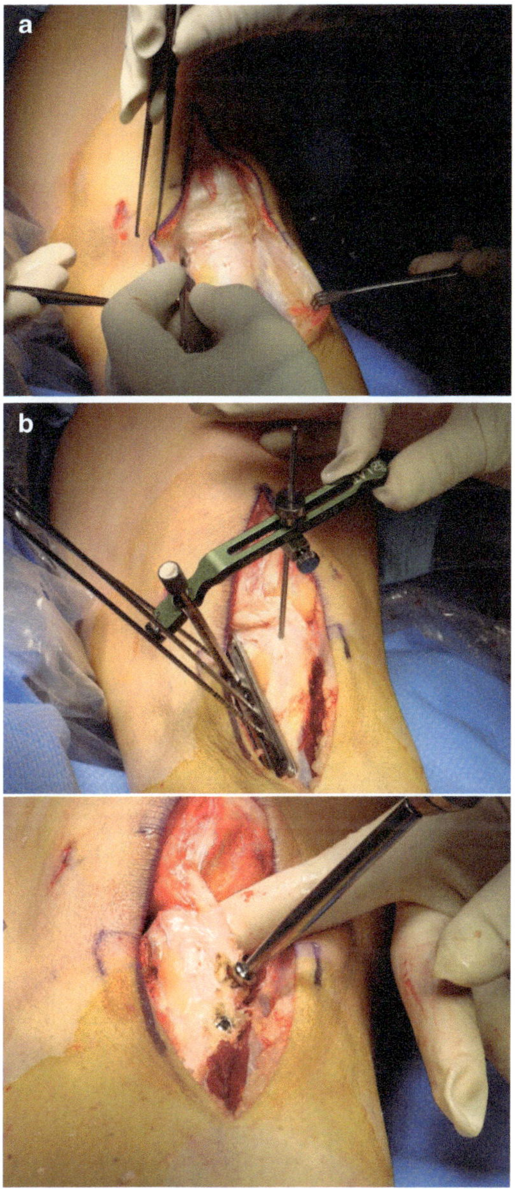

Fig. 13.1 Exposure for an associated anteromedialization procedure. (a) Exposure. (b) Anteromedialization of the tibial tubercle

periphery of the defect. All damaged tissue will be removed to but not through the level of the subchondral bone using a ring curette. At this point, the tourniquet is deflated, and hemostasis is achieved with a combination of epinephrine soaked sponges and small amounts of fibrin glue. A sterile paper or thin aluminum foil template is then used to size the defect.

13.6.4 Implantation

CAIS

After diagnostic arthroscopy, hyaline cartilage is arthroscopically harvested from the lateral wall of the intercondylar notch or trochlear ridge with an amount similar to that for ACI (200–300 mg) using a unique device that minces cartilage into 1–2 mm pieces. After harvest, this device (DePuy/Mitek, Raynham, MA) uniformly disperses the minced cartilage onto the aforementioned 3D scaffold to which fixation is achieved using fibrin glue (Fig. 13.2). The scaffold/cartilage construct is cut and sized according to the paper or foil template. After this, the trimmed CAIS scaffold implant is transferred to the defect with the cartilage fragments facing the subchondral bone and is affixed in situ with 2–4 PDO staples placed circumferentially around the edges of the graft construct (Advanced Technologies and Regenerative Medicine, Raynham, MA) (Fig. 13.2) [7, 9].

DeNovo NT

Thin aluminum foil is pressed into the defect to create a 3D mold. Once formed, the mold is removed and its surface area is calculated – one package of DeNovo NT covers 2.5 cm^2. Following this, the medium in which the DeNovo NT is contained is aspirated, and the particulate cartilage fragments are transferred to the mold spaced 1–2 mm apart. Fibrin glue is subsequently applied to the fragments of cartilage until the mold is filled to within 1 mm of its total depth. After a curing time of 3–10 min, fibrin glue is also applied to the base of the defect; the cartilage-fibrin glue construct is separated off the foil and is pressed into the defect. The total curing time for the final construct (Fig. 13.3) is approximately 10 min [6, 9, 11].

13.7 Potential Complications and Troubleshooting

Prior to proceeding with surgical repair of any chondral defect, it is imperative to address concomitant pathology in the form of malalignment, ligamentous instability, or an absent or functionally deficient meniscus. Failure to address such

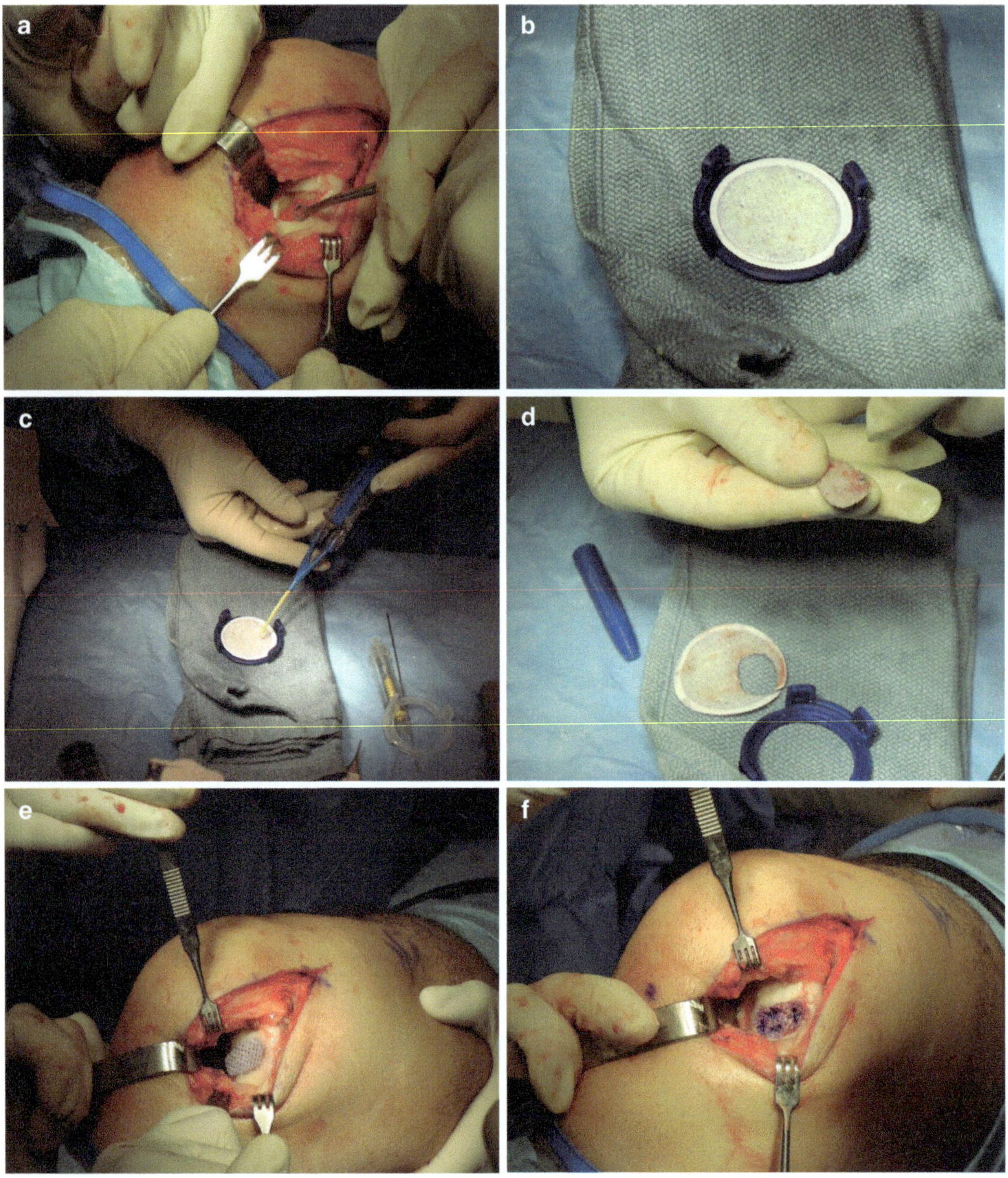

Fig. 13.2 CAIS procedure. (**a**) Defect preparation and sizing. (**b**) Harvested cartilage placed on the copolymer scaffold. (**c**) Application of fibrin glue. (**d**) The scaffold is sized and cut according to the prepared defect. (**e**) CAIS scaffold implant placed and fixed in situ. (**f**) In situ fixation with PDO staples

pathology can lead to premature failure of any cartilage repair treatment option.

For the DeNovo NT procedure, it is also important to note that the fibrin glue-cartilage tissue construct is recessed relative to the surrounding cartilage shoulders in order to minimize the potential for shear or compressive forces [11].

13.8 Rehabilitation

A comprehensive postoperative rehabilitation program is performed according to established protocols [19]. In general the rehabilitation program is focused initially on protection of the cartilage repair process and then progressed towards

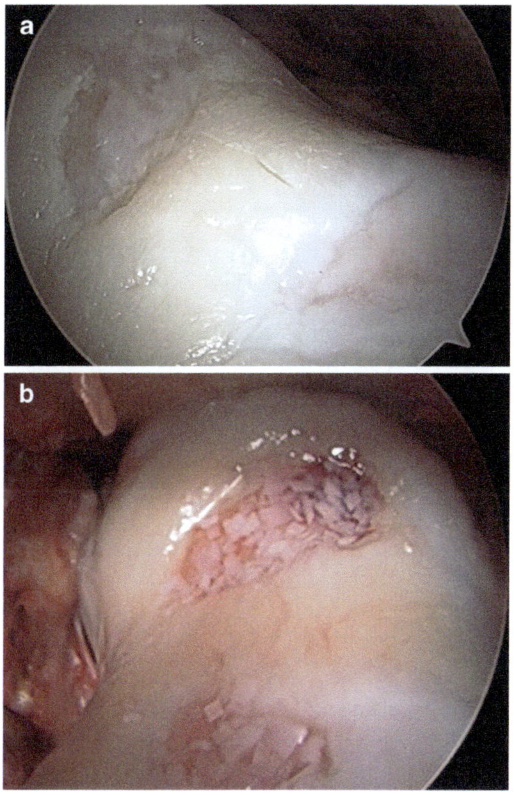

Fig. 13.3 DeNovo NT procedure. (**a**) Arthroscopic visualization of two trochlear defects. (**b**) Application of DeNovo NT after debridement and sizing

controlled loading, increased range of motion, and progressive muscle strengthening [7]. Specifically, the patient with condylar lesions are kept toe-touch weight bearing for a period of 6 weeks, whereas individuals with patellofemoral lesions can weight bear as tolerated in extension. Furthermore, a hinged knee brace is locked in extension postoperatively. Continuous passive motion is started on the first postoperative day for 8 h/day [13, 19, 21]. For condylar defects, range of motion from 0° to 45° is permitted for the first four weeks and is subsequently increased as tolerated to 90° over the ensuing 3 weeks. For patellar or trochlear defects, range of motion from 0° to 30° is allowed for the first 2 weeks and is increased by 30° increments up to the 6 week mark. After 6 weeks, patients may progress to full weight bearing and full range of motion as tolerated. Muscle strength is maintained through isometric quadriceps sets, straight leg raises, isometric contraction of the hamstrings, hip abductors, and hip adductors. Return to low-load activities at weeks 6–8 is permitted, and progression in activity is based on strength and comfort [7].

13.9 Postoperative Follow-Up

Patients are seen postoperatively at 2 weeks for a clinical and radiological (x-ray) exam. Following this, we routinely evaluate our patients at 6 weeks and then at 3, 6, and 12 months. Postoperative MRI is obtained for patients enrolled in clinical trials at 6 or 12 months or if patients have persistent pain despite physical therapy and conservative treatment (in the absence of trauma) at a minimum of 6 months postoperatively. Assuming patients achieve progressive relief in pain, activities can increase over time to full release without restrictions no sooner than 8 months.

13.10 Comparison to Other Techniques

Cole et al. conducted a proof-of-concept and safety randomized controlled trial in 29 patients where patient-reported outcomes and MRI findings were compared at a minimum of 2-year follow-up among patients treated with CAIS and microfracture [7]. This study demonstrated that the Short Form 36 (SF-36), International Knee Documentation Committee (IKDC) score, and Knee Injury and Osteoarthritis Outcome Score (KOOS) improved in both groups over a 24-month period. However, patients who were treated with CAIS had significantly higher overall IKDC score at 12 months postoperatively and had significantly higher scores on all five KOOS subscales at 24 months after surgery. Although MRI scores did not differ in terms of fill of the graft bed, tissue integration, or presence of subchondral cysts, patients treated with microfracture had a higher incidence of intralesional osteophytes at 6 and 12 months postoperatively. Furthermore, there were no differences in adverse events or complications between the two study groups. Although this initial pilot study is limited by small sample size and an increased number of cases with an acute onset of symptoms in the CAIS group, the findings are encouraging. A larger multicenter randomized trial comparing CAIS and microfracture is currently in progress.

The use of DeNovo NT in a clinical setting was first reported by Bonner et al. [6] where a patellar defect was successfully treated at 2-year follow-up as measured by the IKDC and post-op MRI which demonstrated fill of the defect with repair tissue and near full resolution of preoperative subchondral bone edema. Subsequently, Farr and Yao [11] reported the results from the first 4 of 25 patients enrolled in a prospective single-arm cohort study investigating the use of DeNovo NT in patients with one or two chondral lesions on the femoral condyles or trochlea. Initial results demonstrated improvements in IKDC and KOOS scores at 2 years compared to baseline as well as defect filling that persists to at least 2 years following surgery. There were also no complications and no evidence of graft rejection phenomena.

Although the clinical evidence which supports the use of particulated articular cartilage is limited in quantity, the initial results are encouraging. Further prospective comparative studies with microfracture and ACI are required to determine the long-term efficacy of such techniques. Both patient-reported outcome measures and objective parameters as measured by MRI and histological examination will ultimately determine whether particulated grafts will become a preferred treatment methods for specific subgroups of patients with chondral lesions.

References

1. Adkisson HD 4th, Martin JA, Amendola RL et al (2010) The potential of human allogeneic juvenile chondrocytes for restoration of articular cartilage. Am J Sports Med 38(7):1324–1333
2. Albrecht FH (1983) Closure of joint cartilage defects using cartilage fragments and fibrin glue. Fortschr Med 101(37):1650–1652
3. Alford JW, Cole BJ (2005) Cartilage restoration, part 1: basic science, historical perspective, patient evaluation, and treatment options. Am J Sports Med 33(2): 295–306
4. Alford JW, Cole BJ (2005) Cartilage restoration, part 2: techniques, outcomes, and future directions. Am J Sports Med 33(3):443–460
5. Beck PR, Thomas AL, Farr J, Lewis PB, Cole BJ (2005) Trochlear contact pressures after anteromedialization of the tibial tubercle. Am J Sports Med 33(11):1710–1715
6. Bonner KF, Daner W, Yao JQ (2010) 2-year postoperative evaluation of a patient with a symptomatic full-thickness patellar cartilage defect repaired with particulated juvenile cartilage tissue. J Knee Surg 23(2):109–114
7. Cole BJ, Farr J, Winalski CS et al (2011) Outcomes after a single-stage procedure for cell-based cartilage repair: a prospective clinical safety trial with 2-year follow-up. Am J Sports Med 39(6):1170–1179
8. Farr J, Cole B, Dhawan A, Kercher J, Sherman S (2011) Clinical cartilage restoration: evolution and overview. Clin Orthop Relat Res 469(10): 2696–2705
9. Farr J, Cole BJ, Sherman S, Karas V (2012) Particulated articular cartilage: CAIS and DeNovo NT. J Knee Surg 25(1):23–29
10. Farr J, Schepsis A, Cole B, Fulkerson J, Lewis P (2007) Anteromedialization: review and technique. J Knee Surg 20(2):120–128
11. Farr J, Yao JQ (2011) Chondral defect repair with particulated juvenile cartilage allograft. Cartilage 2:346–353
12. Frisbie DD, Lu Y, Kawcak CE, DiCarlo EF, Binette F, McIlwraith CW (2009) In vivo evaluation of autologous cartilage fragment-loaded scaffolds implanted into equine articular defects and compared with autologous chondrocyte implantation. Am J Sports Med 37(Suppl 1):71S–80S
13. Howard JS, Mattacola CG, Romine SE, Lattermann C (2010) Continuous passive motion, early weight bearing, and active motion following knee articular cartilage repair: evidence for clinical practice. Cartilage October 2010:(1)4276–286
14. Jones DG, Peterson L (2006) Autologous chondrocyte implantation. J Bone Joint Surg Am 88(11): 2502–2520
15. Lu Y, Dhanaraj S, Wang Z et al (2006) Minced cartilage without cell culture serves as an effective intraoperative cell source for cartilage repair. J Orthop Res 24(6):1261–1270
16. McCormick F, Yanke A, Provencher MT, Cole BJ (2008) Minced articular cartilage–basic science, surgical technique, and clinical application. Sports Med Arthrosc 16(4):217–220
17. McNickle AG, Provencher MT, Cole BJ (2008) Overview of existing cartilage repair technology. Sports Med Arthrosc 16(4):196–201
18. Namba RS, Meuli M, Sullivan KM, Le AX, Adzick NS (1998) Spontaneous repair of superficial defects in articular cartilage in a fetal lamb model. J Bone Joint Surg Am 80(1):4–10
19. Nho SJ, Pensak MJ, Seigerman DA, Cole BJ (2010) Rehabilitation after autologous chondrocyte implantation in athletes. Clin Sports Med 29(2): 267–282, viii

20. Reinold MM, Wilk KE, Macrina LC, Dugas JR, Cain EL (2006) Current concepts in the rehabilitation following articular cartilage repair procedures in the knee. J Orthop Sports Phys Ther 36(10):774–794
21. Salter RB, Simmonds DF, Malcolm BW, Rumble EJ, MacMichael D, Clements ND (1980) The biological effect of continuous passive motion on the healing of full-thickness defects in articular cartilage. An experimental investigation in the rabbit. J Bone Joint Surg Am 62(8):1232–1251

Part VI

Cultured Cells for Cartilage Tissue Engineering

Classical ACI for Chondral and Osteochondral Defects

14

James B. Richardson

Contents

14.1 Introduction

Classic ACI gives good results in around 80 % of patients out to the 15th year if the correct patient is chosen and all underlying abnormalities are corrected. No alternative technique has been shown to be better. Of particular importance are the surgical techniques used and an understanding that cell engineering has particular requirements compared to other surgery. The cells are delicate seeds to be handled like replanting growing plants. A bit of heat or a little dehydration will quickly kill a cell, whereas vascular pieces of tissue we move at will in surgery are quite resistant to our surgical onslaught, fortunately.

Firstly, do keep your mind alert to the clinical situation. 'A surgeon must be a physician first and last. Otherwise he is little more than a meddler, an amateur mechanic, and often an indifferent one at that' (McEwan 1848–1924) [2]. You will learn to plan full reconstruction with an '**à** la carte' approach where a combination of different techniques provides full reconstruction. A thorough assessment of the patient is essential. Not only must a chondral defect be symptomatic, but it must be giving enough trouble for the patient to have two-part extensive surgery with prolonged rehabilitation. Do not embark on ACI unless your patient is committed to all the rehabilitation required.

The patient needs full information to make a reasoned choice. Present several options to your patient. The first must always be to use analgesia and modify activities and so avoid surgery.

J.B. Richardson, MBChB, FRCS, MD
Institute of Orthopaedics, Institute of Science and Technology in Medicine (Keele University) and Robert Jones and Agnes Hunt Orthopaedic Hospital, Oswestry, Shropshire SY10 7AG, UK
e-mail: james.richardson@nhs.net

A.A. Shetty et al. (eds.), *Techniques in Cartilage Repair Surgery*,
DOI 10.1007/978-3-642-41921-8_14, © ESSKA 2014

A second might be even a repeat of more conservative surgery. The third option might be ACI with other appropriate procedures.

14.2 Prospective Data and Audit

Science requires numbers. Ensure a preoperative score on every patient. The Lysholm score has been modified and validated as an ordinal scale for this type of patient as a self-assessment score [7].

'Hot audit' is where the patient either uses the Internet before coming to clinic or has a questionnaire entered into a database in the clinic. This database can then provide a printout of scores over time and thus good feedback both to the patient and to the surgeon. On this basis, my practice at Oswestry finds almost 79 % of patients improve with ACI over their preoperative score, with better outcomes in men and in younger patients. It is useful to explain to patients that their score has been falling over time and that if the score continues to fall, then this is probably what the situation would have been without attempts of repair. In due course by having data collected routinely by your patients, you will over time have the feedback to identify improvements from changes in your patient selection, technique and rehabilitation.

14.3 Chondrocyte Culture

I was fortunate to grow a range of skeletal cells during my MD thesis. This gave me an insight into what your biologist needs. Mats Brittberg, Lars Petersen and Anders Lindahl all undertook extensive research studies also in growing cells before treating their first patients, as did most orthopaedic surgeons in Japan who use a cell therapy. Thus, a good start to set up a local cell therapy service is for the surgeon to learn to grow cells!

Good cartilage cells come from good cartilage. The starting material your laboratory receives is probably the most crucial determinant of which cells will be produced. Cells produce growth factors in the medium and so a small biopsy leads to a loss of initial number of cells and so low levels of growth factors in the early media and a low initial starting count.

Chondrocytes lose the ability to form cartilage with each cell division. Professor Charlie Archer explains that it is important to keep the number of cell divisions below a total of 7. Fortunately, exponential growth allows large numbers of cells to be grown, but with a limit of seven divisions and requirement perhaps for ten million cells you need in theory to start with 80,000 cells. Some cells in the biopsy will not adhere to the culture plate and so a biopsy of at least 200 mg is necessary. This is the size of a peanut. Do not include any synovial tissue.

Cartilage contains a mix of cells: surface, middle and deep. I therefore use a full-thickness biopsy down to bleeding bone, and by 3 weeks you will see healing already under way and a healed defect by 1 year. There is a lot of debate as to which cell is the 'best' chondrocyte. My understanding is that a mix is good, and I trust the 'cleverness of the cells' to enable a full repair.

The aim of the laboratory is to minimally modify cells. Autologous serum does seem the best option for culture. Cells particularly respond to autologous serum, and indeed one method of culture is to place finely chopped up cartilage in autologous serum. Chondrocytes will actually mobilise from their chondrons and exit from the cartilage. They will only do this in the presence of autologous serum.

Patients are happy to provide serum for their own cells, and it helps the laboratory to know that you will work on their behalf to get a good supply of serum in addition to the good quality biopsy. No opiate must be present in the serum as this inhibits cell growth [5] and so patients must stop taking tramadol and codeine. Avoid taking serum under anaesthesia as usually there is opiate given as part of the anaesthetic. Other factors in the diet of the patient prior to serum being collected are probably important. Insulin helps chondrocyte growth and this may explain why we observe better results for serum that is taken after a meal.

We have examined our data for an effect of cell density on the outcome of ACI but failed to find a correlation. The application of drug manufacturing quality controls has driven a rigid approach to this issue of 'dose' of cells. I suspect many cells are lost from the defect soon after surgery in any case. A general target is for one million chondrocytes per square cm, but not much attention is paid to the quality of these chondrocytes. In the future, I would hope that fine tuning the number of chondrocytes to the size of defect would allow a supply of chondrocytes that have undergone as few divisions as possible. The ability to form cartilage reduces with each division of the cells, so it is good to work with your laboratory in reducing the number of divisions.

There may also be a disadvantage of excess numbers of chondrocytes. There will be a limit of resources in the closed defect such as the glucose that chondrocytes need for metabolism. Too many in a confined space will also produce an excess of metabolites. Finally there are only so many attachment points for chondrocytes in a defect. ACI depends on chondrocytes attaching to the freshly cut surfaces or cartilage and bone through their CD44 integrins. These special proteins on the cell surface allow cells to attach within 20 min to the hyaline surface of freshly cut cartilage.

14.4 Consent

Pain can be a significant problem in a patient who has had previous multiple surgeries. Pain syndromes can cause severe pain for many years and I have seen one follow an injection of steroid to a patient's knee. This is usefully included in the full explanation a patient needs before they freely consent to a procedure.

In the USA, it appears that every possible complication must be explained for full consent. In the UK, a valid consent involves providing information on the common complications and the serious if rare ones. In my practice I include infection, failure to improve, increased pain, deep vein thrombosis and a possible fatal outcome. It is important to explain the positive steps that will be taken to minimise the risks you are explaining. I ask each patient if they would wish further information, and if they do, then I continue with rarer complications such as a compartment syndrome, numbness and stiffness. I document the details given together with an explanation that these complications are only indicative of the sort of problems that can occur and are not a comprehensive list. New complications can arise from any procedure, but if a patient is aware of the major ones, and accepts that risk, then they will find it easier to accept the rare complication that was not considered and discussed preoperatively.

A relaxed patient will feel less pain postoperatively and have a better outcome.

The implications of each complication must be explained. Alternatives always include the option of managing their disability conservatively and alternative options so the patient is able to make a fully informed decision whether to choose the option of ACI.

A GMP laboratory can accept your patient's harvest biopsy if it does not have evidence that the patient does not harbour a significant and communicable infection. This is an additional part of the consent process. The patients will understand that if everyone has tests for syphilis, hepatitis and HIV, then this makes the laboratory a safer place for all concerned. Sometimes a false-positive result will be obtained and the ability for the laboratory to be informed and for you to be contacted is an important part of good clinical practice. Where the first blood tests have been done in good time, it does not then cause difficulties as usually simply a repeat blood test is required.

14.5 The Surgery

14.5.1 Theatre Team

A high-quality theatre team is central to this second procedure. We are fortunate at Oswestry to have a special open-plan operating theatre suite with the highest quality of filtered air and a good working environment. As a specialist unit, there are a full range of equipment available and second options should there be a problem. Theatre time must not be restricted. Despite having an 'à la carte' approach, each part of the procedure preferably should be standardised and preplanned. Requirements for each option are best in a personal standard operating procedure folder. As far as possible, all procedures should be planned in advance and be on the theatre list. A team meeting first thing at the start of a list allows the team to double-check that all materials and equipment will be available and a plan of the sequence of procedures.

Personal preparation is important. This is not an operation to rush. Good theatre time must be available. This is an operation where a course in microvascular technique is useful and some surgeons use operating loupes for the fine sutures used. A seated position is best with the wrist supported wherever possible. A good assistant is essential. Good music helps!

The sequence of procedures is important. If a tibial tuberosity is to be undertaken (and this is almost inevitable for patellofemoral ACI), then this is undertaken early as it will contribute to improved exposure. A meniscal transplant needs to be performed in sequence following ACI of the tibial surface as the suturing of the meniscus itself will help to seal the often difficult tibial surface patch. An ACL procedure is best left to last for obvious reasons as are repair of collateral ligaments or the patellofemoral ligament. All releases are done widely at the beginning.

Do not use a tourniquet and your patients will have less pain postoperatively and less risk of a haematoma. In the arthroscopic harvest procedure, the tourniquet can be applied, but not inflated unless required. Add adrenaline to the irrigation fluid. For the second procedure, you will undertake excellent haemostasis and not need a drain postoperatively.

14.5.2 First Stage: Harvest Biopsy

Routine arthroscopy allows confirmation of the diagnosis and an assessment of alignment of the patella, the condition of the menisci and the cruciate ligaments, as all problems must be corrected for the transplanted chondrocytes to survive in the long term. The new cartilage will not be better than the original.

Harvest biopsies can be partial thickness and from the least important areas of the knee, but all cartilage is there for a reason. There is no non-weight-bearing cartilage. I take a full-thickness harvest from the central proximal trochlea down to bleeding sub-articular bone, with a second favourite, the notch. The former has better quality cartilage, and the latter contributes fewer symptoms postoperatively. I have followed a few patients who had harvest from normal knees to treat the hip and ankle. Their Lysholm scores fell by about 15 points for a year. The healing of harvest biopsy sites is evidence that chondral defects generally heal.

A very sharp gouge must be used as crushing of cartilage at the edges of your biopsy will lead to apoptosis of those cells. Do not complete the cut and a then very large pituitary rongeur can capture the harvest readily in one or two large pieces. About the size of a half peanut, 200 mg of synovial-free cartilage is the goal.

Significant bleeding from the defect at the time of cell implantation will prevent the chondrocytes from adhering to the surface of the defect or in the worst case will flush them out of the pouch. If extensive debridement is needed such as removal of an internal osteophyte or reshaping the trochlea where cartilage is lost, then this is best undertaken at the harvest biopsy stage. You will then find that at Stage II, there is a stable cellular membrane covering the defect. This may be vascular and pink if a lot of bone has been removed. If the bone is left in the base of a defect that is eburnated and sclerotic, then this can become a residual source of pain.

Preoperative prerequisites for the second stage are (1) the cells have grown and (2) the previous wounds have healed free of infection. In 450 cases at Oscell, we have had three problems with wound healing. On two occasions an infection followed the first arthroscopy. In one case, the patient went canoeing very soon after the arthroscopy and so the wound was contaminated. In the second, a young soldier arranged a lot of travelling between the two procedures but ended up with infection. Patients who present for ACI are generally highly motivated and active individuals. They need particular explanation to take good care of the knee following the first arthroscopy. It is wise to advise they stay at home and rest for 3 or 4 days after arthroscopy and longer if the wounds seep.

14.5.3 Second Stage: Cell Implantation

Good exposure makes for easy surgery. In the hip, there is a case for arthroscopy as this maximises the view without requiring the healing of an open approach. For the ankle, a chevron osteotomy of the medial malleolus gives good stability and the best exposure medially. On the lateral side of the ankle, an oblique osteotomy immediately above the ankle joint line can be combined with quite radical release to the point of having just a distal pedicle attached to the distal fibula, if necessary.

In the knee, previous scars must be considered and future knee replacement also. There is a division of opinion in trochleoplasty as to medial or lateral para-patellar approaches, but where possible a lateral approach causes least upset to sensation postoperatively and can be extended distally to allow osteotomy of the patellar tendon, which nearly always benefits from being medialised and sometimes distalised slightly.

14.6 Preparation of the Defect

Debride the edges of the defect vertically, and abrade the underlying calcified cartilage. Chondral defects where the original cartilage has been separated are generally exposing the calcified zone, not the bone. This must be abraded down to the bone, but not to the point that there is significant bleeding. Be very critical of the edges. There can be delamination of cartilage from the calcified zone that is hard to see and so test the edges critically and remove more cartilage as necessary.

Some chondral defects are old with fibrocartilage repair that has subsequently been eroded. In these patients, there may be sclerotic bone in the base of the defect, or an internal osteophyte best seen on imaging. These defects are best abraded at the time of harvest biopsy by a high-speed burr. At that time, examine the defect repeatedly with the fluid flow turned off to see that dead bone has been removed but avoid taking more bone than necessary so that the subchondral plate is preserved. Three weeks later at implantation, this debrided bone will have healed with a thin smooth cover and probably should then only have minimal debridement by a swab, or it will bleed vigorously. Bleeding can also usefully be controlled by intravenous tranexamic acid. Flush the defect clean of debris with autologous serum.

14.7 Application of the Chondrogide Patch

Cut a template to fit your defect and then a patch of chondrogide. Do not get blood on the patch and transfer to smooth-side up. This membrane was designed to prevent cells moving through it, so I soak it in autologous serum with perhaps 10 % of the available cells so some cells reach the surface. Apply it rough-side down. I avoid putting fibrin in the base of the defect unless it is needed for haemostasis but put fibrin around the edge on top of the intact cartilage so that the seal between the patch and cartilage is maximised. I do not expect it to usefully hold the patch in place, as it is not strictly a glue, but a sealant.

I use a top-down approach with a series of continuous sutures, making use of the tail of each suture to tie off the last one, and so minimise knots. I use a 'backstitch' so there is an almost continuous line of suture holding down the chondrogide patch. Where necessary, the sutures can use tissue in the notch, for example, or drill 1 mm holes at the edge of an uncontained defect. Where possible, reach the edge of an articular zone to minimise the patch from being knocked off. The leading edge of a medial femoral condyle is at risk and so a double row of sutures here is advisable.

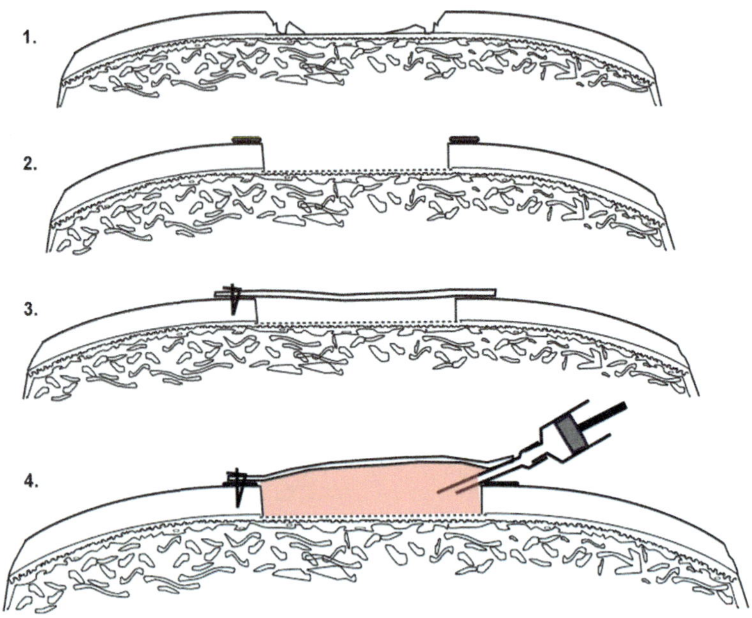

Fig. 14.1 A chondral defect undergoing autologous chondrocyte implantation. The defect in *step 1* is debrided by sharp dissection back to stable edges and the calcified cartilage is debrided down to the deepest part of the cartilage but only just into the subchondral bone plate so no significant bleeding occurs. In *step 2*, a strip of fibrin is place around the edges of the defect. *Step 3* shows the 'top-down' suturing which is a continuous backstitch to provide a continuous pressure down on the chondrogide. In *step 4*, the cells are inserted usually though the uppermost side of the defect, and then this access is closed by suture and fibrin sealant

14.8 Testing and Cell Insertion

There is probably only a certain amount of nutrition available in the covered defect, but chondrocytes produce the best cartilage when they are in high concentration. The aim is therefore that the defect should hold the cells well and in the face of motion so that nutrition is maximised. You will have an estimate of the security of your sutures. Water tightness is tested not to the point of blowing off the patch, but it will give you feedback on your suturing technique. It is important to use autologous serum when testing as saline is toxic to cells. Do not aspirate strongly or blood will be sucked into the defect.

Mobilise cells in their syringe by leaving a small bubble in place and they can be gently resuspended. I use a spare plastic cannula from the fibrin system to both test and then leaving it in place to inject cells. A suture is then used to close the entry area after removing the cannula. In certain cases, a yellow spinal needle can be used passed into the defect through intact cartilage. Take care not to inject cells quickly along a fine needle, as this will disrupt the cells (Fig. 14.1).

14.9 Use of Air

Some surgeons are using air to replace irrigation fluid in cartilage surgery. Allowing air to enter by draining fluid is used by R Villar and also Fontana for the hip, for example [4]. Great care must be taken not to inflate a joint under pressure with a gas as life-threatening gas embolism can ensue if there should be a direct communication of a large vein to the joint. This has happened with CO_2, with air and in a veterinary case with helium. N_2O in the anaesthetic gas exacerbates the problem as this gas expands air in the circulation.

Use of a fibrin spray has very rarely led to cases of air embolism in various anatomic sites. Due to these problems, many fibrin sprays now use carbon dioxide as the carrier gas, and this greatly reduces the risks as the venous system is highly adapted for the absorption and removal of dissolved CO_2 [1].

14.10 Osteochondral Defects

The commonest problem is an osteochondral defect of the lateral part of the medial femoral condyle. Up to the age of 18, there is often good healing with debridement and microfracture. Bone graft with a layer of chondrogide to stabilise the graft is an option with autologous chondrocytes in a pouch under a second layer, known as the 'sandwich technique' and described by the Gothenberg team.

Another option is to combine mosaicplasty and ACI to treat bone loss. The mosaic plugs can be separated to get good stable support, and the bone contour prioritised as the chondrocytes will fill in the other areas to give a smooth finish without the problem of fluid gaining access between the plug and surrounding cartilage [6].

14.11 Postoperative Care

The patient is in a splint for 4 h following surgery and then placed in a CPM for 3 days. Good analgesia is important throughout this period. A femoral catheter as previously discussed will help in allowing a patient to supply their own local anaesthetic. Preferably pain is controlled, but not muscle power blocked. Patients are then partial weight bearing from Day 3.

Continuous motion is essential postoperatively. A Continuous Passive Motion machine at home is a good option and these devices can be hired from companies on the Internet. A cheaper option is the use of small exercise pedals, also bought over the Internet. An exercise bike must be available from week four then there should be sufficient knee flexion.

14.12 Rehabilitation

For patellofemoral reconstruction, it is usual to encourage full weight bearing immediately and to limit flexion under load for 6 weeks. For tibiofemoral compartments of the knee gradually increase weight bearing to 20 kg at 2 weeks, 30 kg at 3 weeks, 40 kg at 4 weeks and 50 kg at 5 weeks and full weight bearing at 6 weeks.

The general target is then to run at 6 months and return to sport between 1 and 2 years.

14.13 Biomarkers

The future improvements in case selection, I believe, will come from improvements in assessment of biology of the injured joint. Evidently, cell therapy depends on the biological milieu of the joint. If arthritis is to be considered 'organ failure' of a joint, then the follow-up Lysholm score parallels progressive failure of function.

There is consensus that at some point the ability of a joint to heal itself is lost and in due course even with the insertion of cells fails to lead to improvement. Eventually there is a 'point of no return' where deterioration progresses and a joint replacement marks final failure of the knee as an organ.

Our recent experience and research in the role of biomarkers and cartilage degradation is an exciting area of development. We have looked at a range of biomarkers in ACI patients' knee joint fluid. In a study of 107 patients, we have identified a correlation between postoperative nonresponders ($n=29$) who have been shown to have high levels of aggrecanase (ADAMTS-4) activity. See Fig. 14.2.

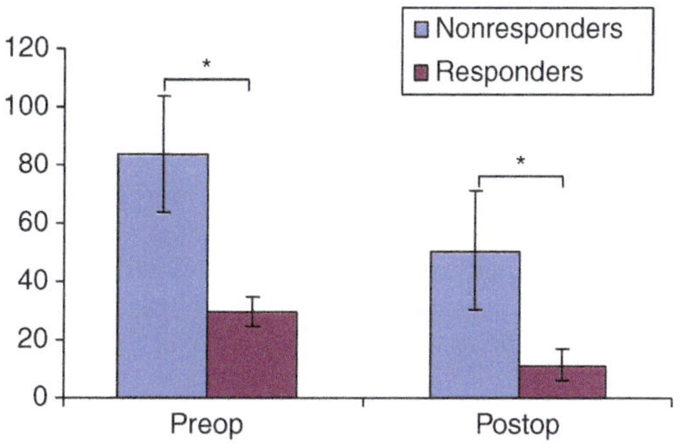

Fig. 14.2 A histogram of the preoperative measures of aggrecanase-1 activity predicted those who respond from those who will not respond to autologous chondrocyte implantation. The high levels of aggrecanase-1 (ADAMTS-4) activity persisted in the knee postoperatively

In the future, such markers will be used to predict and improve those who will benefit from ACI.

14.14 Cost-Effectiveness

As ACI is relatively expensive compared to alternatives, it is important that the cost-effectiveness of ACI receives due consideration. Compared to other forms of treatment, it does remain a very cost-effective treatment as the benefit continues for many years. A 10–20 % improvement over alternative treatments makes this treatment cost-effective if the benefit is continued over 10 years [3].

References

1. Bhosale AM, Kuiper JH, Johnson WE, Harrison PE, Richardson JB (2009) Midterm to long-term longitudinal outcome of autologous chondrocyte implantation in the knee joint: a multilevel analysis. Am J Sports Med 37(Suppl 1):131S–138S, *Background*: Autologous chondrocyte implantation is a cell therapeutic approach for the treatment of chondral and osteochondral defects in the knee joint. The authors previously reported on the histologic and radiologic outcome of autologous chondrocyte implantation in the short- to midterm, which yields mixed results. *Purpose*: The objective is to report on the clinical outcome of autologous chondrocyte implantation for the knee in the midterm to long term. *Study Design*: Cohort study; Level of evidence, 3. *Methods*: Eighty patients who had undergone autologous chondrocyte implantation of the knee with mid- to long-term follow-up were analyzed. The mean patient age was 34.6 years (standard deviation, 9.1 years), with 63 men and 17 women. Seventy-one patients presented with a focal chondral defect, with a median defect area of 4.1 cm (2) and a maximum defect area of 20 cm (2). The modified Lysholm score was used as a self-reporting clinical outcome measure to determine the following: (1) What is the typical pattern over time of clinical outcome after autologous chondrocyte implantation; and (2) Which patient-related predictors for the clinical outcome pattern can be used to improve patient selection for autologous chondrocyte implantation? *Results*: The average follow-up time was 5 years (range, 2.7–9.3). Improvement in clinical outcome was found in 65 patients (81 %), while 15 patients (19 %) showed a decline in outcome. The median preoperative Lysholm score of 54 increased to a median of 78 points. The most rapid improvement in Lysholm score was over the 15-month period after operation, after which the Lysholm score remained constant for up to 9 years. The authors were unable to identify any patient-specific factors (i.e., age, gender, defect size, defect location, number of previous operations, preoperative Lysholm score) that could predict the change in clinical outcome in the first 15 months. *Conclusion*: Autologous chondrocyte implantation seems to provide a durable clinical outcome in those patients demonstrating success at 15 months after operation. Comparisons between other outcome measures of autologous chondrocyte implantation should be focused on the clinical status at 15 months after surgery. The patient-reported clinical outcome at 15 months is a major predictor of the mid- to long-term success of autologous chondrocyte implantation
2. Bowman AK (1942) The life and teaching of Sir William McEwan. William Hodge and Co, London
3. Clar C, Cummins E, McIntyre L, Thomas S, Lamb J, Bain L, Jobanputra P, Waugh N (2005) Clinical and cost-effectiveness of autologous chondrocyte implantation for cartilage defects in knee joints: systematic review and economic evaluation. Health Technol Assess 9(47):iii–iv, ix–x, 1–82. *Objective*: To support a review of the guidance issued by the National Institute for Health and Clinical Excellence (NICE) in December 2000 by examining the current clinical and cost-effectiveness evidence on autologous cartilage transplantation. *Data Sources*: Electronic databases. *Review methods*: Evidence on clinical effectiveness was obtained from randomised trials, supplemented by data from selected observational studies for longer term results, and for the natural history of chondral lesions. Because of a lack of long-term results on outcomes such as later osteoarthritis and knee replacement, only illustrative modelling was done, using a range of assumptions that seemed reasonable, but were not evidence based. *Results*: Four randomised controlled trials were included, as well as observational data from case series. The trials studied a total of 266 patients and the observational studies up to 101 patients. Two studies compared autologous chondrocyte implantation (ACI) with mosaicplasty, the third compared ACI with microfracture, and the fourth compared matrix-guided ACI (MACI) with microfracture. Follow-up was 1 year in one study, and up to 3 years in the remaining three studies. The first trial of ACI versus mosaicplasty found that ACI gave better results than mosaicplasty at 1 year. Overall, 88 % had excellent or good results with ACI versus 69 % with mosaicplasty. About half of the biopsies after ACI showed hyaline cartilage. The second trial of ACI versus mosaicplasty found little difference in clinical outcomes at 2 years. Disappointingly, biopsies from

the ACI group showed fibrocartilage rather than hyaline cartilage. The trial of ACI versus microfracture also found only small differences in outcomes at 2 years. Finally, the trial of MACI versus microfracture contained insufficient long-term results at present, but the study does show the feasibility of doing ACI by the MACI technique. It also suggested that after ACI, it takes 2 years for full-thickness cartilage to be produced. Reliable costs per quality-adjusted life-year (QALY) could not be calculated owing to the absence of necessary data. Simple short-term modelling suggests that the quality of life gain from ACI versus microfracture would have to be between 70 and 100 % greater over 2 years for it to be more cost-effective within the 20,000–30,000 pounds sterling per QALY cost-effectiveness thresholds. However, if the quality of life gains could be maintained for a decade, increments relative to microfracture would only have to be 10–20 % greater to justify additional treatment costs within the cost-effectiveness band indicated above. Follow-up from the trials so far has only been up to 2 years, with longer term outcomes being uncertain. *Conclusions*: There is insufficient evidence at present to say that ACI is cost-effective compared with microfracture or mosaicplasty. Longer term outcomes are required. Economic modelling using some assumptions about long-term outcomes that seem reasonable suggests that ACI would be cost-effective because it is more likely to produce hyaline cartilage, which is more likely to be durable and to prevent osteoarthritis in the longer term (e.g. 20 years). Further research is needed into earlier methods of predicting long-term results. Basic science research is also needed into factors that influence stem cells to become chondrocytes and to produce high-quality cartilage, as it may be possible to have more patients developing hyaline cartilage after microfracture. Study is also needed into cost-effective methods of rehabilitation and the effect of early mobilisation on cartilage growth

4. Fontana A, Bistolfi A, Crova M, Rosso F, Massazza G (2012) Arthroscopic treatment of hip chondral defects: autologous chondrocyte transplantation versus simple debridement – a pilot study. Arthroscopy 28(3):322–329, *Purpose*: To compare the effectiveness of simple arthroscopic debridement versus arthroscopic autologous chondrocyte transplantation (ACT) for the treatment of hip chondral lesions. *Methods*: We carried out a controlled retrospective study of 30 patients affected by a post-traumatic hip chondropathy of the third or fourth degree, according to the Outerbridge classification, measuring 2 cm (2) in area or more. Of these patients, 15 underwent arthroscopic ACT, whereas the other 15 underwent arthroscopic debridement. The two groups were similar in age, sex, degree, and location of the pathology. All the patients were assessed before and after the procedure with the Harris Hip Score (HHS). *Results*: In both groups the mean follow-up was approximately 74 months (range, 72–76 months). The mean size of the defect was 2.6 cm (2). The patients who underwent ACT (group A) improved after the procedure compared with the group that underwent debridement alone (group B). The mean HHS preoperatively was 48.3 (95 % confidence interval [CI], 45.4–51.2) in group A and 46 (95 % CI, 42.7–49.3) in group B (*P*=.428 [no significant difference]). The final HHS was 87.4 (95 % CI, 84.3–90.5) in group A and 56.3 (95 % CI, 54.4–58.7) in group B (*P*<.001 [significant difference]). *Conclusions*: This study indicates that an ACT procedure can be used in the hip for acetabular chondral defects. *Level of evidence*: Level III, retrospective comparative study
5. Harrison PE, Pfeifer PM, Turner SL, Richardson JB, Jones PW, Ashton BA (2003) Serum from patients anesthetized with opiates less effective in the support of chondrocyte growth in vitro. Tissue Eng 9(1):37–39, Risk of viral and/or prion disease transmission associated with the use of fetal bovine serum in clinical cell culture has led to the increasing use of autologous human serum in tissue engineering. A relatively large volume of blood is needed and so, to decrease patient discomfort, we have investigated the feasibility of taking blood when the patient is anesthetized. Two serum samples were prepared from each of 22 patients: (1) from the awake patient (PRE) and (2) from the patient 5 min after induction of general anesthesia (PER). The sera were compared for their ability to support the in vitro proliferation of primary human chondrocytes, determined by cell counting. The effects of anesthetic agents on the PER/PRE cell number ratio were established by analysis of variance and stepwise multilinear regression analysis. The PER sample supported higher growth in 2 of 22 patients, equivalent growth in another 11, and significantly lower growth in the remaining 8. Only the opiate analgesics (fentanyl [Sublimaze], alfentanyl [Rapifen], and diamorphine) had a significant and inhibitory effect on chondrocyte proliferation. It is suggested that opiate analgesics be avoided when blood is taken to support the in vitro growth of human cells
6. Smith GD, Richardson JB, Brittberg M, Erggelet C, Verdonk R, Knutsen G, Ashton BA, Ashton IK, Harrison PE (2003) Autologous chondrocyte implantation and osteochondral cylinder transplantation in cartilage repair of the knee joint. J Bone Joint Surg Am 85-A(12):2487–2488, author reply 2488
7. Smith HJ, Richardson JB, Tennant A (2009) Modification and validation of the Lysholm Knee Scale to assess articular cartilage damage. Osteoarthritis Cartilage 17(1):53–58, *Objective*: The Lysholm Knee Scale is an 8-item questionnaire originally designed as an outcome measure for ligament reconstruction but is commonly used as a measure for knee chondral damage. This study tests the scale's

internal construct validity using the Rasch model, a measurement model which sets strict standards for the quality of measurement derived from the scale. The study also investigates the level of agreement between scores from patients and physiotherapists; and reviews the present weighting system. *Design*: One hundred and fifty-seven patients with knee chondral damage awaiting surgery completed the Lysholm as part of a multicentre clinical trial based in 16 UK and two Norwegian hospitals. The patients were assessed by a physiotherapist who independently completed the Lysholm on the same day. *Results*: Fit to the Rasch model was achieved [mean item fit −0.26, standard deviation (SD) 1.01] after removal of one item (Swelling). With no differential item functioning (DIF) by rater, the intraclass correlation coefficient was 0.9 [95 % confidence interval (CI): 0.86–0.93] and a Bland-Altman plot showed no consistent difference in rating. *Conclusions*: The Lysholm Knee Scale satisfies Rasch model expectations after removal of the swelling item. Generally there is a high degree of agreement between the patient and professional ratings. By removing the swelling item and using unweighted scores, a modified version of the Lysholm Knee Scale is recommended as an outcome measure for knee chondral damage

Gel ACI (GACI): Articular Cartilage Repair Technique

15

Seok-Jung Kim, Asode Ananthram Shetty, and Vishvas A. Shetty

Contents

S.-J. Kim, MD, PhD, FRCS (✉)
Department of Orthopedic Surgery, Uijeongbu St. Mary's Hospital, College of Medicine, The Catholic University of Korea, 480-717 Gyeonggi-do, Republic of (South Korea)

Faculty of Stem Cell Research and Regenerative Medicine, NITTE University, Mangalore, India
e-mail: orthopland@naver.com

A.A. Shetty, MD, MCh, PhD, FRCS Ed., FRCS Eng., FRCS Orth
Department of Minimally Invasive Surgery, Faculty of Health and Social Sciences, Canterbury Christ Church University, Pembroke Court 30, ME4 4UF Chatham Maritime, Kent, UK

Faculty of Stem Cell Research and Regenerative Medicine, NITTE University, Mangalore, India

Vishvas A. Shetty
Department of Minimally Invasive Surgery, Faculty of Health and Social Sciences, Canterbury Christ Church University, Pembroke Court 30, ME4 4UF, Chatham Maritime, Kent, UK

15.1 Introduction

As articular cartilage has only limited ability to regenerate, various treatment options have been developed during the past several decades to treat symptomatic articular cartilage injuries [1, 2]. Among these treatment options available, autologous chondrocyte implantation (ACI), an advanced, cell-based, biologic technology, has become a standard technique used to repair symptomatic, full-thickness, chondral injuries [2]. The traditional ACI technique involves injection of cultured autologous chondrocyte cells into the prepared cartilage defect covered by a periosteal flap. This was the first generation of ACI. However, complications such as periosteal hypertrophy and, less commonly, calcification and delamination have been encountered when periosteum is used as a cover material [3]. Furthermore, improvements in tissue engineering have resulted in a new generation of ACI techniques in which cells are combined with bioactive resorbable biomaterials such as a bilayer type I/III collagen membranes, hyaluronan polymer, and copolymers of polylactin and polyglactin [3]. However, all these techniques require open arthrotomy for the second stage of cell implantation, which has associated patient morbidity and complications [4].

Latest is fourth generation of ACI in which gel-based autologous chondrocytes are inserted into a three-dimensional scaffold provided by fibrin gel at defect site without using any patches. This composite combines cultured chondrocytes

A.A. Shetty et al. (eds.), *Techniques in Cartilage Repair Surgery*, DOI 10.1007/978-3-642-41921-8_15, © ESSKA 2014 with a three-dimensional biocompatible scaffold which provides better structural stability and durability [5]. Hence, it can be done through a mini-arthrotomy.

15.2 Indications and Preoperative Planning

After a history and thorough clinical examination, all lesions are assessed by MRI scan. For axial alignment a long leg X-ray is performed and, where indicated, a patellofemoral joint is assessed by CT tracking scans. MRI scan helps accurately determine the location and size of the chondral lesions. The International Cartilage Repair Society (ICRS) criterion is reliable and relevant tool for gradation of cartilage defects in patients on the basis of macroscopic evaluation of cartilage defect site [6]. Cartilage defects can be classified from grade 0 to grade 4 according to ICRS criteria [6].

15.2.1 Surgical Technique

Autologous chondrocytes implantation is a two-step procedure. The first step of ACI is to perform an arthroscopic surgery to identify the area of cartilage damage and determine whether an ACI procedure and collection of chondrocytes cells will be appropriate [1].

15.2.2 GACI First Stage

Biopsy and Chondrocyte Harvest

During the arthroscopic procedure, a biopsy of healthy cartilage plug attached to some subchondral bone is taken from a non-weight-bearing area (6 mmØ; 100–200 mg). The most common sites to obtain samples of healthy cartilage are the superomedial and superolateral edges of the femoral condyles and on the lateral wall of the intercondylar notch (Figs. 15.1, 15.2, and 15.3) [4]. The biopsy is placed directly into the media solution (Fig. 15.4). This is to be supplied to a cell expansion GMP laboratory, along with a vacutainer containing a blood sample (8.5 ml) for testing (HIV, VDRL, hepatitis B). The biopsy has a good viability for up to 72 h and must be kept at a temperature of 2–8 °C. At the laboratory, these cells are multiplied by growing in culture.

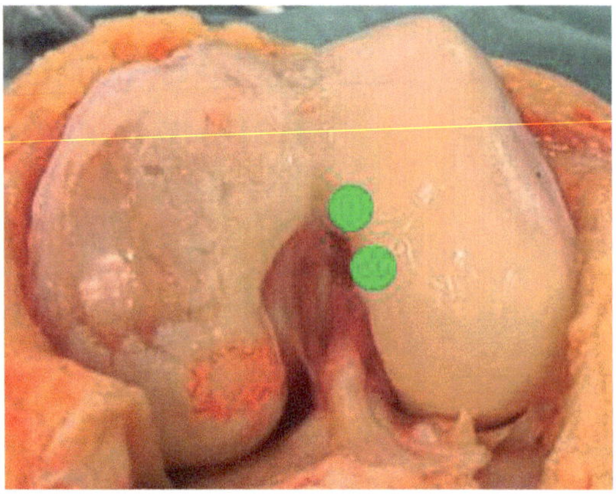

Fig. 15.1 Cartilage biopsy site

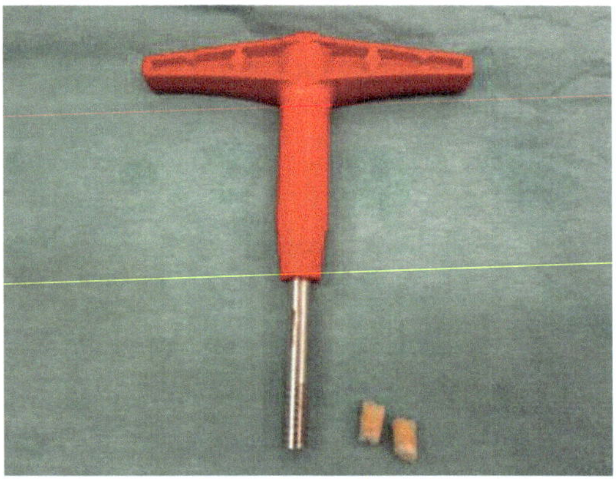

Fig. 15.2 Biopsy harvester and cartilage plug

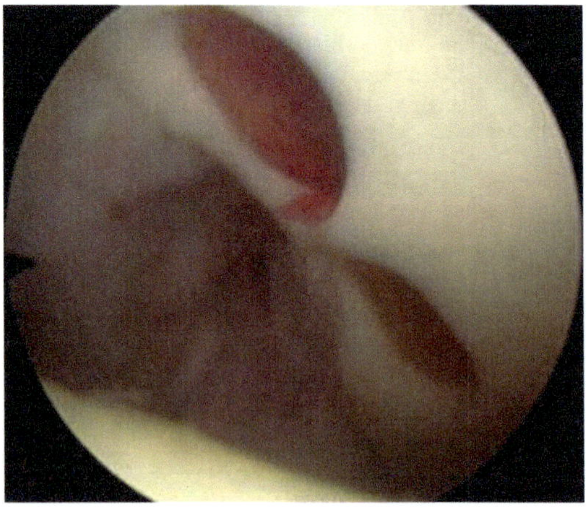

Fig. 15.3 Arthroscopic notch view of biopsy site

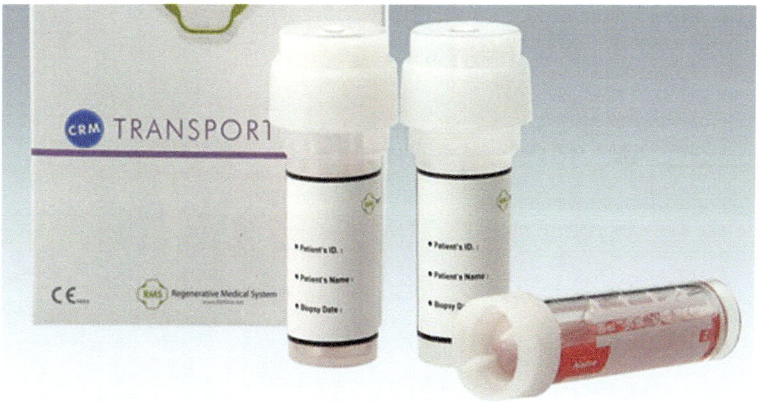

Fig. 15.4 Transport Kit (RMS Innovations, UK) and vacutainer for blood sample

Culture Process

Chondrocytes are isolated from the cartilage biopsy using an enzyme digest. The isolated cells are grown in a carbon dioxide-rich atmosphere and gradually expanded in vitro, from 25-cm^3 flasks gradually up to 150-cm^3 flasks. Once the desired cell number has been reached, the cells are enzymatically stripped from the flasks. The cells are then cleaned and packed in sterile ampoules ready for implantation. The overall process takes between 6 and 8 weeks.

Once the biopsy is received from the hospital, the tissue sample is tested for the presence of viral infections. After each subculture of the individual cell lines, a small portion of the sample is taken in order to ensure that sample is free of bacterial and fungal contamination. Prior to the release of the final product, the quantification and viability tests are conducted. Moreover, the final stage product is also assessed for the presence of the any microbial contamination (Fig. 15.5).

Transportation of Cultured Cells

Once produced, the cells will remain a high viability for 72 h. Within this time constraint they must be implanted. They are transported in up to 4 vials, each containing at least 12 million cells (0.5 ml). These vials are housed for protection and put into the Delivery Kit (Fig. 15.6). Mixing vials and vials of media are also included. The Delivery Kit has everything needed to be combined with the contents of the fibrin glue and produce the finished product.

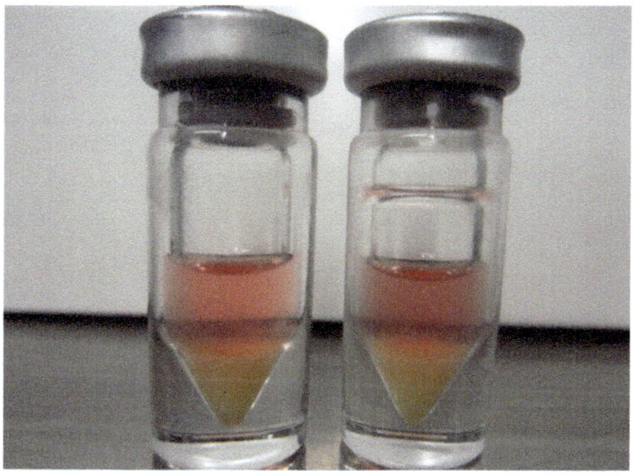

Fig. 15.5 Cultured chondrocytes (12 million cells/vial)

15.2.3 GACI Second Stage

In-Theater Mixing Procedure

Preparation for first syringe: 1 ml of supplied culture media is transferred to the fibrinogen powder vial and 1 ml transferred to the thrombin powder vial, where they are warmed and stirred until fully dissolved.

Preparation for second syringe: 0.1 ml of the thrombin solution is then transferred into an empty mixing vial. The contents of 2 cell vials (12 million cells per vial) are also transferred to the mixing vial (Fig. 15.7).

Dual-syringe assembly: In the aseptic area, the scrub nurse will withdraw 1 ml of the solution from the mixing vial. In a separate syringe 1 ml of the fibrinogen solution is taken. These two syringes are then assembled on to the dual-syringe body, and the nozzle is held in place by a tether strap (Fig. 15.8).

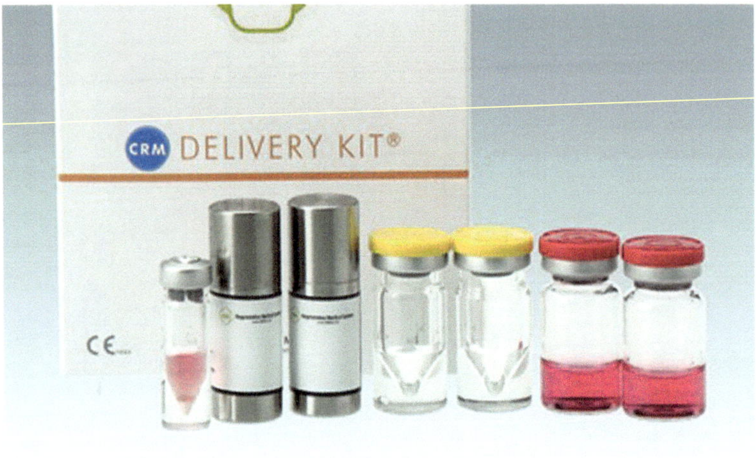

Fig. 15.6 Delivery Kit (RMS Innovations, UK) For delivery of cells for implantation. Media and mixing vials are also included. Contents: up to 4x (encased) vials of at least 12 million cells each, 2x mixing vials, 2x media vials

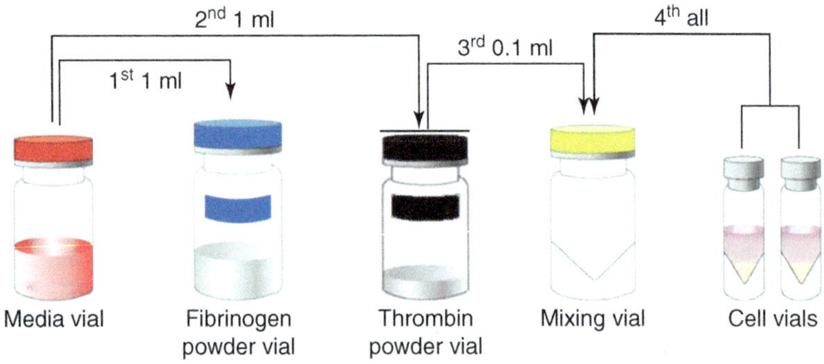

Fig. 15.7 Diagrammatic representation of mixing procedure for gel ACI (RMS Innovations, UK)

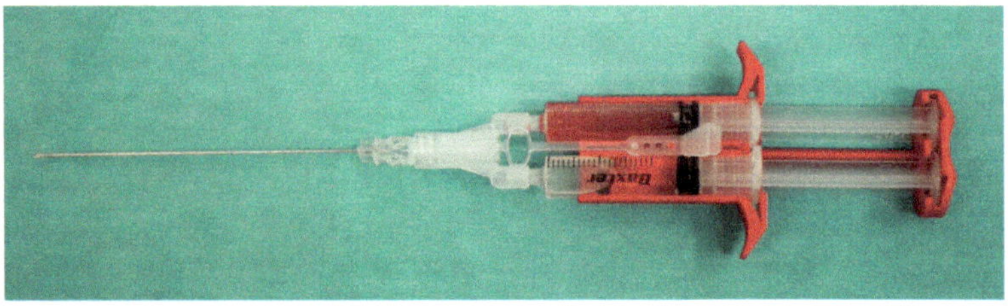

Fig. 15.8 Double syringe (DUPLOJECT) loaded with cells in thrombin and fibrinogen, ready for implantation

Application: Upon contact between the contents of the two chambers, the mixture will set within 5 min. If the lesion is particularly large, the remaining 2 cell vials may also be used. For this, the same process is used as outlined above.

Theater Setup

Patient is positioned supine with the table horizontal at an appropriate height. Leg is placed in appropriate flexion with lateral thigh support and foot holder (Fig. 15.9a). A tourniquet is applied as high up on the thigh as possible and inflated to 100 mg above systolic blood pressure.

Patient is anesthetized using general or spinal anesthesia. NSAIDs are withheld as these drugs are known to be chondrotoxic. Appropriate antibiotic is administered intravenously prior to inflation of tourniquet.

Implantation of Cells

Once the sufficient cartilage cells have been grown, patient is called back for the second

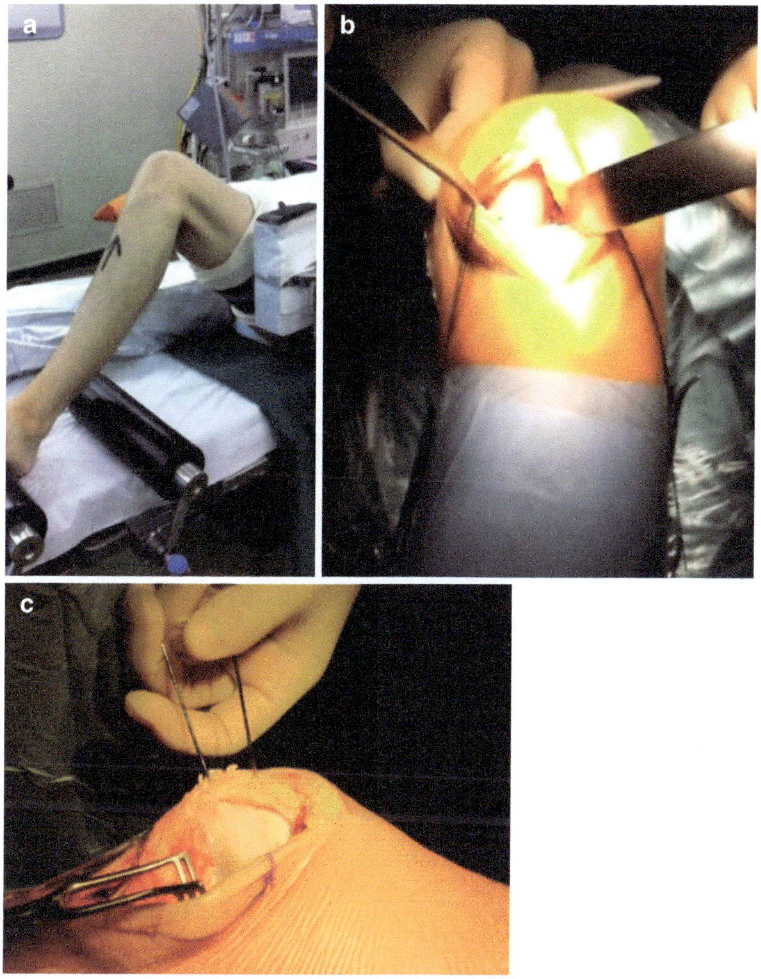

Fig. 15.9 (**a**) Position for arthrotomy. (**b**) Stay sutures and retractor placement for exposure of lesion. (**c**) K-wire insertion for eversion and exposure of patella

surgery which involves implantation of cultured chondrocytes. During this surgery, standard parapatellar, medial, or lateral incision is made, and the knee is opened up by means of mini-arthrotomy. Two stay sutures are applied to the synovium at the opposite edges of the middle of the arthrotomy. For patellar lesions, two 1.8 K-wires are inserted from the lateral margin; this acts as a retractor and holds the position of the patella for application of the gel. Hyperextension of knee in extended position makes the retraction of patella easier (Fig. 15.9).

After achieving adequate exposure of defective site, for removing unviable tissue, the lesion should be debrided. A no. 11 blade is used to cut the margin of the lesion sharply with slight obliquity towards the lesion (Fig. 15.10a). The damaged cartilage in lesion is removed, the chondral fissures and erosions inside the defect are regularized, and the fibrous tissue present at the base of the lesion is debrided [1, 2, 8].

Multiple holes of 3 mm depth are made using 1.5-mm drill bit so that holes would provide a stable base. These holes increase the surface area of raw bone and also provide rotational stability for the gel (Fig. 15.10b, c, d). For the injection procedure, two 1-ml syringes and a Y-shaped mixing adapter are used. In one syringe, fibrinogen filled with medium and, on the other, 1 ml of cells (24 million) and thrombin are mixed [1, 2].

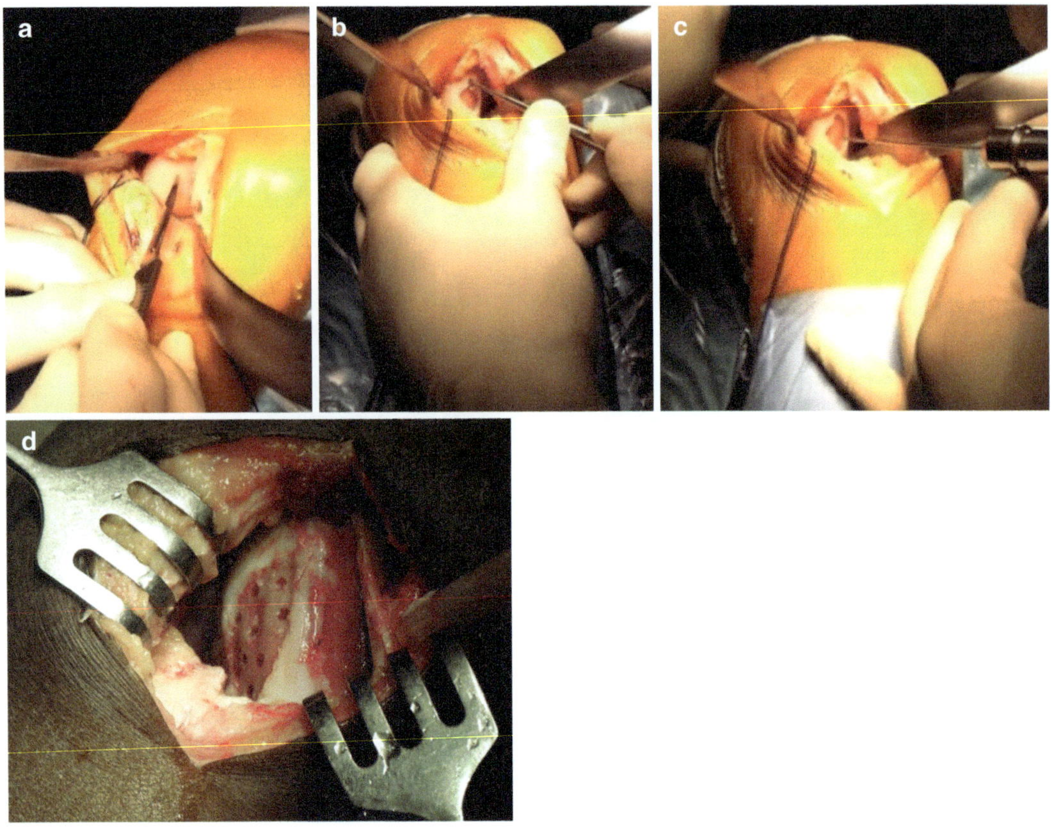

Fig. 15.10 (a) Preparation of edge of lesion with no. 11 blade. (b) Curettage of lesion to subchondral bone. (c) Multiple drill holes up to 3 mm depth into the subchondral bone. (d) Lesion prepared for implantation of cells

After preparing the autologous chondrocytes-fibrin mix, the affected knee is flexed so as to position the surface of lesion parallel to the floor in a gravity-dependent position (Fig. 15.11a). Autologous cultured chondrocytes mixed with fibrin gel is slowly injected onto the defect area starting from filling the holes, then the periphery and then to the center [1, 8]. The injected mix of chondrocytes-fibrin gel fills and sticks to defect site and replicates the convexity of the condylar surface [2] (Fig. 15.11b, c). In order to avoid overflow of ACI-fibrin gel mixture into the surrounding area, the gravity-dependent position of the defect site should be maintained for 5–6 min. Flexion and extension motion of the knee is performed three to five times in order to check for any graft stability [8]. After implantation, appropriate measures should be taken to close the incision made to knee (Fig. 15.12) [1, 8].

15.3 Postoperative Rehabilitation

The rehabilitation program after GACI varies with size and location of the area of cartilage damage [7]. The basic principles for success of the postoperative GACI rehabilitation program should be focused on the safeguard of graft, joint mobilization exercises, muscle strengthening, and load progression.

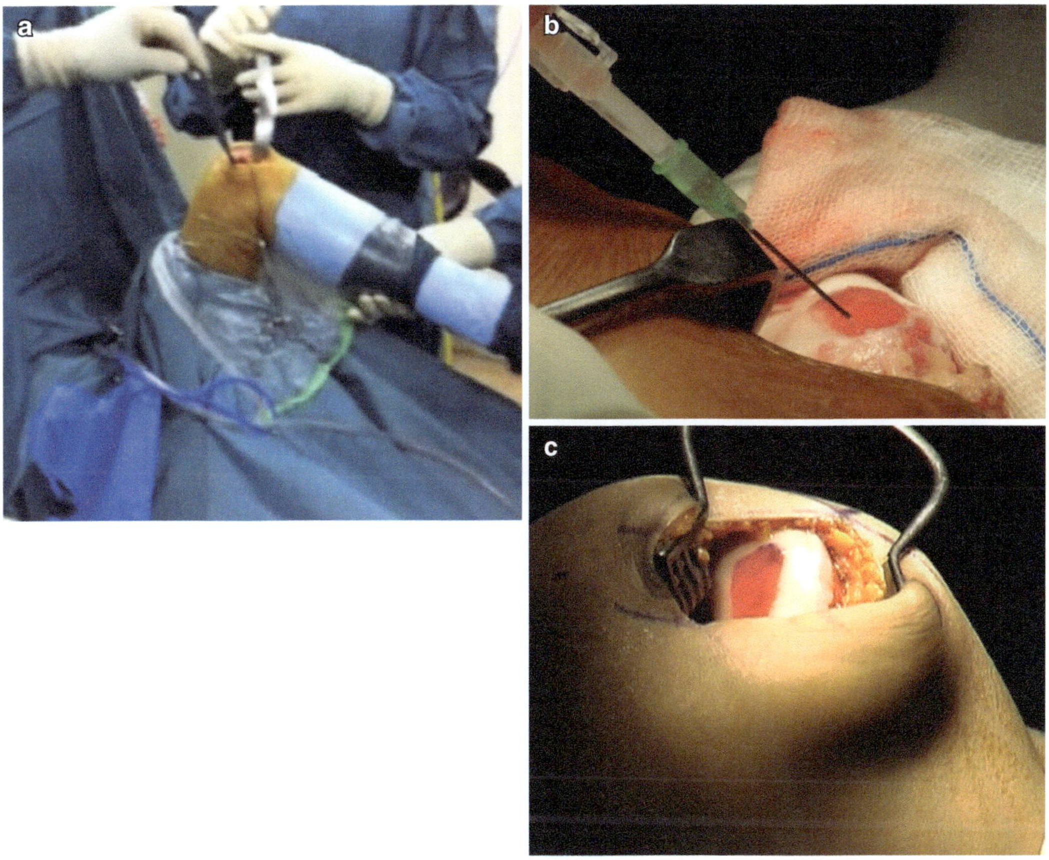

Fig. 15.11 Clinical photographs taken during autologous chondrocytes implantation: (**a**) Position of leg for implantation with surface of lesion parallel to the floor. (**b**) Injection of fibrin gel mixed autologous chondrocyte cells on defect. (**c**) Graft of autologous chondrocytes cells with fibrin gel on defect site after implantation

15.3.1 Weight Bearing

Following surgery, Continuous Passive Motion (CPM) is initiated for 4–6 h while the patient remains in the hospital. Patients need to avoid excessive weight-bearing activities immediately after surgery. Partial weight bearing is advised for at least 6 weeks following surgery and then steadily progressed over time. After 3–6 months, training can increase in load bearing and intensity, and sporting activities can begin about 9–12 months after surgery [7, 8].

15.3.2 Range of Motion

Range of motion is usually initiated early on after surgery. However, if the area of GACI treatment is within the patellofemoral joint, flexion is increased by 20° a week, up to 6 weeks, when the brace is removed [7, 8]. The reason for starting motion as early as possible is that the movement helps to stimulate healthy cartilage development. However, this motion must be balanced with the pressure caused by motion [7].

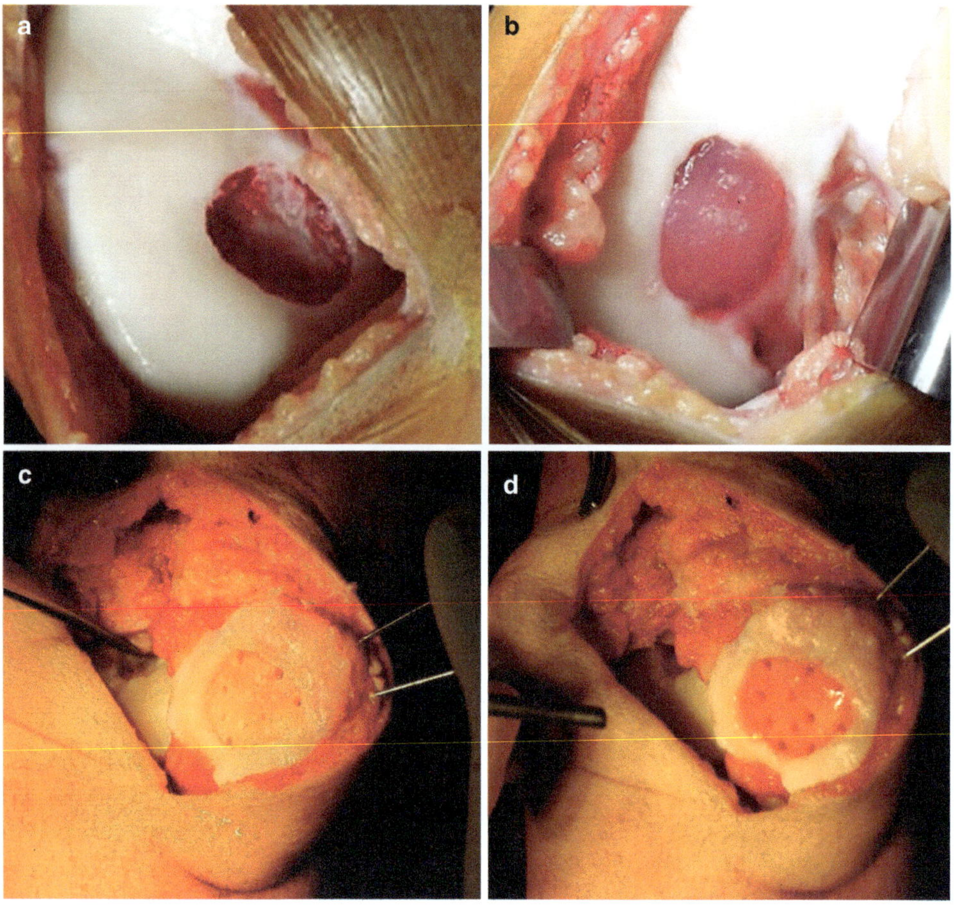

Fig. 15.12 Clinical photographs: (**a**, **b**) Pre- and post-implant medial femoral condylar lesion. (**c**, **d**) Pre- and post-implant patellar lesion

15.4 Complications

Few complication associated with ACI are symptomatic hypertrophy, inadequate fusion of the regenerative cartilage to the healthy surrounding cartilage, insufficient regenerative cartilage, formation of fibrous cartilage, and delamination. Adaptations of newer techniques, trained surgeons, and compliance with postoperative rehabilitation have reduced the failure and complication associated with traditional ACI procedures (Fig. 15.13).

15.5 Results

The MTT assay showed that the viability of the cells in the gel remained above 90 % of the initial viability for 72 h (Fig. 15.14a). The cells were found to be well mixed with fibrin and evenly distributed within the gel (Fig. 15.14b). The viable status and distribution of chondrocytes in the gel were also confirmed based on the Calcein-AM/Ethidium homodimer-1 staining. The viability of the cells in the cell-gel mixture, according to the fluorescence staining, was found to exceed 90 % after 72 h of

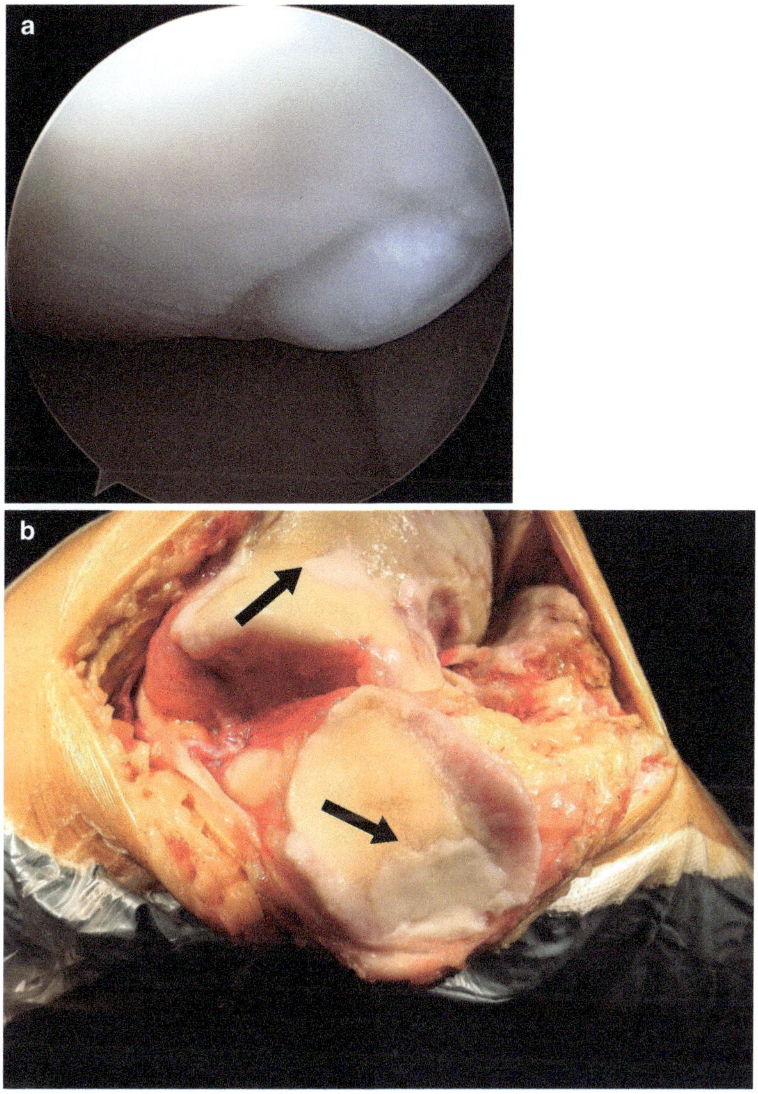

Fig. 15.13 (**a**) Hypertrophy of implanted cartilage. (**b**) Failure due to fibrous cartilage formation (*Arrows*: trochlear and patellar lesions)

culturing the mixture, as shown in the MTT assay (Fig. 15.15). We found that the pores were evenly present within the fibrin gel. We also noted that the chondrocytes were evenly distributed and maintained a round shape within the pores on the scanning electron microscopy (SEM) (Fig. 15.16).

Clinician evaluations showed significant mean improvement in the tKSS-A and tKSS-B scores for all of the data of the three, postoperative, follow-up periods (95 % confidence interval, P-value <0.05) (Fig. 15.17).

The tKSS-A score showed improvement from 43.52 ± 20.20 to 89.71 ± 13.69 ($P<0.05$), while according to the tKSS-B scores, knees were shown to have improved from 50.66 ± 20.05 to 89.38 ± 15.76 ($P<0.05$). The total improvement was from 94.18 ± 31.43 to 179.10 ± 24.69 ($P<0.05$). Clinical evaluations showed significant mean improvement in the tKSS-A and tKSS-B scores for each postoperative follow-up period (95 % confidence interval, P-value <0.05) (Table 15.1).

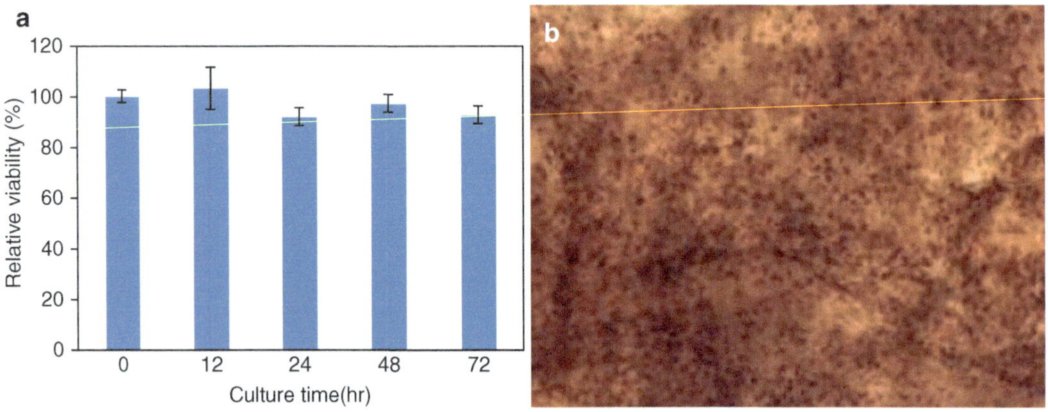

Fig. 15.14 The viability and distribution of chondrocytes within the cell-fibrin gel. (**a**) The relative cell viability profiles assayed by MTT assay. (**b**) The distribution of chondrocytes within the gel

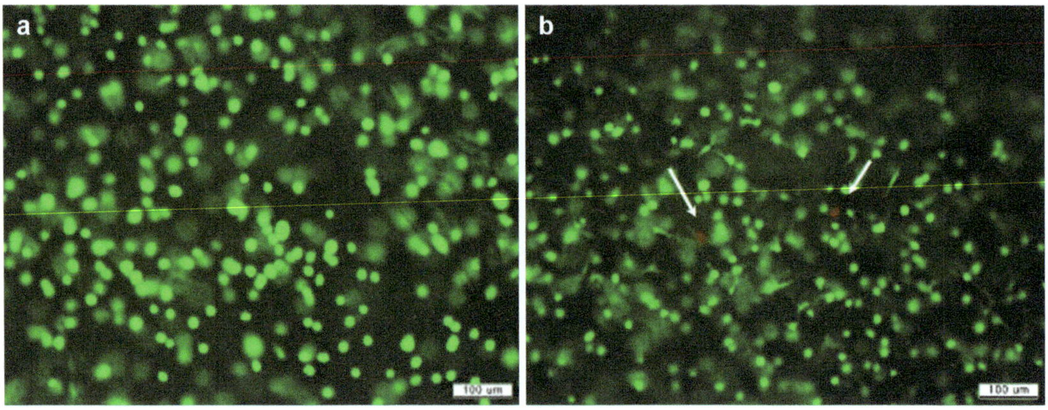

Fig. 15.15 The viable chondrocytes within the cell-gel mixture on Calcein-AM/Ethidium homodimer-1 staining: (**a**) A 0-h and (**b**) a 72-h culture (×100). The *white arrows* in (**b**) denotes the dead cells which appear as a reddish color

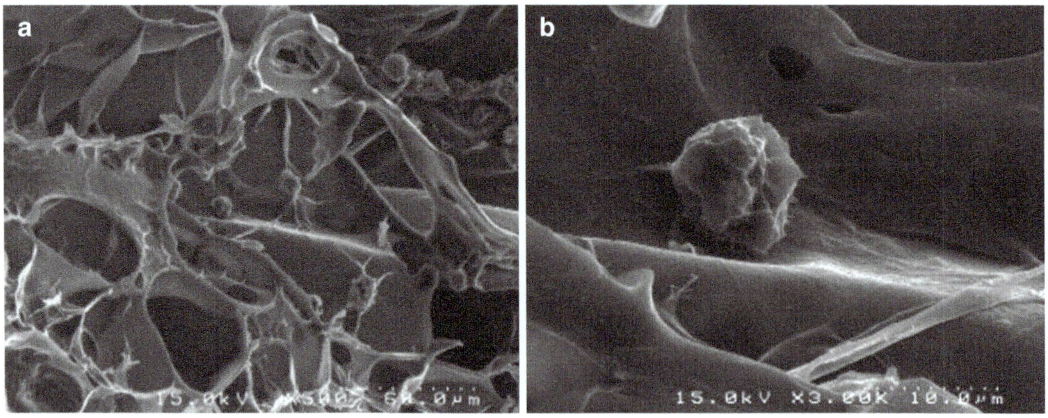

Fig. 15.16 A scanning electron microscopy picture showing the morphological structure of chondrocytes within the cell-fibrin gel. The cell-fibrin gel was incubated in a CO_2 incubator and was freeze-dried in order to reveal the scaffold structure. (**a**) ×500, (**b**) ×3,000

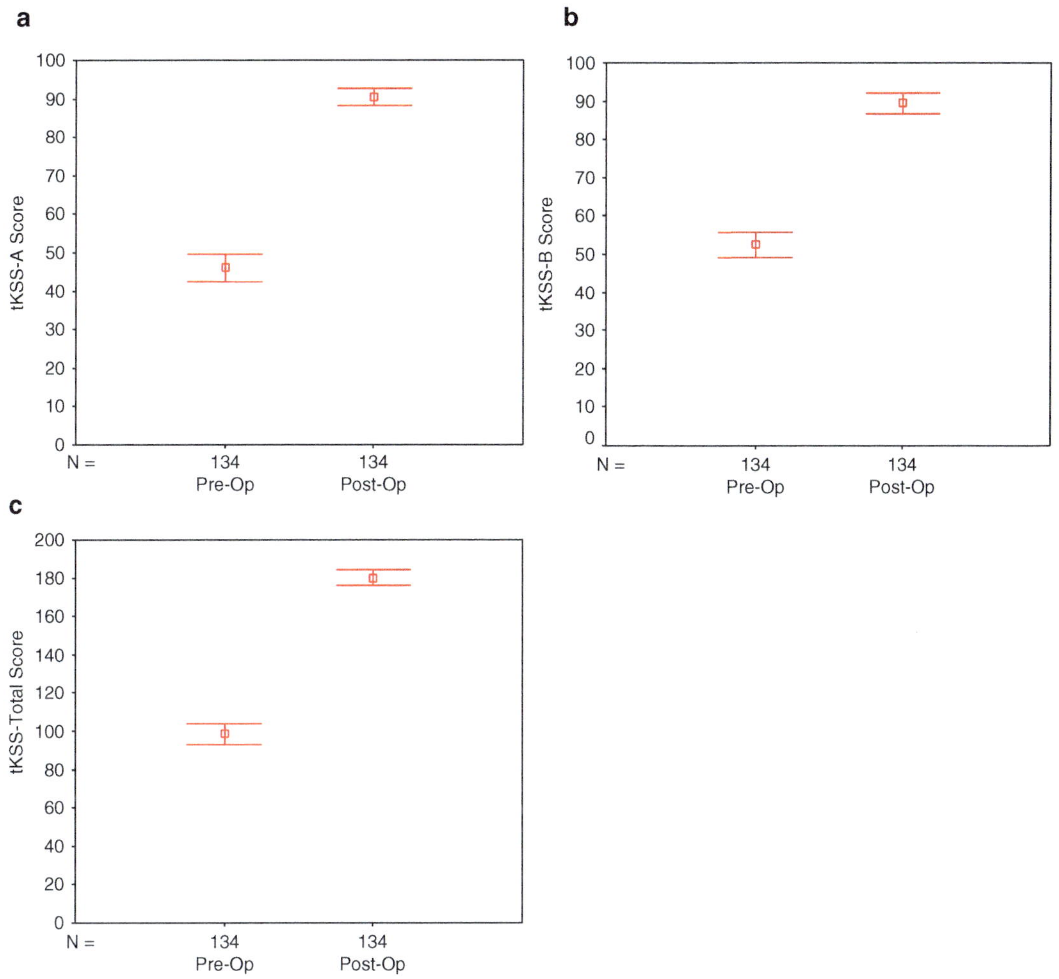

Fig. 15.17 The *error-bar graph* illustrating the tKSS-A, tKSS-B, and tKSS-total scores (95 % confidence intervals)

Table 15.1 Overall KSS scores [1]

		Pre-op (mean ± std)	Post-op (mean ± std)	*P*-value[a]
tKSS-A		43.52 ± 20.20	89.71 ± 13.69	<0.05
tKSS-B		50.66 ± 20.05	89.38 ± 15.76	<0.05
tKSS-total		94.18 ± 31.43	179.10 ± 24.69	<0.05
Post-op 13–24 months	tKSS-A	47.37 ± 20.56	88.58 ± 15.04	<0.05
	tKSS-B	53.70 ± 18.62	88.70 ± 16.39	<0.05
	tKSS-total	101.08 ± 30.22	177.29 ± 27.19	<0.05
Post-op > 25 months	tKSS-A	37.92 ± 18.53	91.35 ± 11.44	<0.05
	tKSS-B	46.25 ± 21.44	90.37 ± 14.95	<0.05
	tKSS-total	84.17 ± 30.78	181.72 ± 20.57	<0.05

[a]Statistical significance was evaluated using the Wilcoxon signed-rank test

Table 15.2 The tKSS score difference in each group [1]

	Post-op 13–24 months ($n=58$)	Post-op >25 months ($n=40$)	P-value[a]
tKSS-A difference (mean ± std)	41.20 ± 22.75	53.42 ± 17.95	<0.05
tKSS-B difference (mean ± std)	35.00 ± 20.32	44.12 ± 25.69	<0.05
tKSS-total difference (mean ± std)	76.20 ± 35.97	97.55 ± 31.41	<0.05

[a]Statistical significance was tested using the Mann-Whitney test in each group

According to the follow-up period, improvement of the score of the "greater than 25 months" group was statistically greater than that of the other group (Table 15.2). Improvements in tKSS-A and B scores were not found to be related to age, gender, defect size, defect location, the number of vials of chondrocyte used for implantation, or the time interval between cartilage harvesting and ACI.

References

1. Choi N-Y, Kim B-W, Yeo W-J, Kim H-B, Suh D-S, Kim J-S, Kim Y-S, Seo Y-H, Cho J-Y, Chun C-W, Park H-S, Shetty AA, Kim S-J (2010) Gel-type autologous chondrocyte (Chondron™) implantation for treatment of articular cartilage defects of the knee. BMC Musculoskelet Disord 11:103. doi:10.1186/1471-2474-11-103
2. Kim MK, Choi SW, Kim SR, Oh IS, Won MH (2010) Autologous chondrocyte implantation in the knee using fibrin. Knee Surg Sports Traumatol Arthrosc 18:528–534. doi:10.1007/s00167-009-0905-y
3. Filardo G, Kon E, Di Martino A, Iacono F, Marcacci M (2011) Arthroscopic second-generation autologous chondrocyte implantation: a prospective 7-year follow-up study. Am J Sports Med 39(10):2153–2160
4. Ipach I, Schäfer R, Lahrmann J, Kluba T (2011) Stiffness after knee arthrotomy: evaluation of prevalence and results after manipulation under anaesthesia. Orthop Traumatol Surg Res 97(3):292–296. doi:10.1016/j.otsr.2011.01.006, Epub 2011 Apr 11
5. Barreto RB, Pécora JR, Gobbi RG, de Rezende MU, Camanho GL (2011) Autologous chondrocyte implantation. Acta Ortop Bras 19(4):219–225
6. Van den Borne MP, Raijmakers NJ, Vanlauwe J, Victor J, de Jong SN, Bellemans J, Saris DB (2007) International Cartilage Repair Society (ICRS) and Oswestry macroscopic cartilage evaluation scores validated for use in Autologous Chondrocyte Implantation (ACI) and microfracture. Osteoarthritis Cartilage 15(12):1397–1402, Epub 2007 Jul 2
7. Reinold MM, Wilk KE, Macrina LC, Dugas JR, Cain EL (2006) Current concepts in the rehabilitation following articular cartilage repair procedures in the knee. J Orthop Sports Phys Ther 36:774–794
8. Kim S-J, Chang C-H, Suh D-S, Ha H-K, Suhl K-H (2009) Autologous chondrocyte implantation for rheumatoid arthritis of the knee: a case report. J Med Case Reports 3:6619

A Scaffold-Free Mesenchymal Stem Cells-Based Implant to Repair a Three-Dimensional Chondral Lesion

16

Kazunori Shimomura, Wataru Ando, Hideki Yoshikawa, and Norimasa Nakamura

Contents

K. Shimomura, MD, PhD
H. Yoshikawa, MD, PhD
Department of Orthopaedics, Osaka University Graduate School of Medicine, 2-2 Yamadaoka, Suita, Osaka 565-0871, Japan
e-mail: kazunori-shimomura@umin.net; yhideki@ort.med.osaka-u.ac.jp

W. Ando, MD, PhD
Department of Orthopaedics, Kansai Rosai Hospital, 3-1-69 Inabasou, Amagasaki, Hyogo 660-8511, Japan
e-mail: w-ando@umin.ac.jp

N. Nakamura, MD, PhD (✉)
Institute for Medical Science in Sports, Osaka Health Science University, 1-9-27 Tenma, Kita-ku, Osaka City, Osaka 530-0043, Japan

Center for Advanced Medical Engineering and Informatics, Osaka University, 2-2 Yamadaoka, Suita, Osaka 565-0871, Japan
e-mail: norimasa.nakamura@ohsu.ac.jp

16.1 Introduction

The articular cartilage does not usually heal spontaneously due to its avascular surroundings and unique matrix organization. Therefore, a variety of approaches have been tested to improve cartilage healing [1, 2]. Among them, chondrocyte-based therapies have been extensively studied since the successful report of autologous chondrocyte implantation [3–5]. However, this procedure may have limitations including the sacrifice of undamaged cartilage within the same joint and alterations associated with the in vitro expansion of the cells. Furthermore, due to the degenerative changes in the cartilage accompanying aging, the availability of the cells may be limited in elderly individuals [6].

A.A. Shetty et al. (eds.), *Techniques in Cartilage Repair Surgery*,
DOI 10.1007/978-3-642-41921-8_16, © ESSKA 2014

To overcome such potential problems, stem cell therapy has been tested to facilitate regenerative tissue repair. Mesenchymal stem cells (MSCs) have the capability to differentiate into a variety of connective tissue cells including the bone, cartilage, tendon, muscle, and adipose tissue [7]. These cells may be isolated from various tissues such as the bone marrow, skeletal muscle, synovial membrane, adipose tissue, and umbilical cord blood [7–12]. Pluripotent cells isolated from the synovium may be well suited for cell-based therapies for the cartilage because of the relative ease of harvest and their strong capability of chondrogenic differentiation [9]. Synovium-derived cells are reported to exhibit the greatest chondrogenic potential among the other mesenchymal tissue-derived cells examined [10].

In addition to the selection of cell source, local delivery of cells to chondral lesions has been another area of concern. It is widely accepted that the appropriate three-dimensional (3D) environment is important to optimize cell proliferation and chondrogenic differentiation [13]. Therefore, a 3D scaffold, which is seeded with cells, is usually utilized to repair the defect. A scaffold generally consists of synthetic polymers such as poly(L-lactide) (PLLA), poly(glycolide) (PGA), poly(DL-lactide-co-glycolide) (PLGA), and alginate [14–17] or of biological materials such as collagen, fibrin, hyaluronan, and chitosan [18–21]. Various scaffolds have been approved for clinical use by some governmental institutions [22]. However, there are still several issues associated with the long-term safety of the material. Synthetic polymers may have potential problems regarding retention and degradation in situ [23, 24]. Biological materials potentially carry the risk of transmission of infectious agents and precipitating immunological reactions [25, 26]. Taken together, in order to avoid unknown risk, such materials should ideally be excluded throughout the treatment procedure, and in this regard, a scaffold-free cell delivery system could be an excellent alternative.

Meanwhile, due to its unique matrix organization, articular cartilage has anti-adhesive properties and therefore, integration of implanted tissue to adjacent cartilage matrix has been an issue in the treatment of chondral injuries [2]. To overcome this problem, most implantation procedures into chondral lesions have required enzyme treatment of the surface of the cartilage matrix [27] or reinforcement of the initial fixation by suturing [28, 29] or by the use of absorbable pins [30]. However, an animal study revealed that a suture track in the surrounding articular cartilage remains unhealed and thus a defect which could potentially be a trigger site for subsequent degradation of matrix around the margin between the implant and the adjacent cartilage tissue [28]. Therefore, an implantable tissue that possesses highly adhesive properties to the cartilage tissue is needed for secure tissue integration.

Additionally, another one of the crucial factors that may affect the results of cell-based therapies is the age of the donors and recipients. Regarding the cell proliferation and differentiation capacities of MSCs, it is controversial as to whether they are age-dependent [31–34] or not [9, 35–38]. In terms of the host tissue reaction, natural healing responses of osteochondral defects has been compared between immature and mature animals using rabbit models, and in this species, the studies demonstrated better healing responses in immature animals [39–42]. On the other hand, there have been no studies which compared the results of cell-based repair of chondral defects between immature and mature animal models. Regarding the clinically relevant animal models for cartilage repair, it is difficult to create a chondral injury which does not breach the subchondral bone in small animals such as rabbits, rats, and mice due to the limited thickness of their articular cartilage. Therefore, in consideration of clinical relevance, it is preferable to utilize a large animal model to investigate the influence of maturity on the results of cell-based therapy in chondral lesions.

To address these issues, several methods using bone marrow MSCs or synovial MSCs for chondral repair have been developed in our country [43–46]. Especially, we have developed a novel scaffold-free three-dimensional tissue-engineered construct (TEC) that is composed of either human or porcine MSCs derived from the synovium and the extracellular matrices (ECMs) synthesized by

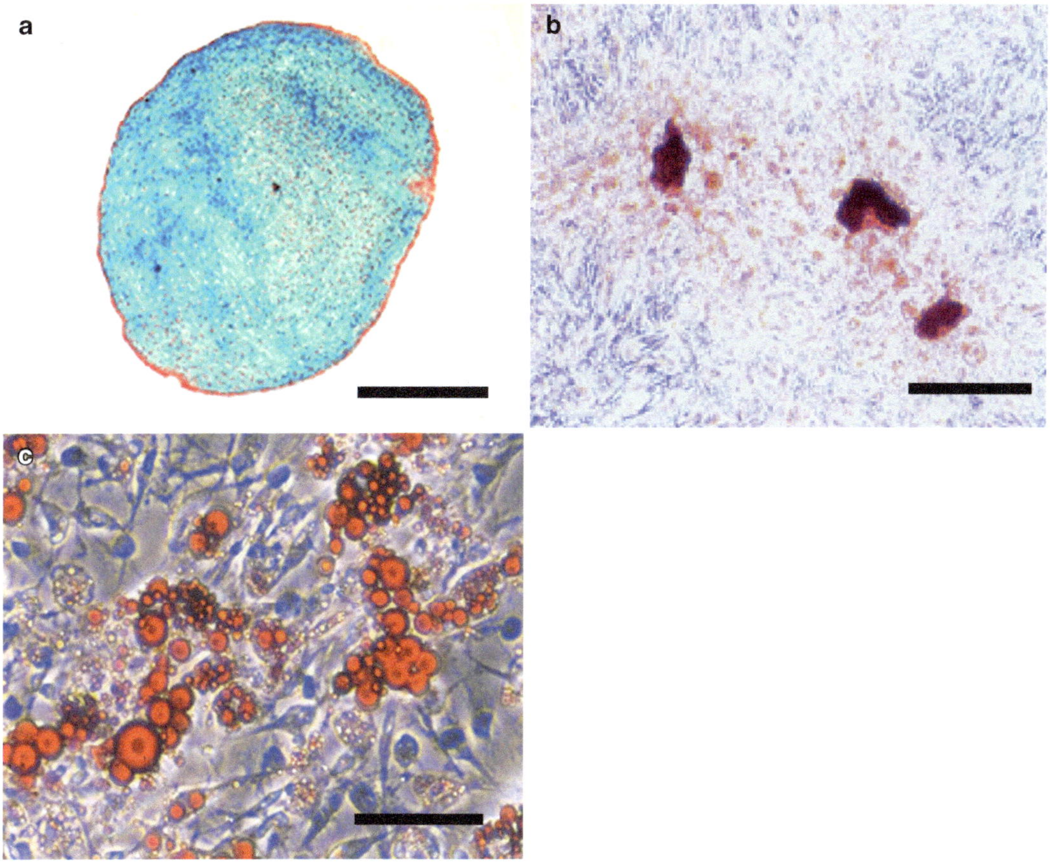

Fig. 16.1 Pluripotency of the synovial cells. (**a**) Alcian blue staining of the cultured synovial cells under pellet culture system in chondrogenic medium. There is intense blue staining observed. Bar = 500 μm. (**b**) Alizarin red staining of the synovial cells (at passage 5) under osteogenic medium. These synovial cells form mineralized matrix as evidenced by Alizarin red staining. Bar = 100 μm. (**c**) Oil-red O staining of synovial cells (at passage 5) under adipogenic medium. Morphological changes in cells as well as the formation of neutral lipid vacuoles are noticeable. Bar = 100 μm

the cells [47–49]. In the present chapter, the suitability and effectiveness of the TEC in cartilage repair and regeneration will be discussed.

16.2 Characterization of Cultured Cells Derived from the Human Synovium

The cultured cells isolated from the human synovium displayed a long-term self-renewal capacity and expanded over at least 10 passages in basal medium with consistent growth kinetics (data not shown). The cell surface phenotypic marker analyses showed that the cells were consistently positive (>80 %) for CD13, CD44, and CD90; weakly positive (3–80 %) for CD29, CD34, CD54, CD105, and CD166; and negative (<3 %) for CD14, CD31, and CD45. Although there were slight changes in expression levels of markers between cells at passages 4 and 7, these profiles were generally similar to those of MSCs from various tissues such as the bone marrow, adipose tissue, and synovial membrane [10, 30, 50], except that the expression of CD105 was lower in the present results. The differentiation capacity of the cultured human cells to chondrogenic, osteogenic, and adipogenic lineages at either passage were confirmed by in vitro differentiation assays (Fig. 16.1a–c). Based on these findings, the cultured cells derived from the human synovium were considered to be MSCs.

16.3 Development of the Basic TEC

When synovium-derived MSCs were cultured to confluence in the basic growth medium, they did not synthesize an abundant collagenous matrix. In contrast, in the presence of >0.1 mM ascorbic acid-2 phosphate (Asc-2P), collagen synthesis significantly increased with time in culture (Fig. 16.2a, b). Subsequently, the monolayer cell-matrix complex cultured in Asc-2P became a stiff sheet-like structure, which could be easily

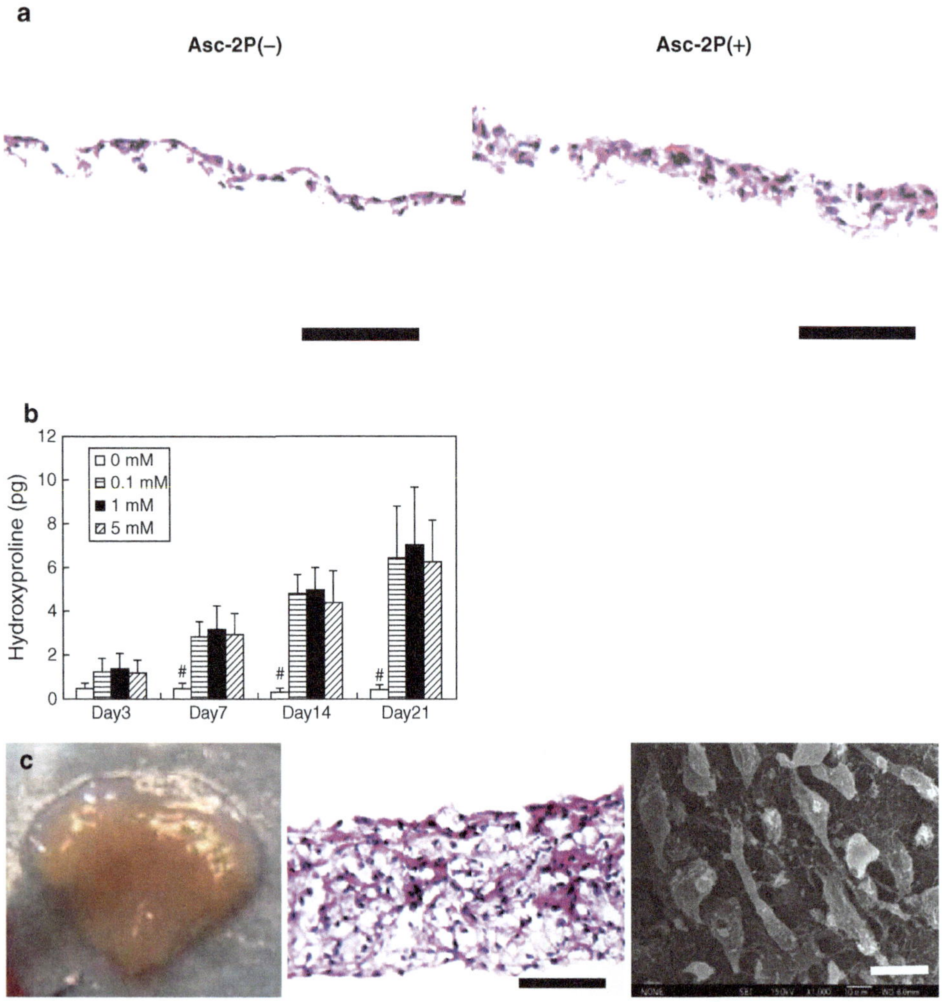

Fig. 16.2 Development of the TEC. (**a**) Photomicrograph of monolayer culture in the absence (*left*) or presence (*right*) of 0.2 mM ascorbic acid 2-phosphate (Asc-2P). Bar = 100 μm. (**b**) The hydroxyproline contents of the TEC (1.6×10^6 cells/12 well culture plate) cultured in the growth medium in the absence or presence of Asc-2P (0.1, 1, and 5 mM). There is a significant increase in collagen synthesis when Asc-2P is added at the concentration of more than 0.1 mM over 7 days ($N=4$, # $p<0.001$, compared to 0 mM). There is no significant dose effect of Asc-2P at more than 0.1 mM. In the presence of Asc-2P, collagen synthesis was significantly increased with time-dependency ($p<0.001$). (**c**) Macroscopic view (*left*: Bar = 1 cm), photomicrograph (*middle*: Bar = 100 μm), and SEM view (*right*: Bar = 20 μm) of the TEC. (**d**) Immunohistochemical analysis of the TEC stained with type I collagen (Col I), type II collagen (Col II), type III collagen (Col III), fibronectin, vitronectin, and negative IgG (control). Red is nuclei and green is target antibody. Adhesion molecules such as fibronectin and vitronectin are diffusely distributed within the TEC. Bar = 100 μm. (**e**) Macroscopic view of the TEC (8.0×10^6 cells//6 cm dish, 14 days culture) which was integrated to one spherical body. The diameter of this TEC was 5 mm and the thickness was 2 mm. (**f**) HE staining (*right*) and fibronectin staining (*right*) of the TEC which was integrated to one spherical body with additional 7 days culture. Bar = 100 μm

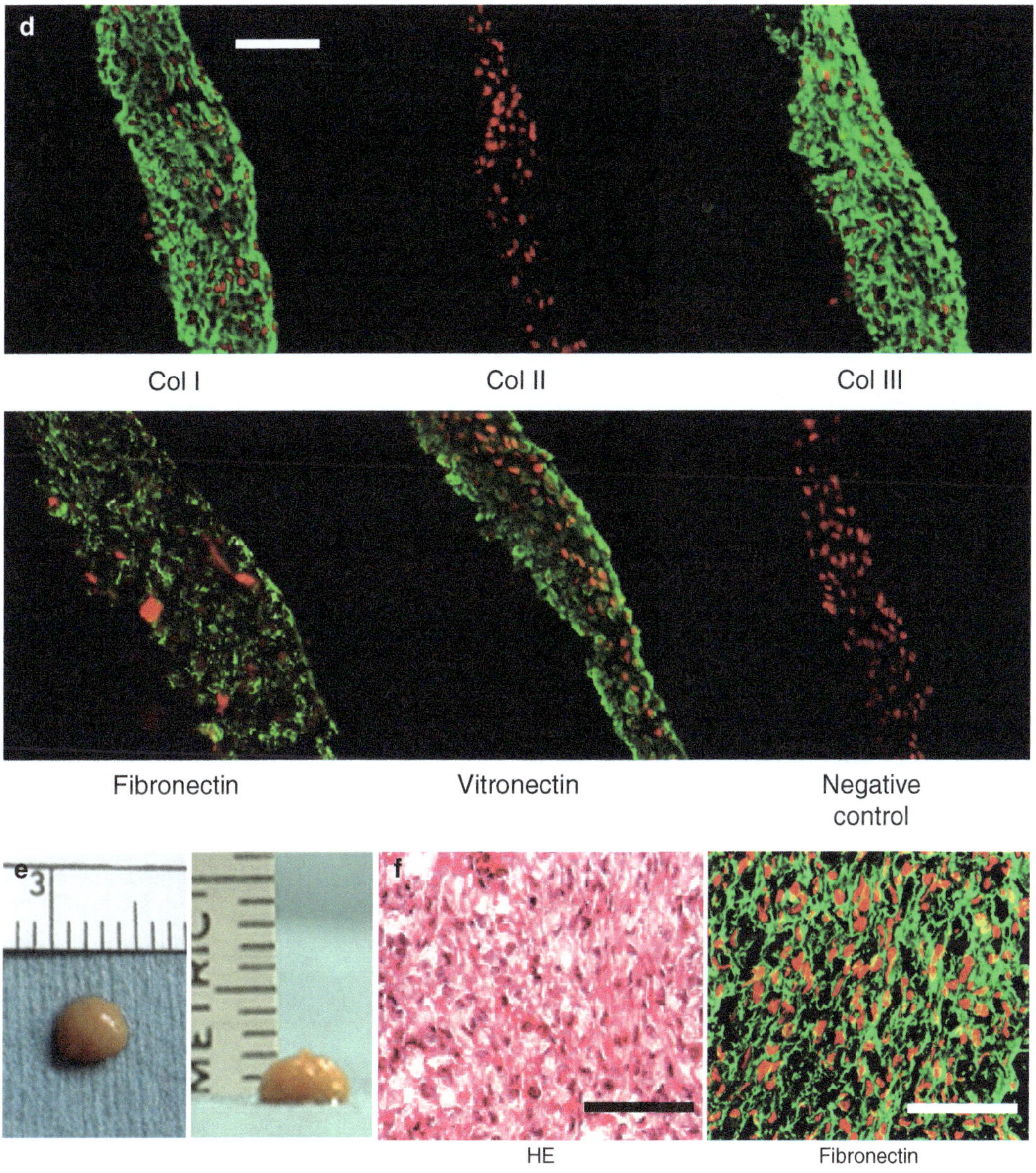

Fig. 16.2 (continued)

detached from the substratum by exerting mild shear stress at the cell-substratum interface using gentle pipetting. After detachment, the monolayer sheet immediately began to actively contract and evolved into a thick 3D tissue (Fig. 16.2c). Histology and scanning electron microscope (SEM) assessment of the 3D tissue showed that the cells and the ECM were three dimensionally integrated together at high cell density. Immunohistochemical analysis showed that the TEC was rich in collagen I and III. In contrast, there was no expression of collagen II within the TEC. Fibronectin and vitronectin were also abundant in the TEC (Fig. 16.2d). Notably, all the molecules were diffusely distributed throughout the matrix and there was no overt polarity in matrix organization within the TEC. When the TEC was folded within the matrix, it was apparent that the layers were integrated into each other and a series of foldings led to development of one spherical body several millimeters thick (Fig. 16.2e, f).

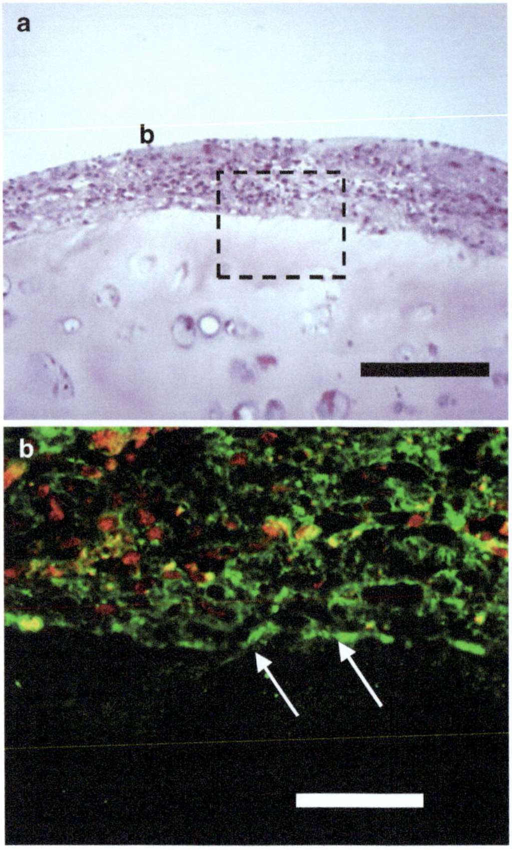

Fig. 16.3 The TEC had adhesiveness to cartilage matrix. (**a**) Photomicrograph (HE staining) of the cultured chondral fragment for 7 days after the implantation of the TEC on the injured surface. As can be seen, the bioengineered tissue is closely attached to the injured surface. Bar = 200 μm. (**b**) Immunohistochemical analysis stained with fibronectin in area enclosed by a *dotted rectangle* in (a). Bar = 50 μm

This contracted tissue was termed a tissue-engineered construct (TEC) derived from MSCs.

16.4 The Basic Human TEC Has Adhesive Properties Which Facilitate Association and Adhesion to Cartilage Matrix

To test the adhesive property of the TEC to an established intact cartilage matrix, basic human TECs were placed on the injured surface of a fresh-frozen human chondral fragment. Within 5 min, the TEC had adhered to the chondral fragments. When the TEC-chondral complexes were further cultured for 7 days, they remained stably associated for the entire time. Histology at day 7 showed close adhesion of the TEC to the injured surface of the chondral fragments (Fig. 16.3a). Immunohistochemistry showed that fibronectin (Fig. 16.3b) and vitronectin (data not shown) were localized at the interface between the TEC and the injured surfaces of chondral fragments.

16.5 Chondrogenic Differentiation Capacity of a Human TEC

Human TEC cultured in a chondrogenic medium containing BMP-2 showed increased glycosaminoglycan (GAG) synthesis and deposition as evidenced by intense Alcian blue staining (Fig. 16.4a). The quantification of GAGs indicated that GAG synthesis was significantly higher in the TEC exposed to the chondrogenic medium compared to those generated in the absence of such components (Fig. 16.4b, c). Detection of cartilage-specific markers, collagen II (Col2a1), aggrecan, and sox9 messenger RNA (m-RNA) by semiquantitative RT-PCR confirmed the cartilage phenotype of the treated TEC. Untreated TEC, as well as monolayer cell cultures, showed only a weak expression of cartilage-specific markers (Fig. 16.4d).

16.6 A Basic Porcine TEC Can Effectively Repair Chondral Defects In Vivo and Inhibit the Progression of Chondral Defects to Overt Osteoarthritis for a Wide Range of Ages

In order to assess the efficacy of the TEC in an in vivo model, a porcine model was chosen as the physiology of the pig is similar to that of humans in many respects [51], and porcine articular cartilage of the knee is sufficiently thick as to allow creation of a chondral defect without damaging the subchondral bone. Prior to performing

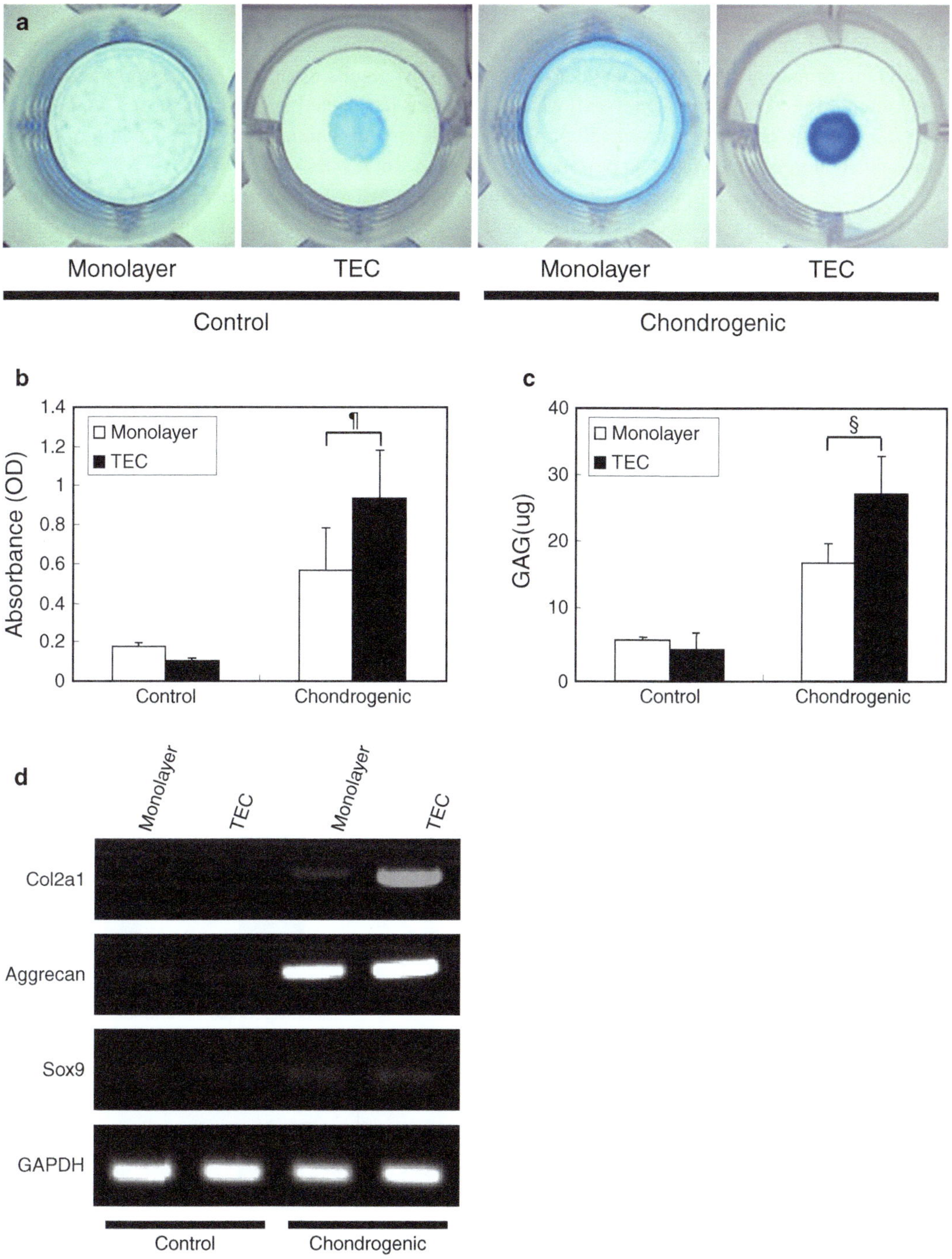

Fig. 16.4 Chondrogenesis of the TEC. (**a**) Alcian blue staining of the monolayer cultured synovial cells or the TEC in the control medium or in the chondrogenic medium for 14 days, respectively. (**b**, **c**) The quantification of Alcian blue staining (**b**) and GAG contents (**c**) of monolayer culture complex or the TEC in the control medium or in the chondrogenic medium. GAG synthesis is significantly higher in the TEC treated by chondrogenic medium ($N=8$, ¶ $p=0.047$, § $p=0.016$). (**d**) Semiquantitative reverse transcription-PCR (RT-PCR) analysis for chondrogenic marker genes, type II collagen (Col2a1), aggrecan, Sox 9, and GAPDH

such studies, a preliminary characterization of the ability of porcine-derived MSC from the synovium comparable to that discussed above for the human MSC was undertaken. Next, we compared the in vitro characteristics of cell proliferation and chondrogenic capacity in porcine MSCs isolated from skeletally immature animals with mature animals. Cell number assessments, as well as WST-1 assays, demonstrated that there were no significant differences in the proliferation capacity of porcine synovial MSCs derived from immature or mature animals (Fig. 16.5a, b). In addition, there were no significant differences in chondrogenic capacities between MSCs isolated from immature and mature animals, based on the results of mRNA expression level of collagen II detected by RT-PCR, GAG synthesis, or Alcian blue staining using a pellet culture system (Fig. 16.5c–f).

To test the feasibility of using a porcine TEC for a wide range of ages without chondrogenic manipulation to repair a chondral injury, immature as well as mature porcine chondral injury model was used. After implantation, the TEC firmly adhered to the injured joint surface without suture. To confirm the early adhesion

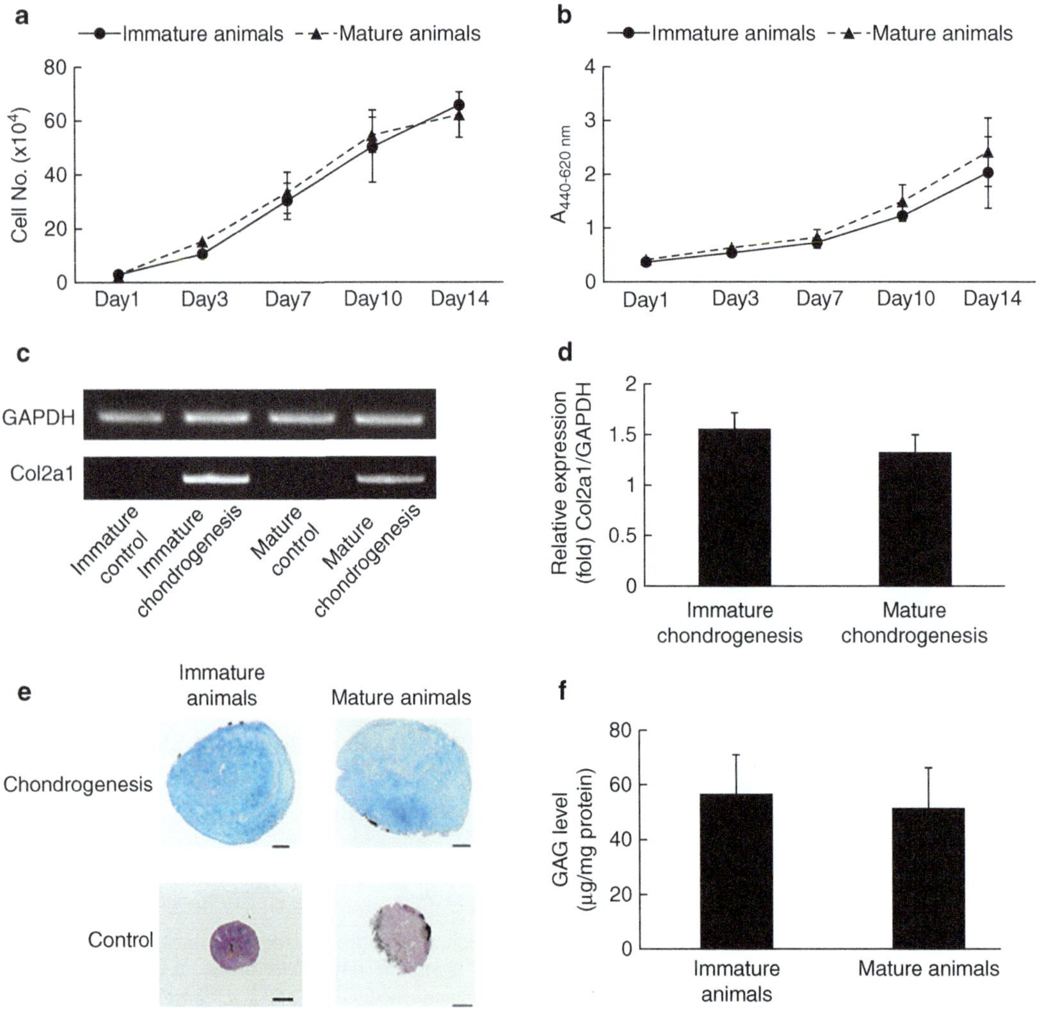

Fig. 16.5 Cell Proliferation assay assessed by cell counting (**a**) and the WST-1 method (**b**). There are no significant differences in proliferative capacity between immature ($N=3$) and mature porcine synovial MSCs ($N=3$). Chondrogenic potential of porcine MSCs derived from immature and mature animals assessed by collagen II expression by RT-PCR (**c**, **d**), alcian blue staing (**e**), and GAG synthesis (**f**). Bar = 200 mm. There are no significant differences detected between immature-pellets ($N=3$) and mature-pellets ($N=3$) in RT-PCR (**d**) and GAG synthesis (**f**)

mode of the TEC to the injured surface, histology at Day 7 was examined. The TEC was tightly adhered to the injured chondral surfaces (Fig. 16.6a). Higher magnification revealed that the adhesion was mediated by matrix-to-matrix interaction (Fig. 16.6b) and, as shown in the in vitro culture study, fibronectin was localized to the interface between the TEC and the surface of the defects (Fig. 16.5c). At 6 months postimplantation, regardless of ages, untreated lesions had no or only partial tissue coverage, while the defects treated with the TEC were totally or partially covered with repaired tissue (Fig. 16.6d). The mean macroscopic score for the TEC group (1.50 ± 0.50, immature group, and 1.50 ± 0.50, mature group) was significantly higher than that for the untreated group (0.25 ± 0.50, immature group, and 0.67 ± 0.75, mature group) ($p = 0.017$ and $p = 0.034$, respectively) (Fig. 16.6e), where a lower score is suggestive of a failure to resolve and progression towards osteoarthritis. Histologically, the chondral lesions in the nontreatment control group showed evidence of osteoarthritic changes with loss of cartilage and destruction of subchondral bone in both skeletally immature and mature animals (Fig. 16.6f). Conversely, when treated with the TEC, the defects were filled with repair tissue exhibiting good integration to the adjacent cartilage and the restoration of a smooth surface, regardless of ages (Fig. 16.6f). Higher-magnification views showed that there was good tissue integration to the adjacent cartilage obtained when the TEC were implanted in both immature and mature animals (Fig. 16.6g, h, arrows). The repair tissue exhibited predominantly spindle-shaped fibroblast-like cells in the superficial area of the repair tissue, while the majority of the remaining repair matrix contained round-shaped cells in the lacuna (Fig. 16.6i, j). Following implantation, no histological findings were obtained that suggested either central necrosis of the implanted TEC or that an abnormal inflammatory macrophage and lymphocyte response consistent with immunological rejection had occurred in this allogenic situation, regardless of ages. In histological scoring, the TEC group exhibited significantly higher scores than did the control group in all criteria categories in the immature animals (Fig. 16.6k). In mature animals, the TEC group had significantly higher scores than did the corresponding control group in all categories except the "Matrix" and "Cell distribution" categories (Fig. 16.6l). Comparing the repair tissues by the TEC in immature and mature animals, there was no significant difference detected (Fig. 16.6m).

16.7 The Mechanical Properties of Porcine Chondral Defects Treated with a Porcine-Derived TEC Approximates Those of Normal Cartilage 6 Months Postimplantation

It is accepted that the articular cartilage is a biphasic viscoelastic material which indicates a strain-rate-dependent mechanical behavior [52]. It means that the viscoelasticity of the cartilage which retains interstitial water might be mainly reflected in faster compression test, while the matrix viscoelasticity without interstitial water could be mainly reflected in slower compression test.

In the tissue localized in the defects of the untreated control group, the tangent modulus (defined as the slope of the curve at 5 % of strain) in immature animals was significantly lower than that for normal cartilage at a compression rate of either 4 mm/s (Fig. 16.7a) or 100 mm/s (Fig. 16.7b). In contrast, there were no significant differences detected between the tangent modulus for the repair tissue by the TEC and that for normal cartilage at either 4 mm/s (Fig. 16.7a) or 100 mm/s (Fig. 16.7b) in immature animals. Similarly, the mean tangent modulus in the untreated mature animals was significantly lower than that for normal cartilage at a compression rate of 4 mm/s (Fig. 16.7a), while there were no significant differences detected between the tangent modulus for repaired tissue in mature recipients treated by the TEC and that for normal cartilage at either 4 mm/s (Fig. 16.7a) or 100 mm/s (Fig. 16.7b). These results suggest that the viscoelastic properties of the tissue in defects repaired by the TEC are likely similar to those of normal cartilage, regardless of ages.

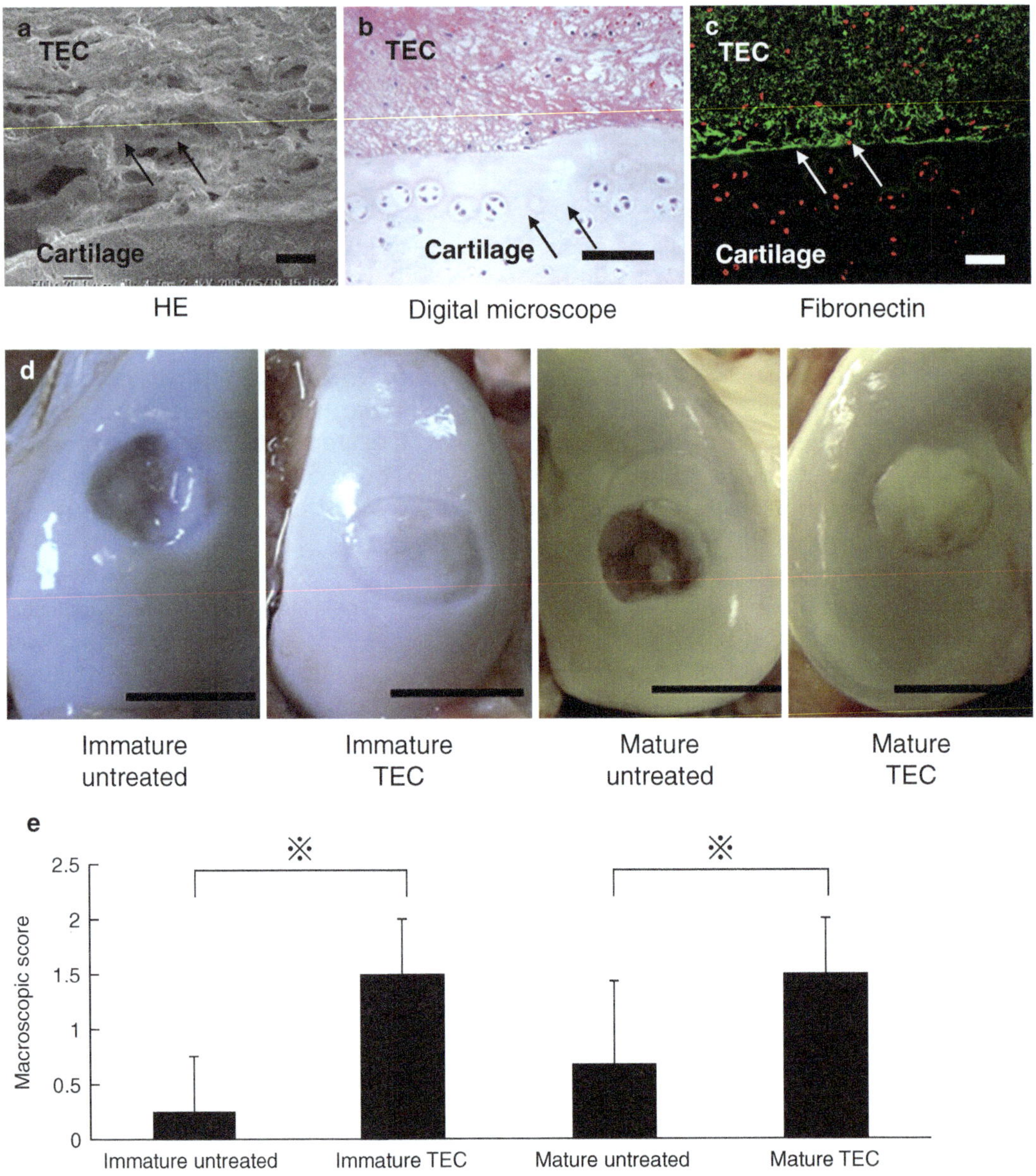

Fig. 16.6 Macroscopical and histological assessment of in vivo TEC implantation on chondral defect. (**a–c**) Photomicrograph (HE staining; **a**), the interface view by digital microscope (**b**), and fibronectin staining (**c**) of porcine chondral defect treated with TEC at day 7. *Arrows* indicate interface between the TEC and the cartilage defect. Bar=50 μm. (**d**) Macroscopic view of immature or mature porcine chondral lesion treated without or with the TEC at 6 months after operation. Bar=10 mm. (**e**) Macroscopic score of the chondral lesion treated with the TEC (immature animals, $N=8$; mature animals, $N=6$) or untreated (immature animals, $N=4$; mature animals, $N=6$) at 6 months. Regardless of ages, the TEC group shows significantly higher score than the untreated group. ※; $p<0.05$. (**f**) Safranin-O staining of untreated chondral lesions or lesions repaired by the TEC. Bar=1 mm. (**g–j**) Higher magnification view at the border area (**g**, **h**) and central area (**i**, **j**) of the repaired tissue by the TEC. Bar=200 mm. Regardless of ages, the defects treated with the TEC are completely filled with Safranin-O-positive repaired tissue (**i**, **j**) with good tissue integration (**g**, **h**, *arrow*). (**k–m**) Modified ICRS score in repaired cartilage immature (**k**) and mature animals (**l**). The TEC group ($N=8$) exhibits significantly higher scores than does the untreated control group ($N=4$) in all the criteria categories in the immature animals. ※; $p<0.05$. Likewise, the TEC group ($N=6$) exhibits significantly higher scores than does the untreated control group ($N=6$) in the criteria categories except for the "Matrix" and "Cell distribution" categories in the mature recipients. ※; $p<0.05$. (**m**) As to the quality of repaired cartilage by the TEC, there is no significant difference observed in any criteria category between the immature ($N=8$) and mature animals ($N=6$)

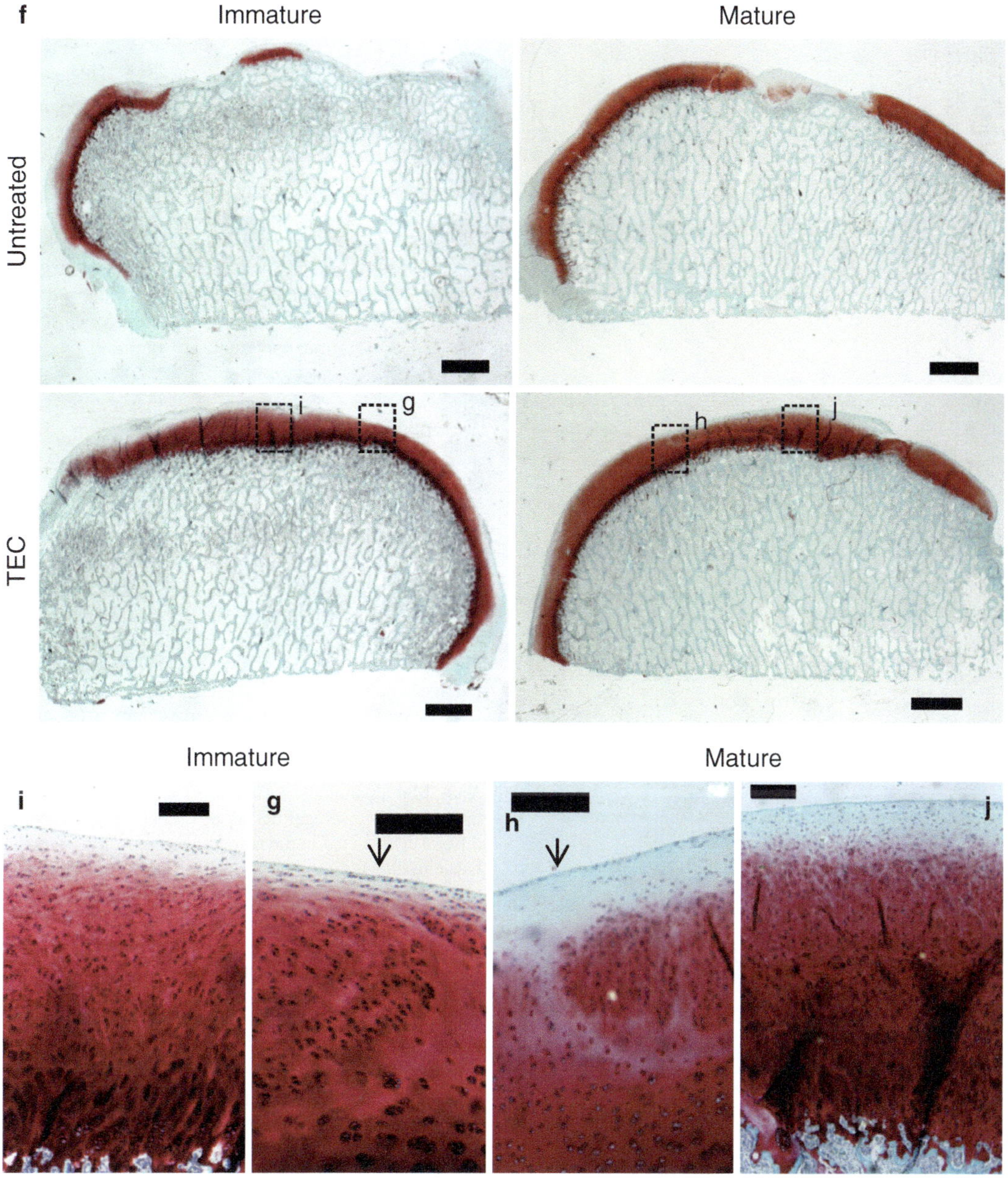

Fig. 16.6 (continued)

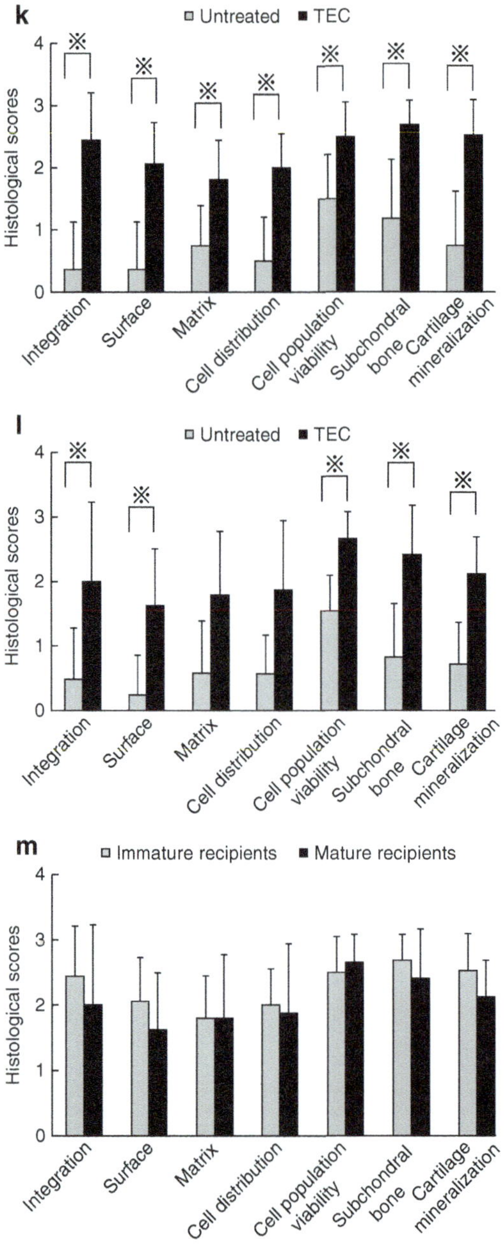

Fig. 16.6 (continued)

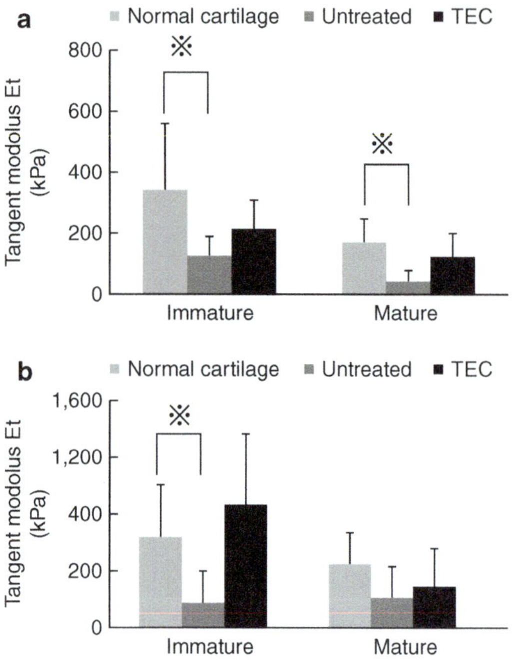

Fig. 16.7 Mechanical assessment of in vivo TEC implantation on chondral defect. (**a**, **b**) The results of compression tests at slower compression speed (4 mm/s) (**a**) and at faster compression speed (100 mm/s) (**b**). (Immature animals: normal cartilage, $N=11$, TEC, $N=7$, untreated, $N=4$; Mature animals: normal cartilage, $N=5$, TEC, $N=5$, untreated, $N=5$.) Regardless of ages, there is no significant difference detected in the tangent modulus of the repaired tissue by the TEC and of normal cartilage at either slower or faster compression speed. Conversely, the untreated cartilage, whether immature or mature, showed significantly lower tangent modulus than the normal cartilage at either slower or faster compression speed. ※; $p<0.05$

16.8 The TEC Derived from Synovial MSCs

16.8.1 The Next-Generation Cell-Based Strategy to Regenerate Cartilage

The present chapter has demonstrated the feasibility of using a unique scaffold-free tissue-engineered construct (TEC) generated from MSCs for effective cell-based cartilage repair. The cultured synovial-derived cells had high self-renewal capacity and stable expression profiles of surface antigen, similar to that observed in bone marrow-derived MSCs, through passages 4–7. Furthermore, they had the capability of osteogenic, chondrogenic, and adipogenic differentiation as previously reported [9]. Thus, the cultured synovial-derived cells have characteristics similar to those of MSCs and consequently, the in vitro-generated TEC could be regarded as an MSC-based 3D bioengineered tissue.

The development of a 3D tissue without an artificial scaffold could be the crucial center of this tissue-engineering technology, which is based on the active contraction of a cultured monolayer cell/matrix complex. The phenomenon of active tissue contraction is similar to that observed with the contraction of cultured collagen gels [53, 54]. As reported in previous collagen gel studies [55], negative regulators of the actin cytoskeleton significantly inhibit the contraction of the monolayer sheet (data not shown). Contractile forces generated within the actin cytoskeleton of the cultured MSCs may be at least partially involved in this active tissue contraction. Importantly, the TEC can be developed without any exogenous scaffold and therefore, implantation of the TEC would have a minimal risk of potential side effects induced by artificial or extrinsic biological materials contained in the scaffold. Furthermore, we confirmed that human serum is no less effective than bovine serum in promoting proliferation of synovium-derived MSCs without losing the differentiation potential of the cells (data not shown). Accordingly, with the use of autologous human serum, it is technically possible to develop the TEC in a xeno-free system, a factor which could minimize the risk of immune reactivity developing to the TEC [26].

Since the active contraction of a monolayer cell/matrix complex could be expected as a natural course when the culture conditions of the complex converts from a conventional adherent culture to a suspension culture, as has been reported in previous collagen gel contraction studies [53], the safe and reproducible detachment of the cultured monolayer cell/matrix complex is crucial for this tissue-engineering technology. Previous studies have shown the feasibility of using a temperature-sensitive culture dish to detach a cultured cell sheet from the substratum [56]. Conversely the present method does not require any special equipment and thus could be an easier and more direct method to accomplish this purpose.

Another further structural advantage of the TEC is that the MSCs and the ECM synthesized by the cells are integrated together into a 3D structure with a uniform cellular distribution. Thus, there is no need to modify or adjust the cellular distribution within the TEC. It is also notable that the TEC possesses sufficiently self-supporting mechanical properties in spite of the fact that it does not contain any artificial scaffold. The tensile strength of the TEC, which is developed in the presence of Asc-2P for 14 or 21 days, is comparable with that of healing ligament tissue at 1–2 weeks after injury [57]. Therefore, the TEC can be readily handled without causing overt damage to the matrix during implantation procedures.

Another important biological characteristic of the TEC described in this report is its tissue adhesiveness. This property contributes to a rapid and secure adhesion of the TEC to a natural cartilage matrix and thus, simple implantation procedures for the placement of the TEC into chondral lesions or defects could be expected to proceed without augmentation of the initial fixation. Moreover, such adhesiveness also enables rapid self-association internally with its own matrix, a factor which also contributes to the tissue plasticity of the TEC. In reality, it is possible to develop a spherical-shaped tissue of several millimeters in thickness by folding up the tissue in series. Thus, it is possible to develop the TEC that matches the size and the shape of a chondral defect more than several millimeters in thickness. Although we have not yet identified the crucial factor(s) which determine the tissue adhesiveness of the TEC, immunohistochemical analysis has shown that fibronectin and vitronectin are localized at the interface between the TEC and the base of the chondral lesions. Therefore, fibronectin and vitronectin may likely be, at least partially, involved in the adhesive properties of the in vitro-generated TEC.

It is known that a 3D culture environment at high density, such as micromass culture [58] and pellet culture [59], is an important variable to promote chondrogenesis. However, these methods cannot be directly applied to most clinical situations due to limitations in the mass size of the materials [13]. The present study revealed that the TEC overcomes this problem of tissue size while providing a three-dimensional and highly dense environment for the MSCs to differentiate towards a chondrogenic phenotype without causing cell and tissue necrosis. The TEC originally does not contain chondrogenic marker molecules such as collagen II and instead is rich in collagen I and III. However, after implantation in vivo, the basic TEC which did not receive ex vivo stimulation towards chondrogenic differentiation appears to have evolved the matrix composition to that of a more chondrogenic tissue. The findings from in vitro chondrogenesis experiments suggest that local biological and mechanical environment factors may facilitate degradation of the "old" matrix followed by the synthesis of a new chondrogenic matrix, thus leading to an overall phenotypic change of the matrix within the TEC during chondrogenic differentiation in vivo.

The series of in vitro experiments reported in the present study suggest that the TEC may be plastic, adhesive, and capable of chondrogenic differentiation and could be a unique and promising implant for cartilage repair. This possibility was confirmed following assessment of TEC implanted in vivo into porcine chondral defects. The TEC firmly attached to the surface of the injured cartilage at the initial stage of implantation, and thus a sutureless implantation was possible. Hereafter, the TEC maintained good tissue integration to the adjacent cartilage matrix and the repair tissue exhibited chondrogenic differentiation without any evidence of central necrosis or immunological rejection up to 6 months after implantation, regardless of ages. This biological integration was already evident 3 months after implantation. Using the modified International Cartilage Repair Society (ICRS) histological score [60], it was shown that the repair tissue with the TEC implants was histologically superior compared to that of the control lesions in all aspects, regardless of ages and implantation of the TEC appeared to prevent progression of the defects towards overt osteoarthritis. In addition, there is no significant difference observed in any criteria category between the immature and mature animals, as to the quality of repaired cartilage by the TEC. Moreover, biomechanical analysis also revealed that the tissue repaired with the TEC implant exhibited modulus properties similar to the properties of normal cartilage in both immature and mature animals. Therefore, the results of the present studies would support the clinical application of this strategy to promote cartilage repair and regeneration in patients over a wide range of patient ages.

It is notable that the implantation of the TEC without any pretreatment to promote a specific differentiation pathway resulted in tissue repair associated with an active chondrogenic differentiation response, although the repaired tissue still contained fibrous tissue, mainly at the surface or superficial zone. Obviously, one caveat in the therapeutic use of progenitor cells is that such use involves the potential risk of unintended differentiation and formation of tissues inappropriate for the application intended.

However, the implanted TEC did not exhibit any such inappropriate phenotypic changes. While the mechanisms underlying the successes obtained thus far are still not clearly delineated, it should be noted that the animal model used in the present study involves a chondral injury which does not breach the subchondral plate and thus, a relatively bleeding-free environment at the site of the lesion might be involved in such specific chondrogenic differentiation in vivo rather than fibrocartilage development. However, to attain a more extensive chondrogenic differentiation response including surface area, some biological manipulation of the TEC may be required before implantation to further optimize the rate and extent of repair, and this approach is one of our next steps. In addition, the use of TEC in the repair of osteochondral defects is currently underway.

In conclusion, we have demonstrated the characteristics of a scaffold-free three-dimensional synthetic tissue (TEC) derived from the cultured synovial-derived MSCs as a unique and promising implant for cartilage repair for the patients over a wide range of ages [47–49]. Due to the scaffold-free nature of the in vitro-generated structure, implantation of the TEC could yield more long-term safety and efficacy than that derived from scaffold-based cell therapies. Being a collagen I-rich matrix, the basic TEC construct could be suitable for augmenting repair of compromised skin or enhancing the repair of ligaments or tendons which are also collagen I-rich. Since the TEC also has osteogenic or adipogenic differentiation capacity, the basic TEC could also be used for other applications. Moreover, the TEC can be developed from MSCs derived from other tissues, such as adipose tissue, and these have characteristics similar to those of the synovium-derived TEC. Therefore, tissue engineering using the TEC technology could potentially provide a variety of therapeutic interventions in regenerative medicine for a variety of tissue applications using MSC from different sources.

Acknowledgment This work is supported by the grant of New Energy and Industrial Technology Development Organization, Japan, and the Grants-in-Aid for Scientific Research, Japan Society for the Promotion of Science.

References

1. Buckwalter JA (2002) Articular cartilage injuries. Clin Orthop Relat Res 402:21–37
2. Hunziker EB (2002) Articular cartilage repair: basic science and clinical progress. A review of the current status and prospects. Osteoarthritis Cartilage 10(6):432–463. doi:10.1053/joca.2002.0801, S1063458402908010 [pii]
3. Brittberg M, Peterson L, Sjogren-Jansson E, Tallheden T, Lindahl A (2003) Articular cartilage engineering with autologous chondrocyte transplantation. A review of recent developments. J Bone Joint Surg Am 85-A(Suppl 3):109–115
4. Ochi M, Adachi N, Nobuto H, Yanada S, Ito Y, Agung M (2004) Articular cartilage repair using tissue engineering technique – novel approach with minimally invasive procedure. Artif Organs 28(1):28–32, doi:7317 [pii]
5. Marcacci M, Berruto M, Brocchetta D, Delcogliano A, Ghinelli D, Gobbi A, Kon E, Pederzini L, Rosa D, Sacchetti GL, Stefani G, Zanasi S (2005) Articular cartilage engineering with Hyalograft C: 3-year clinical results. Clin Orthop Relat Res (435):96–105. doi:00003086-200506000-00015 [pii]
6. Hickery MS, Bayliss MT, Dudhia J, Lewthwaite JC, Edwards JC, Pitsillides AA (2003) Age-related changes in the response of human articular cartilage to IL-1alpha and transforming growth factor-beta (TGF-beta): chondrocytes exhibit a diminished sensitivity to TGF-beta. J Biol Chem 278(52):53063–53071. doi:10.1074/jbc.M209632200, M209632200 [pii]
7. Pittenger MF, Mackay AM, Beck SC, Jaiswal RK, Douglas R, Mosca JD, Moorman MA, Simonetti DW, Craig S, Marshak DR (1999) Multilineage potential of adult human mesenchymal stem cells. Science 284(5411):143–147
8. Jankowski RJ, Deasy BM, Huard J (2002) Muscle-derived stem cells. Gene Ther 9(10):642–647. doi:10.1038/sj.gt.3301719
9. De Bari C, Dell'Accio F, Tylzanowski P, Luyten FP (2001) Multipotent mesenchymal stem cells from adult human synovial membrane. Arthritis Rheum 44(8):1928–1942. doi:10.1002/1529-0131(200108)44:8<1928::AID-ART331>3.0.CO;2-P
10. Sakaguchi Y, Sekiya I, Yagishita K, Muneta T (2005) Comparison of human stem cells derived from various mesenchymal tissues: superiority of synovium as a cell source. Arthritis Rheum 52(8):2521–2529. doi:10.1002/art.21212
11. Wickham MQ, Erickson GR, Gimble JM, Vail TP, Guilak F (2003) Multipotent stromal cells derived from the infrapatellar fat pad of the knee. Clin Orthop Relat Res 412:196–212. doi:10.1097/01.blo.0000072467.53786.ca
12. Lee OK, Kuo TK, Chen WM, Lee KD, Hsieh SL, Chen TH (2004) Isolation of multipotent mesenchymal stem cells from umbilical cord blood. Blood 103(5):1669–1675. doi:10.1182/blood-2003-05-1670, 2003-05-1670 [pii]
13. De Bari C, Dell'Accio F, Luyten FP (2004) Failure of in vitro-differentiated mesenchymal stem cells from the synovial membrane to form ectopic stable cartilage in vivo. Arthritis Rheum 50(1):142–150. doi:10.1002/art.11450
14. Vunjak-Novakovic G, Martin I, Obradovic B, Treppo S, Grodzinsky AJ, Langer R, Freed LE (1999) Bioreactor cultivation conditions modulate the composition and mechanical properties of tissue-engineered cartilage. J Orthop Res 17(1):130–138. doi:10.1002/jor.1100170119
15. Andriano KP, Tabata Y, Ikada Y, Heller J (1999) In vitro and in vivo comparison of bulk and surface hydrolysis in absorbable polymer scaffolds for tissue engineering. J Biomed Mater Res 48(5):602–612. doi:10.1002/(SICI)1097-4636(1999)48:5<602::AID-JBM3>3.0.CO;2-6 [pii]
16. Guo JF, Jourdian GW, MacCallum DK (1989) Culture and growth characteristics of chondrocytes encapsulated in alginate beads. Connect Tissue Res 19(2–4): 277–297. doi:10.3109/03008208909043901
17. Masuda K, Takegami K, An H, Kumano F, Chiba K, Andersson GB, Schmid T, Thonar E (2003) Recombinant osteogenic protein-1 upregulates extracellular matrix metabolism by rabbit annulus fibrosus and nucleus pulposus cells cultured in alginate beads. J Orthop Res 21(5):922–930. doi:10.1016/S0736-0266(03)00037-8, S0736026603000378 [pii]
18. Lee CH, Singla A, Lee Y (2001) Biomedical applications of collagen. Int J Pharm 221(1-2):1–22, doi:S0378517301006913 [pii]
19. Homminga GN, Buma P, Koot HW, van der Kraan PM, van den Berg WB (1993) Chondrocyte behavior in fibrin glue in vitro. Acta Orthop Scand 64(4):441–445
20. Brun P, Cortivo R, Zavan B, Vecchiato N, Abatangelo G (1999) In vitro reconstructed tissues on hyaluronan-based temporary scaffolding. J Mater Sci Mater Med 10(10/11):683–688, doi:238447 [pii]
21. Lahiji A, Sohrabi A, Hungerford DS, Frondoza CG (2000) Chitosan supports the expression of extracellular matrix proteins in human osteoblasts and chondrocytes. J Biomed Mater Res 51(4):586–595. doi:10.1002/1097-4636(20000915)51:4<586::AID-JBM6>3.0.CO;2-S [pii]
22. O'Grady JE, Bordon DM (2003) Global regulatory registration requirements for collagen-based combination products: points to consider. Adv Drug Deliv Rev 55(12):1699–1721, doi:S0169409X03001893 [pii]
23. Daniels AU, Andriano KP, Smutz WP, Chang MK, Heller J (1994) Evaluation of absorbable poly(ortho

esters) for use in surgical implants. J Appl Biomater 5(1):51–64. doi:10.1002/jab.770050108
24. van der Elst M, Klein CP, de Blieck-Hogervorst JM, Patka P, Haarman HJ (1999) Bone tissue response to biodegradable polymers used for intra medullary fracture fixation: a long-term in vivo study in sheep femora. Biomaterials 20(2):121–128, doi:S0142-9612(98)00117-3 [pii]
25. Yang C, Hillas PJ, Baez JA, Nokelainen M, Balan J, Tang J, Spiro R, Polarek JW (2004) The application of recombinant human collagen in tissue engineering. BioDrugs 18(2):103–119, doi:1824 [pii]
26. Martin MJ, Muotri A, Gage F, Varki A (2005) Human embryonic stem cells express an immunogenic nonhuman sialic acid. Nat Med 11(2):228–232, doi:nm1181 [pii]. 10.1038/nm1181
27. Hunziker EB, Rosenberg LC (1996) Repair of partial-thickness defects in articular cartilage: cell recruitment from the synovial membrane. J Bone Joint Surg Am 78(5):721–733
28. Lee CR, Grodzinsky AJ, Hsu HP, Spector M (2003) Effects of a cultured autologous chondrocyte-seeded type II collagen scaffold on the healing of a chondral defect in a canine model. J Orthop Res 21(2):272–281. doi:10.1016/S0736-0266(02)00153-5, S0736026602001535 [pii]
29. Dorotka R, Bindreiter U, Macfelda K, Windberger U, Nehrer S (2005) Marrow stimulation and chondrocyte transplantation using a collagen matrix for cartilage repair. Osteoarthritis Cartilage 13(8): 655–664. doi:10.1016/j.joca.2005.04.001, S1063-4584(05)00097-X [pii]
30. Nakamura N, Horibe S, Iwahashi T, Kawano K, Shino K, Yoshikawa H (2004) Healing of a chondral fragment of the knee in an adolescent after internal fixation. A case report. J Bone Joint Surg Am 86-A(12): 2741–2746, doi:86/12/2741 [pii]
31. Murphy JM, Dixon K, Beck S, Fabian D, Feldman A, Barry F (2002) Reduced chondrogenic and adipogenic activity of mesenchymal stem cells from patients with advanced osteoarthritis. Arthritis Rheum 46(3):704–713. doi:10.1002/art.10118 [pii]
32. Quarto R, Thomas D, Liang CT (1995) Bone progenitor cell deficits and the age-associated decline in bone repair capacity. Calcif Tissue Int 56(2):123–129
33. Bergman RJ, Gazit D, Kahn AJ, Gruber H, McDougall S, Hahn TJ (1996) Age-related changes in osteogenic stem cells in mice. J Bone Miner Res 11(5):568–577
34. Kretlow JD, Jin YQ, Liu W, Zhang WJ, Hong TH, Zhou G, Baggett LS, Mikos AG, Cao Y (2008) Donor age and cell passage affects differentiation potential of murine bone marrow-derived stem cells. BMC Cell Biol 9:60. doi:10.1186/1471-2121-9-60, 1471-2121-9-60 [pii]
35. Oreffo RO, Bennett A, Carr AJ, Triffitt JT (1998) Patients with primary osteoarthritis show no change with ageing in the number of osteogenic precursors. Scand J Rheumatol 27(6):415–424
36. Leskela HV, Risteli J, Niskanen S, Koivunen J, Ivaska KK, Lehenkari P (2003) Osteoblast recruitment from stem cells does not decrease by age at late adulthood. Biochem Biophys Res Commun 311(4):1008–1013, doi:S0006291X0302179X [pii]
37. De Bari C, Dell'Accio F, Luyten FP (2001) Human periosteum-derived cells maintain phenotypic stability and chondrogenic potential throughout expansion regardless of donor age. Arthritis Rheum 44(1): 85–95.doi:10.1002/1529-0131(200101)44:1<85::AID-ANR12>3.0.CO;2-6
38. Scharstuhl A, Schewe B, Benz K, Gaissmaier C, Buhring HJ, Stoop R (2007) Chondrogenic potential of human adult mesenchymal stem cells is independent of age or osteoarthritis etiology. Stem Cells 25(12):3244–3251, doi:2007-0300 [pii] 10.1634/stemcells.2007-0300
39. Rudert M (2002) Histological evaluation of osteochondral defects: consideration of animal models with emphasis on the rabbit, experimental setup, follow-up and applied methods. Cells Tissues Organs 171(4):229–240, doi:cto71229 [pii]
40. Bos PK, Verhaar JA, van Osch GJ (2006) Age-related differences in articular cartilage wound healing: a potential role for transforming growth factor beta1 in adult cartilage repair. Adv Exp Med Biol 585:297–309
41. Yamamoto T, Wakitani S, Imoto K, Hattori T, Nakaya H, Saito M, Yonenobu K (2004) Fibroblast growth factor-2 promotes the repair of partial thickness defects of articular cartilage in immature rabbits but not in mature rabbits. Osteoarthritis Cartilage 12(8):636–641. doi:10.1016/j.joca.2004.04.007, S1063458404000706 [pii]
42. Wei X, Gao J, Messner K (1997) Maturation-dependent repair of untreated osteochondral defects in the rabbit knee joint. J Biomed Mater Res 34(1):63–72. doi:10.1002/(SICI)1097-4636(199701)34:1<63::AID-JBM9>3.0.CO;2-L [pii]
43. Wakitani S, Goto T, Pineda SJ, Young RG, Mansour JM, Caplan AI, Goldberg VM (1994) Mesenchymal cell-based repair of large, full-thickness defects of articular cartilage. J Bone Joint Surg Am 76(4): 579–592
44. Wakitani S, Imoto K, Yamamoto T, Saito M, Murata N, Yoneda M (2002) Human autologous culture expanded bone marrow mesenchymal cell transplantation for repair of cartilage defects in osteoarthritic knees. Osteoarthritis Cartilage 10(3):199–206. doi:10.1053/joca.2001.0504, S1063458401905047 [pii]
45. Koga H, Shimaya M, Muneta T, Nimura A, Morito T, Hayashi M, Suzuki S, Ju YJ, Mochizuki T, Sekiya I (2008) Local adherent technique for transplanting mesenchymal stem cells as a potential treatment of cartilage defect. Arthritis Res Ther 10(4):R84. doi:10.1186/ar2460, ar2460 [pii]
46. Nakamura T, Sekiya I, Muneta T, Hatsushika D, Horie M, Tsuji K, Kawarasaki T, Watanabe A, Hishikawa S, Fujimoto Y, Tanaka H, Kobayashi E (2012) Arthroscopic, histological and MRI analyses of cartilage repair after a minimally invasive method of transplantation of allogeneic synovial mesenchymal

stromal cells into cartilage defects in pigs. Cytotherapy 14(3):327–338. doi:10.3109/14653249.2011.638912
47. Ando W, Tateishi K, Hart DA, Katakai D, Tanaka Y, Nakata K, Hashimoto J, Fujie H, Shino K, Yoshikawa H, Nakamura N (2007) Cartilage repair using an in vitro generated scaffold-free tissue-engineered construct derived from porcine synovial mesenchymal stem cells. Biomaterials 28(36): 5462–5470. doi:10.1016/j.biomaterials.2007.08.030, S0142-9612(07)00672-2 [pii]
48. Ando W, Tateishi K, Katakai D, Hart DA, Higuchi C, Nakata K, Hashimoto J, Fujie H, Shino K, Yoshikawa H, Nakamura N (2008) In vitro generation of a scaffold-free tissue-engineered construct (TEC) derived from human synovial mesenchymal stem cells: biological and mechanical properties and further chondrogenic potential. Tissue Eng Part A 14(12):2041–2049. doi:10.1089/ten.tea.2008.0015
49. Shimomura K, Ando W, Tateishi K, Nansai R, Fujie H, Hart DA, Kohda H, Kita K, Kanamoto T, Mae T, Nakata K, Shino K, Yoshikawa H, Nakamura N (2010) The influence of skeletal maturity on allogenic synovial mesenchymal stem cell-based repair of cartilage in a large animal model. Biomaterials 31(31): 8004–8011. doi:10.1016/j.biomaterials.2010.07.017, S0142-9612(10)00858-6 [pii]
50. De Ugarte DA, Alfonso Z, Zuk PA, Elbarbary A, Zhu M, Ashjian P, Benhaim P, Hedrick MH, Fraser JK (2003) Differential expression of stem cell mobilization-associated molecules on multi-lineage cells from adipose tissue and bone marrow. Immunol Lett 89(2-3):267–270, doi:S0165247803001081 [pii]
51. Vodicka P, Smetana K Jr, Dvorankova B, Emerick T, Xu YZ, Ourednik J, Ourednik V, Motlik J (2005) The miniature pig as an animal model in biomedical research. Ann N Y Acad Sci 1049:161–171. doi:10.1196/annals.1334.015, 1049/1/161 [pii]
52. Huang CY, Soltz MA, Kopacz M, Mow VC, Ateshian GA (2003) Experimental verification of the roles of intrinsic matrix viscoelasticity and tension-compression nonlinearity in the biphasic response of cartilage. J Biomech Eng 125(1):84–93
53. Bell E, Ivarsson B, Merrill C (1979) Production of a tissue-like structure by contraction of collagen lattices by human fibroblasts of different proliferative potential in vitro. Proc Natl Acad Sci USA 76(3): 1274–1278
54. Sheetz MP, Felsenfeld DP, Galbraith CG (1998) Cell migration: regulation of force on extracellular-matrix-integrin complexes. Trends Cell Biol 8(2):51–54, doi:S0962892497012166 [pii]
55. Yanase M, Ikeda H, Matsui A, Maekawa H, Noiri E, Tomiya T, Arai M, Yano T, Shibata M, Ikebe M, Fujiwara K, Rojkind M, Ogata I (2000) Lysophosphatidic acid enhances collagen gel contraction by hepatic stellate cells: association with rho-kinase. Biochem Biophys Res Commun 277(1):72–78. doi:10.1006/bbrc.2000.3634, S0006-291X(00)93634-9 [pii]
56. Okano T, Yamada N, Okuhara M, Sakai H, Sakurai Y (1995) Mechanism of cell detachment from temperature-modulated, hydrophilic-hydrophobic polymer surfaces. Biomaterials 16(4):297–303, doi:014296129593257E [pii]
57. Provenzano PP, Hayashi K, Kunz DN, Markel MD, Vanderby R Jr (2002) Healing of subfailure ligament injury: comparison between immature and mature ligaments in a rat model. J Orthop Res 20(5):975–983. doi:10.1016/S0736-0266(02)00036-0
58. Denker AE, Nicoll SB, Tuan RS (1995) Formation of cartilage-like spheroids by micromass cultures of murine C3H10T1/2 cells upon treatment with transforming growth factor-beta 1. Differentiation 59(1):25–34. doi:10.1046/j.1432-0436.1995.5910025.x, S0301-4681(09)60787-8 [pii]
59. Lennon DP, Haynesworth SE, Arm DM, Baber MA, Caplan AI (2000) Dilution of human mesenchymal stem cells with dermal fibroblasts and the effects on in vitro and in vivo osteochondrogenesis. Dev Dyn 219(1):50–62. doi:10.1002/1097-0177(2000)9999:9999<::AID-DVDY1037>3.0.CO;2-7
60. Mainil-Varlet P, Aigner T, Brittberg M, Bullough P, Hollander A, Hunziker E, Kandel R, Nehrer S, Pritzker K, Roberts S, Stauffer E (2003) Histological assessment of cartilage repair: a report by the Histology Endpoint Committee of the International Cartilage Repair Society (ICRS). J Bone Joint Surg Am 85-A(Suppl 2):45–57

Injectable Autologous Bone-Marrow-Derived Mesenchymal Stem Cells for Cartilage Repair: The Singapore Technique

17

Derrick Lam, Keng Lin Wong, Ping Law, and James H.P. Hui

Contents

D. Lam
Yong Loo Lin School of Medicine, National University of Singapore, Singapore

K.L. Wong • J.H.P. Hui (✉)
Department of Orthopaedic Surgery, University Orthopaedic, Hand and Reconstructive Microsurgery Cluster, National University Health System, Singapore
e-mail: james_hui@nuhs.edu.sg

P. Law
Tissue Engineering and Cell Therapy (GMP) Laboratory, National University Health System, Singapore

17.1 Introduction

The cartilage, which is mesodermal in origin, provides excellent lubrication and wear characteristics required for continuous gliding motion. It serves to absorb mechanical shock and spread the applied load onto the bony supporting structures below. But its limited capacity for repair can cause severe and progressive disability of the joint, such as osteoarthritis. Osteoarthritis is the leading cause of chronic disability in large developed countries like the United States [3], and Singapore is no exception. According to the Singapore Ministry of Health National Health Surveillance [16], 10.1 % of residents between the ages of 18 and 69 have arthritis and chronic joint symptoms. The prevalence increased with age and was highest among older residents aged 60–69 years (19.8 %). At present, current treatments reduce pain and inflammation, but do not retard the destruction of cartilage [15]. One of the most well-known and utilized treatments is the total knee replacement (TKR). While it has been successful for the older, less-active patient [21], the degradation of these replacements over time makes it less suitable for younger active patients [14]. As TKRs usually last for no more than 20 years, they are only recommended for patients greater than 60 years of age.

A.A. Shetty et al. (eds.), *Techniques in Cartilage Repair Surgery*,
DOI 10.1007/978-3-642-41921-8_17, © ESKKA 2014

Among older adults in the United States, nearly 1.5 million of those with a primary total knee replacement are 50–69 years old, indicating a large population is at risk for cost revision surgery and long-term complications of total knee replacement [20]. This has called for a look into the viability of stem cell engineering as a solution.

17.2 The Proposed Solution

Bone-marrow-derived mesenchymal stem cells (BMSCs) with its chondrogenic potential have been proven in both in vivo and in vitro studies to be capable of enhancing chondral healing. It has been demonstrated through in vitro research that human bone marrow (BM) is a better source of mesenchymal stem cells (MSCs) than adipose tissue [1]. In the study, BM and adipose MSC were cultured from the same sets of donors. Results showed that BM MSC produced significantly more collagen II and s-GAG. It was further demonstrated in small and large animals that MSC were capable of enhancing cartilage repair [4, 6, 17]. Especially in porcine, biomechanical testing showed that meniscus repaired with the addition of MSC was significantly stronger than that of the control animals.

Regarding physical stimulation of MSC, adult stem cell fraction is present in nucleated cells of the marrow; however few are actually BMSCs capable of differentiating into bone, cartilage or muscle. Physical methods of marrow stimulation such as microfracture have been clinically shown to produce significant results in terms of chondral healing; however when done as an isolated procedure, fibrous cartilage dominates the regenerated cartilage and results in decrease in clinical scores after 24 months [7, 11].

Clinically, comparisons have been made between autologous BMSCs implantation and autologous chondrocyte implantation. In an observational cohort study led by James Hui et al. [13], 72 matched (lesion site and age) patients underwent cartilage repair using chondrocytes ($n=36$) or BMSCs ($n=36$).

Patients were evaluated at 3, 6, 9, 12, 18 and 24 months postoperatively. Trained research staff assessed them using the International Cartilage Repair Society (ICRS) Cartilage Injury Evaluation Package [2] which included questions from the Short-Form (SF-36) Health Survey, International Knee Documentation Committee (IKDC) subjective knee evaluation form, Lysholm knee scale and Tegner activity level scale. Second-look arthroscopy was performed in seven patients (four in the BMSC group and three in the ACI group) 9–12 months after implantation. A biopsy sample of the repair tissue was obtained in two cases (one in each group).

The study showed a significant improvement in the patients' quality of life (physical and mental components of the Short Form-36 questionnaire included in the ICRS package) after cartilage repair in both groups. There was, however, no difference in terms of clinical outcome, except BMSCs were better for physical role functioning, with a greater improvement over time in the BMSC group ($P=0.044$ for interaction effect). The IKDC subjective knee evaluation ($P=.861$), Lysholm ($P=.627$) and Tegner ($P=.200$) scores did not show any significant difference between groups over time. Men performed generally better than women. For BMSCs, all ages performed about the same, whereas for chondrocytes, those below 45 did better while those above 45 did worse. BMSC treatment requires one less knee surgery, reduced costs and minimized donor-site morbidity. Overall, the study shows BMSCs to be as effective as chondrocytes, while offering additional advantages.

While the bulk of patients with cartilage defects belong to the older age group, the young and active could also benefit from effective cartilage repair. A study involving young patients was led by Hui et al. [19]. The team recognized that although recent advances have been made in using chondrocytes and other cell-based therapy to treat cartilage defects in adults, it is unclear whether they should be extended to the adolescent and young adult-aged patients. They retrospectively reviewed 23 patients between 12 and 21 years of age treated for osteochondritis dissecans (OCD) lesions involving the patella from 2001 to 2008 and found out that cell-based therapy was associated with short-term improvement in function in adolescents and young adults with patellar OCD. Therefore, the transplantation of autologous BM stromal cells can promote the repair of large focal articular cartilage defects in young, active patients.

After these multiple basic science and clinical trials conducted by our institution (National

University Hospital (NUH) in Singapore) to evaluate the safety and efficiency of autologous BMSCs in cartilage repair, we propose a protocol for cartilage repair with a combination of microfracture and cultured injectable autologous BMSCs. Our hypothesis centres around our belief that the injected MSCs have the ability to home in on the site of injury/microfracture and adhere to the site of lesion. The homing ability of MSCs have been proven by many other authors such as [5, 8, 12].

Multiple (single institution) trials (Institutional Review Board approved) are now open and accruing patients at our institution to evaluate the safety and efficiency of autologous BM MSC in cartilage repair. Since 2003, 365 patients from NUH have been offered cultured stem cell therapy.

17.3 Patient Selection: Indications and Contraindications

All patients undergo a thorough preoperative assessment via clinical and radiological methods. The inclusion criteria consist of patients aged 55 years old or less, presence of uni-compartmental osteoarthritis with minimal mechanical axis deformity, no cruciate or collateral ligament instability and no fixed flexion deformity of the knee. The exclusion criteria consist of patients older than 55 years old, significant mal-alignment of the knee and bi-compartmental and tri-compartmental osteoarthritis. Patients who were unable tolerate magnetic resonance imaging (MRI) scans, unable to answer subjective questionnaires or are not mentally fit to give informed consent were also excluded. Cartilage repair was conducted with the informed consent of the patients.

17.4 Preoperative Preparation

The orthopaedic surgeon will assess the clinical condition of the affected knee via a detailed clinical evaluation. This is carried out through a review of his medical history, a complete physical examination of the knee, previous documentation of his joint condition and physical examinations such as X-ray or MRI scanning.

17.5 Patient Setup and Surgical Approach

Surgery was performed under general anaesthesia and tourniquet control. Patients were positioned supine with side support on the lateral aspect of the hip on the operating side to facilitate arthroscopy. Incisions made for arthroscopic access to the knee are of the standard medial and lateral arthroscopic portals.

17.6 Arthroscopic Evaluation and Initial Surgical Treatment

All patients underwent a full arthroscopic examination to grade the cartilage status based on the ICRS classification. The size, number and stage of the chondral ulcers were documented.

After assessing and recording the details of the chondral ulcers, patients undergo a microfracture followed by bone marrow harvesting in the same setting (Fig. 17.1). Marrow stimulation was achieved by performing microfracture as described by Steadman et al. [18]. With the patient under the same setting of general anaesthesia, 60 ml of bone marrow was aspirated using a Jamshidi needle from the iliac crest of each patient into heparinized syringes and transferred into sterile containers (Fig. 17.2). Seventy to 80 ml of each patient's blood was collected as well. The bone marrow aspirate was processed

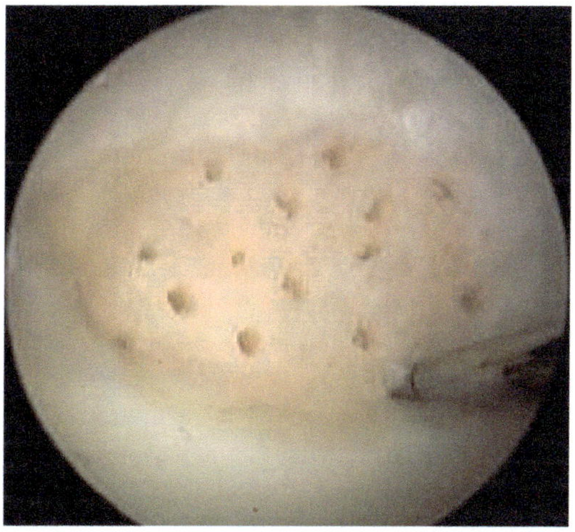

Fig. 17.1 Arthroscopic photograph of microfracture performed on chondral defect

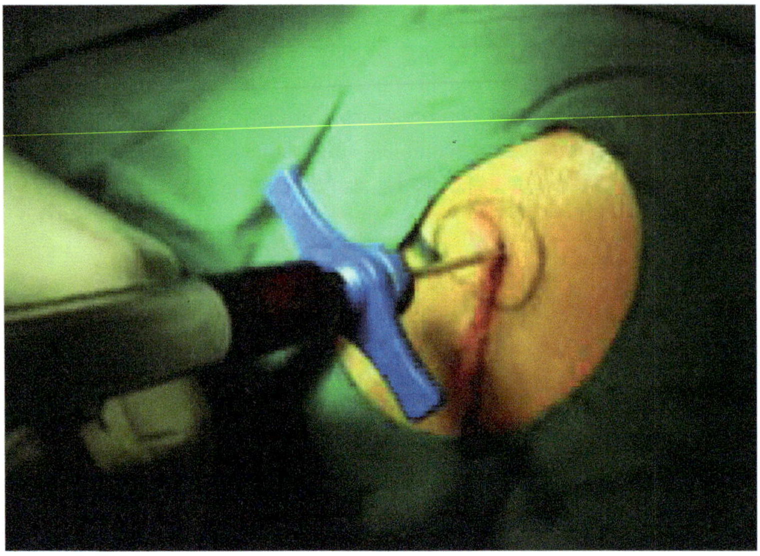

Fig. 17.2 Bone marrow harvesting via anterior iliac crest using Jamshidi needle for aspiration

within 1 h in a clean room environment (GMP cell processing facility at the National University Hospital) and cultured for 3 weeks until there is sufficient concentration of cells present. The cultured BMSCs (approximately 10–15 million cells, with a viability rate of 96 %) are then suspended in 2 ml of hyaluronic acid (which help to fill up spaces between collagen fibres and deliver the stem cells into the joint) and are injected under local anaesthesia into the knee joint 3 weeks after the initial surgery.

17.7 Bone Marrow-Derived Mesenchymal Stem Cell Preparation

A summary of the preparation is shown in Fig. 17.3. Autologous BMSCs are cultured from bone marrow in a class B clean room environment. Briefly, between 35 and 74 ml of marrow (median = 49 ml) were collected from the hip of the patients under general anaesthesia during microfracture surgery in the operating theatre. Un-coagulated whole blood was also collected (from which autologous serum was prepared and stored at −20 °C). A majority of the red blood cells were removed from the marrow by dextran sedimentation and the leukocyte-rich fraction was washed and cultured for BMSCs in DMEM plus 10 % fetal bovine serum and ascorbic acid (50 μg/ml) (all from Invitrogen) in 5–6 T-75 flasks. Culture medium was completely replaced every 2–3 days until harvest. BMSCs were passaged when they reached >30 % confluency (usually after 10–13 days, median = 12) by treating with trypsin (Invitrogen) and washes. Between 9 and 11 days, culture supernatant was sent for assays for mycoplasma as well as microbial contamination (aerobic and anaerobic bacteria as well as fungus). BMSC release criteria (for administration) include no growth on mycoplasma and microbial culture, confluency >70 %, normal BMSC morphology and >75 % viable (by fluorescent acridine orange and propidium iodide staining). Between 19 and 23 days (medium = 22), BMSCs were trypsinized, washed and resuspended in 0.5–1 ml autologous serum and delivered to the clinic for administration directly into the knee within 4 h. A small fraction from each sample was removed (prior to resuspension in serum) for cell count, viability and flow cytometry (MSC phenotyping kit, Miltenyi Biotec) using FACSCanto II with FACSDiva software (BD). All patients were administered with p1 BMSC except in the rare situations (e.g. patient could not make the appointment) when p2 BMSCs were used. Characteristics of the BMSCs were (average ± SD): total cells: $1.46 \pm 0.29 \times 10^7$; viability: 87.1 ± 6.4 %; lineage negative (CD14, CD20, CD34 & CD45): 93.0 ± 5.5 %; CD73+: 95.2 ± 4.2 %; CD90+: 88.9 ± 6.7 %; and CD105+: 89.7 ± 6.3 % (Figs. 17.4 and 17.5).

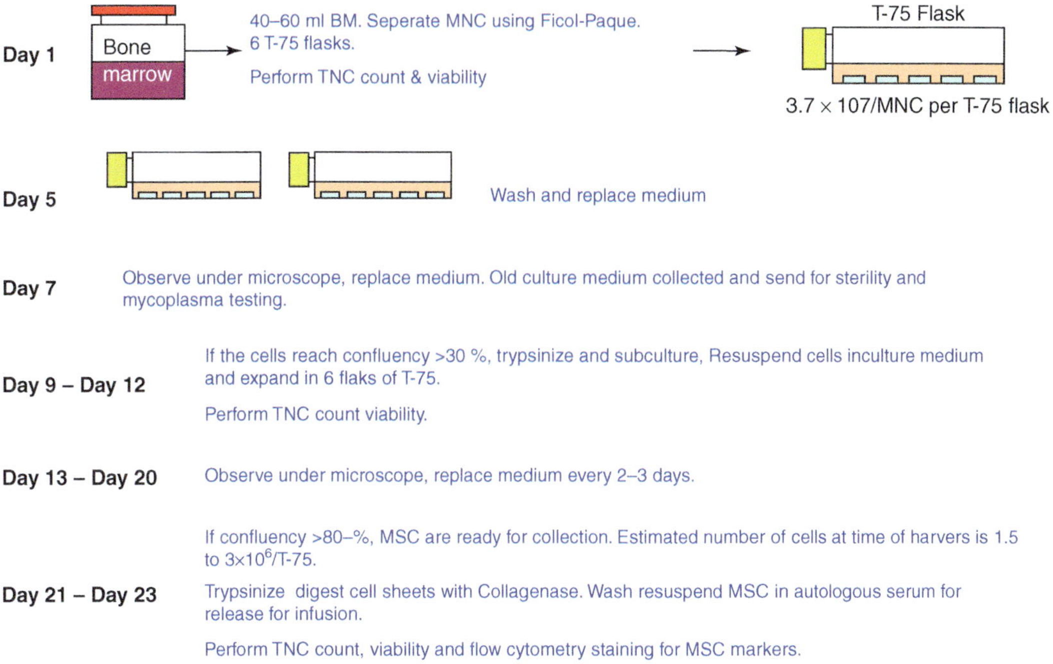

Fig. 17.3 Preparation process for bone-marrow-derived mesenchymal stem cells

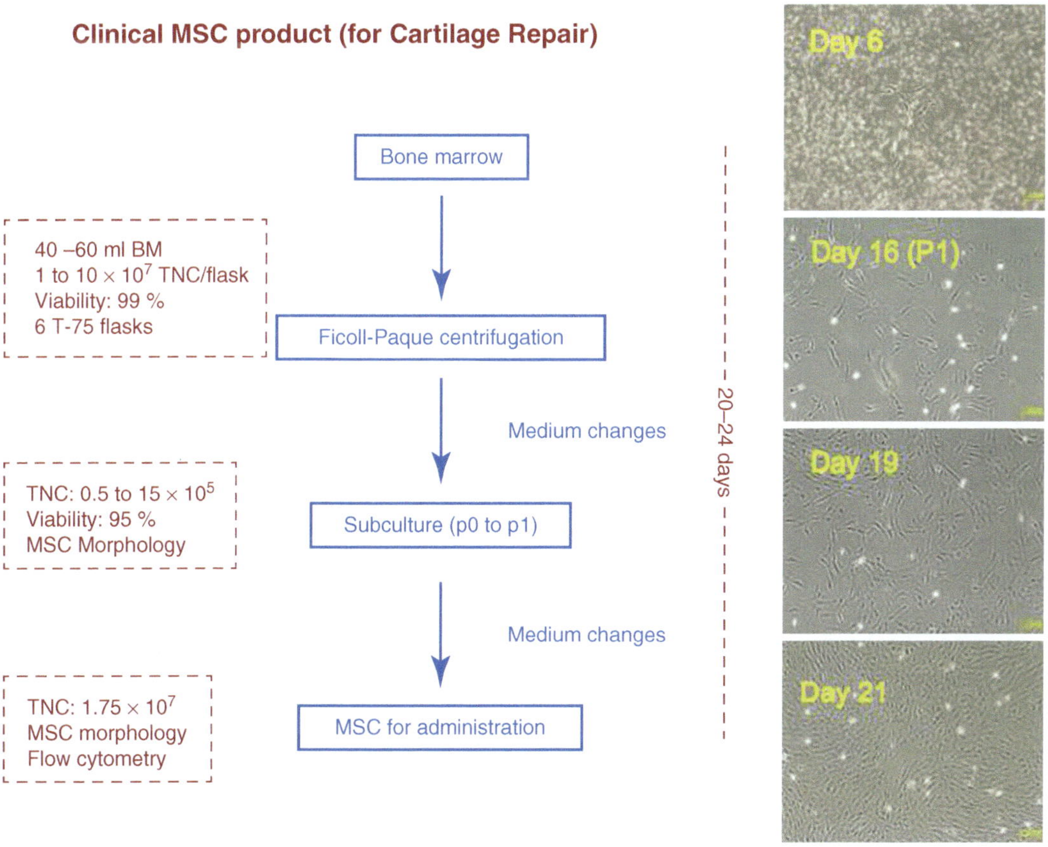

Fig. 17.4 Histological characteristics of the clinical product of bone marrow-derived mesenchymal stem cells

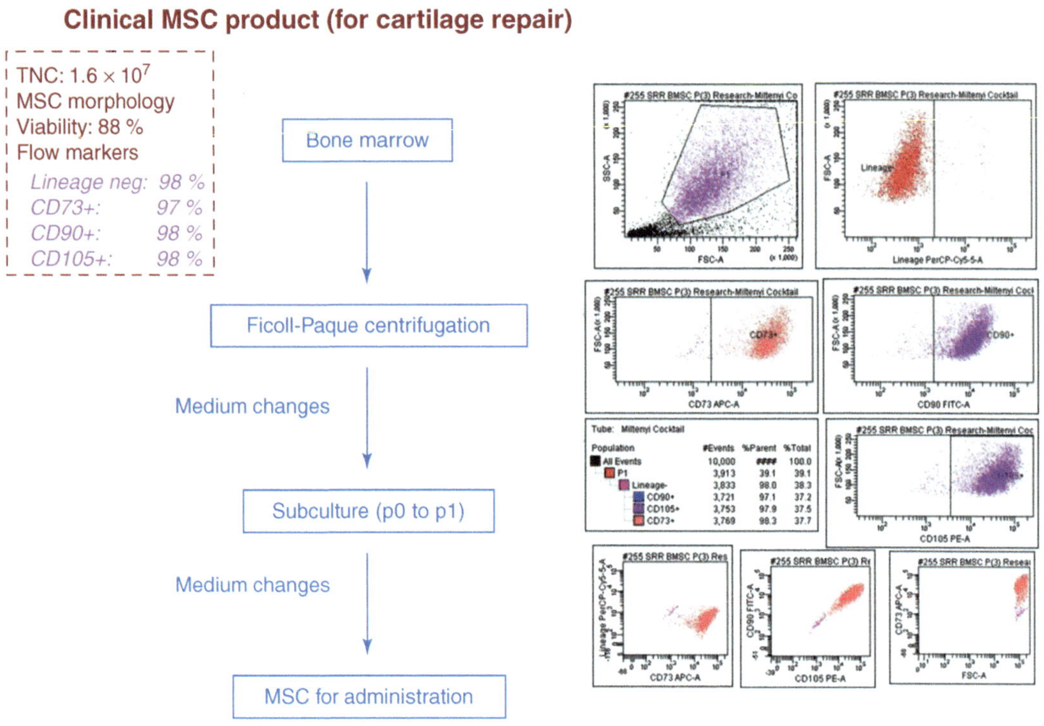

Fig. 17.5 Cellular lineage of the clinical product of bone-marrow-derived mesenchymal stem cells

17.8 Complications

Preliminary results showed that MSC injection is a safe procedure (in terms of serious adverse events during administration of MSC) and the rate of microbial contamination is low (1 in 218 processes during a 6-year span from 2006 to 2011).

17.9 Postoperative Follow-Up

Patients were reviewed on the 14th postoperative day for wound inspection followed by another review at 3 weeks. During the second review, MSC injection with 2 ml hyaluronic acid (HA) was injected into the intra-articular space using a 19-gauze needle (under local anaesthesia) (Fig. 17.6). Two more doses of 2 ml HA injection were repeated at weekly intervals for all patients.

Patients were followed up at 6 weekly intervals thereafter for the first 6 months. At 6 months, 1 year and 2 year reviews, Tegner and Lysholm knee scores and IKDC scores were documented for all patients.

MRI was performed after 1 year to look for cartilage regeneration based on the magnetic resonance observation of cartilage repair tissue (MOCART) scoring system [10]. MRI was performed on a 1.5 T Sigma HDxt MRI scanner (GE Healthcare, Milwaukee, WI, USA) with a dedicated extremity surface coil (HD TR knee PA). Normal knee sequences used were axial T2, coronal PD fat-saturated, coronal T1, Sagittal PD and sagittal T2 fat-saturated. Cartilage sequences used were axial SPGR, sagittal SPGR, Axial FIESTA and Sagittal FIESTA. Each MRI scan consists of 19 slices for the normal knee protocol and 32 slices for cartilage sequences. All patients were positioned consistently with the joint space in the middle of the coil and the knee extended in the coil.

17.10 Rehabilitation

The rehabilitation process is one of the most important parts of recovery. However, it takes a year or more to receive the maximum benefits of the surgery, and patients need to appreciate that

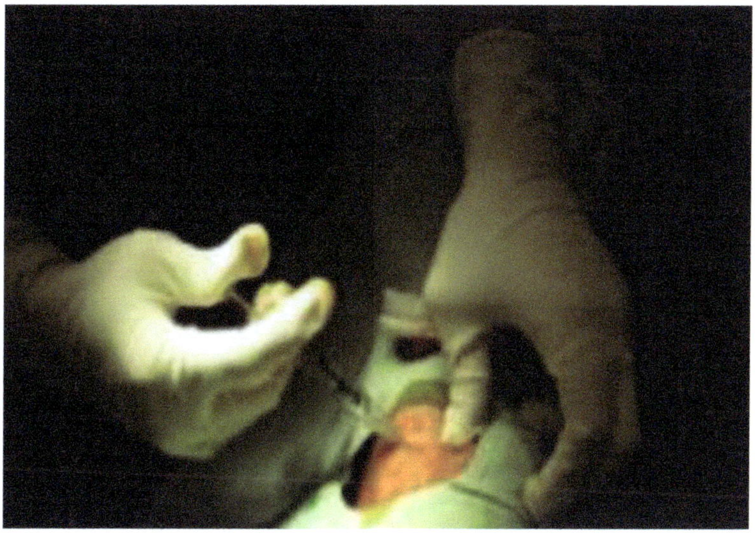

Fig. 17.6 Clinical picture of MSC injection with 2 ml hyaluronic acid (HA) injection in syringe to be injected into the intra-articular space using a 19-gauze needle

much hard work is required in the months following the surgery to derive the maximum benefit from the treatment. They are advised to adhere tightly to the rehabilitation protocol. The protocol focuses on four key areas of walking/weightbearing, range of motion, strength and cardiovascular capacity. It began on the actual day of surgery and encompassed isometric muscle contractions and passive range of motion. Patients are placed on initial touchdown weightbearing for 6 weeks and then progressed to partial weightbearing and active motion at 6 weeks, before finally embarking on full weightbearing exercise after 12 weeks. Once full weightbearing and good range of motion are achieved for the knee, the patient undergoes a comprehensive rehabilitation programme with the aims of restoring muscular function. This includes the usage of stationary bicycles, elliptical trainers and treadmills along with closed chain exercises. The protocol is customized according to the location and size of the lesion, concomitant procedures, and patient's age and previous activity level.

17.11 Initial Results and Future Directions

An initial prospective comparative study on the safety and efficacy of our injectable autologous BMSC technique was carried out by a team led by James Hui et al. [9]. The open technique of cartilage repair, where MSCs were implanted beneath a sutured periosteal patch over the defect, was compared against the technique of arthroscopic microfracture and outpatient intra-articular injections of autologous BMSCs and HA. There were 35 patients in each arm. Patients were evaluated with the IKDC, Tegner and Lysholm scores, and postoperative MRI evaluation was performed at 1 year.

The initial results were promising. There were significant improvements in the mean IKDC, Lysholm and SF-36 physical component scores and visual analogue pain scores in both treatment groups (Figs. 17.7, 17.8, 17.9, and 17.10). There were no clinically significant adverse side effects reported during the course of the study. MRI findings were encouraging with formation of neo-cartilage with good fill and integration demonstrated in the injectable group of patients (Fig. 17.11). This has led to the conclusion that our technique of arthroscopic microfracture and outpatient intra-articular injections of autologous BMSCs and HA was comparable to the open technique, with the added advantages of only being minimally invasive and requiring only a single operation under general anaesthesia. Its safety has been validated in this study, and clinically efficacy is currently evaluated in an ongoing randomized controlled trial.

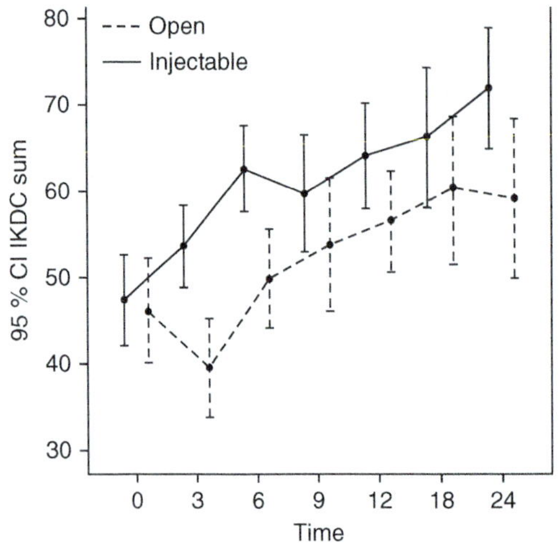

Fig. 17.7 A graph showing the International Knee Documentation Committee (IKDC) sum score: injectable vs open technique

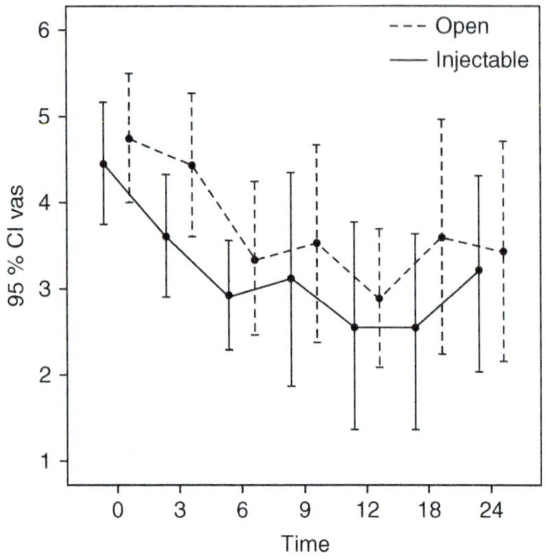

Fig. 17.9 A graph showing the visual analogue scale (VAS): injectable vs open technique

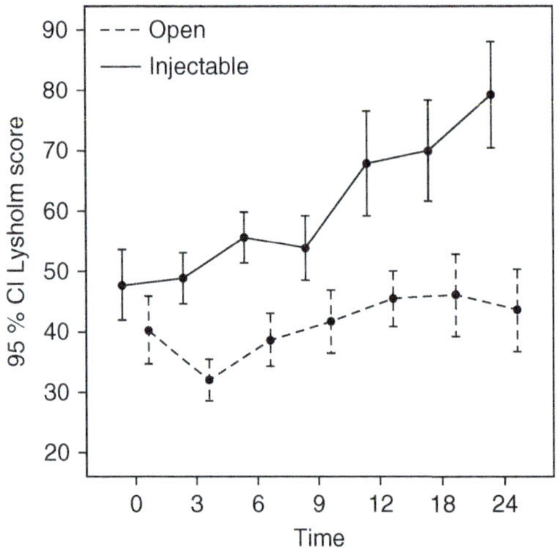

Fig. 17.8 A graph showing the Lysholm score: injectable vs open technique

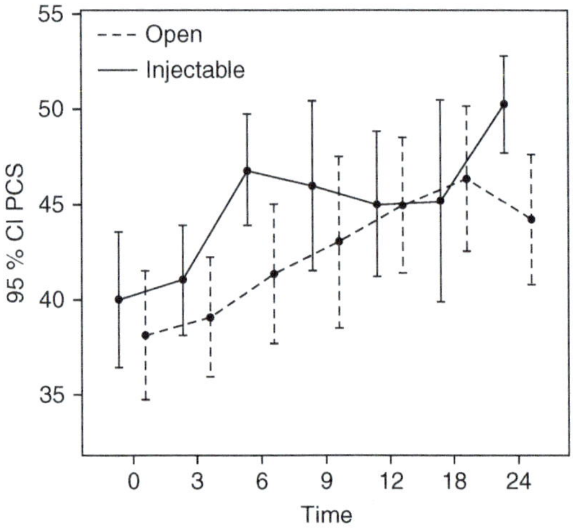

Fig. 17.10 A graph showing SF-36 (PCS): injectable vs open technique

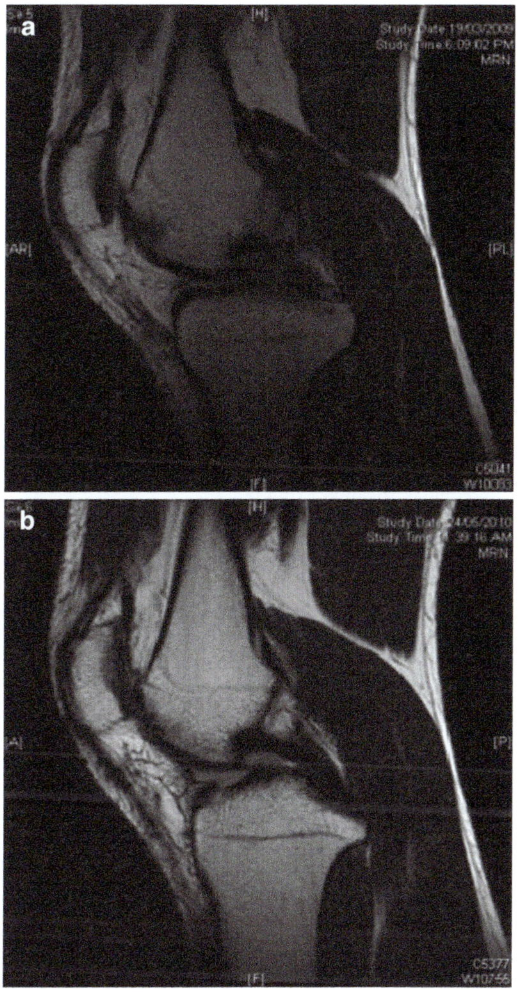

Fig. 17.11 (a) Preoperation MRI (SAG FSE PD) showing a large full thickness chondral ulcer with discontinuity of the subchondral bone and significant underlying marrow oedema. (b) One year postoperation MRI (SAG FSE PD) showing neo-cartilage formation with good fill and significant reduction in the underlying marrow oedema

Conclusion

Our research has demonstrated that, in the setting of cartilage repair, it is feasible to translate longitudinally from laboratory to clinical studies (bench to bedside), using animal models (small and large) to validate in vitro results prior to the design and initiation of human trials. The efficacy of autologous MSC in cartilage repair awaits the completion of patient accrual and final analysis of the trials.

References

1. Afizah H, Yang Z, Hui JH, Ouyang HW, Lee EH (2007) A comparison between the chondrogenic potential of human bone marrow stem cells (BMSCs) and adipose-derived stem cells (ADSCs) taken from the same donors. Tissue Eng 13(4):659–666
2. Brittberg M, Winalski CS (2003) Evaluation of cartilage injuries and repair. J Bone Joint Surg Am 85-A(Suppl 2):58–69
3. Centers for Disease Control and Prevention (2009) Prevalence and most common causes of disability among adults -United States, 2005. MMWR Morb Mortal Wkly Rep 58:421–426
4. Fortier LA, Potter HG, Rickey EJ, Schnabel LV, Foo LF, Chong LR, Stokol T, Cheetham J, Nixon AJ (2010) Concentrated bone marrow aspirate improves full-thickness cartilage repair compared with microfracture in the equine model. J Bone Joint Surg Am 92(10):1927–1937
5. Horie M, Sekiya I, Muneta T, Ichinose S, Matsumoto K, Saito H, Murakami T, Kobayashi E (2009) Intra-articular injected synovial stem cells differentiate into meniscal cells directly and promote meniscal regeneration without mobilization to distant organs in rat massive meniscal defect. Stem Cells 27(4):878–887
6. Koga H, Muneta T, Ju YJ, Nagase T, Nimura A, Mochizuki T, Ichinose S, von der Mark K, Sekiya I (2007) Synovial stem cells are regionally specified according to local microenvironments after implantation for cartilage regeneration. Stem Cells 25(3):689–696
7. LaPrade RF, Bursch LS, Olson EJ, Havlas V, Carlson CS (2008) Histologic and immunohistochemical characteristics of failed articular cartilage resurfacing procedures for osteochondritis of the knee: a case series. Am J Sports Med 36:360–368
8. Lee KB, Hui JH, Song IC, Ardany L, Lee EH (2007) Injectable mesenchymal stem cell therapy for large cartilage defects – a porcine model. Stem Cells 25(11):2964–2971, Epub 2007 Jul 26
9. Lee KB, Wang VT, Chan YH, Hui JH (2012) A novel, minimally-invasive technique of cartilage repair in the human knee using arthroscopic microfracture and injections of mesenchymal stem cells and hyaluronic acid – a prospective comparative study on safety and short-term efficacy. Ann Acad Med Singapore 41(11): 511–517
10. Marlovits S, Striessnig G, Resinger CT et al (2004) Definition of pertinent parameters for the evaluation of articular cartilage repair tissue with high-resolution magnetic resonance imaging. Eur J Radiol 52:310–319
11. Mithoefer K, Williams RJ III, Warren RF et al (2005) The microfracture technique for the treatment of articular cartilage lesions in the knee. A prospective cohort study. J Bone Joint Surg Am 87:1911–1920
12. Motoyama M, Deie M, Kanaya A, Nishimori M, Miyamoto A, Yanada S, Adachi N, Ochi M (2010) In vitro cartilage formation using TGF-beta-immobilized

magnetic beads and mesenchymal stem cell-magnetic bead complexes under magnetic field conditions. J Biomed Mater Res A 92(1):196–204
13. Nejadnik H, Hui JH, FengChoong EP, Tai BC, Lee EH (2010) Autologous bone marrow–derived mesenchymal stem cells versus autologous chondrocyte implantation. Am J Sports Med 38:1110–1116
14. Parsons IM, Sonnabend DH (2004) What is the role of joint replacement surgery? Best Pract Res Clin Rheumatol 18:557–572
15. Simon L (1999) Osteoarthritis: a review. Clin Cornerstone 2:26–37
16. Singapore Ministry of Health National Health Surveillance (2007) http://www.moh.gov.sg/content/dam/moh_web/Publications/Reports/2009/nhss2007.pdf
17. Soon MY, Hassan A, Hui JH, Goh JC, Lee EH (2007) An analysis of soft tissue allograft anterior cruciate ligament reconstruction in a rabbit model: a short-term study of the use of mesenchymal stem cells to enhance tendon osteointegration. Am J Sports Med 35(6):962–971
18. Steadman JR, Rodkey WG, Rodrigo JJ (2000) Microfracture: Surgical technique and rehabilitation to treat chondral defects. Clin Orthop Relat Res 391(suppl):S362–S369
19. Teo BJ, Buhary K, Tai BC, Hui JH (2013) Cell-based therapy improves function in adolescents and young adults with patellar osteochondritis dissecans. Clin Orthop Relat Res 471(4):1152–8. doi:10.1007/s11999-012-2338-z
20. Weinstein AM, Rome BN, Reichmann WM, Collins JE, Burbine SA, Thornhill TS, Wright J, Katz JN, Losina E (2013) Estimating the burden of total knee replacement in the United States. J Bone Joint Surg Am 95(5):385–392. doi:10.2106/JBJS.L.00206
21. Yarashi T, Rutherford-Davies J, Anand S, Johnson DS (2008) Knee outcome scores — do we get people back to normal?", British Orthopaedic Association Annual Meeting, Liverpool

Stem Cell Research in Orthopaedic and Trauma Surgery

18

Seok-Jung Kim and Asode Ananthram Shetty

Contents

S.-J. Kim, MD, PhD, FRCS (✉)
Department of Orthopedic Surgery, Uijeongbu St. Mary's Hospital, College of Medicine, The Catholic University of Korea, 480-717 Gyeonggi-do, Republic of (South Korea)

Faculty of Stem Cell Research and Regenerative Medicine, NITTE University, Mangalore, India
e-mail: orthopland@naver.com

A.A. Shetty, MD, PhD, MCh, FRCS Ed., FRCS Eng., FRCS Orth
Department of Minimally Invasive Surgery, Faculty of Health and Social Sciences, Canterbury Christ Church University, Pembroke Court 30, ME4 4UF Chatham Maritime, Kent, UK

Faculty of Stem Cell Research and Regenerative Medicine, NITTE University, Mangalore, India
e-mail: aashetty@hotmail.com

18.1 Cartilage Injury

Cartilage cells are present in all of the articular cartilages, they form the matrix, and function to maintain the cartilages. As articular cartilages are avascular, superficial injury can therefore not induce a sufficient inflammatory reaction in other to cause regeneration. Upon injury, the regeneration capacity of cartilage is limited and injury induces degeneration of the fibrillar organization of collagens.

The incidence of chondral lesions is unclear, and in patients with knee joint problems, it has been estimated that approximately 5–10 % patients have full-thickness cartilage lesions [5]. Nevertheless, the incidence of cartilage lesions in asymptomatic patients is unknown. In addition, the natural history after articular cartilage injury is also unclear. However, it is generally accepted as the natural history of cartilage injury that once articular cartilages are injured, their ability to regenerate is limited and the injury thus progresses to arthritis with time [5]. For its treatment, various methods have been developed and are used, with the representative treatment methods being arthroscopic debridement, microfracture, multiple drilling, osteochondral transfer, and ACI. Among these treatment methods, arthroscopic debridement has been shown to have limited effects and thus the remaining treatment methods, excluding this method, could be

A.A. Shetty et al. (eds.), *Techniques in Cartilage Repair Surgery*,
DOI 10.1007/978-3-642-41921-8_18, © ESSKA 2014

divided into treatment methods which apply cells and those which apply tissue. Some of the treatment methods which apply cells include abrasion chondroplasty, microfracture, multiple drilling, and ACI. Some of the treatment methods which apply tissues include osteochondral transfer and allograft. Treatment methods which apply both cells and tissues are new-generation ACI and microfracture using biomaterials.

18.2 Microfracture

As full-thickness injury invades the subchondral bone, a slight healing response in which bone marrow cells are recruited can be anticipated. When the subchondral bone is broken, clots are formed by leaked marrow components containing mesenchymal stem cells, and these cells differentiate and form fibrocartilages. Differing from hyaline cartilages, these fibrocartilages contain abundant type I collagen; however, as the proteoglycan content is minimal, they thus show poor wear characteristics.

Prior to the development of the concept of tissue engineering, biomaterials were not used, and surgery to treat cartilage injury by simply stimulating bone marrow or debridement was used as the basic treatment method. Numerous, successful results with relatively small articular cartilage defects were reported; however, it was long recognized that this treatment was limited to the treatment of large defects.

In 1959, Pridie described the formation of cartilages in arthritic knees using subchondral drilling for the first time [21]. Subsequently, Rodrigo et al. introduced the arthroscopic microfracture technique in which, to avoid thermal necrosis, awls were used rather than drills [23]. Such techniques have been readily used for articular cartilage defect areas since the 1990s.

Based on several reports noting that in lesions larger than 2 cm^2, the patients' clinical outcomes were poor, the size has been suggested as the upper limit of microfracture in many cases. Therefore, microfracture has primarily been used as the treatment for small-size articular cartilage injury or for partial injury, and as successful results were reported during the short-term follow-ups, it is now regarded as the first-line treatment for post-traumatic, femoral cartilage defects. Although poor outcomes are expected, surgeons often use microfracture for relatively large lesions (Fig. 18.1).

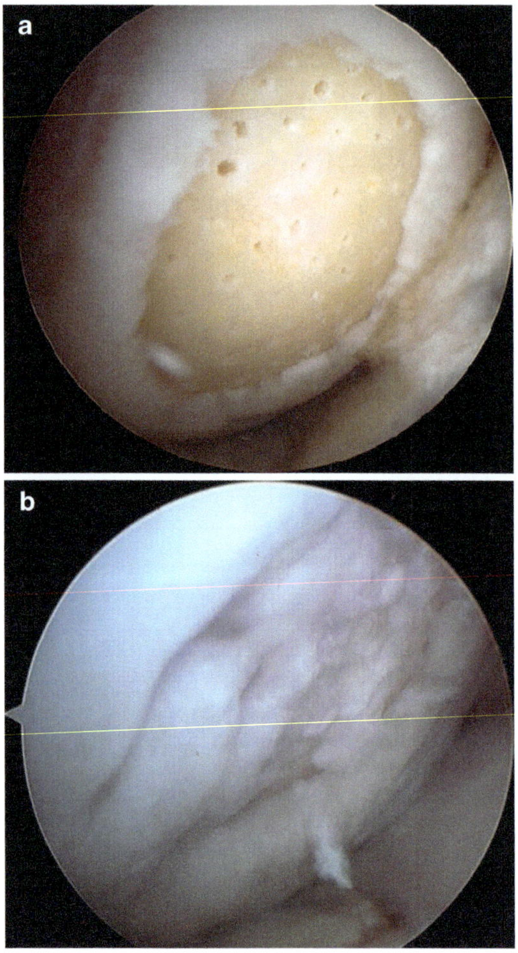

Fig. 18.1 (**a**) Microfracture; (**b**) postoperative 1 year (Courtesy Dr. J.H. Cho)

Author's recommended treatments in biocytotherapy

Cartilage defect size	Small(2 cm^2)	Medium (<10 cm^2)	Large (>10 cm^2)
Author-recommended treatment	1. Microfracture 2. Microfracture with biomaterial	1. Microfracture with biomaterial 2. ACI	1. ACI 2. Microfracture with biomaterial

18.3 ACIC (Autologous Collagen-Induced Chondrogenesis)

For the past several decades, as the treatments for the damage of articular cartilage, there have been treatment methods such as arthroscopic debridement, microfracture, drilling, osteochondral transplantation, and autologous chondrocyte implantation (ACI). Of these, autologous chondrocyte implantation (ACI) has been established as the most definite method for attempting a recovery to the normal articular cartilage. To date, however, ACI gives a lot of burden to patients in that patients should undergo two surgeries where some part of normal articular cartilage is extracted and it is transplanted following the culture [2, 19].

Besides, for the treatment of small-sized defects of the articular cartilage, the morbidity which is exerted for the cellular transplantation has been reported to be relatively higher. In this regard, as the treatment methods for chondromalacia or small-sized cartilaginous lesions, with the application of the previous surgical methods, the necessity for creating the simplified technique has been increasing.

Even if regenerated cartilages through microfracture are not hyaline cartilages but are mechanically weak fibrocartilages, considering the favorable, short-term results, cost-effectiveness, and ease of the method, it is not a technique that will become readily obsolete. Rather, efforts to improve the outcomes by emphasizing existing advantages will be required. Because of this necessity, to facilitate the regeneration of articular cartilages after the microfracture procedure using a bioscaffold, several procedures have begun to be developed.

Recently, a procedure known as Autologous Matrix-Induced Chondrogenesis (AMIC), which is a procedure performed to improve chondrogenesis by covering cartilage defect with a collagen membrane after microfracture, has been developed and is actively used. This method facilitates marrow-derived stem cells remaining in cartilage defect areas after microfracture, using a collagen scaffold; it also improves cartilage production through this technique [25]. Such a procedure is suitable for the treatment for focal lesions such as osteochondral defects. Given the above background, following the microfracture, while using a mixture of atelocollagen and fibrin as a scaffold, attempts were made to examine the possibility for the treatment of cartilaginous defects.

There have been various types of surgical methods to treat articular cartilage due to limitation of the regenerative potential of the cartilage [8]. Among the treatments, ACI has become a standard treatment. It provides patients with a burden for the decision on the surgical operation, however, to undergo surgical operations twice for the extraction of the normal cartilage and the transplantation of cartilage following the culture of it. Besides, in cases in which the damage of articular cartilage was not of severe degree and the size of defect areas was relatively smaller, ACI can be stated to be a type of overtreatment.

It is therefore necessary to review a one-stage procedure and then to develop it. Of the previous surgical methods, the treatment methods using stem cells representatively include a microfracture. There are many reports describing the good clinical outcomes after microfracture. At present, however, new treatment modalities as well as criticism for the above methods have been proposed [15].

Besides, in cases in which a microfracture was simply performed, as the time elapsed, the degeneration of the articular cartilage occurs. Accordingly in these cases, the additional revision is needed. Recent studies have shown the good experimental results with a concomitant use of scaffold with a microfracture [20].

For the procedure where a solid-form scaffold is transplanted to the cartilage defect, the depth of the defect area should be relatively greater and the press fit should be created accordingly. In cases in which the depth of defect areas is smaller, with the use of a suture or a membrane, the scaffold should be maintained at the site of transplantation. Atelocollagen and fibrin mixture do not need this process. According to the coagulation cascades, they can be maintained at the sites where a scaffold is shallow. Accordingly, the cartilage defect can easily be applied to even the posterior condyle to which a surgical access cannot be made.

Collagen is the connective tissue protein which plays a key role in maintaining the morphology of tissue, and atelocollagen is a highly purified type I collagen which was obtained following the treatment of pepsin from skin dermis. This atelocollagen is obtained following the removal of telopeptide which is immunologically problematic, and it is used for a wide variety of areas such as wound healing, vessel prosthesis, bone substitute, and hemostatic agent [1].

On the other hand, fibrin sealants are biological adhesives that mimic the final step of the coagulation cascade and thus help with the bone bleeding control [4], and it is a very safe combination. Fibrin gel is recently attracting attention as a good material for cartilage reconstruction. Fibrin has high biocompatibility, biodegradability, no toxicity, and has long been used as a clinical material for bleeding control. Fibrin is known for its use as an injectable carrier for generating neo-cartilage [3, 10]. The fibrin can maintain the shape of the articulation approximately 5 min after injection, thus causing the atelocollagen to stay in the injected sites.

In the current experiment, in the group where atelocollagen and fibrin mixture were transplanted, there was good cartilage regeneration. Besides, type II collagen was well formed. These results indicate that the cartilage was well formed with the actions of bone marrow stromal cells. At this time, the scaffold well maintained the shape of the articular cartilage which was formed from the stem cells. It is also assumed to play a key role in making the effective connectivity between the cells.

The clinical applicability of this procedure can be seen during AMIC (Autologous Matrix-Induced Chondrogenesis). This is a procedure where a microfracture is priorly performed for the damage articular cartilage and it is covered by the collagen membrane. Thus attempts are made to consistently perform the chondrogenesis [13]. During the joint movement, however, there is a possibility for a graft detachment. In this procedure, however, with the use of atelocollagen and fibrin mixture, the defect sites were covered. Then, the joint movement was performed. Thus, a lack of graft detachment was confirmed. Accordingly in cases in which this procedure was directly applied to the clinical practice, despite the application to a small-sized lesion, or those in which ACI could not be performed due to several reasons despite the presence of large-sized lesions, it is highly probable that the current procedure would be accepted as a good alternative treatment regimen. Atelocollagen using fibrin for articular cartilage defects of the knee appears to be an effective method for cartilage regeneration and also has many potential surgical advantages.

18.3.1 Surgical Procedure

The patient is anesthetized under general anesthesia or reginal and was placed in a supine position. All preparations are the same as other arthroscopic operations. The operation can be done by open procedure or arthroscopically.

For open procedure, arthrotomy is performed on the medial or lateral portion of the patella along the chondral defects. To ensure that the implanted collagen gel merged well with normal cartilaginous tissue when exposed to defective areas, damaged cartilage is removed from the edges of the chondral defects. Multiple holes of 5-mm depth and 2.5-mm diameter were made at 1–2-cm intervals using a 2.5-mm drill bit or microfracture awl so that the holes of the defect would act as the passage of bone marrow stem cells.

18.3.2 Injection of Atelocollagen and Fibrin Mixture

For the injection procedure, two 1-ml syringes and a Y-shaped mixing catheter were used. In one syringe, 1 ml of fibrinogen (Tisseel, Baxter Inc., Korea) was filled with medium, and the other syringe was filled with 0.9 ml of atelocollagen (TheraFill, Sewon Cellontech, Seoul, Korea) and 0.1 ml of thrombin (50 IU). Atelocollagen mixed with fibrin was then slowly injected into the defect area.

In order not to overflow the margin, the dependent position of the defect site was maintained for 5 min. Flexion and extension motion of the knee was performed three to five times in order to check for any graft failure. The wound was then closed layer by layer.

The use of continuous passive motion (CPM) machines was recommended for rehabilitation after surgery, followed by full weight bearing beginning 6–8 weeks postoperatively.

18.4 Autologous Chondrocyte Implantation (ACI)

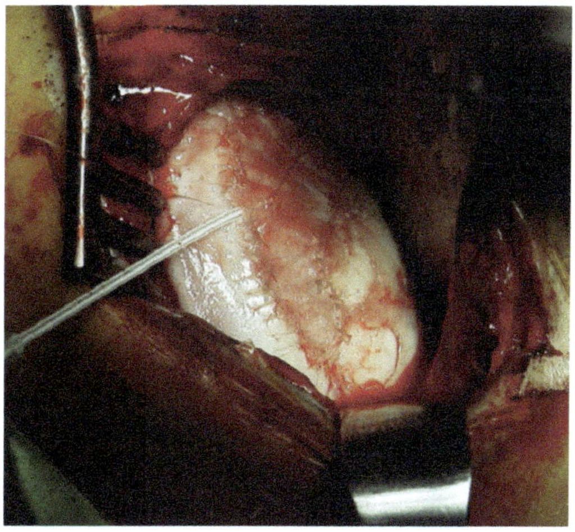

Fig. 18.2 Conventional ACI (Courtesy Dr. J.H. Cho)

18.4.1 Conventional ACI

Periosteum using ACI was first introduced in 1987 in Sweden and subsequently became a major procedure for the regeneration of normal articular cartilages [17]. The steps of this conventional ACI surgery can be summarized as debridement of the cartilage defect, harvesting of periosteum, suturing the periosteum, and chondrocyte implantation. During this surgical procedure, cartilage defect areas are covered with the periosteum, and the success or failure of the surgery is determined by the dense suturing of the periosteum in the vicinity of the cartilage defect area in order to prevent leakage of injected cells. Many clinicians currently feel pressured to use this procedure.

In addition, for adequate suturing the periosteum, the lesion area should be exposed sufficiently. Even for the small defect, the procedure requires large incision (Fig. 18.2). Despite this limitation, the short- and long-term results of this surgery are relatively successful.

18.4.2 Gel AGI (GACI)

The surgical procedure of conventional ACI can be summarized as consisting of debridement of the cartilage defect, harvesting of the periosteum, suturing the periosteum, and chondrocyte implantation [7]. Among these procedures, periosteum suturing is a difficult and time-consuming procedure for the surgeon, and periosteal harvesting and periosteum suturing procedures have some risk of patient morbidity. Conventional ACI is not preferred because of the periosteal grafting component which requires an additional operation to harvest the periosteum. In addition, for watertight suturing of the periosteal graft to the surrounding cartilage, a large surgical incision is required, thus presenting the potential problem of subsequent leakage of injected cells from the defect as well as graft detachment [8].

To overcome these potential problems, some researchers have proposed using collagen membrane rather than the periosteum [8, 15, 18]. If the surgeon's preference is to not use the periosteum, methods using collagen membrane can eliminate the need for a second incision for periosteal harvest as well as reducing the long surgical time and extensive suturing. However, with this approach, there are also some potential problems such as the loss of critical chondrocytes caused by the cutting and repeated manipulation of the seeded membrane. There is also the possibility of detachment of the collagen membrane from the cartilage defect. Therefore, it is becoming increasingly evident that it is necessary to develop a new method.

In the gel-type ACI (GACI), the fibrin can already maintain the shape of the articulation approximately 5 min after injection, thus allowing the cells to remain at the injected sites. And even if there is a defect along the chondral margin, fibrin helps to maintain the shape of the graft according to the articulation [20]. The 5-mm-deep holes serve an important function by increasing the adhesive force of the graft to the defect during knee motion. In the surgical procedures, in order to prevent both the formation of fibrocartilaginous tissue [1] and detachment of the injected cell and fibrin mixture, bleeding control is very important. Fortunately, fibrin sealants are biological adhesives that mimic the final step of the coagulation cascade and therefore help with the bone bleeding control [4]. Also, any commercially available fibrin product can be used because of the similar range of the amounts of fibrinogen and thrombin. Following surgery, we check the stability of the graft by flexion and extension knee-motion exercise. If the graft adequately remains in the defect site, we finish the surgery.

The number of cells introduced in initial explants is important as the seeded chondrocyte number is linearly related to biosynthetic activity [3]. In that respect, GACI can have an advantage over other treatments such as ACIC and MACI. The collagen membrane occupies quite a substantial amount of space in a cartilage defect, although the cell–gel mixture occupies the space in the GACI. Although the optimal number of required cells has not been determined, high cell densities seem to be desirable [10] and one vial of Chondron™ could cover a total condyle defect. The 96 patients (98.0 %) we treated achieved measurable postoperative improvement and only two patients (2.0 %) showed deterioration of their "no change." One patient required repeat surgery, and all of the patients who underwent surgery showed substantial improvement during the follow-up period. The authors regard these as encouraging results compared with those of other reports regarding marrow stimulation or ACI [13]. In fact, our repeat surgery rate is far less than that associated with other forms of knee surgery [9, 14].

However, it is difficult to conclude that this technique is superior to other techniques, such as ACIC or MACI, as this study is not a comparative study. Many successful results have also been reported using other techniques [6, 12, 16]. In this study, the authors used a telephone-based scoring system. If the patient does not feel any discomfort, he/she would not need to come to the hospital as job and time limitations frequently prevent patients from checking in with their doctors. Therefore, the necessity and benefits of telephone or Internet consultation are increasing. There is also a continuing necessity to develop a new, remote scoring system which can handle the other knee condition evaluations.

Swedish researchers have reported improvements for longer than 2 years following ACI [26]; similarly, in our study, improvements were more apparent after 24 months. However, the preoperative score of greater than 25-month follow-up group was lower than that of 13–24-month follow-up group. Therefore, it is difficult to insist the same result as Swedish report.

An even more positive aspect of this study is that clinical improvement was apparent even during the short-term, post-op follow-up period of less than 2 years following surgery.

With respect to the surgical success based on the size of the articular cartilage defects, there was no statistical difference in the results. There was one case of 1 cm^2 of cartilage defect and the others were over 2 cm^2. A small cartilage defect can cause severe discomfort and pain if a patient's activity level is high. The pressure generated during weight bearing is so high that it stimulates a weak articular cartilage area even though the defect size may be very small. Therefore, covering a cartilage defect with healthy cartilage is very important, and GACI offers a successful treatment option for both small and large cartilage defects.

To resolve the problems of conventional ACI using the periosteum, the ACI method using a collagen membrane was designed [24]. This currently widely used method uses a membrane onto which chondrocytes are seeded and cultured for several days before the membrane is cut to the correct size and shape of the defect. If the surgeon's preference is to not use the periosteum, methods using collagen membrane can eliminate the need for a second incision for periosteal harvest as well as reducing the long surgical time and extensive suturing. Such methods have substantially eliminated the discomfort of conventional surgical techniques and have thus been used in several countries; the results are also encouraging [24].

Recently, as a new cartilage cell graft technique, a method using the cell–gel mixture was introduced as gel-type autologous chondrocyte implantation (GACI, Chondron). The natural substance fibrin gel appears to be an excellent material for cartilage reconstruction. As fibrin has the characteristics of high biocompatibility, nontoxicity, and excellent biodegradable properties, it has long been used as a clinical material. As an injectable carrier to produce neo-cartilage, fibrin has many advantages [2]. In addition, fibrin matrix in a 3-dimensional scaffold has excellent cell attachment properties, cell proliferation and migration within the matrix can occur readily, and it thus provides an environment in which cells can effectively develop into tissues; its biodegradable property is excellent, and thus with the formation of new tissue by cells contained within the matrix, it can be replaced by complete tissues [11].

At operation, fibrin can already maintain the shape of the articulation approximately 5 min following its injection, thus allowing the cells to remain at the injected sites. And even if there is a defect along the chondral margin, fibrin helps to maintain the shape of the graft according to the articulation [2]. Recently, some very successful results have been reported (Fig. 18.3).

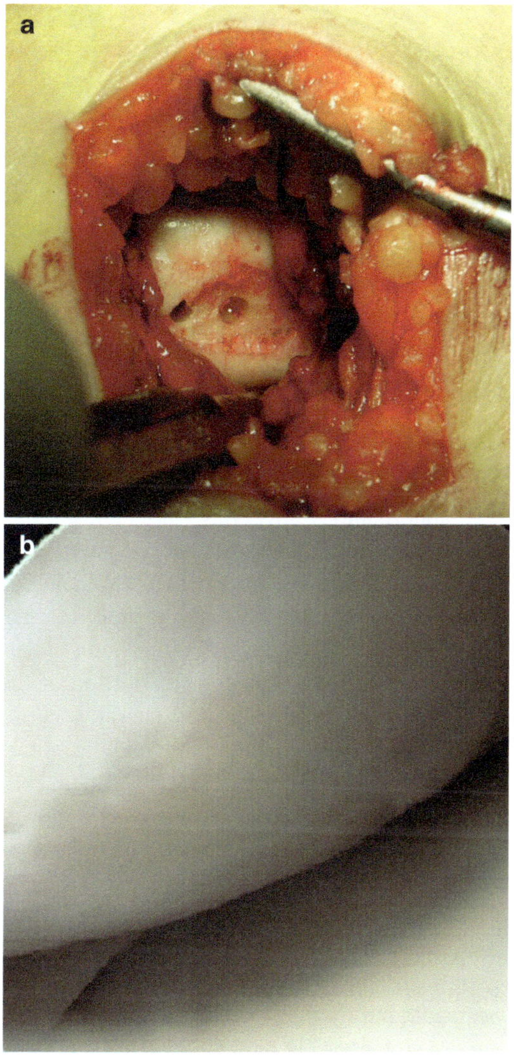

Fig. 18.3 (**a**) Chondral defect; (**b**) postoperative 1 year (GACI)

18.4.3 Evaluation of Patient Suitability for Study Participation (Inclusion and Exclusion Criteria)

The indications for ACI were clinically significant, symptomatic, cartilaginous defects (Outerbridge III–IV) of the knee joint in patients with one or more cartilage defects not exceeding 15 cm^2 for a single defect or 20 cm^2 for multiple defects. The knee joint must be stable and without a severe deformity greater than 5–10° of the valgus or varus.

The exclusion criteria included advanced osteoarthritis (Kellgren–Lawrence Grading Scale >2) and inflammatory arthritis with severe deformity exceeding the above range. Patellofemoral instability, drug abuse history, and psychological problems were also included as patient exclusion criteria.

18.4.4 Surgical Techniques

We used a two-stage surgical technique. After completing the clinical and radiological assessments, arthroscopy was performed in order to measure the positions, sizes, and depths of the chondral defects and to identify chondral defects

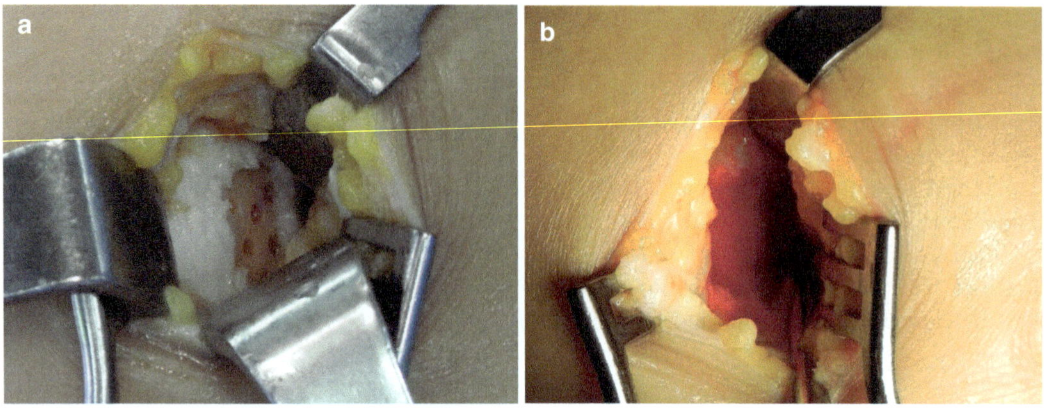

Fig. 18.4 (**a**) Preparation of the lesion. (**b**) Post injection of mixture (cell and gel)

and abnormalities involving the menisci and ligaments. Knee standing AP, lateral, and tangential radiographs were obtained to evaluate the knee joint deformity and the potential presence of osteoarthritis. In addition, 200–300 mg of cartilage from a non-weight-bearing portion of the knee, generally the medial or lateral superior ridge of the condyle or the intercondylar notch, was collected and sent to the GMP-certified, cell-culturing facility (Sewon Cellontech, Korea) for processing using the CE/MDD-certified, human-cell-processing kit (CRM kit™, Sewon Cellontech, Korea).

Autologous chondrocyte implantation was performed when 1.2×10^7 chondrocytes/vial had been cultured for 4–6 weeks after the initial surgery. Autologous chondrocytes were aseptically processed. The cell viabilities of all supplied products were greater than 80 % prior to the final packaging.

During the second surgical procedure, arthrotomy was performed on the medial or lateral portion of the patella along the chondral defects. To ensure that the implanted chondrocytes merged well with normal cartilaginous tissue when exposed to defective areas, damaged cartilage was removed from the edges of the chondral defects. Multiple holes of 5-mm depth and 2.5-mm diameter were made at 1–2-cm intervals using a 2.5-mm drill bit so that the holes of the defect would receive the holding force of the graft (Fig. 18.4a). After release of the tourniquet, bone bleeding control was achieved using compression force applied to the holes using epinephrine-soaked gauze packing. For the injection procedure, two 1-ml syringes and a Y-shaped mixing adapter were used. In one syringe, 1 ml of fibrinogen (Greenplast, Green Cross, Korea) was filled with medium (CRM kit™, Sewon Cellontech, Korea), and the other syringe was filled with 0.9 ml of cell suspension and 0.1 ml of thrombin. Cultured autologous chondrocytes mixed with fibrin (1:1) were then slowly injected into the defect area (Fig. 18.4b).

In order not to overflow the margin, the dependent position of the defect site was maintained for 5 min. Flexion and extension motion of the knee was performed three to five times in order to check for any graft failure. The wound was then closed layer by layer. The use of continuous passive motion (CPM) machines was recommended for rehabilitation after surgery, followed by full weight bearing beginning 6–8 weeks postoperatively.

18.4.5 Cell and Gel Mixture Ex Vivo Evaluation

Fibrin glue was used to develop the implantation protocol of gel-type cultured autologous chondrocytes. The order and ratio of mixing the major constituents of the fibrin glue with the cultured autologous chondrocytes were optimized in order to guarantee maximal cellular viability and the ability to solidify within a practical length of time after implantation.

To measure the viability of chondrocytes mixed with fibrin according to the established protocol, cultured human chondrocytes (1.2×10^7cells/vial) proliferated ex vivo were collected. The collected cell suspension was mixed with the same volume of fibrin glue used to prepare 2 ml of cell–fibrin mixture gel. This gel was cultured for 3 days at 37 in an 8 % CO_2 incubator. The viability of chondrocytes within the fibrin gel which was cultured for 0, 12, 24, 48, and 72 h was measured using MTT (3-(4,5-Dimethyl-2-thiazolyl)-2,5-diphenyl-2H-tetrazolium bromide, Sigma, USA.) assay.

In addition, the viable status of chondrocytes within the cell–fibrin matrix was grossly examined using Calcein-AM/Ethidium homodimer-1 (Invitrogen, USA) staining. Live cells were expressed as a green color and dead cells were expressed as a red color under fluorescent microscopy following the staining. A scanning electron microscope (Hitachi, Japan) was used to confirm the morphological structure of the mixture of chondrocytes and fibrin. The material safety of autologous chondrocytes mixed with fibrin was confirmed as lacking the toxicity seen in a subcutaneous toxicity study using C57BL/6 mice (Korea Institute of Toxicology, 2006).

18.4.6 Gel ACI for RA or OA

Rheumatoid arthritis (RA) is an autoimmune disease that causes chronic inflammation of the joints. To date, pharmacologic treatment remains the primary form of treatment. However, if pain and limitation of joint function become severe and debilitating, surgical treatment should be considered [19].

Joint pain and loss of mobility are among the most common causes of impairment in middle-aged and older people. This occurs frequently in the clinical syndrome of osteoarthritis. Over the last few decades, artificial joint replacement has developed very rapidly and many arthritic conditions have been successfully treated. However, total joint arthroplasty does not last so long, revisional operation is inevitable. A need increasingly exists for a method that biologically regenerates the arthritic lesion of knee as the life span of man is increasing.

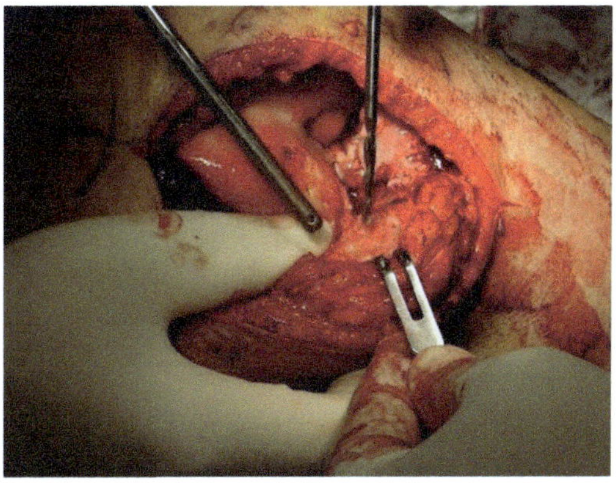

Fig. 18.5 Arthritic lesion exposure

Surgical Technique

With the patient under general or spinal anesthesia, a longitudinal midline incision was made, extending 5 cm above superior pole of the patella to the level of the tibia tubercle. The subcutaneous tissue was divided in the line of the skin incision. A medial skin flap was developed to expose the quadriceps tendon, medial border of the patella, and the medial border of the patellar tendon. Medial parapatellar capsular incision was made, and the patella was dislocated laterally to expose the arthritic chondral lesions (Fig. 18.5). The overhanging osteophytes were resected. Deformed and degenerated articular cartilage tissue was resected and debrided to the margin of the femoral condyles and patella. Multiple holes of 2-mm depth and 2.5-mm diameter using 2.5-mm drill bit are made at 1–2-cm interval, so that holes of the defect should get a holding force of the graft. After release of the tourniquet, bone bleeding control was achieved using bone wax and compression force to the holes with epinephrine-soaked gauze packing. Cultured autologous chondrocytes mixed with fibrin (1:1) were injected slowly to defect area. The dependent position of defect site not to flow over the margin was maintained

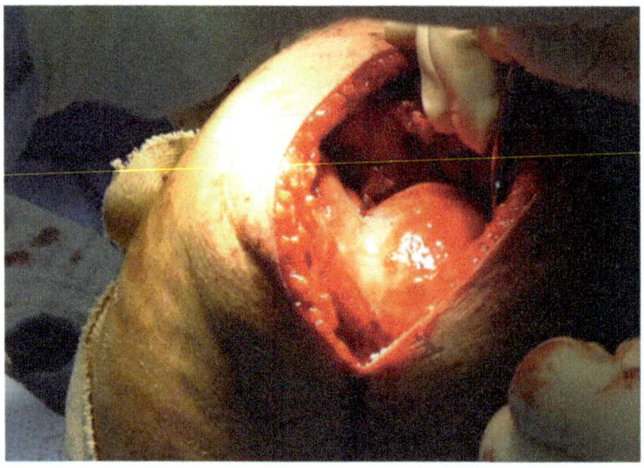

Fig. 18.6 Post injection of arthritic lesion

for 5 min. Three or five times flexion and extension motion of the knee was performed to check any graft failure (Fig. 18.6). The wound was closed layer by layer.

18.4.7 Rehabilitation

The patient remained non-weight bearing for 6 weeks postoperatively, began bearing weight of approximately 10–15 kg from the 7th week, and gradually progressed to full weight bearing at 12 weeks. The range of motion exercise from 0° to 40° was started at the next day of operation by using CPM (continuous passive motion) for 4–6 h. After a week, the angle was increased by 5° per day and was limited to as little as 0° to as much as 120° from the fourth to eighth week. During this period, quadriceps strengthening exercise and stretching of the hamstring and calf were continued.

18.5 Summary

Once it is damaged articular cartilage has limited potential for repair. Many treatment modalities introduced to repair the cartilage.

In the past, the main treatments were passive mode, and it was dependent only on the regeneration potential of bone marrow itself.

However, at present, many options have been developed using cell culturing, applying new biomaterial, and devising new application methods. These options are more of an active mode for cartilage regeneration, not just waiting for natural regeneration potential. These methods enhance the cartilage repair ability and are proved by many researchers and the publications.

The clinical applications of stem cell therapy is still at an early stage. Therefore more experiments and clinical trials are necessary for setting this as a formal treatment option.

References

1. Ashton BA, Allen TD, Howlet CR, Eaglesom CC, Hatori A (1980) Maureen Owen: formation of bone and cartilage by marrow stromal cells in diffusion chambers in vivo. Clin Orthop 151:294–307
2. Choi NY, Kim BW, Yeo WJ, Kim HB, Suh DS, Kim JS, Kim YS, Seo YH, Cho JY, Chun CW, Park HS, Shetty AA, Kim SJ (2010) Gel-type autologous chondrocyte (Chondron) implantation for treatment of articular cartilage defects of the knee. BMC Musculoskelet Disord 11:103
3. Connolly JF (1998) Clinical use of marrow osteoprogenitor cells to stimulate osteogenesis. Clin Orthop Relat Res (355 supplement):S257–S266
4. Connolly JF, Shindell R (1986) Percutaneous marrow injection for an ununited tibia. Nebr Med J 71(4): 105–107
5. Curl WW, Krome J, Gordon ES, Rushing J, Smith BP, Poehling GG (1997) Cartilage injuries: a review of 31,516 knee arthroscopies. Arthroscopy 13:456–460
6. Gangji V, Hauzeur JP, Matos C, De Maertelaer V, Toungouz M, Lambermont M (2004) Treatment of osteonecrosis of the femoral head with implantation of autologous bone-marrow cells. A pilot study. J Bone Joint Surg Am 86-A(6):1153–1160
7. Gluckman E, Broxmeyer HA, Auerbach AD, Friedman HS, Douglas GW, Devergie A, Esperou H, Thierry D, Socie G, Lehn P, Cooper S, English D, Kurtzberg J, Bard J, Boyse EA (1989) Hematopoietic reconstitution in a patient with Fanconi's anemia by means of umbilical-cord blood from an HLA-identical sibling. N Engl J Med 321:1174–1178
8. Gronthos S, Graves SE, Ohta S, Simmons PJ (1994) The STRO-1+ fraction of adult human bone marrow contains the osteogenic precursors. Blood 84(12): 4164–4173
9. Hernigou P, Beaujean F (2002) Treatment of osteonecrosis with autologous bone marrow grafting. Clin Orthop Relat Res (405):14–23
10. Hernigou PH, Poignard A, Beaujean F, Rouard H (2005) Percutaneous autologous bone-marrow grafting for nonunions: influence of the number and concentration of progenitor cells. J Bone Joint Surg Am 87(7):1430–1437

11. Ho W, Tawil B, Dunn JC, Wu BM (2006) The behavior of human mesenchymal stem cells in 3D fibrin clots: dependence on fibrinogen concentration and clot structure. Tissue Eng 12:1587–1595
12. Kim SJ, Bahk WJ, Chang CH, Jang JD, Suhl KH (2008) Treatment of osteonecrosis of the femoral head using autologous cultured osteoblasts: a case report. J Med Case Reports 2:58
13. Kim SJ, Jang JD, Lee SK (2007) Treatment of long tubular bone defect of rabbit using autologous cultured osteoblasts mixed with fibrin. Cytotechnology 54:115–120
14. Kim S-J, Shin Y-W, Yang K-H et al (2009) A multicenter, randomized, clinical study to compare the effect and safety of autologous cultured osteoblast (Ossron) injection to treat fractures. BMC Musculoskelet Disord 10:Article 20
15. Long MW, Robinson JA, Ashcraft EA, Mann KG (1995) Regulation of human bone marrow-derived osteoprogenitor cells by osteogenic growth factors. J Clin Invest 95(2):881–887
16. Majors AK, Boehm CA, Nitto H, Midura RJ, Muschler GF (1997) Characterization of human bone marrow stromal cells with respect to osteoblastic differentiation. J Orthop Res 15(4):546–557
17. Marlovits S, Zeller P, Singer P, Resinger C, Vécsei V (2006) Cartilage repair: generations of autologous chondrocyte transplantation. Eur J Radiol 57:24–31
18. Muschler GF, Boehm C, Easley K (1997) Aspiration to obtain osteoblast progenitor cells from human bone marrow: the influence of aspiration volume. J Bone Joint Surg Am 79(11):1699–1709
19. Nehrer S, Breinan HA, Ramappa A, Shortkroff S, Young G, Minas T, Sledge CB, Yannas IV, Spector M (1997) Canine chondrocytes seeded in type I and type II collagen implants investigated in vitro. J Biomed Mater Res 38:95–104
20. Pitaru S, Kotev-Emeth S, Noff D, Kaffuler S, Savion N (1993) Effect of basic fibroblast growth factor on the growth and differentiation of adult stromal bone marrow cells: enhanced development of mineralized bone-like tissue in culture. J Bone Miner Res 8(8):919–929
21. Pridie KH (1959) A method of resurfacing osteoarthritic knee joints. J Bone Joint Surg Br 41:618–619
22. Regenerative medicine glossary (2009) Regen Med 4 (4s):S30. doi:10.2217/rme.09.s1
23. Rodrigo JJ, Steadman JR, Silliman JF, Fulston HA (1994) Improvement of full thickness chondral defect healing in the human knee after debridement and microfracture using continuous passive motion. Am J Knee Surg 7:109–116
24. Steinwachs M (2009) New technique for cell-seeded collagen-matrix-supported autologous chondrocyte transplantation. Arthroscopy 25:208–211
25. Steinwachs MR, Guggi T, Kreuz PC (2008) Marrow stimulation techniques. Injury 39:S26–S31
26. Vashishth D, Gibson G, Kimura J, Shcaffler MB, Fyhrie DP (2002) Determination of bone volume by osteocyte population. Anat Rec 267:292–295

Knee Cartilage Repair with Hyalograft® (Hyaff-11 Scaffold with Seeded Autologous Chondrocytes)

19

Mats Brittberg

Contents

M. Brittberg, MD, PhD
Cartilage Research Unit, Orthopaedic Department, University of Gothenburg, Kungsbacka, Sweden

Region Halland Orthopaedics, Kungsbacka Hospital, Kungsbacka, Sweden
e-mail: mats.brittberg@telia.com

19.1 Introduction

Autologous chondrocyte implantation (ACI) was first introduced clinically in October 1987 as a new method of repairing damaged cartilage [2]. Regarded as a second line of treatment when other techniques have failed [4], the methodology now could present good long-term results up to 25 years follow-up [16].

The ACI methodology related to the first-generation ACI is based on harvest of 200–300 mg of cartilage from a less loaded area in the knee. The cartilage is sent to a laboratorium for processing. The cartilage is digested; the isolated chondrocytes are expanded in vitro during 2–3 weeks. The expanded final amount of cells is resent to the surgeon as a suspension.

The cells are to be injected into the defect covered with a membrane, periosteum (first generation) or collagen membrane (second generation). However, the two first generations of ACI are used as arthrotomy procedures.

In order to improve and facilitate the implantation of cultured chondrocytes and make it possible to perform an autologous chondrocyte implantation (ACI) procedure transarthroscopically, different porous scaffolds have been tested. One such material is based on the benzylic ester of hyaluronic acid (Hyaff-11, Fidia Advanced Biopolymers Laboratories, Padova, Italy) and consists of a network of 20-μm-thick fibres with interstices of variable sizes [7, 8].

Hyaluronan is one of the main components of the extracellular matrix, and it contributes

A.A. Shetty et al. (eds.), *Techniques in Cartilage Repair Surgery*,
DOI 10.1007/978-3-642-41921-8_19, © ESSKA 2014

significantly to cell proliferation and migration [17]. In embryology, it is proposed that joint cavitation is facilitated by a rise in local hyaluronan concentration [9]. Furthermore, hyaluronan is an important component of articular cartilage where aggrecan monomers bind to hyaluronan in the presence of link protein and large highly negatively charged aggregates form [10]. These aggregates bind water molecules and are responsible for the resilience of cartilage (its resistance to compression).

Hyaluronan has been demonstrated to be an optimal physical support to allow cell-cell contacts, cluster formation, and extracellular matrix deposition and to deliver differentiated chondrocytes [1]. Ultrastructural observations have supported the evidence that chondrocytes grown onto a hyaluronan-derived three-dimensional scaffold maintain their unique phenotype and organization in a cartilage-like extracellular matrix. These findings support the further pursuit of a transplantable engineered cartilage using human chondrocytes for the repair of chondral lesions. As the Hyaff-scaffold material is easy to use, fold and recoil again, it is of great interest to use for endoscopic delivery. Today, there exist medium to long term follow ups with both open and arthroscopic implantations of hyaluronic cell seeded implants [5, 11, 14, 15].

19.2 Cell Isolation, Expansion and Scaffold Culture

The harvested cartilage biopsy is transported to the cell culture lab in sterile saline solution (0.9 % NaCl, Fresenius Kabi, Uppsala, Sweden) supplemented with gentamicin sulphate (0.05 μg/ml, Gibco, Invitrogen, Paisley, UK) and amphotericin B (0.5 μg/ml, Gibco, Invitrogen). After removal of contaminating subchondral bone and connective tissue, the chondrocytes are isolated from the surrounding matrix by mechanical mincing of the tissue with a scalpel followed by enzymatic treatment with collagenase (0.8 mg/ml, Worthington Biochemical Corp, Lakewood, NJ, USA) in Ham's F-12 (Gibco, Invitrogen), overnight at 37 °C in 7 % CO_2/90 % air. The isolated cells are

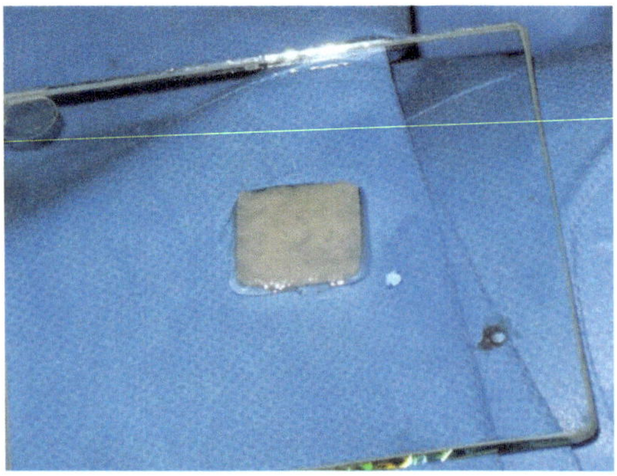

Fig. 19.1 A 2×2 cm large Hyalograft scaffold prior to sizing for implantation

then seeded at a density of $10–16 \times 10^3$ cells/cm^2 in culture flasks (Primaria®, Falcon, BD, New Jersey, USA) in DMEM/F12 (Gibco, Invitrogen) supplemented with ascorbic acid (0.08 mg/ml, Apotekets produktionsenhet, Umeå, Sweden), gentamicin sulphate (0.05 mg/l), amphotericin B (0.5 μg/ml) and L-glutamine (2 mM, Gibco, Invitrogen) with addition of 10 % autologous serum. The first medium change is made at day 6 and thereafter twice a week. When the cells reach 80 % confluence, they are subcultured or frozen. Thawed cells are subcultured into new flasks (Costar, Corning scientific, USA) at a density of $3–4 \times 10^3$ cells/cm^2. The culture expanded cells (passage 1 or 2) are seeded on 2×2 cm autologous serum pre-coated Hyaff-11® scaffolds (Anika Therapeutics, USA) at a density of 1.5×10^6–$2.0 \times 10^6/cm^2$. The scaffolds are then cultured for 13–15 days in a differentiation medium, i.e. DMEM/F12 medium (Gibco, Invitrogen) supplemented with 10 % autologous serum, ascorbic acid (0.8 mg/ml), L-glutamine (2 mM), transforming growth factor β1 ((10 ng/ml, R&D Systems Europe Ltd., Abingdon, UK), dissolved in reconstitution solution containing recombinant human albumin (G-MM, Vitrolife, SE)), insulin (10 μg/ml, Actrapid, Novo Nordisk A/S, Bagsværd, DK) and dexamethasone (10–7 M, Fluka, Sigma-Aldrich, Gillingham, UK). The media is changed three times per week. The cell-seeded scaffold (Fig. 19.1) is aseptically packed and sent for implantation in a two-container system (NUNC/AS, Roskilde, Denmark).

19.3 Patient Selection

19.3.1 Indications

The ideal patient to be treated with autologous chondrocyte implantation is a symptomatic patient with a full-thickness chondral or osteochondral defect surrounded by healthy, normal cartilage in an otherwise healthy joint. However, the ideal lesion is more the exception than the rule, as many lesions occur in joints with concomitant pathology and some degree of uncontainment.

Subsequently, a patient that has been treated before with another cartilage repair technique that has failed is most often the patient that is considered for ACI [4].

All areas besides the patella surface might be considered for transarthroscopic ACI. The patella surface is most often treated by open ACI, but in a few patients with a lax patella, a transarthroscopic ACI could be tried.

As mentioned above, the cartilage defects are typically focal or localized defects, while even though with Hyalograft more widespread cartilage damage could be treated if the compartment is unloaded post surgery with a temporary unloader brace or a definite unloading osteotomy.

Osteochondritis dissecans patients can be done transarthroscopic with Hyalograft with or without bone grafting depending on the depth of the osteochondral lesion

Also bipolar lesions are OK to treat if the defects are well contained with good quality surrounding cartilage.

Malalignment must be addressed.

There is no definite age limit. Instead, the biological age and the quality of the joint tissues decide if the patient should be included as an ACI candidate or not.

19.3.2 Contraindications

ACI is not indicated as a treatment option for advanced osteoarthritis.

Other contraindications are active rheumatoid arthritis, active autoimmune connective tissue diseases and concomitant malignancies.

19.4 The Operative Technique

The ACI technique includes, as mentioned above, two-stage procedures with an initial cartilage biopsy, which is sent for chondrocyte culture, followed by a second stage operation, which includes the procedure for cell implantation.

Implantation of a hyaluronan-based scaffold seeded with chondrocytes consists of an arthrotomy or in 90–95 % as a transarthroscopic procedure, defect preparation, implantation of the chondrocyte-seeded scaffold and wound closure.

19.4.1 Harvest of Cartilage for Cell Expansion

The chondrocytes that are harvested most often originates from a full-thickness biopsy through all layers down to the subchondral bone. However, here seem to be a chondrocyte subpopulation with progenitor-like characteristics in the surface layer of cartilage indicating that it might be enough to harvest the superficial layers for chondrocyte isolation and expansion [13, 18].

The most common sites for a cartilage biopsy is the superomedial edge of the femoral condyle and the lateral intercondylar notch in the same location in which a notchplasty is performed during anterior cruciate ligament (ACL) reconstruction [2]. The other recommended area is the super lateral edge of the femoral condyle that is non-articulating with the tibia or patella. Furthermore of interest, Biant and Bentley [3] have shown that chondrocytes from the damaged cartilage within the lesion itself could be viable alternatives to harvest-derived cells. An arthroscopic gouge or ring curette is used to obtain two or three small slivers of partial- to full-thickness cartilage depth the size of a fingernail clipping (200–300 mg). It is often helpful to try to leave an end of the biopsy attached to the subchondral bone so it can be grasped with an arthroscopic grasper and torn off.

Simultaneously, 10×6 ml of autologous venous blood is collected for preparation of serum to be used together with the culture medium.

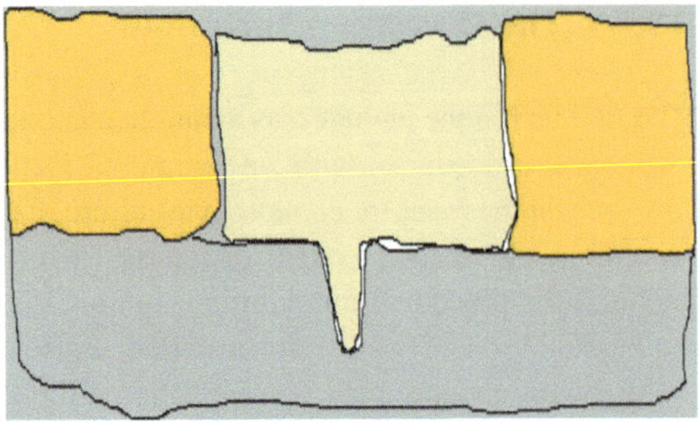

Fig. 19.2 A Hyalograft scaffold has been implanted and secured in the bottom of the defect via a small anchoring bone defect made by an awl; "mushroom" technique

The cells harvested from the patient are expanded and then seeded onto the scaffold where the cells are able to re-differentiate and retain a chondrocytic phenotype even after a long period of in vitro expansion in monolayer culture [6].

The Hyalograft with cultured chondrocytes may be implanted by press fitting directly into the lesion as described by Marcacci et al. [12]. The scaffold has self-adhesive properties, but most often additional fibrin glue is needed for a secure positioning.

In this chapter, the author describes *a slightly modified implantation technique*: the "folded blanket" technique for the knee.

19.4.2 Operative Technique for the Knee

Transarthroscopic Technique

A high anteromedial or anterolateral portal is created and a standard arthroscopy is performed in supine position.

The transarthroscopic Hyalograft®-chondrocyte technique is applicable for defects at the medial and lateral femoral condyle, trochlea, and tibial plateau and in some rare cases when reachable also for the patella.

The direct implantation and positioning of the cell-seeded scaffold into a well-prepared chondral or osteochondral defect is per se same if done open or via the arthroscope.

For a defect at the medial femoral condyle a medial suprameniscal portal is created. This portal is needed to introduce the cell-seeded scaffold into the joint. A half pipe introducer may be used to facilitate the introduction of the scaffold into the joint.

The defect is debrided into vertical walls and a clean bone surface. The central part of the defect is treated by a microfracture awl to get a fixation point (*mushroom fixation*) (Fig. 19.2).

The chondrocyte-seeded matrix is then cut with a scissor or scalpel to the size of the defect. It is often enough with an approximate size (Fig. 19.3). The scaffold is covered with a thin fibrin glue layer, grasped with an arthroscopic grasp instrument with plain surfaces (Fig. 19.4), *and* introduced into the joint along the half pipe to reach the defect or directly through a well-prepared arthroscopic portal.

The pressure controlled pump inflow may be partly reduced intermittently during the procedure. The scaffold is released from the grasper and with a smooth arthroscopy obturator caught and moved into the defect. The central part of the scaffold is pressed gently into the fixation point (Figs. 19.5, 19.6, 19.7 and 19.8).

Some extra fibrin glue is injected over the implanted scaffold and the scaffold is compressed towards the defect bottom with a curved smooth tonsil elevator or with a small Howarth instrument. If the scaffold is oversized, the edges may be folded like a blanket into the defect to fill it up entirely (Fig. 19.9).

If an implanted graft is too small, additional cut pieces of the scaffold are implanted to fill the defect like a patchwork quilt.

If the defect is quite deep, several layers of Hyalograft® may be needed to fill the defect up to surrounding cartilage (*millefeuille technique*) (Fig. 19.10).

Excess glue is taken away with a gentle move with the shaver. Be careful not to catch the implant with the shaver.

Graft adherence and integration are controlled by moving the knee joint with flexion and extension movements. The scaffold should either be in level with surrounding cartilage or slightly below.

The Tibial Plateau

In a defect that is situated on the tibial plateau and often depressed, the repair can be done in a retrograde direction. With a vector guide, a channel is drilled from the proximal tibia to the defect

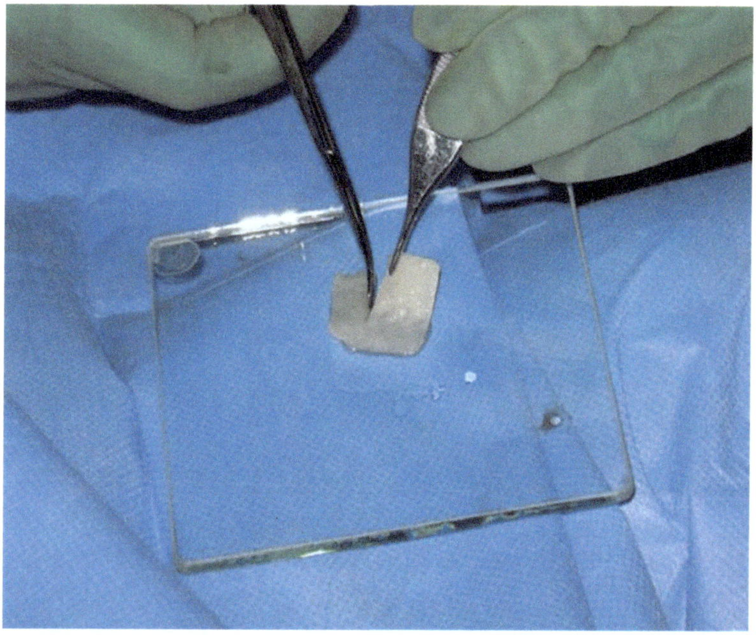

Fig. 19.3 The Hyalograft is sized to fit into the defect that should be treated

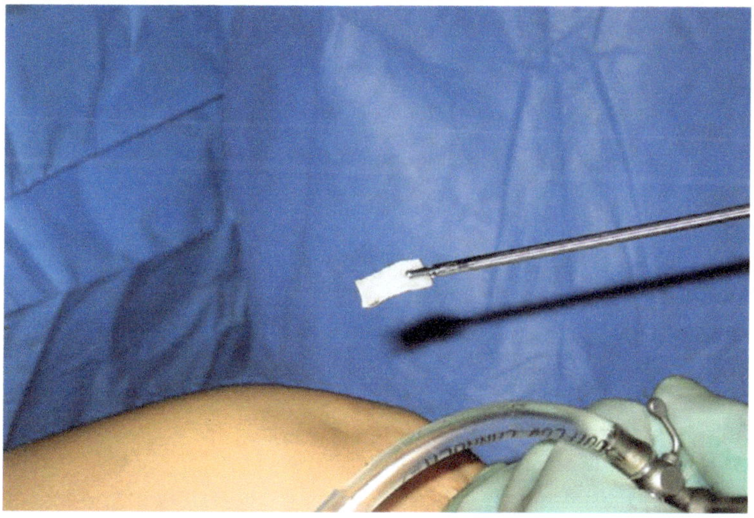

Fig. 19.4 The Hyalograft has been grasped with an arthroscopic grasp instrument with plain surfaces to be introduced via the anteromedial portal

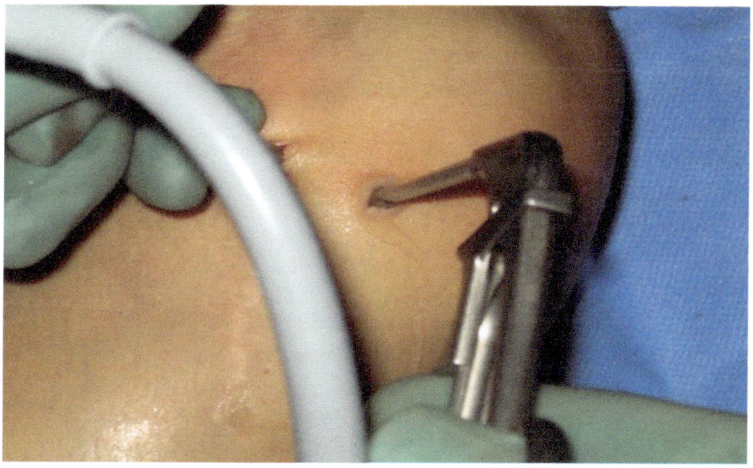

Fig. 19.5 The Hyalograft scaffold is introduced into the joint directly through a well-prepared arthroscopic portal

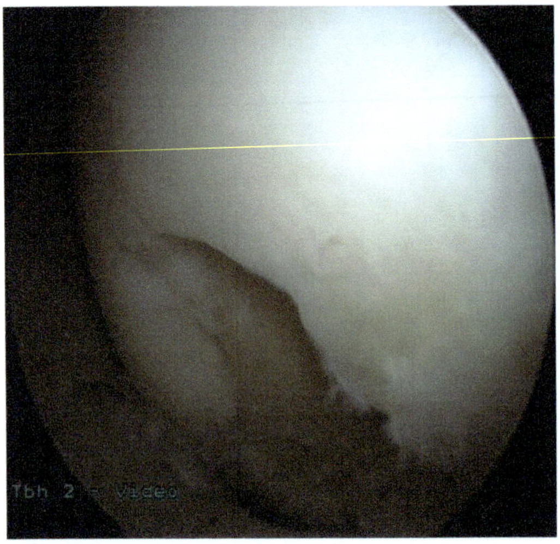

Fig. 19.6 The femoral condylar defect has been well debrided into a defect with vertical walls and a clean bare bone bottom surface

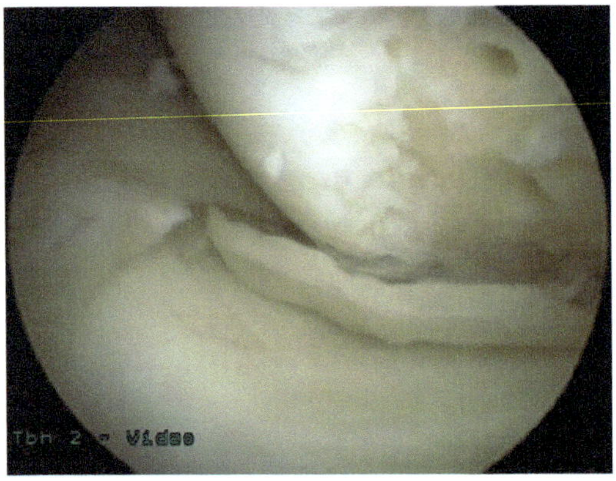

Fig. 19.7 The scaffold has just been released from the grasper and should now be caught by a smooth arthroscopy obturator to be moved into the defect

area. A Hyalograft scaffold is pushed through the channel to the cartilage defect surface followed by a bone graft filling of the channel. From the inside, a pusher or a curved tonsil elevator keeps the implant in place, while from the channel, the bone paste is compressed against the implant with counterpress (Fig. 19.11).

The Patella

If the patella is fairly lax, an attempt to implant the cell-seeded scaffold may be done transarthroscopically. Drill two k-wires to either medial or lateral bony edges of the patella. The K-wires are used to tilt the patella in order to expose the cartilage surface. The cartilage defect is debrided as described above and the graft is introduced into the joint and put in place with a curved tonsil elevator (Fig. 19.12). Most often several layers of the graft are needed to fill up a deep patella defect.

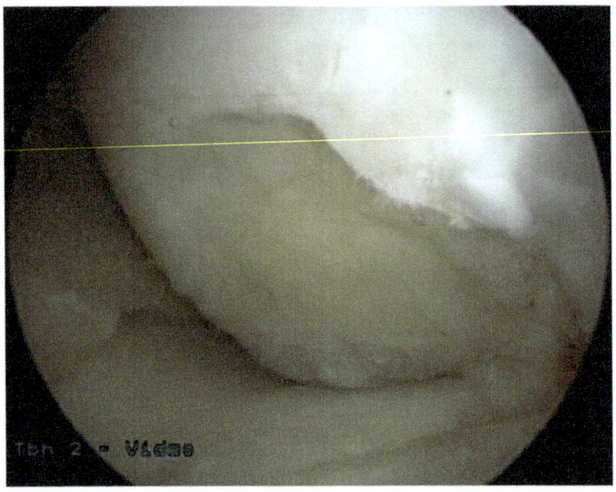

Fig. 19.8 The Hyalograft scaffold has been put place and fixated with fibrin glue

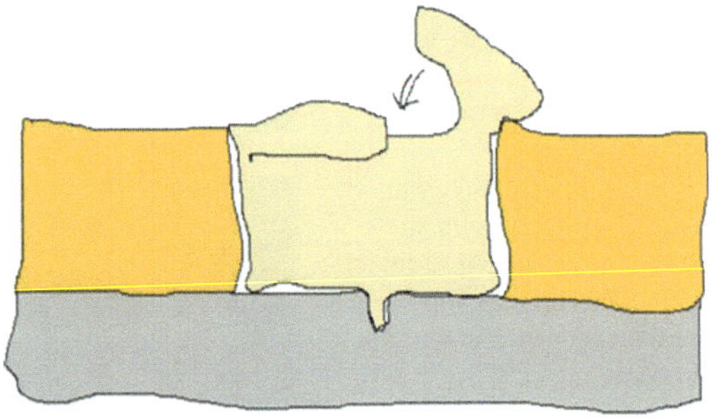

Fig. 19.9 When a scaffold is a little too oversized, the edges may be folded like a blanket into the defect to fill it up entirely

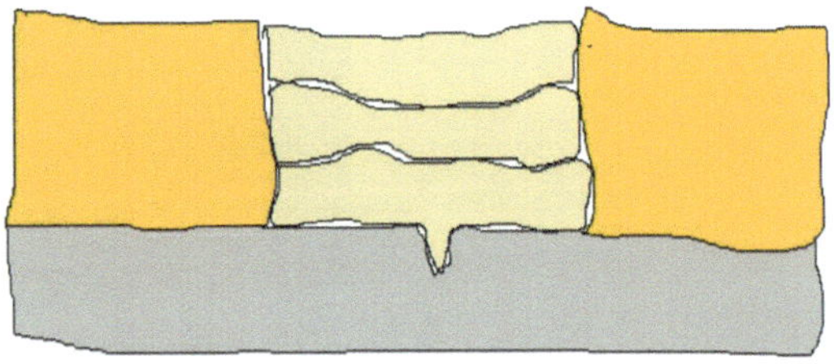

Fig. 19.10 Deep chondral defects are treated by several layers of the graft; "millefeuille" technique

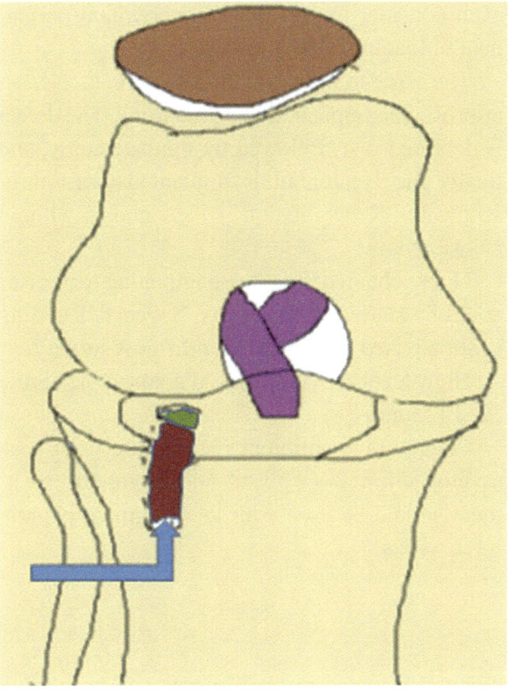

Fig. 19.11 Tibial plateau defects are treated by transarthroscopic retrograde drilling with a vector guide. The Hyalograft scaffold is pushed through the tibial channel to the tibial plateau surface and below the graft; the channel is then afterwards filled with bone grafts

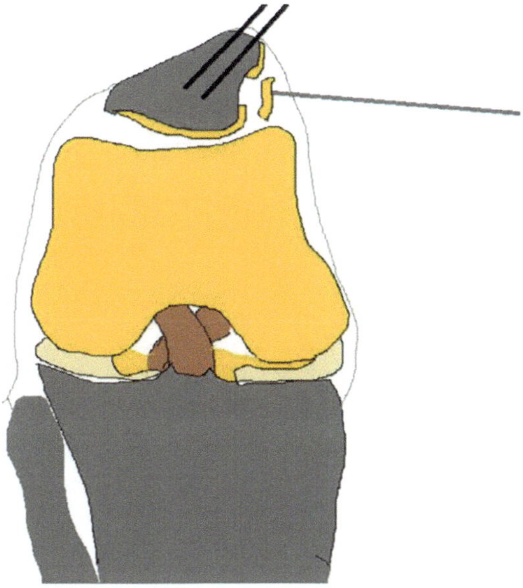

Fig. 19.12 Transarthroscopic patella Hyalograft implantation

Hyalograft with Seeded Chondrocytes + Bone Grafting for Osteochondral Defects

When a bone grafting is needed for deep and large osteochondral defects such as osteonecrosis and osteochondritis dissecans, the seeded scaffold may be used directly in combination with bone grafts.

The bone grafts may be harvested from crista iliaca anterior superior region or from the proximal tibia.

The bone grafts are mixed with fibrin glue to receive a putty consistence, bone paste. The bone grafts are put into a 2 ml syringe where the top of syringe has been cut off leaving a round opening. The bone grafts may be mixed with an artificial bone substitute if needed.

The bony defect has been prepared by excision and subchondral drilling to stimulate the sclerotic bone region.

Finally, the bone paste is implanted via the syringe into the osteochondral defect. The bone paste is compressed to fill the osseous part of the defect.

The cell-seeded scaffold is implanted and put over the top of the bone grafts, saturated with fibrin glue (Fig. 19.13). The stability of the dual graft is tested by extension-flexion motions.

Open Surgery Hyalograft Implantation

The access to the joint is via a mini-arthrotomy and often a subvastus incision. The debridement of the lesion as well as the implantation of the graft is identical as to the transarthroscopic description (Fig. 19.14).

19.5 Postoperative Rehabilitation for an Implanted Knee Joint

The extremity is immobilized in a brace locked in extension for 2 weeks. Full weight bearing is allowed in the brace as to a level what pain allows. After 2 weeks, the brace is used outdoors unlocked for another 4 weeks.

A very large defect may be protected by an unloader brace for a longer period, or one may

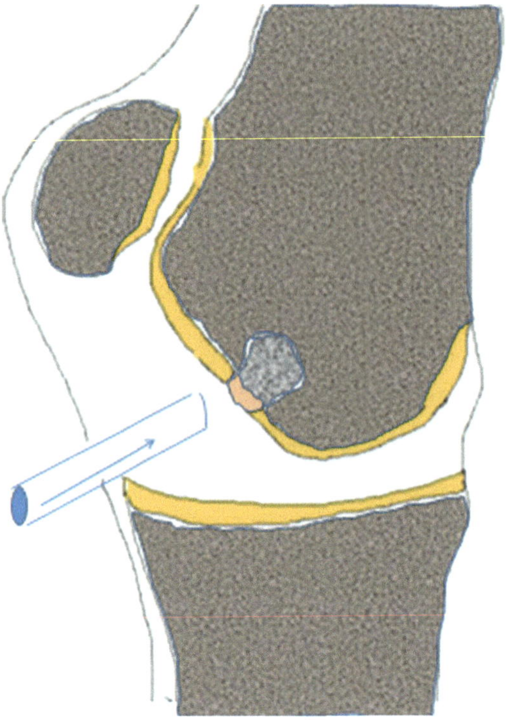

Fig. 19.13 Osteochondral defects treated by a one-stage bone grafts and Hyalograft implantation

even consider to perform a concomitant permanent unloading with osteotomy.

The osteotomy can be performed as an arthroscopic implantation + osteotomy. The defect is debrided first, followed by the osteotomy, and finally the Hyalograft is implanted transarthroscopically. Rehabilitation is the same as without an osteotomy.

Open chained knee strengthening exercises could be started from approx. 8 weeks. Running is not advised until 9–10 months post surgery.

High-level activities should not be done before 12–14 months.

Preoperative antibiotics should be used such as cloxacillin 2 g×3 and antithrombotic treatment should be used with low fragment heparin for 2 weeks.

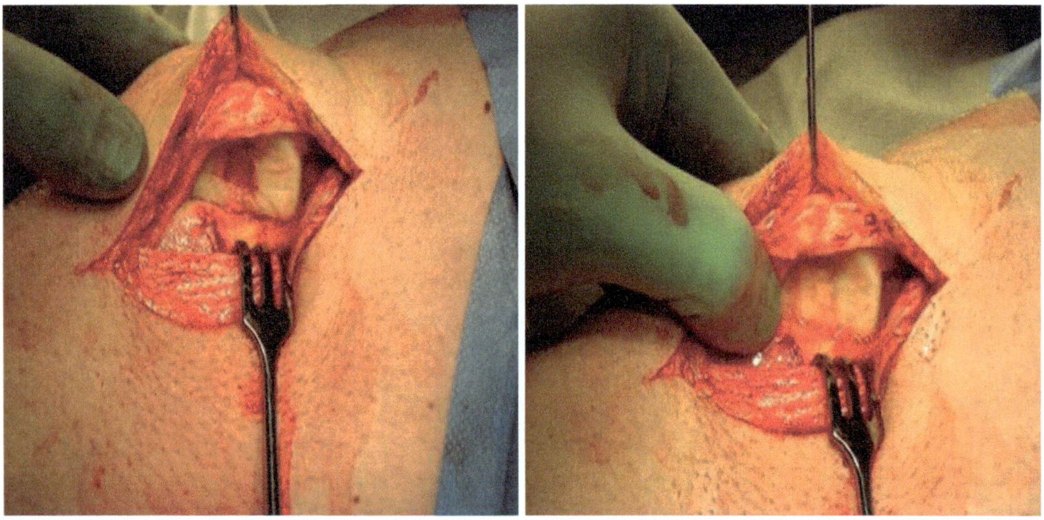

Fig. 19.14 Open Hyalograft implantation on a patellar defect via mini-arthrotomy

References

1. Astachov L, Vago R, Aviv M, Nevo Z (2012) Hyaluronan and mesenchymal stem cells: from germ layer to cartilage and bone. Front Biosci 16:261–276, Review
2. Brittberg M, Lindahl A, Nilsson A, Ohlsson C, Isaksson O, Peterson L (1994) Treatment of deep cartilage defects in the knee with autologous chondrocyte transplantation. N Engl J Med 331(14): 889–895
3. Biant LC, Bentley G (2007) Stem cells and debrided waste: two alternative sources of cells for transplantation of cartilage. J Bone Joint Surg Br 89(8):1110–1114
4. De Windt TS, Concaro S, Lindahl A, Saris DB, Brittberg M (2012) Strategies for patient profiling in articular cartilage repair of the knee: a prospective cohort of patients treated by one experienced cartilage surgeon. Knee Surg Sports Traumatol Arthrosc(Jan 14)
5. Filardo G, Kon E, Di Martino A, Iacono F, Marcacci M (2011) Arthroscopic second-generation autologous chondrocyte implantation: a prospective 7-year follow-up study. Am J Sports Med 39(10): 2153–2160
6. Girotto D, Urbani S, Brun P, Renier D, Barbucci R, Abatangelo G (2003) Tissue-specific gene expression in chondrocytes grown on three-dimensional hyaluronic acid scaffolds. Biomaterials 24(19): 3265–3275
7. Grigolo B, Lisignoli G, Piacentini A, Fiorini M, Gobbi P, Mazzotti G, Duca M, Pavesio A, Facchini A (2002) Evidence for redifferentiation of human chondrocytes grown on a hyaluronan-based biomaterial (HYAff 11): molecular, immunohistochemical and ultrastructural analysis. Biomaterials 23(4):1187–1195
8. Grigolo B, Roseti L, Fiorini M, Fini M, Giavaresi G, Aldini NN, Giardino R, Facchini A (2001) Transplantation of chondrocytes seeded on a hyaluronan derivative (hyaff-11) into cartilage defects in rabbits. Biomaterials 22(17):2417–2424
9. Khan IM, Redman SN, Williams R, Dowthwaite GP, Oldfield SF, Archer CW (2007) The development of synovial joints. Curr Top Dev Biol 79:1–36, Review
10. Knudson CB, Knudson W (2001) Cartilage proteoglycans. Semin Cell Dev Biol 12(2):69–78, Review
11. Kon E, Gobbi A, Filardo G, Delcogliano M, Zaffagnini S, Marcacci M (2009) Arthroscopic second-generation autologous chondrocyte implantation compared with microfracture for chondral lesions of the knee: prospective non randomised study at 5 years. Am J Sports Med 37(1):33–41
12. Marcacci M, Berruto M, Brocchetta D, Delcogliano A, Ghinelli D, Gobbi A, Kon E, Pederzini L, Rosa D, Sacchetti GL, Stefani G, Zanasi S (2005) Articular cartilage engineering with Hyalograft C: 3-year clinical results. Clin Orthop Relat Res 435:96–105
13. McCarthy HE, Bara JJ, Brakspear K, Singhrao SK, Archer CW (2012) The comparison of equine articular cartilage progenitor cells and bone marrow-derived stromal cells as potential cell sources for cartilage repair in the horse. Vet J 192:345–351
14. Nehrer S, Chiari C, Domayer S, Barkay H, Yayon A (2008) Results of chondrocyte implantation with a fibrin-hyaluronan matrix: a preliminary study. Clin Orthop Relat Res 466(8):1849–1855
15. Pavesio A, Abatangelo G, Borrione A, Brocchetta D, Hollander AP, Kon E, Torasso F, Zanasi S, Marcacci M (2003) Hyaluronan-based scaffolds (Hyalograft C) in the treatment of knee cartilage defects: preliminary clinical findings. Novartis Found Symp 249:203–217
16. Peterson L, Vasiliadis HS, Brittberg M, Lindahl A (2010) Autologous chondrocyte implantation: a long-term follow-up. Am J Sports Med 38(6):1117–1124
17. Toole BP, Jackson G, Gross J (1972) Hyaluronate in morphogenesis: inhibition of chondrogenesis in vitro. Proc Natl Acad Sci U S A 69(6):1384–1386
18. Williams R, Khan IM, Richardson K, Nelson L, McCarthy HE, Analbelsi T, Singhrao SK, Dowthwaite GP, Jones RE, Baird DM, Lewis H, Roberts S, Shaw HM, Dudhia J, Fairclough J, Briggs T, Archer CW (2010) Identification and clonal characterisation of a progenitor cell sub-population in normal human articular cartilage. PLoS One 5(10):e13246

Matrix-Induced Autologous Chondrocyte Implantation

20

L. Johnston, M. Faimali, P.D. Gikas, and Timothy W.R. Briggs

Contents

L. Johnston (✉) • M. Faimali
Royal National Orthopaedic Hospital,
Stanmore, London, UK
e-mail: ljohnston@doctors.org.uk

P.D. Gikas • T.W.R. Briggs
Royal National Orthopaedic Hospital,
Stanmore, London, UK

Institute of Orthopaedic and Musculoskeletal
Science, University College London, London, UK

20.1 Background

20.1.1 Chondral Injuries

Chondral and osteochondral injuries of the knee are common injuries, with a prevalence of isolated, focal articular cartilage defects of approximately 5 % [1]. Articular cartilage is avascular and aneural with limited potential for repair [2]. Chondrocytes have minimal migratory ability and so normal cartilage cells surrounding a defect are not able to fill it. These factors, combined with persistent use of the extremity by the patient, create a poor environment for spontaneous repair following injury.

20.1.2 Chondrocyte Implantation

The use of isolated chondrocytes as a treatment for chondral injuries began in 1971 when Bentley and Greer [3] showed that isolated chondrocytes could be used to treat osteochondral defects on the articular surface of rabbit knees. Aston and Bentley [4] then showed that chondrocytes could be grown and cultured whilst maintaining type II collagen and proteoglycans of the matrix.

Chondrocyte implantation following cultured growth of chondrocytes allowed the development of autologous chondrocyte implantation (ACI), which has since become an established technique

A.A. Shetty et al. (eds.), *Techniques in Cartilage Repair Surgery*,
DOI 10.1007/978-3-642-41921-8_20, © ESSKA 2014

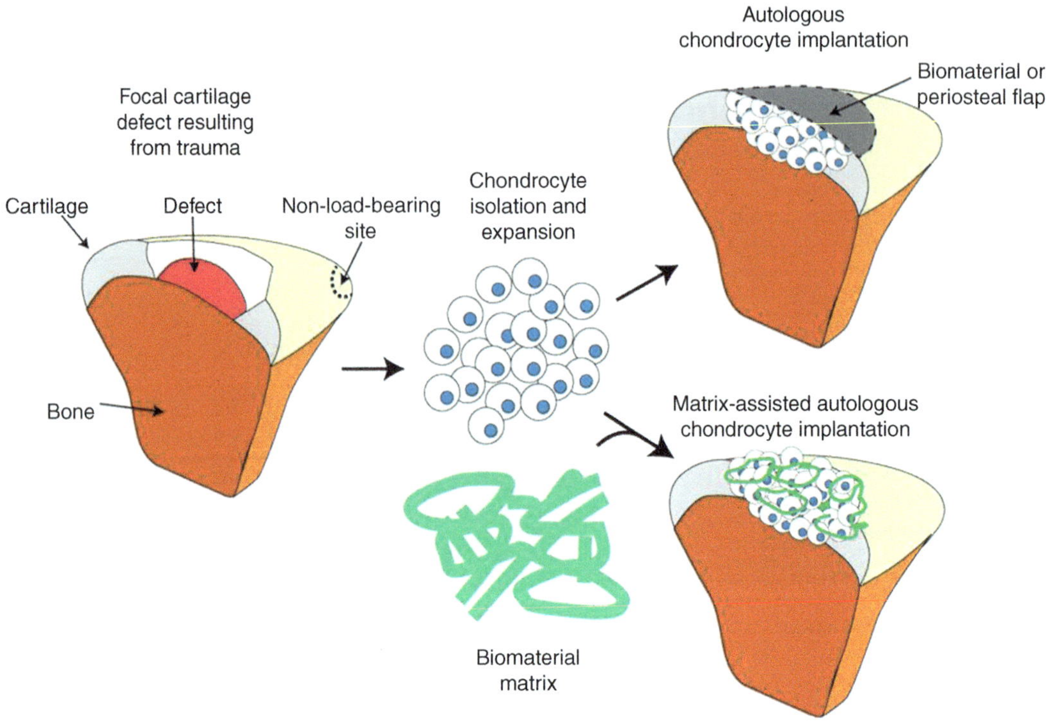

Fig. 20.1 Traditional autologous chondrocyte implantation and third-generation matrix-assisted techniques (Image from http://www.nature.com/nmat/journal/v11/n8/images/nmat3392-f2.jpg. Accessed on 26/11/2013)

for the repair of full-thickness chondral defects in the knee. Matrix-induced ACI (MACI) is the third and current generation of this technique, developed to reduce both operating times and to allow ACI to be performed using minimally invasive surgery.

Traditional ACI techniques require suturing of a membrane to keep the implanted chondrocytes in their desired location. Either periosteal covers (ACI-P) or porcine-derived collagen covers (ACI-C) are used to cover the defect before the chondrocytes are injected underneath. These techniques risk uneven distribution and leakage of chondrocytes, as well as requiring more extensive exposure and, for ACI-P, harvesting of a periosteal graft. These factors led to the development of MACI.

MACI uses a porcine type I/III collagen bilayer seeded with chondrocytes that is secured in place with fibrin glue [5]. This can be performed arthroscopically, thereby reducing both the extent of the exposure and operating times (Fig. 20.1).

20.2 Patient Selection

20.2.1 Indications

Autologous chondrocyte implantation is a treatment option for symptomatic International Cartilage Repair Society (ICRS) grade III and IV lesions of between 1 and 12 cm^2 located on the femoral condyle or trochlear regions (Table 20.1, Fig. 20.2). The patient may have undergone failed mosaicplasty or microfracture. If the bone is deeper than 6–8 mm, then autologous bone grafting should be undertaken.

Potential candidates should be well motivated and willing and able to comply with both pre- and post-operative rehabilitation regimens.

20.2.2 Contraindications

Reciprocal or “kissing” lesions are considered a contraindication for the technique. MACI is also contraindicated in both osteoarthritis and inflammatory arthritis. Whilst not contraindicated, results following ACI in patella lesions have been less promising and so patients presenting with such lesions should be considered carefully.

Table 20.1 ICRS grade of cartilage injuries

Grade	Title	Description
0	Normal	Normal cartilage
1	Nearly normal	Superficial lesions A. Soft indentation B. Superficial fissures and cracks
2	Abnormal	Lesions extending down to <50 % of cartilage depth
3	Severely abnormal	Cartilage defects A. >50 % of calcified layer B. Down to calcified layer C. Down to but not through subchondral bone D. Blisters
4	Severely abnormal	Cartilage defect exposing underlying subchondral bone

Associated malalignment, ligamentous instability or meniscal lesions are relative contraindications due to the negative effects they place on the cartilage and as such should be repaired in combination with MACI surgery where indicated.

20.3 Assessment

20.3.1 Patient Assessment

In order to be considered for MACI, the patient should be well motivated and otherwise in good health, to enable them to participate actively in both pre- and post-operative rehabilitation programmes. Several factors may affect potential

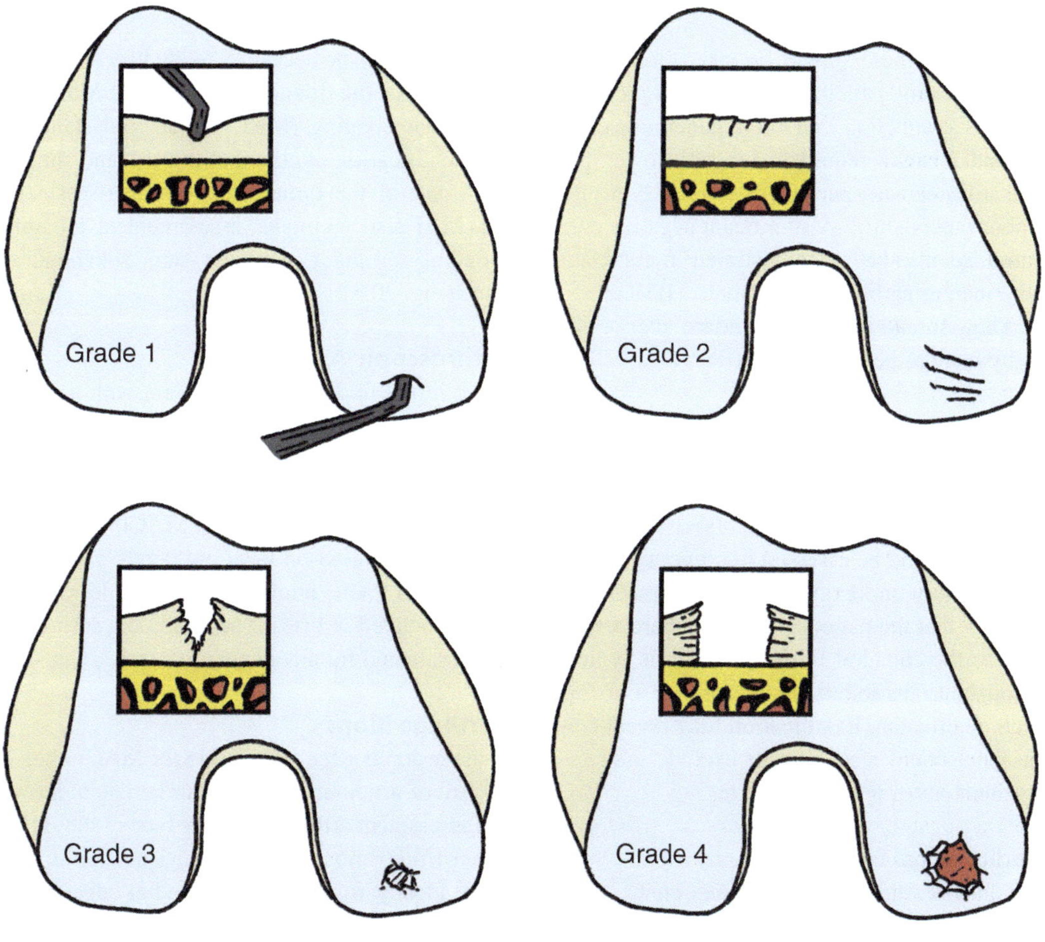

Fig. 20.2 Diagram of the pathogenesis of osteoarthritis, modified from the Outerbridge classification

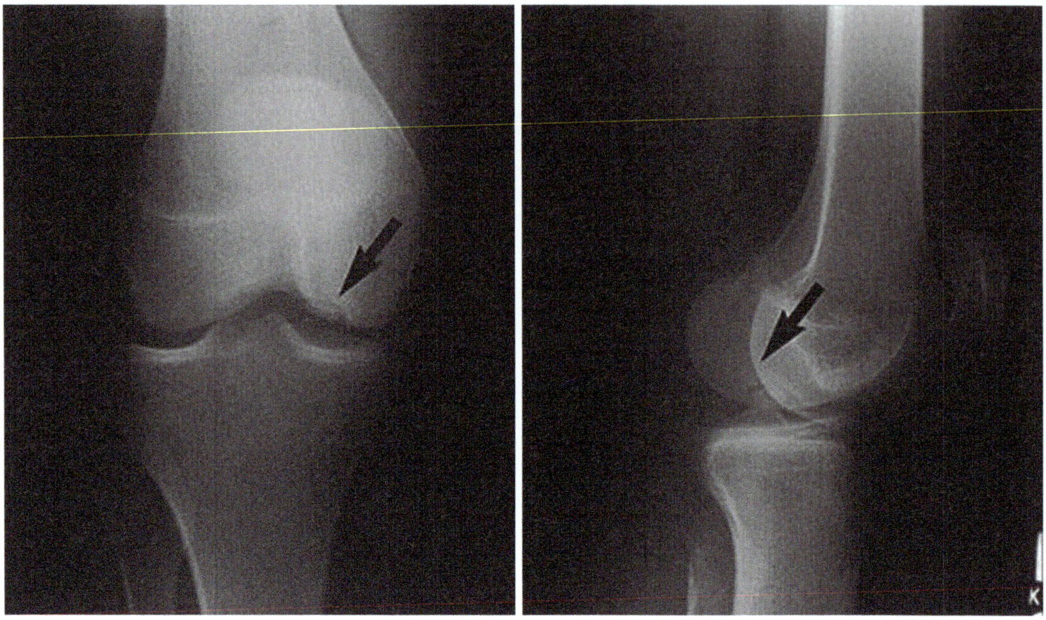

Fig. 20.3 Osteochondral defect

success and these should be taken into account when assessing patient suitability. Advancing age leads to a reduction in tissue regenerative capacity and so may require a longer, slower post-operative recovery period and ultimately result in a poor outcome [6]. A significant negative correlation has also been demonstrated in association with increasing body weight index (BMI).

They should undergo standard preoperative assessment as per NICE guidelines [7].

20.3.2 Assessment of Injury

History and Examination

Patients should be assessed in clinic with a thorough history and examination. It is essential to confirm that the patient's symptoms are attributable to the chondral lesion [8]. Pain is typically localised to the joint line and may be associated with an effusion. Examination may reveal crepitus but should also look to exclude associated ligamentous or meniscal injuries.

Radiological Evaluation

AP, lateral, flexed and skyline views of the affected knee should be obtained, along with weight-bearing radiographs. Long-leg alignment views may also be necessary to identify abnormal alignment of the tibiofemoral joint [8]. Magnetic resonance imaging (MRI) is the gold standard for identification of chondral injuries and should form part of the initial radiological assessment [9]. MRI also facilitates assessment of the surrounding articular cartilage and subchondral bone (Fig. 20.3).

Arthroscopic Assessment

If the initial findings are consistent with a chondral injury, the patient then progresses to arthroscopic assessment. Arthroscopic assessment allows direct visualisation of the lesion and assessment of its suitability for MACI. The lesion is evaluated based on location, depth, size, margins, ICRS grade, number and type of lesion and any associated injuries. The reciprocal surface is also evaluated for any damage.

Cartilage Biopsy

If the lesion is deemed suitable for MACI, then a biopsy of articular cartilage can be taken during the assessment arthroscopy. The biopsy should be taken from a non-weight-bearing portion of the joint, ideally from the superomedial edge of the femoral trochlea, the superolateral trochlear edge or the lateral aspect of the inter-condylar notch.

The biopsy specimen should weigh 200–300 mg and should include a small portion of underlying subchondral bone [10]. Pathological cartilage such as femoral osteophytes or loose intra-articular fragments should not be used.

The harvested cells are then maintained at 4 °C until transfer to an appropriate laboratory for processing. The laboratory will suspend the cells in a scaffold of type I/III collagen. This scaffold acts as a carrier for the chondrocytes, ensuring even distribution of one million cells/cm^2.

20.4 Preoperative Management

20.4.1 Patient Education

Preoperative patient education plays an important role in preparing the patient both mentally and physically. Describing the operative technique and explaining how certain knee movements might compromise the outcome of their graft is likely to improve patient compliance with the lengthy post-operative restrictions and physiotherapy.

20.4.2 Preoperative Physiotherapy

Edwards et al. [6] describe a detailed preoperative physiotherapy protocol designed to optimise patient strength, mobility and function. The protocol not only builds strength around the knee but also aims to improve upper body and trunk strength in order to facilitate transfers and crutch ambulation in the early post-operative period. Alongside strength building exercises, improving cardiovascular fitness and weight loss are encouraged to optimise post-operative recovery and reduce excess load on the affected knee.

20.5 Surgical Technique

20.5.1 Exposure

Traditional ACI is performed via a medial parapatellar approach. MACI can be performed under much more limited exposure, and as such smaller incisions can be used on both medial and lateral sides. It is important that care is taken to avoid damage to the bodies and anterior horns of the menisci.

20.5.2 Preparation of the Defect

All fibrillated, partially damaged cartilage must be debrided back to reveal normal cartilage margins. This may be performed by first demarcating the boundaries of the chondral lesion using a number 15 blade before subsequently removing the damaged cartilage using a small curette. Damage to subchondral bone must be minimised in order to avoid excessive bleeding into the defect.

20.5.3 Implantation of Cultured Chondrocytes

The defect is measured and the preprepared membrane trimmed to fit (Fig. 20.4). The membrane can then be inserted directly into the defect with the cells (rough side) lying against the intact subchondral bone and secured in situ with fibrin glue (Fig. 20.5). Light digital pressure is applied whilst the glue sets [10]. If the implant is unstable or the lesion is uncontained, then additional suture anchors may be used in addition to the fibrin glue to minimise the risk of delamination.

Following wound closure, the wounds are dressed and a Robert-Jones bandage applied.

20.6 Post-operative Management

20.6.1 Graft Maturation

Maturation of the MACI graft occurs in several stages. The first is termed the "implantation and early protection" phase and lasts 0–6 weeks following surgery. During this stage the graft may be partially protected by the adjacent healthy native cartilage. The second phase covers the period from 6 to 12 weeks post-operative and is the "transition and proliferation" phase. Over this period the chondrocytes migrate through the fibrin glue to the subchondral bone. They start to

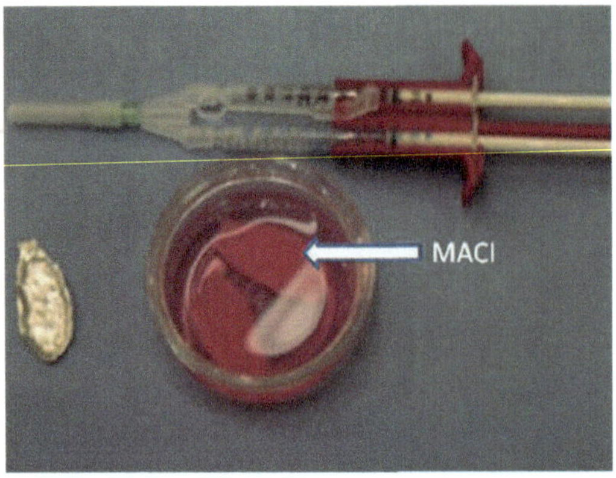

Fig. 20.4 MACI membrane with attached cartilage cells in petri dish ready for cutting to the size of the defect

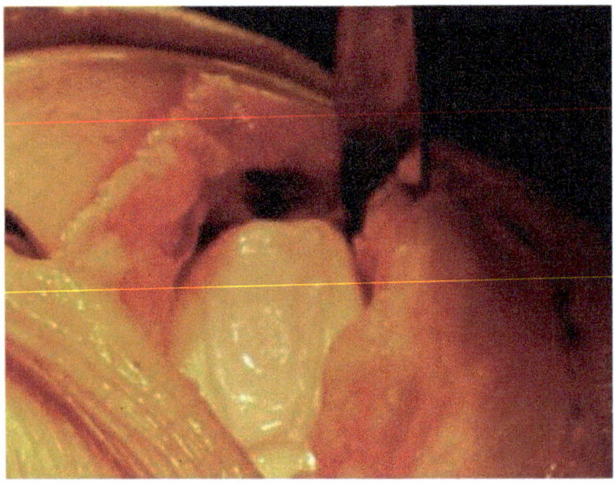

Fig. 20.5 MACI implant in position secured with glue

produce soft, primitive repair tissue that starts to fill the defect. The third, "remodelling" phase, lasts from 12 to 26 weeks post-operatively. During this phase the graft becomes firmer as the chondrocytes produce a matrix of type II collagen, aggrecan and other matrix proteins. The final phase is that of graft "maturation". This stage begins 6 months after surgery and lasts up to 3 years. The chondrocytes and matrix continue to mature, integrating with the native cartilage and underlying bone, resulting in a hardened graft.

20.6.2 Rehabilitation

Edwards et al. [6] describe a detailed and comprehensive protocol for post-operative rehabilitation following MACI surgery with various stages from day 1 to 18 months post-operatively. They recommend that the initial post-operative period focuses on the management of pain, swelling and inflammation by following the "PRICE" (protect, rest, ice, compression, elevation) protocol [11]. Edwards et al. [6] go on to describe a protocol of increasing movement and weight bearing, culminating in the return to pre-injury sports. They emphasise that the speed at which patients return to weight bearing and increasing range of movement will vary depending on several factors relating to the patient, the lesion and the repair.

The protocol at the Royal National Orthopaedic Hospital is designed to avoid impact loading and twisting or shearing forces. These forces may damage the repair and displace the implanted cartilage cells. Patients are fitted with a knee brace in fixed extension for the first week, following which the patient is kept toe-touch weight bearing until 6 weeks. During this period progressive flexion-extension exercises provide chondrogenic stimulus and a full range of movement. Weight bearing is increased to partial for 6–10 weeks, before progressing to full weight bearing from 10 weeks.

Other regimens advocate the use of continuous passive movement as early as 6 h after surgery as it is thought early mobilisation may aid differentiation of mesenchymal cells. Partial weight bearing is recommended for between 6 and 12 weeks. The protocol for the autologous chondrocyte transplantation/implantation versus existing treatment trial (ACTIVE) suggests patients should be capable of low-impact exercise such as cycling by 12 weeks.

20.7 Post-operative Evaluation

20.7.1 Assessment of the Defect

Arthroscopic assessment remains the optimum method of post-operative evaluation and, in some centres during ethically approved trials, was carried out routinely during follow-up. The repair is directly visualised, stiffness is assessed by probing and a biopsy may be taken to allow histological evaluation of the repair.

MRI assessment is an increasingly important, non-invasive method of assessing the repair. The use of delayed gadolinium-enhanced scans may prove to be useful in the assessment of the graft matrix and in predicting the histological phenotype.

20.7.2 Assessment of Clinical Outcomes

Evidence suggests that MACI is a successful method to treat symptomatic isolated cartilage defects. Visna et al. [12] found MACI to produce significantly larger improvements when compared with microfracture as part of a 1-year randomised controlled trial of 50 patients. Basad et al. [13] found similar results in a 60-patient (40 MACI, 20 microfracture) randomised controlled trial at 2 years.

Bartlett et al. [10] compared MACI with traditional ACI in a randomised controlled trial of 44 ACI-C patients and 47 MACI patients. They found significant improvements in both groups at 1 year after surgery, with an increased frequency of good to excellent functional outcomes after MACI than with ACI-C. Arthroscopic review was performed at 1 year on 42 of the patients demonstrating excellent or good ICRS scores in 79.2 % of ACI-C patients and 66.6 % of MACI patients. Biopsies taken at review arthroscopy showed hyaline-like cartilage or mixed hyaline-like and fibrocartilage in 42.9 % of ACI-C patients and 36.4 % of MACI patients. Neither the arthroscopic outcomes nor the histological outcomes were significantly different. They also found that outcomes were negatively affected by previous failed mosaicplasty or a history of more than two surgical procedures.

Gikas et al. [14] reported a prospective study of 332 patients treated with either ACI or MACI and an average follow-up of 32 months (12 months to 9 years). They describe statistically significant sequential annual improvements in functional scores for both ACI and MACI. Initial score at 1 year showed outcomes with ACI were statistically better than with MACI ($p=0.454$); however, there was no significant difference in subsequent years.

This is supported by other evidence, such as the randomised controlled trial performed by Zeifang et al. [15], which suggests there is no significant difference between MACI and conventional ACI at 12 or 24 months following surgery.

Overall, evidence is consistently indicating favourable outcomes following MACI. However, a significant advantage when compared with traditional ACI has yet to be clearly demonstrated. Further studies with longer-term assessment are required to establish difference in outcomes between the two techniques.

References

1. Curl WW, Krome J, Gordon ES, Rushing J, Smith BP, Poehling GG (1997) Cartilage injuries: a review of 31,516 knee arthroscopies. Arthroscopy 13:456–460
2. Buckwalter JA, Mankin HJ (1998) Articular cartilage repair and transplantation. Arthritis Rheum 41:1331–1342
3. Bentley G, Greer RB (1971) Homotransplantation of isolated epiphyseal and articular cartilage chondrocytes into joint surfaces of rabbits. Nature 230(5293):385–388
4. Aston JE, Bentley G (1986) Repair of articular surfaces by allografts of articular and growth-plate cartilage. J Bone Jonit Surg Br 68(1):29–35
5. Barlett W, Gooding CR, Carrington RWJ, Skinner JA, Briggs TWR, Bentley G (2005) Autologous chondrocyte implantation at the knee using a bilayer collagen membrane with bone graft. J Bone Joint Surg Br 87(3):330–332
6. Edwards PK, Ackland T, Ebert JR (2014) Clinical rehabilitation guidelines for matrix-induced autologous chondrocyte implantation (MACI) on the tibiofemoral joint. J Orthop Sports Phys Ther 44(2):102–19
7. NICE guidelines for pre-op assessment. http://wwwnice.org.uk/nicemedia/live/10920/29090/29090.pdf
8. Dunkin BS, Lattermann C (2013) New and emerging techniques in cartilage repair: matrix-induced autologous chondrocyte implantation. Oper Tech Sports Med 21:100–107
9. Potter HG, Chongle R (2009) Magnetic resonance assessment of chondral lesions and repair. J Bone Joint Surg Am 91(suppl 1):126–131
10. Bartlett W, Skinner JA, Gooding CR, Carrington RW, Flanagan AM, Briggs TW, Bentley G (2005) Autologous chondrocyte implantation versus matrix-induced autologous chondrocyte implantation for osteochondral defects of the knee: a prospective randomised study. J Bone Joint Surg Br 87(5):640–645
11. Hambly K (2006) Autologous chondrocyte implantation postoperative care and rehabilitation: science and practice. Am J Sports Med 34:1020–1038

12. Visna P, Pasa L, Cizmar I, Hart R, Hoch J (2004) Treatment of deep cartilage defects of the knee using autologous chondrograft transplantation and by abrasive techniques – a randomized controlled study. Acta Chir Belg 104(6):709–714
13. Basad E, Ishaque B, Bachmann G, Sturz H, Steinmeyer J (2010) Matrix-induced autologous chondrocyte implantation versus microfracture in the treatment of cartilage defects in the knee: a two-year randomised study. Knee Surg Sports Traumatol Arthrosc 18:519–527
14. Gikas PD, Baylis L, Bentley G, Briggs TWR (2009) An overview of autologous chondrocyte implantation. J Bone Joint Surg Br 91-B(8):997–1006
15. Zeifang F, Oberle D, Nierhoff C, Richter W, Moradi B, Schmitt H (2010) Autologous chondrocyte implantation using the original periosteum-cover technique versus matrix-associated autologous chondrocyte implantation: a randomized clinical trial. Am J Sports Med 38(5):924–933

CaReS®, Cartilage Regeneration System: Autologous Chondrocyte Transplantation in a Collagen Gel

21

Stefan Nehrer, Florian Halbwirth, and Thomas Luksch

Contents

S. Nehrer, MD (✉) • F. Halbwirth, MA
Center for Regenerative Medicine and Orthopedics, Department for Biomedicine and Health, Danube University Krems, Austria
e-mail: stefan.nehrer@donau-uni.ac.at

T. Luksch, MD, MSc
Department of Orthopedic, Hospital Krems, Austria

21.1 Background

Articular cartilage is a white, shiny, moisture tissue comprising less than 5 % cells, about 35 % extracellular matrix of mostly collagen type II and proteoglycans and about 60 % water, and provides outstanding biomechanics. Hence the tissue looks simple in its structure; the biomechanical properties are linked to the complex nanostructured architecture of the tissue, which partly relates to the high water content bound to macromolecules [26]. Since the composition of articular cartilage is not restored by natural healing, many attempts have been made to improve the quality of the repair tissue including microfracture [13] or osteochondral autografting; both methods are limited due to tissue quality or resources of grafts [3, 8, 10, 16]. Autologous chondrocyte transplantation has changed the paradigm of the treatment of cartilage defects from repair to regeneration, and this has been demonstrated in randomised trials proving the concept of regenerating tissue in a cell-based therapy approach [21]. However, the limitations of the periosteal flap concerning size and thickness and surgical demands with suturing and the variability of biological reaction including hypertrophy, calcification and delamination [2, 16, 17, 20, 27], as well as the uncontrolled cell transplantation in a cell suspension [25], have supported the introduction of the use biomaterials as a scaffold. The first attempt was to replace the periosteal flap by a collagen membrane which were sutured or glued to the defect combined with the cell

A.A. Shetty et al. (eds.), *Techniques in Cartilage Repair Surgery*,
DOI 10.1007/978-3-642-41921-8_21, © ESSKA 2014

suspension injected or seeded onto the membrane during the surgery before implantation [2, 4, 9, 15, 19]. Concerns about the phenotype of the cultured cells led to preculturing techniques on biomaterials in sponges or gels to maintain the chondrocytic function of the cells and allow a more controlled dispersion of the chondrocytes throughout the defect [22]. The matrix characteristics concerning biochemical composition, biophysical appearance in gel, foams or sponges, degradation dynamics and products, toxicity, immunological reactions and general biocompatibility are important parameters of biomaterial development [1, 5, 9, 15, 18]. The cell-biomaterial interaction in a biological environment is the decisive process of successful cartilage regeneration.

A 3D aqueous gel seeded with cells seems to simulate perfectly the real situation chondrocytes in cartilage, and also the high water content allows the cells to arrange the extracellular matrix in a more free way than in a preformed sponge or foam. The 3D culture system in gels allows the chondrocytes to maintain the chondrocytic phenotype, especially when P0 cells are used. The distribution of the cells in a gel resembles more the sparsely cell dispersion in natural cartilage, and a high bioactivity of the cells is achieved with vigorous cartilage-specific protein production. Various studies have shown that dedifferentiated chondrocytes can regain the chondrocytic phenotype in gel-like biomaterials like agarose or collagen gels. Gels also allow to support the cultured cells with nutrients in a bioreactor and expose them to growth factors [11]. Also after the implantation there is an immediate exposure to modulating factors which penetrate the gel by diffusion especially when continuous passive motion is applied early. Findings in our laboratory have shown that collagen type I is highly expressed at the time of implantation; however, cartilage-specific markers like sox 9 and aggrecan also remain highly expressed. Experimental studies from our lab have shown that mechanical stimulation increases type II collagen production and sGAG synthesis immediately and also induces a shift from the catabolic to an anabolic situation of the chondrocytes [6, 7, 12, 14, 24]. This findings support that a gel provides an optimal environment for chondrocytes, but early mobilisation after the implantation is necessary to achieve a mechanical impact on the chondrocytes.

21.2 Patient Selection

As other studies have shown, the most promising indication for autologous chondrocytes with various biomaterials is in patients with well-defined cartilage defects from about 2 cm^2 to 8 cm^2 on the medial or lateral femoral condyle [4, 20]. Prerequisite for a successful cartilage treatment is a well-aligned joint with stable well-balanced ligaments, no prior surgery and injury within the last year. The maximal age of the patients is 50 years. Further inclusion criteria are that the opposing cartilage surface has a maximum defect of Outerbridge II, no kissing lesion, intact menisci or a maximum partial resection of one third of the meniscus. A leg axis must be of more than 5° and has to be corrected by means of high tibial osteotomy. Chronic onset of cartilage problems over the years, prior microfracture or other cartilage treatment reduces the prognosis of the cartilage therapy. The gel-like mechanical characteristics of the gel must be respected in the choice of the defect size and localisation. Moreover the gel needs a well-defined defect to achieve a stable fixation just by gluing the gel into the defect site. Osteoarthritic conditions in all joint compartments, inflammatory, immunological or infectious diseases like HIV and hepatitis are excluded from any type of cell therapy.

The preoperative workup has to include an MRI with cartilage-specific sequences to rule out the area of the damaged cartilage, ligament status, effusion and synovitis. Furthermore adjacent structures, especially the subchondral bone, have to be evaluated: extensive subchondral necrosis or oedema also limits the implantation of a gel or has to be treated with autologous bone augmentation at the same time. In our hands the combination of osseous cylinder grafting from the iliac crest and CaReS implantation has shown good results.

21.3 Surgical Procedures and Techniques

21.3.1 Biopsy

After evaluation of the patient and imaging of the defect, the final decision for the implantation is done during an arthroscopy. The patient is consented to a cartilage biopsy, if the defect is eligible for cell-based therapy. We perform a thorough assessment of the defect concerning size of the damaged cartilage area as well as bone quality. If the damaged area is unclear to define, the defects are debrided immediately with removal of flaps or partial fixed osteochondral fragments. If debrided or clear defect margins are larger than 1.5 cm^2, a CaReS implantation is considered. If the bone stock is damaged or sclerotic resulting in an osteochondral defect deeper than 0.5 cm, an osseous reconstruction by autografts from the iliac crest is planned for the second surgery. All concomitant damage in meniscus is treated at this time including resections and sutures of the meniscus. Instability related to ACL rupture and varus or valgus alignment is addressed at the second surgery during implantation. After the decision for CaReS implantation is made, a biopsy is taken from the non-weight-bearing area of the knee, mostly from the intercondylar notch area with a cartilage basket grasper. Usually we take four to six bites with the grasper which relates to about 150–250 mg of cartilage. We select carefully the area of the biopsy with regard to firm cartilage surface and take a full-thickness biopsy down to the subchondral bone, including all layers of the articular cartilage. The specimens are immediately placed in buffered serum-free media in small wells which allow sterile closure on the table. Afterwards these wells are put in small boxes which are finally placed in a cooling box providing a 2–10 °C environment and are labelled accordingly to clearly identify the biopsy. Furthermore 120–140 ml of whole blood is taken from the patient in 10 ml tubes that are also put into the cooler. The biopsy box including the blood samples are then sealed with the necessary information and documentation and sent to the good manufacturing practice (GMP) facility (Arthro Kinetics, Krems Austria) for further processing. Tests have shown that a biopsy transport time up to 72 h in the cooling box does not influence the quality or yield of the cell process.

21.3.2 Cell Processing

In the GMP-certified Tissue and Cell Bank, the cartilage biopsies are minced and digested by collagenase; the released cells are centrifuged, washed and finally analysed for viability and cell count. The cell viability must be more than 50 % direct after digestion. The autologous blood is centrifuged and serves as autologous serum for the culture period, which also optimises outcome of the cell culture. Chondrocytes are then placed in a 2-fold gel neutralisation solution with 20 % serum and gently mixed with type I collagen (6 mg/ml) to obtain a final concentration of 3 mg type I collagen/ml. The collagen type I is obtained from rat-tail tendons by collagen extraction in a standardised controlled process to avoid contamination. The collagen-cell mixture is allowed to polymerise at 37 °C in a humidified atmosphere. The cell seeded collagen implants are produced in a round shape with a diameter of 34 mm and 6–8 mm thickness, which relates to double thickness of the treated cartilage, since the aqueous gel loses water and therefore height during implantation. The implants are cultured at 37 °C, 5 % CO_2 for about 12 days (10–13 days). Autologous culture media with 10 % serum is changed every 3–4 days. Before transport for implantation a quality control is performed, assuring a sterility of the implant, a cell density of at least 3×10^4 cells per implant, a doubling time per day for at least 0.250, a cell viability of more than 80 % and expression of type II collagen by rt-PCR (real-time polymerase chain reaction). Since autologous serum is used, the cell proliferation and bioactivity of the cells are supported; however, the cell doubling time in a gel is lower than in monolayer culture, and few quantities of cartilage matrix is produced during the short culture period. The implants are usually shipped within 24 h in a cooling box providing a 2–10 °C environment but also sustain transporting time of 48–72 h without decreased cell quality [23].

21.3.3 Implantation Procedure

At the time of the scheduled second surgery – about 14 days after the biopsy – the implantation box including two implants with about 3 cm diameter is delivered in sterile conditions in a sealed box to the operating theatre. Identity of the patient and the number of the cell graft are checked before opening of the boxes comprising the implant in media at a temperature of 6–8 °C.

The patient is placed in a supine position, intravenous antibiotics applied and sterile draped. A tourniquet is applied, but it is usually not activated to avoid unexpected bleeding after the implantation, for this reason meticulous bleeding control is mandatory. Depending on the location of the defect, a medial or lateral parapatellar approach is used to assess the defect. Spreaders are used to expose the index condyle after the fat pad is cut gently avoiding meniscal damage. A 5–7 cm approach is usually sufficient. By bending and stretching the knee, more anterior or posterior areas can be addressed. However in more complex lesions in the trochlea or combined medial and lateral lesions, we do not hesitate to open the joint like a minimal invasive total joint approach.

A special implantation set is available for the optimal sizing of the graft. There are three sizes with oval and round shape of punches. The surgeon chooses the best fitting puncher to include the damaged area of the cartilage. These cartilage punchers are matched to the defect site and then firmly pressed into the soft chondral layer. The punch should include all damage tissue and can then be used as a template to clean the defect vigorously with a curette. This allows a very fast and secure way to clean the defect without damaging adjacent cartilage and provides a very clear delineation of the defect borders. After removal of the punch, a final cleaning of the subchondral bone is done by using a low-speed burr not only to roughen the subchondral surface, without opening of the subchondral bone, but to secure complete removal of the calcified layer. The soft collagen gel needs a well-debrided defect with stable walls to allow a press-fit stabilisation supported by fibrin glue.

Each of this defect punches relates to an implant punch which is about 1 mm wider to provide a slightly bigger implant. The implant puncher is softly pressed into the collagen-cell graft to cut out the fitting size of the implant. We administer fibrin glue (Tissucol, Baxter, Vienna, Austria) to the bottom of the defect in a thin layer and then place the graft into the defect with a spatula. For defects on the condyle, we bend the knee and hip 90° to provide a horizontal plane in the condyle and avoid shifting of the graft. In this way the graft shows a complete fill of the defect and a perfect bonding to the adjacent cartilage. If the graft is still too thick, a soft pressure with a spatula helps to press water out of the gel to achieve a levelled graft thickness. After that the spreaders are removed and the knee is moved to check implant stability. After final blood control the wound is closed in layers with no drainage in a stretched position. A knee brace with an elastic bandage underneath is put on after wound closure in a stretched position allowing 10° of range of motion.

21.3.4 Concomitant Surgery

In about one third of the cases, osteotomies or ACL grafting has to be performed at the same time. With osteotomies in varus situations, we perform a high tibial osteotomy in an open-wedge technique by using an angle-stable plate (TomoFix, Synthes, Swiss) to provide a stable situation for early mobilisation protocols. A single-incision anteromedial approach allows to address the defect and the medial open-wedge osteotomy. In this case we start with the preparation of the defect, continue with the osteotomy by extending the incision more distally and finally place the collagen graft and close in a stretched position. In an ACL procedure we do a semiopen ACL after having prepared the defect for implantation and also end with the graft implantation after the joint has a stable situation. Also patellofemoral realignment is crucial at the time of graft implantation: medialisation of the tuberositas tibiae by Elmslie or Fulkerson as well as MPFL reconstruction can be performed with the CaReS procedure but always the implantation of the soft gel has to be done at the end of the procedure.

21.3.5 Rehabilitation

Depending on size and localisation of the defect, the rehabilitation programme has to be adjusted. Postoperatively compression and cryotherapy is administered as well as isometric muscle training. Generally we allow a flexion of 30° from the second day after surgery on a CPM machine. After 2 weeks the ROM is increased 10° every week until the sixth week where the brace is removed and full range of motion is allowed. The patients walk on crutches for 6 weeks, where in the first 2 weeks, only touchdown mobilisation is allowed. From week 2–4 weight bearing is gradually increased, and from week 4 we allow full weight bearing with crutches in a 4-point manner. We also prefer to use active muscle movement; starting at week 4 a CAMOPED active muscle training machine is used and replaces the continuous passive motion. Between week 6 and 8 the patients start to train on stationary bikes and coordinative training including resistance exercises. Running starts usually around 4 months and sport specific exercises in 6 months; competition level of stop and go sports takes around 1 year. Important is that there are no effusion or synovitis and no pain on loading during or after exercise to allow sports on a competitional level.

21.3.6 Postoperative Follow-Up

Patients are followed in a standardised programme beginning with the preoperative documentation with IKDC and Lysholm score as well as KOOS and VAS pain scale. Clinical results are documented at 3, 6, 12 and 24 months with MRI documentation at 12 and 24 months. Only in studies these protocol may be varied according to special study design.

21.4 Clinical Studies

Schneider et al. [23] reported a first case-controlled study comparing classic ACT with periosteum to CaReS technology using the cell-augmented collagen gel. The study shows similar clinical results for both groups, with significant reduced OR time and less adverse events like effusions in the CaReS group. The authors conclude that the collagen gel allows safe and secure implantation in less time and no periosteal troubles like hypertrophy, graft displacement or synovitis. These statements are generally found in studies using biomaterials opposed to periosteal patching. Schneider also reported on a group of more challenging patients with complex lesions also with comparable results to ACT.

Lately a prospective multicentre study on the outcome of the CaReS technique was published including 116 patients in 9 different centres. The follow-up using standardised evaluations scores revealed a significant improvement of patients within 12–60 months of follow-up period. The overall satisfaction was 88 % good and excellent by the surgeons and 80 % by the patients. Given the mean defect size of above 5 cm and inclusion of 22 patella/trochlea defects and 10 patients with more than one defect, the result is quite respectable for a multicentre study; however, control group and randomisation are missing. Our own series of 35 patients with follow-up between 1 and 3 years reveals similar results.

Compared to other biomaterial-augmented chondrocyte transplantation (MACI) like hyaluronan (Hyalograft C®) [18], collagen membrane (MACI, Chondro-Gide®) or polyglycan/polylactides (Bioseeds®), CaReS® reveals similar results. Defects smaller than 4 cm, single circumscribed lesions in patients less than 40 years generally show success rates about 90–95 % in all these reports. Multiple prior surgeries, long-term onset of symptoms, osteoarthritic lesions and patients aged over 40 show worse results. However the implantation of the CaReS implant seems to be a safe and effective technique of chondrocyte transplantation. The instrumentation allows the creation of a well-defined defect which allows a stable implantation of the soft implant. No sutures are necessary to stabilise the gel, and surgical handling is comfortable when used correctly; however, in complex situations with shallow defect margins or more degenerative lesions, the fixation can be demanding and request the covering by a membrane, which can be difficult.

Although no comparative study is available up to date, case studies show promising results up to 5 years follow-up, with sparsely records of adverse effects or complications. However, further long-term follow-up studies are required to demonstrate which MACI technique delivers the best results.

References

1. Albrecht C, Tichy B, Nürnberger S et al (2011) Gene expression and cell differentiation in matrix-associated chondrocyte transplantation grafts: a comparative study. Osteoarthritis Cartilage 19:1219–1227
2. Bartlett W, Skinner JA, Gooding CR et al (2005) Autologous chondrocyte implantation versus matrix-induced autologous chondrocyte implantation for osteochondral defects of the knee. J Bone Joint Surg Br 87:640–645
3. Bentley G, Biant LC, Carrington RW et al (2003) A prospective, randomized comparison of autologous chondrocyte implantation versus mosaicplasty for osteochondral defects in the knee. J Bone Joint Surg Br 85:223–230
4. Brittberg M, Lindahl A, Nilsson A, Ohlsson C, Isaksson O, Peterson L (1994) Treatment of deep cartilage defects in the knee with autologous chondrocyte transplantation. N Engl J Med 331:889–895
5. Browne JE, Branch TP (2000) Surgical alternatives for treatment of articular cartilage lesions. J Am Acad Orthop Surg 8:180–189
6. Buschmann MD, Gluzband YA, Grodzinsky AJ, Hunziker EB (1995) Mechanical compression modulates matrix biosynthesis in chondrocyte/agarose culture. J Cell Sci 108(Pt 4):1497–1508
7. Demarteau O, Wendt D, Braccini A et al (2003) Dynamic compression of cartilage constructs engineered from expanded human articular chondrocytes. Biochem Biophys Res Commun 310:580–588
8. Gudas R, Kalesinskas RJ, Kimtys V et al (2005) A prospective randomized clinical study of mosaic osteochondral autologous transplantation versus microfracture for the treatment of osteochondral defects in the knee joint in young athletes. Arthroscopy 21:1066–1075
9. Haddo O, Mahroof S, Higgs D et al (2004) The use of chondroguide membrane in autologous chondrocyte implantation. Knee 11:51–55
10. Horas U, Pelinkovic D, Herr G, Aigner T, Schnettler R (2003) Autologous chondrocyte implantation and osteochondral cylinder transplantation in cartilage repair of the knee joint: a prospective, comparative trial. J Bone Joint Surg Am 85:185–192
11. Kim IL, Mauck RL, Burdick JA (2011) Hydrogel design for cartilage tissue engineering: a case study with hyaluronic acid. Biomaterials 32:8771–8782
12. Kisiday JD, Jin M, DiMicco MA et al (2004) Effects of dynamic compressive loading on chondrocyte biosynthesis in self-assembling peptide scaffolds. J Biomech 37:595–604
13. Kreuz PC, Steinwachs MR, Erggelet C et al (2006) Results after microfracture of full-thickness chondral defects in different compartments in the knee. Osteoarthritis Cartilage 14:1119–1125
14. Lee DA, Bader DL (1997) Compressive strains at physiological frequencies influence the metabolism of chondrocytes seeded in agarose. J Orthop Res 15:181–188
15. Marcacci M, Berruto M, Brocchetta D et al (2005) Articular cartilage engineering with Hyalograft C: 3 year clinical results. Clin Orthop Relat Res 435:96–105
16. Marcacci M, Kon E, Zaffagnini S et al (2005) Multiple osteochondral arthroscopic grafting (mosaicplasty) for cartilage defects of the knee: prospective study results at 2-year follow-up. Arthroscopy 21:462–470
17. Minas T, Peterson L (1999) Advanced techniques in autologous chondrocyte transplantation. Clin Sports Med 18:13–44
18. Nehrer S, Dorotka R, Domayer S et al (2009) Treatment of full-thickness chondral defects with hyalograft C in the knee: a prospective clinical case series with 2 to 7 years' follow-up. Am J Sports Med 37(Suppl 1):81S–87S
19. Ochi M, Uchio Y, Kawasaki K, Wakitani S, Iwasa J (2002) Transplantation of cartilage–like tissue made by tissue engineering in the treatment of cartilage defects of the knee. J Bone Joint Surg Br 84:571–578
20. Peterson L, Minas T, Brittberg M, Nilsson A, Sjogren-Jansson E, Lindahl A (2000) Two-to 9-year outcome after autologous chondrocyte transplantation of the knee. Clin Orthop Relat Res 374:212–234
21. Saris DB, Vanlauwe J, Victor J et al (2008) Characterized chondrocyte implantation results in better structural repair when treating symptomatic cartilage defects of the knee in a randomized controlled trial versus microfracture. Am J Sports Med 36:235–246
22. Schneider U, Andereya S (2003) Erste Ergebnisse einer prospektiven randomisierten Klinischen Studie zur traditionellen Autologen Chondrocytentransplantation versus CaReS-technologie. Z Orthop Ihre Grenzgeb 141:496–497
23. Schneider U, Rackwitz L, Andereya S et al (2011) A prospective multicenter study on the outcome of type I collagen hydrogel-based autologous chondrocyte implantation (CaReS) for the repair of articular cartilage defects in the knee. Am J Sports Med 39:2558–2565
24. Shelton JC, Bader DL, Lee DA (2003) Mechanical conditioning influences the metabolic response of cell-seeded constructs. Cells Tissues Organs 175:140–150
25. Sohn DH, Lottman LM, Lum LY et al (2002) Effect of gravity on localization of chondrocytes implanted in cartilage defects. Clin Orthop Relat Res 394:254–262
26. Stockwell RA (1967) The cell density of human articular and costal cartilage. J Anat 101:753–763
27. Ueno T, Kagawa T, Mizukawa N, Nakamura H, Sugahara T, Yamamoto T (2001) Cellular origin of endochondral ossification from grafted periosteum. Anat Rec 264:348–357

Part VII

Cartilage Repair of Other Joints

Autologous Matrix-Induced Chondrogenesis (AMIC)-Aided Repair of Osteochondral Lesions of the Talus

22

Martin Wiewiorski and Victor Valderrabano

Contents

M. Wiewiorski, MD (✉) • V. Valderrabano, MD, PhD
Orthopaedic Department, University Hospital of Basel, Spitalstrasse 21, Basel 4031, Switzerland
e-mail: wiewiorskim@googlemail.com

22.1 Historical Development

The autologous matrix-induced chondrogenesis (AMIC) technique was first reported by Behrens in 2005 [1, 2] and has been initially described for treatment of full-thickness cartilage defects in the knee joint [3, 4]. This one-step procedure combines debridement of the cartilage lesion and microfracturing of the subchondral bone to release bone marrow, containing mesenchymal stem cells (MSCs). The defect is then covered by a commercially available collagen I/III matrix to cover and stabilise the resulting blood clot. The scaffold is fixed with autologous or partial autologous fibrin glue [5].

The challenge in surgical treatment of osteochondral lesions (OCL) of the talus is to reconstruct the frequently found bony defect underlying the cartilage lesion. The modified AMIC technique for treatment of talar OCL was first described by Wiewiorski and Valderrabano in 2010 [6]. In addition to microfracturing, cancellous bone is added for reconstruction of the osseous defect [7]. The objective of this modified AMIC-aided procedure is to repair the osteochondral talar defect in an economically efficient single-step procedure and obtain a pain-free joint with physiological range of motion.

22.2 Technical Details

The bilayer collagen type I/III matrix (Chondro-Gide®, Geistlich Surgery, Wolhusen, Switzerland) has a compact and a porous side.

A.A. Shetty et al. (eds.), *Techniques in Cartilage Repair Surgery*,
DOI 10.1007/978-3-642-41921-8_22, © ESSKA 2014

The compact layer consists of a cell-occlusive surface, preventing the stem-cell-enriched blood coagulate from diffusing into the joint space and protecting it from mechanical stress. The porous layer of the matrix is composed of loose collagen fibres that support cell invasion and ingrowth of newly formed tissue. The arrangement of the fibres provides high tensile strength and resistance to tearing and can therefore be held in position by glue, sutures or pins. On application the coherent collagen fibres swell providing good fit onto the cartilage defect. The matrix is manufactured from porcine collagen, which is naturally resorbed. Collagenases, gelatinases and proteinases are responsible for its breakdown into oligopeptides and finally single amino acids.

22.3 Patient Selection

Inclusion Criteria

- Chondral and osteochondral lesions
- All stages according to the CT classification by Hepple [8]
- Lesion >1.0 cm^2
- Patients aged from 18 to 55 years
- Primary and revision procedure

Exclusion Criteria

- Metabolic arthropathies
- Kissing lesions
- Major, non-reconstructable defects
- Non-correctable hindfoot malalignment
- Chronic inflammatory systemic disorders
- Obesity (BMI >30)

22.4 Preoperative Preparation

Clinical examination of the ankle joint includes documentation of range of motion, sagittal and inversion/eversion stability, location of pressure pain and alignment of the hindfoot.

Initial diagnostic imaging of the foot and ankle consists of conventional radiographs (weight-bearing standard AP/lateral radiographs, Saltzman view) to assess alignment and exclude other pathologies than an OCL. Magnetic resonance imaging (MRI) is performed to examine the condition of the cartilage and accompanying soft tissue pathologies. Computed tomography (CT) adds additional information by assessing the extent of the bone defect. An optional single-photon emission computed tomography–computed tomography (SPECT-CT) can be performed to assess the amount of remodeling activity at the OCL site [9, 10]. In cases of no scintigraphic uptake at the OCL, the lesion should not be surgically addressed, and the focus of surgical treatment should rather be on instability and malalignment correction.

22.5 Patient Setup/Patient Positioning

The procedure can be performed in either spinal or general anaesthesia. The patient is in a supine position. A tourniquet is applied for to improve visualisation. A single-shot antibiotic (cefazolin) is administered intravenously 30 min before incision.

22.6 Surgical Approach

The procedure starts with an arthroscopy of the ankle joint to verify the size and location of the defect and joint stability. A standard anteromedial or anterolateral approach for arthrotomy is used. If the lesion cannot be accessed by arthrotomy alone, we recommend to perform a malleolar osteotomy (oblique medial or Z-shaped lateral osteotomy) (Fig. 22.1a). The defective cartilage and subchondral bone are debrided (Fig. 22.1b). If subchondral cyst(s) is seen on preoperative imaging, it is important to break down the sclerotic subchondral bone underneath the deteriorated cartilage to gain access to the cysts. After debridement of fibrous/necrotic tissue, microfracturing of the underlying bone with a sharp awl is used to release bone marrow (Fig. 22.1c). Because OCL of the talus often involve a large osseous lesion, it needs to be reconstructed to restore the former talar shape. In cases of lesions >1 cm^2 and 0.5 cm of depth, cancellous bone is being harvested (iliac crest, proximal tibia or osteotomy site) which is impacted into the

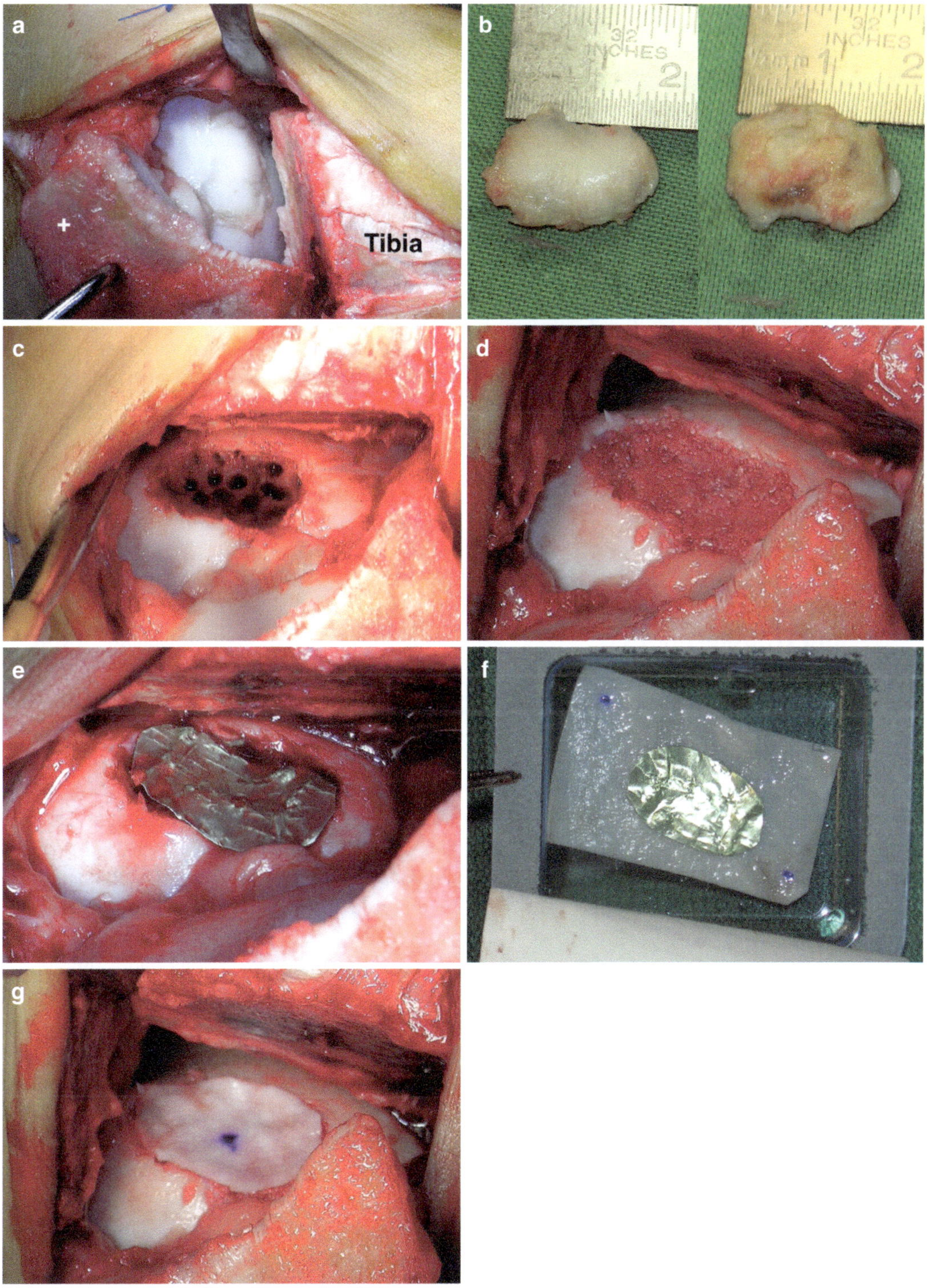

Fig. 22.1 Surgical procedure. An oblique anteromedial osteotomy (+) is performed to gain access to the posterior medial talar edge (**a**). The chondral fragment is sharply removed (**b**). Next debridement and anterograde drilling is performed (**c**). Cancellous bone harvested from the iliac crest is impacted into the defect (**d**). A template is applied (**e**) for sizing of the matrix (**f**). The cut-to-shape collagen matrix is placed on the defect and fixed with fibrin glue (**g**). The ankle is moved several times and position of the matrix is finally controlled

defect (Fig. 22.1d). Next the collagen matrix is being prepared. An aluminium template is used to determine the lesion size (Fig. 22.1e). The cut-to-size matrix (Fig. 22.1f) is glued onto the defect (Tissucol, Baxter, Deerfield, USA) (Fig. 22.1g). Care should be taken not to overlap the surrounding cartilage with the matrix. Finally, the ankle is then moved several times throughout the entire range of motion and correct positioning of the matrix is reassessed.

If malalignment of the hindfoot is present, a corrective osteotomy is recommended. If ankle joint instability is encountered during arthroscopy, ligament repair should be performed. Restoring a healthy biomechanical environment of the ankle joint by correcting the bony architecture and joint stability helps protecting the reconstructed osteochondral defect.

22.7 Potential Complications and Troubleshooting

Though infrequently encountered, potential complications special to this technique include delayed wound healing, delayed consolidation of an osteotomy and an overtight joint after ligament repair.

22.8 Rehabilitation

Postoperative care consists of immobilisation using a walker (e.g. Aircast Walker, DJO Global, Vista, USA) and functional physiotherapy with 15 kg partial weight bearing, maximal range of motion of 20° with a continuous passive motion machine and lymphatic drainage massage for the first 6 weeks. This initial phase is followed by an intensive rehabilitation phase with progression to full weight bearing and strengthening of the ankle joint stabilising lower leg muscles and proprioception training for the following 6 weeks (i.e. up to 12 weeks). After 12 weeks light sports exercising (swimming, cycling) are allowed. Return to competitive sports after 5–6 months. Postoperative care is identical for cases with corrective osteotomy and/or ligament reconstruction.

22.9 Postoperative Follow-Up

The patients are seen in the outpatient clinic 6 and 12 weeks after the surgery for a clinical follow-up examination and conventional radiographs. If a malleolar osteotomy is performed, hardware removal can be done 6 months following cartilage repair. After 1 and 2 years, an MRI is performed to assess cartilage morphology at the repair site.

22.10 Comparison to Other Techniques

Surgical treatment of osteochondral lesions (OCL) of the talus has become an important issue of foot and ankle orthopaedics. Several operative techniques are being routinely employed to address talar OCL: microfracturing, osteochondral autologous transplantation (OATS), matrix-induced autologous chondrocyte implantation (MACI), autologous chondrocyte implantation (ACI) and osteochondral allograft transplantation (mosaicplasty or bulk). Good results for those techniques have been described [11–16]. However, certain disadvantages have been reported. MACI and ACI are two-stage procedures (initial harvesting and culturing of chondrocytes before later implantation) which are expensive and not being reimbursed by an increasing number of health insurances. OATS requires sacrificing healthy cartilage from the knee joint with subsequent donor-site morbidity [16]. Allograft transplantation is not readily available across Europe because of forensic issues [13].

Several reports exist concerning the AMIC technique [6, 7, 17]. Valderrabano et al. reported about 26 patients seen for clinical and radiological follow-up at a minimum of 24 months after surgery (mean, 31 months; range, 24–54 months). The AOFAS ankle score improved significantly from a mean of 60 points preoperatively (range, 17–79 points) to 89 points (range, 61–100 points) postoperatively ($p<.01$). The preoperative pain score averaged 5 (range, 2–8), improving to an average of 1.6 (range, 0–7) postoperatively ($p<.01$). Normal signal intensity of the repair tissue on MRI compared with the adjacent native cartilage was seen in 15 %, with nearly normal activity in 69 % [18]. Those results are comparable to other established techniques [11, 12, 14–16]. Regarding full-thickness cartilage lesions of the knee joint, good clinical outcome results utilising the above-mentioned collagen matrix combined with ACI at 3-year follow-up have been reported [19–21].

We use cancellous bone from the iliac crest to reconstruct the osseous lesion and covering it with a collagen matrix. Cancellous bone grafting for OCL of the talus has been previously described in combination with arthroscopically guided retrograde drilling only [15, 22]. The rationale behind this procedure is to allow cartilage regeneration on the base of healthy bony tissue. In the AMIC process the collagen I/III matrix of porcine origin attracts mesenchymal stem cells from the bone marrow of cancellous bone and provides a suitable environment for formation of cartilaginous repair tissue [23, 24]. Because cancellous bone makes a rather loose nonstructural graft, the authors think that a bony reconstruction can be only successfully achieved with an adequate covering of the graft tissue, as described in our technique.

This novel procedure might offer certain advantages compared to routinely used surgical techniques. The patient has to face only one surgical intervention. No second surgery after initial chondrocyte harvesting and culturing, as required with ACI and MACI, is needed. In contrast to the OATS procedure, vital cartilage of another joint is spared and therefore donor-site morbidity is reduced [16].

From an economic point of view, the AMIC-aided procedure is a very cost-effective, readily available, surgical treatment method. The costs of open ACI surgery for cartilage lesions of the knee joint total 14,000 $ (8,800 $ [6,200 €] for the procedure plus 5,200 $ [3,600 €] for in vitro cell expansion) comparing with 3,800 $ (2,700 €) for microfracturing [25]. A bulk talar allograft is reported to cost about 6,500 $ (4,500 €) [26]. The costs of AMIC-aided treatment are comparable to microfracturing adding the costs for the collagen matrix.

Conclusion

The modified AMIC technique is a promising novel method for operative treatment of osteochondral lesion of the talus. The described technique is cost-effective, is readily available and can be performed as a single surgery for initial operative treatment or revision surgery of osteochondral lesions of the talus.

References

1. Behrens P (2005) Matrixgekoppelte Mikrofrakturierung. Arthroskopie 18:193–197
2. Behrens P, Bitter T, Kurz B, Russlies M (2006) Matrix-associated autologous chondrocyte transplantation/implantation (MACT/MACI)–5-year follow-up. Knee 13:194–202
3. Benthien JP, Behrens P (2010) Autologous matrix-induced chondrogenesis (AMIC): combining microfracturing and a collagen I/III matrix for articular cartilage resurfacing. Cartilage 1:65–68
4. Marlovits S, Singer P, Zeller P, Mandl I, Haller J, Trattnig S (2006) Magnetic resonance observation of cartilage repair tissue (MOCART) for the evaluation of autologous chondrocyte transplantation: determination of interobserver variability and correlation to clinical outcome after 2 years. Eur J Radiol 57: 16–23
5. Gille J, Meisner U, Ehlers EM, Muller A, Russlies M, Behrens P (2005) Migration pattern, morphology and viability of cells suspended in or sealed with fibrin glue: a histomorphologic study. Tissue Cell 37: 339–348
6. Wiewiorski M, Leumann A, Buettner O, Pagenstert G, Horisberger M, Valderrabano V (2011) Autologous matrix-induced chondrogenesis aided reconstruction of a large focal osteochondral lesion of the talus. Arch Orthop Trauma Surg 131:293–296
7. Valderrabano V, Leumann A, Frigg A, Pagenstert G, Wiewiorski M (2011) Autologous matrix-induced chondrogenesis-aided repair of osteochondral lesions of the talus. Tech Foot Ankle Surg 10:159–162. doi:10.1097/BTF.0b013e318237c1b0
8. Hepple S, Winson IG, Glew D (1999) Osteochondral lesions of the talus: a revised classification. Foot Ankle Int 20:789–793
9. Carlsson AM (1983) Assessment of chronic pain. I. Aspects of the reliability and validity of the visual analogue scale. Pain 16:87–101
10. Wiewiorski M, Pagenstert G, Rasch H, Jacob AL, Valderrabano V (2011) Pain in osteochondral lesions. Foot Ankle Spec 4:92–99
11. Assenmacher JA, Kelikian AS, Gottlob C, Kodros S (2001) Arthroscopically assisted autologous

osteochondral transplantation for osteochondral lesions of the talar dome: an MRI and clinical follow-up study. Foot Ankle Int 22:544–551
12. Giannini S, Buda R, Grigolo B, Vannini F (2001) Autologous chondrocyte transplantation in osteochondral lesions of the ankle joint. Foot Ankle Int 22:513–517
13. Raikin SM (2009) Fresh osteochondral allografts for large-volume cystic osteochondral defects of the talus. J Bone Joint Surg Am 91:2818–2826
14. Schneider TE, Karaikudi S (2009) Matrix-induced autologous chondrocyte implantation (MACI) grafting for osteochondral lesions of the talus. Foot Ankle Int 30:810–814
15. Taranow WS, Bisignani GA, Towers JD, Conti SF (1999) Retrograde drilling of osteochondral lesions of the medial talar dome. Foot Ankle Int 20:474–480
16. Valderrabano V, Leumann A, Rasch H, Egelhof T, Hintermann B, Pagenstert G (2009) Knee-to-ankle mosaicplasty for the treatment of osteochondral lesions of the ankle joint. Am J Sports Med 37(Suppl 1):105S–111S
17. Wiewiorski M, Miska M, Nicolas G, Valderrabano V (2012) Revision of failed osteochondral autologous transplantation procedure for chronic talus osteochondral lesion with iliac crest graft and autologous matrix-induced chondrogenesis: a case report. Foot Ankle Spec 5:115–120
18. Valderrabano V, Miska M, Leumann A, Wiewiorski M (2013) Reconstruction of osteochondral lesions of the talus with autologous spongiosa grafts and autologous matrix-induced chondrogenesis. Am J Sports Med 41(3):519–527
19. Steinwachs M, Kreuz PC (2007) Autologous chondrocyte implantation in chondral defects of the knee with a type I/III collagen membrane: a prospective study with a 3-year follow-up. Arthroscopy 23:381–387
20. Niemeyer P, Pestka JM, Kreuz PC, Erggelet C, Schmal H, Suedkamp NP, Steinwachs M (2008) Characteristic complications after autologous chondrocyte implantation for cartilage defects of the knee joint. Am J Sports Med 36:2091–2099
21. Gooding CR, Bartlett W, Bentley G, Skinner JA, Carrington R, Flanagan A (2006) A prospective, randomised study comparing two techniques of autologous chondrocyte implantation for osteochondral defects in the knee: Periosteum covered versus type I/III collagen covered. Knee 13:203–210
22. Lahm A, Erggelet C, Steinwachs M, Reichelt A (2000) Arthroscopic management of osteochondral lesions of the talus: results of drilling and usefulness of magnetic resonance imaging before and after treatment. Arthroscopy 16:299–304
23. Fuss M, Ehlers EM, Russlies M, Rohwedel J, Behrens P (2000) Characteristics of human chondrocytes, osteoblasts and fibroblasts seeded onto a type I/III collagen sponge under different culture conditions. A light, scanning and transmission electron microscopy study. Ann Anat 182:303–310
24. Hamilton WG, Thompson FM, Snow SW (1993) The modified Brostrom procedure for lateral ankle instability. Foot Ankle 14:1–7
25. Clar C, Cummins E, McIntyre L, Thomas S, Lamb J, Bain L, Jobanputra P, Waugh N (2005) Clinical and cost-effectiveness of autologous chondrocyte implantation for cartilage defects in knee joints: systematic review and economic evaluation. Health Technol Assess 9:iii–iv, ix–x, 1–82
26. Brage ME, Reese KA (2009) Techniques for large osteochondral defects of the talus. Tech Foot Ankle Surg 8:43–49. doi:10.1097/BTF.0b013e31819999bb

Cartilage Repair in the Hip

23

Sally Roberts, Andrew McCaskie,
James B. Richardson, and Atanu Bhattacharjee

Contents

23.1 Introduction

Chondropathies of the hip, whether on the femoral head or the acetabulum, are believed to be a frequent cause of hip pain and precedent to osteoarthritis (OA). There are approximately 80,000 hip replacements performed each year in England and Wales, the majority for OA [19]. The incidence of OA is set to double by 2030 with changing demographics and altered lifestyles; it is estimated that one in five OA patients gives up work or retires early because of his or her condition [20]. Over the last 5 years, there has been a 49 % increase in revisions of hip arthroplasty, which are costly, complex and time consuming in theatre usage, in addition to having a less successful outcome than primary arthroplasties. There is a need to develop treatments at an earlier stage which can delay, or better still alleviate, the need for a hip arthroplasty. The treatments must deliver patient benefit and be cost-effective.

Regenerative strategies aim to replace or regenerate human cells, tissue or organs to restore or establish normal function [16]. Such an approach, using the body's own cells, offers an opportunity to repair or regenerate cartilage and

S. Roberts, PhD (✉)
Department of ARC/TORCH Building, Robert Jones and Agnes Hunt Orthopaedic Hospital and Institute of Science and Technology in Medicine (Keele University), Oswestry, Shropshire SY10 7AG, UK
e-mail: sally.roberts@rjah.nhs.uk

A. McCaskie, MB ChB, MMus, MD, FRCS, FRCS (T&O)
Division of Trauma and Orthopaedic Surgery, Department of Surgery, Cambridge University Hospitals NHS Foundation Trust, 180, Addenbrooke's Hospital, CB2 0QQ Cambridge, UK
e-mail: andrew.mccaskie@ncl.ac.uk

J.B. Richardson, MBChB, FRCS, MD
Institute of Orthopaedics, Institute of Science and Technology in Medicine (Keele University) and Robert Jones and Agnes Hunt Orthopaedic Hospital, Oswestry, Shropshire SY10 7AG, UK
e-mail: james.richardson@nhs.net

A. Bhattacharjee
Department of Orthopaedics, Institute of Orthopaedics at RJAH Orthopaedic Hospital and Robert Jones and Keele University, Oswestry, Shropshire, UK

A.A. Shetty et al. (eds.), *Techniques in Cartilage Repair Surgery*,
DOI 10.1007/978-3-642-41921-8_23, © ESSKA 2014

bone in the joint. In this way, the joint 'replacement' would be achieved by cartilage and bone rather than materials such as metals and ceramics. This type of approach is already well described in the knee but much less so in the hip. Imaging techniques, such as magnetic resonance imaging (MRI) with arthrogram and delayed gadolinium-enhanced MRI of cartilage (dGEMRIC), have enabled better study of abnormalities in the young adult hip. In addition, hip arthroscopy has allowed description of relevant pathologies such as hip impingement, labral disease and early osteoarthritic lesions. Baber et al. identified localised OA or an osteochondral defect in 74 patients out of 154 with idiopathic hip pain when they performed arthroscopic examination [2]. Microfracture, osteochondral autologous mosaicplasty (OATS) and cell therapy have been used and reported widely in the knee over the last two decades. This chapter summarises known and reported studies using these approaches in the hip.

23.2 Peculiarities Pertinent to the Hip

There is considerable experience of techniques for cartilage repair in the knee, and some of this knowledge can be transferred directly to the hip. As with the knee, chondral/osteochondral defects commonly coexist with other pathologies of the joint. In the hip, these disorders include labral tears, cam or pincer impingement, hip instability or dislocation, osteonecrosis of the femoral head, slipped femoral epiphysis or hip dysplasia [6]. These coexisting conditions should be treated as appropriate at the same time as the cartilage repair procedure is performed.

The knee has many joint anatomical features that can be palpated at the surface. This has led to well-described operative techniques for regenerative techniques via arthroscopic, arthrotomy and parapatellar approaches. In contrast, anatomically the hip is deeply located and surrounded by large muscle masses [8]. Therefore, chondral or osteochondral defects in the hip can be more difficult in terms of access. Surgical dislocation can certainly provide access. The advantages of surgical hip dislocation are that it provides a wide exposure to allow inspection of the entire femoral head and to treat concomitant labral or acetabular pathology while minimising the risk of avascular necrosis [18]. The blood supply to the femoral head is mainly from the deep branch of the medial femoral circumflex artery (MFCA). Ganz et al. describe how during dislocation of the hip this vessel is protected by the intact obturator externus muscle [11]. Using a trochanteric flip approach, the hip can be exposed anteriorly, subluxated and dislocated in the same direction, if required, while respecting the integrity of the external rotator muscles. This allows a gap of up to 11 cm between the head and the acetabulum, giving a view of the femoral head of almost 360° and a full 360° view of the acetabulum.

Over the last decade, hip arthroscopy has proved useful in treating many conditions, e.g. impingement and labral pathology. The technique (supine or lateral) involves traction applied to the leg to distract the hip. The joint can then be entered safely under fluoroscopic control. Standard portals (2–3) are used to visualise the joint (camera portal) and perform surgery (instrument portal). Instruments include probes, shavers and microfracture awls. Using this type of technique, chondrocyte transplantation has been performed [9].

23.3 Differences with Location in Joints

While articular cartilage has common properties wherever it exists in the body, there are also subtle differences with location, both within a joint and between joints. For example, the proteoglycan content of the maximally loaded region of the femoral condyles in the knee is 50 % greater than that in the lesser loaded posterior tip (Fig. 23.1; [3]).

There are also differences with location in the hip cartilage with the mean value of proteoglycan being higher at the zenith of the femoral head (with a fixed charge density of 0.135 ± 0.017 mEq/g wet weight) than at the anterior-inferior aspect (0.113 ± 0.026 mEq/g wet weight; [24]), probably also related to weight bearing. The anatomy of joints obviously varies hugely, with a different organisation of its molecular components as well

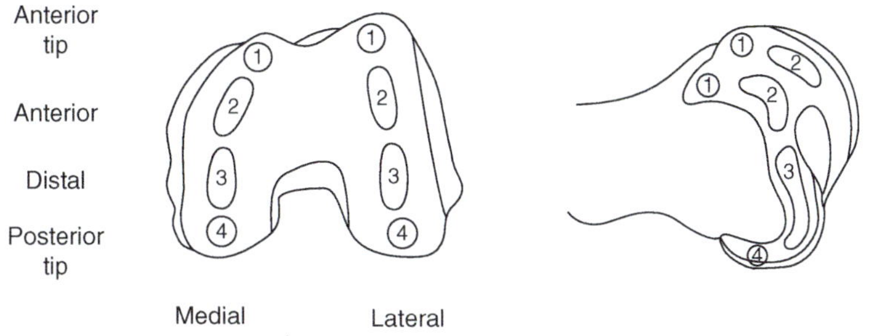

Fig. 23.1 There is significantly less proteoglycan at the posterior tip of the femoral condyle (position 4) than, for example, the anterior condyle (position 2) (Figure reproduced from Brocklehurst et al. [3])

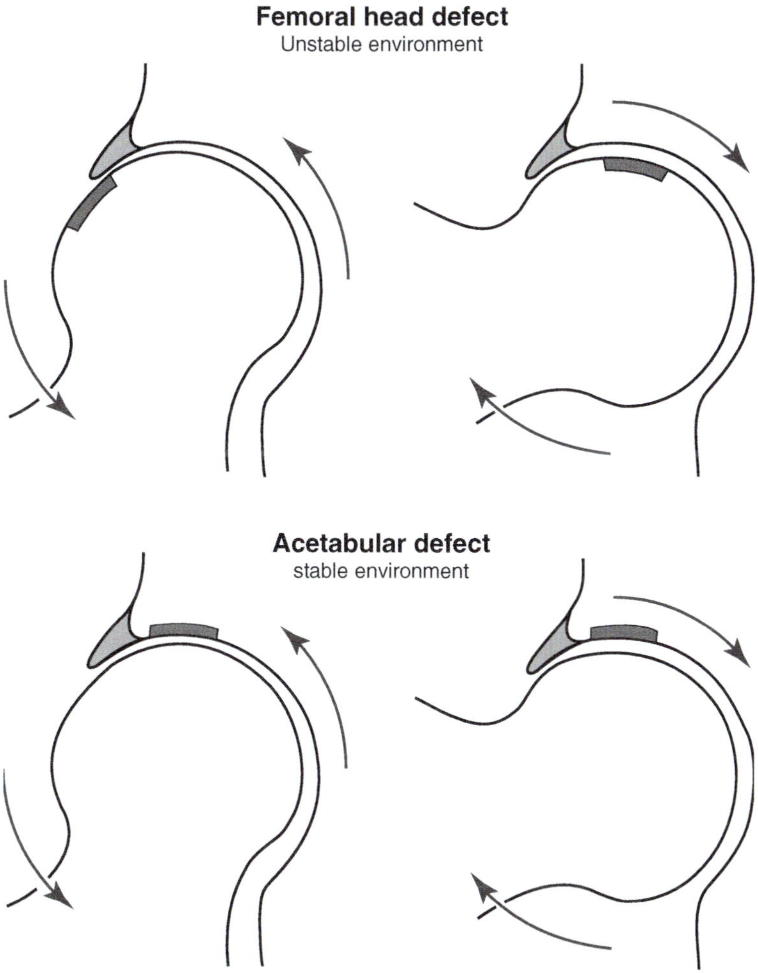

Fig. 23.2 The femoral head provides a more unstable environment for repairing cartilage defects than those in the acetabulum, due to the movement of the joint, allowing the treated defect to 'leave' the protection of the hip socket where it may encounter abrasion or wear from the labrum, osteophytes or other irregularities out of the acetabulum. Defects in the acetabulum, in contrast, normally remain covered by the opposing femoral cartilage

as a difference in quantity [4]. These variations all probably contribute to the different incidence of osteoarthritis in different joints, for example, primary OA of the ankle being a relative rarity compared to in the hip [10]. Hence, what is applicable in one joint is not necessarily true in another and the knowledge and techniques used for cartilage repair in the knee may not transfer to the hip.

In addition there is a difference between the acetabulum and the femoral surfaces. Acetabular defects lend themselves perhaps more to arthroscopic approaches than defects on the femoral head, as they are often smaller and always in contact with the femoral head (Fig. 23.2). Femoral defects, in contrast, may more often require open surgery as they tend to be larger and, due to the articulation of the hip, may undergo abrasion or detachment against the edge of the acetabulum or labrum (Fig. 23.2).

23.4 Microfracture for Repair of Cartilage in the Hip

Microfracture has been used in several studies in the hip. Indications are focal and contained lesions typically of 2–4 cm^2 in size, full thickness loss of cartilage in weight-bearing areas or unstable cartilage flaps overlying intact subchondral bone and with the patient able to undertake adequate postoperative rehabilitation protocol [6]. Karthikeyan et al. [14] have carried out microfracture of the acetabular cartilage on a population of 185 patients with 11 undergoing second look arthroscopies and biopsy. These patients had full thickness cartilage loss, but no underlying bone involvement, in either a weight-bearing area or a region of contact between the femoral head and acetabulum. The microfracture was performed via a lateral approach, unstable cartilage debrided, the calcified layer removed with a curette and microfracture performed with arthroscopic awls at 5 mm intervals. All but one of the patients undergoing the follow-up examination had an average of 95 % fill of the defect at the mean follow-up time of 12 months post-treatment, similar to that reported by Philippon et al. [23]. These authors found that of nine patients undergoing a follow-up arthroscopy between 9 and 36 months after acetabular microfracture, all but one of them had 95 or 100 % fill of the defect, including one with a concomitant defect on the femoral head. One patient with only 25 % fill had diffuse OA at the time of treatment.

23.5 Osteochondral Autograft Transplants in Femoral Head

There are few reports of osteochondral autograft transplants (OATS) or mosaicplasty being performed. Hart et al. reported a case in a 28-year-old who had an osteochondral defect of the femoral head, caused by penetration of a resorbable screw used in a prior open reduction internal fixation of the acetabulum [13]. Two other young patients (aged 15- and 21-year-old) with traumatic focal chondral injuries in the anterior-superior weight-bearing portion of the femoral head were reported to be treated by OATS, using plugs from the ipsilateral knee and inferior femoral head, respectively [18]. In this study, in which the patients underwent surgical dislocation of the hip, they are both reported to demonstrate good autograft incorporation, maintenance of articular surface conformity, no pain and full active range of motion at 1- and 5-year follow-up.

23.6 Autologous Chondrocyte Implantation in the Hip

A trial comparing autologous chondrocyte implantation (ACI) with a group of patients previously treated with debridement for chondral lesions in the hip has been performed by Fontana et al. [9]. Each group contained 15 patients who had suffered traumatic grade 3 or 4 injuries (according to the Outerbridge classification [21]), matched for age, sex and location of the defect. Defect size was a mean of 2.6 cm^2; patients with signs of arthritis, including slightly reduced joint space and small cysts, were included, but those with severely reduced joint space or large cysts were excluded. All 15 patients in each group had acetabular defects, with two in each group having femoral defects also. Both treatments were performed arthroscopically, with debridement only requiring 1 procedure but ACI requiring 2. The first permitted diagnosis and harvesting of cartilage from the pulvinar for cell isolation, while the second arthroscopy, 30 days later, allowed for implantation of the culture-expanded chondrocytes on bioresorbable gel-polymer scaffolds consisting of polyglycolic/polylactic acid and polydioxanone (Bioseed®-C, Biotissue Technologies GmbH, Freiburg). Outcome was assessed via the Harris hip score (HSS; [12]); patients treated with ACI improved significantly more than those who underwent debridement approximately 5 years post-treatment.

In the senior author's centre (JBR), we have treated a much more disparate group of 14 patients with a wide range of large chondral defects (mean 6.2 cm^2) and various pathologies including dislocations, fracture neck of femur, Perthes' disease, epiphyseal dysplasia and OA. In all patients the hip was dislocated, lesions were curetted and chondrocytes (which had been culture expanded from tissue usually harvested from the knee) were implanted with or without a bone plug. The defect was covered by collagen patches (Chondro-Gide®, Geistlich Pharma AG, Switzerland) in 12 patients and periosteum taken from the proximal femur in 2 patients. Ten of the 14 patients showed an improvement in the Harris hip score at 12 months, but 5 patients went on to have a hip arthroplasty within 18 months. Some of the patients in this study had large subchondral cysts prior to treatment, which may prove to be a contra-indication in the future.

There is much interest in the regenerative medicine field in mesenchymal stem/stromal cells (MSCs) as a source of cells for facilitating repair. Autologous adipose-derived mesenchymal stem cells have been used in two patients who had osteonecrosis of the hip [22]. Abdominal adipose tissue was digested with collagenase, and stem cells were administered with hyaluronic acid and platelet-rich plasma to 29- and 47-year-old patients, although there are few details of characterisation of the cells. Infilling of bony defects was reported at 12 weeks, but clinical improvement was variable.

ACI has been applied to a large defect (10 cm^2) on a femoral head, which had been treated previously with autologous osteochondral mosaicplasty [7]. A 19-year-old female, who had had congenital hip dislocation treated with closed reduction as an infant, was treated by transplanting three osteochondral plugs obtained from the lateral trochlea of the ipsilateral knee. Symptoms were resolved for 2 years post-surgery when pain again returned limiting her activity, perhaps due to cartilage loss on the major weight-bearing portion of the femoral head. At this stage it was decided to undertake an ACI on the femoral head at the same time as an osteoplasty. Using an anterolateral approach, the femoral head was dislocated, avoiding branches of the medial circumflex artery, and rotated externally. Twelve million culture-expanded chondrocytes (obtained from the intercondylar notch of the knee) were implanted beneath a porcine collagen membrane. Two years post-treatment the patient was pain-free with maintained joint space.

Probably the largest challenge addressed by cell therapy in the hip is the complete resurfacing of a whole femoral head in a 32-year-old patient who had had failed corrective surgery for a resected femoral head [1]. Twenty-one months after the original injury, cartilage was harvested from the patient's ipsilateral knee and chondrocytes were isolated and culture expanded for ACI. The second stage was undertaken using a Stracathro approach for the hip [17]. An anterior slice of the greater trochanter was removed with proximal medius and distal vastus lateral muscles in continuity. Care was taken to avoid the entry of the medial circumflex artery to the femur at the insertion of the superior gemellus muscle. The screws were removed from the femoral neck and the hip dislocated anteriorly. The femoral head was debrided to healthy bleeding bone using a cibatome (Fig. 23.3a). The defects of the femoral head were filled with bone graft taken from the greater trochanter, and 2 collagen patches (Chondro-Gide; Geistlich Pharma AG, Switzerland) were sutured together with 2.0 Vicryl and placed over the femoral head (Fig. 23.3b). A 'purse string' of polydioxanone suture around the femoral neck was used to shape the patch in order to conform to the head (Fig. 23.3c). Six million chondrocytes were injected under the patch from two entry points. The hip was relocated and the wound was closed. There was significant improvement clinically at 12 months. At 15 months post-ACI, a biopsy was taken showing ~2 mm of cartilage formed which was predominantly fibrocartilaginous. Imaging demonstrated abnormalities remaining within the bony component with cysts and sclerotic areas in the femoral head. The patient remains active and clinically improved at more than 6 years post-operatively, although there is loss of rotation in the hip.

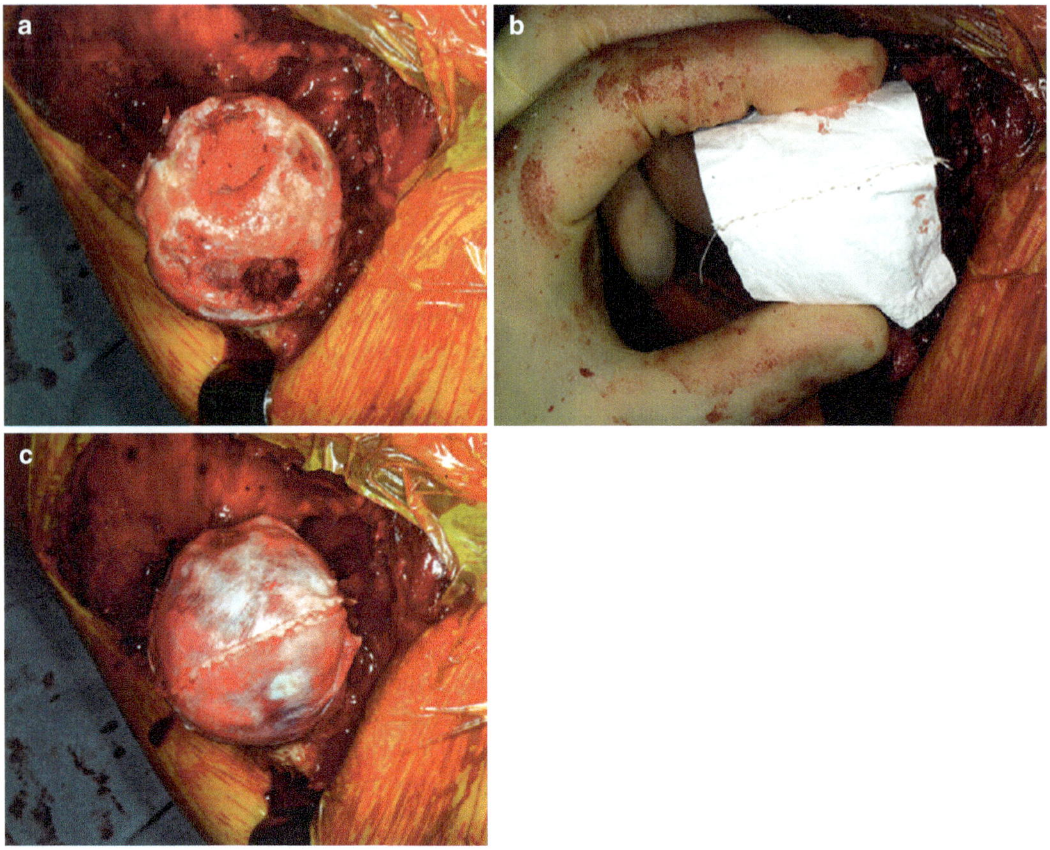

Fig. 23.3 ACI being used in conjunction with a collagen membrane for resurfacing a femoral head. (**a**) A femoral head with excessive chondrolysis prior to being covered with 2 stitched Chondro-Gide patches (**b**); this was pulled tight around the femoral head via a purse-string of stitches and cultured autologous chondrocytes implanted beneath (**c**) (Reproduced from Akimau et al. [1] with permission)

23.7 Post-operative Rehabilitation

Generally similar post-operative rehabilitation procedures are employed as for the relevant procedures carried out in the knee joint. For example, following microfracture, weight bearing was restricted to toe touch for 8 weeks and continuous passive motion used for 8 weeks with return to sport typically 4–6 months post-surgery [23]. The OATS-treated patients reported by Nam et al. [18] were non-weight bearing for 6 weeks, progressing to weight bearing as tolerated, eventually returning to running. Rehabilitation following ACI began from the first day with Fontana et al. [9] but with no weight bearing for 4 weeks. After 7 weeks patients returned to work with a complete return to sports at 12 months post-treatment.

Conclusions

Hip osteoarthritis is a significant clinical problem, but regenerative approaches to repair cartilage are much less common than in the knee. Patients receiving ACI in the knee can now expect good long-term retention of benefit over 20 years (Peterson L, 2012, personal communication), with articular cartilage repair techniques allowing return to sport, although rehabilitation timescales can be lengthy [15]. There is a 78 % average rate of return to sport, varying between 7 and 17 months post-treatment depending on the cartilage repair technique used. It takes the longest to return to sport following ACI, but this method appears to result in the best durability with 96 % of ACI-treated patients continuing sports participation 3 years after treatment [15]. In addition, comparison with microfracture shows statistically significant structural benefit of ACI in terms of the quality of repair tissue formed [25].

It is likely that some of these techniques can be successful when transferred to the hip, although a greater understanding of the pathogenesis of OA in the hip (genetics, impingement and injury) will no doubt help improve that rate of success. In the hip it would appear that ACI on the acetabulum has better promise for successful cartilage repair than on the femoral head. The broad application of ACI, or second or third generation techniques, will be enhanced by the improvements being made in arthroscopic equipment and technology, allowing it to be performed arthroscopically in carefully selected patients, rather than via an open procedure. An arthroscopic approach to treating hip chondropathies reduces risks from arthrotomy [8], such as avascular necrosis of the femoral head, with a reported complication rate in the order of 1.4 % [5]. Cysts within the bone adjacent to the area being treated may be a problem and may prove to be a contra-indication to carrying out ACI in this location. Preliminary results of microfracture appear to indicate that it can be a safe and effective treatment option for certain defects. It is likely that the next few years will see progress in the application of regenerative techniques focused on cartilage and bone repair in the hip.

Acknowledgements We are grateful to the Arthritis Research UK for funding (grant 19429) and to Andrew Biggs (medical illustrator and photographer) for drawing Fig. 23.2.

References

1. Akimau P, Bhosale A, Harrison PE, Roberts S, Richardson JB, Ashton BA (2006) Autologous chondrocyte implantation with bone grafting for osteochondral defect due to posttraumatic osteonecrosis of the hip – a case report. Acta Orthop 77:333–336
2. Baber YF, Robinson AHN, Villar RN (1999) Is diagnostic arthroscopy of the hip worthwhile? J Bone Joint Surg Br 81:600–603
3. Brocklehurst R, Bayliss MT, Maroudas A, Coysh HL, Obst D, Freeman AR, Revell PA, Ali SY (1984) The composition of normal and osteoarthritic articular cartilage from human knee joints. J Bone Joint Surg Am 66:95–106
4. Bullough PG (2012) Normal skeletal structure and development. In: Orthopaedic pathology. Mosby/Elsevier, Missouri, pp 1–79
5. Clarke MT, Aroa A, Villar RN (2003) Hip arthroscopy: complications in 1054 cases. Clin Orthop Relat Res 406:84–88
6. Crawford K, Philippon MJ, Sekiya JK, Rodkey WG, Steadman JR (2006) Microfracture of the hip in athletes. Clin Sports Med 25:327–335
7. Ellender P, Minas T (2008) Autologous chondrocyte implantation in the hip: case report and technique. Oper Tech Sports Med 16:201–206
8. Fontana A (2006) Arthroscopic approach in hip defects. In: Zanasi S, Brittberg M, Maracci M (eds) Basic science clinical repair and reconstruction of articular cartilage defects and current status and prospects. Timeo Editore, Bologna
9. Fontana A, Bistolfi A, Crova M, Rosso F, Massazza G (2012) Arthroscopic treatment of hip chondral defects: autologous chondrocyte transplantation versus simple debridement – a pilot study. Arthroscopy 28:322–329
10. Freeman MAR, Meachim G (1979) Ageing and degeneration. In: Freeman MAR (ed) Adult articular cartilage. Pitman Medical, Bath
11. Ganz R, Gill TJ, Gautier E, Ganz K, Krugel N, Berlemann U (2001) Surgical dislocation of the adult hip: a technique with full access to the femoral head-and acetabulum without the risk of avascular necrosis. J Bone Joint Surg Br 83B:1119–1124
12. Harris WH (1969) Traumatic arthritis of the hip after dislocation and acetabular fractures: treatment by mold arthroplasty. An end-result study using a new method of result evaluation. J Bone Joint Surg Am 51:737–755
13. Hart R, Janecek M, Visna P, Bucek P, Kocis J (2003) Mosaicplasty for the treatment of femoral head defect after incorrect resorbable screw insertion. Arthroscopy 19:e137–e141
14. Karthikeyan D, Roberts S, Griffin DR (2012) Microfracture for acetabular chondral defects in patients with femoro-acetabular impingement: results at second look arthroscopy. Am J Sports Med 40:2725–2730
15. Mandelbaum BR, Mithoefer K, Peterson L, Saris DB, Dvorak J (2012) Cartilage issues in football: an executive summary of the FIFA/ICRS initiative. Cartilage 3:6S–10S
16. Mason C, Dunnill P (2008) A brief definition of regenerative medicine. Regen Med 3(1):1–5
17. McLauchlan J (1984) The stracathro approach to the hip. J Bone Joint Surg Br 66:30–31
18. Nam D, Shindle MK, Buly RL, Kelly BT, Lorich DG (2010) Traumatic osteochondral injury of the femoral head treated by mosaicplasty: a report of two cases. HSS J 6:228–234

19. National Joint Registry 8th Annual Report (2012) www.ntj.org
20. OANation 2012: Survey YouGov (2012) www.arthritiscare.org.uk
21. Outerbridge RE (1961) The etiology of chondromalacia patellae. J Bone Joint Surg Br 43-B:752–757
22. Pak J (2011) Regeneration of human bones in hip osteonecrosis and human cartilage in knee osteoarthritis with autologous adipose-tissue-derived stem cells: a case series. J Med Case Rep 5:296
23. Philippon MJ, Schenker ML, Briggs KK, Maxwell RB (2008) Can microfracture produce repair tissue in acetabular chondral defects? Arthroscopy 24:46–50
24. Roberts S, Weightman B, Urban J, Chappell D (1986) Mechanical and biochemical properties of human articular cartilage in osteoarthritic femoral heads and in autopsy specimens. J Bone Joint Surg 68-B:278–288
25. Saris DBF, Vanlauwe J, Victor J, Haspi M, Bohnsack M, Fortems Y, Vandekerckhove B, Almquist KF, Claes T, Handelberg F, Lagae K, Van der Bauwhede J, Vandenneucker H, Yang KGA, Jelic M, Verdonk R, Veulemans N, Bellemans J, Luyten FP (2008) Characterized chondrocyte implantation results in better structural repair when treating symptomatic cartilage defects of the knee in a randomized controlled trial versus microfracture. Am J Sports Med 36:235–246

Part VIII

Alignment, Stability and Meniscal Replacement

High Tibial Osteotomy in Cartilage Repair

24

Mohammed Shukrimi, Sureshbabu Manivannan, Joel Lee, and James H.P. Hui

Contents

M. Shukrimi • S. Manivannan • J. Lee
J.H.P. Hui (✉)
Department of Orthopaedic Surgery,
University Orthopaedic,
Hand and Reconstructive Microsurgery Cluster,
National University Health System,
Singapore
e-mail: manivannan_suresh_babu@nuhs.edu.sg;
zoelzee@gmail.com; james_hui@nuhs.edu.sg

24.1 Introduction

Deformity of the knee associated with osteoarthrosis (OA) is a common presenting complaint to the orthopedic surgeon. In a normal knee, approximately 60 % of the weight-bearing forces are transmitted through the medial compartment and 40 % through the lateral compartment. The varus knee with unicompartmental OA of the medial compartment has an altered limb alignment and subsequently more load is distributed to the affected compartment. Despite the expanding indications for knee arthroplasty, it is advantageous to delay arthroplasty given the higher wear rate and likelihood of future complex revisions if the primary surgery is performed in patients at a young age [1]. Proximal tibial osteotomy, a joint-preserving procedure, has been reported as a viable surgical option for younger patients with isolated medial compartment arthritis. The aim of the surgery is to shift the weight-bearing axis away from the diseased area, as this relieves the pain and suppresses the disease progression. It has been reported that young active patients with isolated medial compartment disease and varus

A.A. Shetty et al. (eds.), *Techniques in Cartilage Repair Surgery*,
DOI 10.1007/978-3-642-41921-8_24, © ESSKA 2014

knee alignment have the highest likelihood of a good outcome with an osteotomy [2, 3]. This can delay, or potentially avoid, the need for a total knee arthroplasty.

The first report of successful tibial osteotomy in the English literature was written by Jackson and Waugh in 1961 [4]. Coventry et al. [5] and Insall et al. [6] subsequently reported their results with a closing wedge technique. Coventry modified the previously performed procedures by executing the osteotomy proximal to the tibial tubercle, which had several advantages – the osteotomy was performed closer to the area of the deformity, the bone involved was cancellous and tended to heal rapidly, and the patient could bear weight on the leg because the pull of the quadriceps stabilized the osteotomy. However, there are many potential complications of this method. Some complications include neurovascular injury, compartment syndrome, intra-articular fracture, infection, delayed union or nonunion, instability, recurrent varus deformity, and valgus overcorrection [7]. In addition, major corrections cause an offset of the proximal tibia that may compromise placement of the tibial component of a total knee arthroplasty.

An opening wedge technique was initially more popular in Europe, and Hernigou et al. [3] reported their long-term results in 1987. A major advantage of this technique is that it allows precise adjustment of angular correction intraoperatively. This technique may be less invasive, and it does not involve violation of the anterior compartment of the leg. In addition, dissection is away from the peroneal nerve, thereby decreasing the likelihood of injury. The proximal tibiofibular joint is not disturbed during this procedure. HTO has the advantages of maintaining the bone stock and correcting the deformity close to its origin, which may facilitate subsequent arthroplasty [6], and the osteotomy is technically easier. Disadvantages to this technique include the need for the bone graft to fill the osteotomy site. The options are iliac crest graft, allograft, and bone substitutes. Good results have been reported with hydroxyapatite wedges in conjunction with fibula autograft. In comparison with closing wedge osteotomies, there is an increased incidence for delayed union or nonunion and the loss of angular correction as the opening wedge osteotomy heals.

Recently, HTO has gained popularity after meniscal transplantation and cartilage-preserving surgeries. If malalignment is noted in a patient who is considered for meniscal transplantation, the realignment osteotomy is recommended in conjunction with meniscal transplantation. Verdonk et al. [8] published 10-year follow-up data on 42 meniscal allograft transplantations, of which 11 underwent concurrent HTO. Although all subgroups had substantial symptoms, the subgroup of medial meniscal transplant combined with HTO had a greater improvement than did the group undergoing isolated medial meniscal transplantation.

Cartilage-preserving surgery has advanced significantly in the past several years, with techniques such as microfracture, autologous chondrocyte implantation, and autologous osteochondral transplantation becoming more widespread. Good results have been reported, with comparable results for microfracture as well as autologous chondrocyte implantation at medium-term follow-up [9, 10]. However, isolated cartilage-preserving surgery is generally contraindicated in the setting of malalignment. Theoretically, this type of procedure would have a more favorable outcome if the healing cartilage surface was not subjected to the increased mechanical forces present in a malaligned knee. More recent work has shown the combination of HTO and microfracture to have good clinical outcomes at 2-year follow-up [11]. In this chapter, we will discuss the role of HTO in cartilage repair surgery. We routinely do medial-based opening wedge high tibial osteotomy fixed with TomoFix plate.

24.2 Indications and Contraindications of HTO in Cartilage Repair

Osteoarthrosis of the knee has many causative factors. Degenerative changes of the articular cartilage can occur through tension, compression, or shear. Malalignment into a varus position will overload the medial condyles of the femur and tibia. The rationale behind the osteotomy is to correct the angular deformity at the knee and therefore decrease the excessive weight-bearing load across the affected compartment that is the most involved by the degenerative process. The indications for the patients selected for proximal tibial osteotomy should have mostly unicompartmental OA with axial malalignment.

1. Young persons with chondral lesions in the medial compartment of knee with varus deformity and normal lateral compartment and normal patellofemoral joint with intact lateral meniscus are the best candidates for HTO. However, it is contraindicated in a patient with an open growth plate.
2. There is no definite chronological age below which one should undergo high tibial osteotomy. The age of 40–60 is the most suitable, but activity level, lifestyle, and general health must all be considered. Early treatment of the unicompartmental OA in relatively young patients is expected to produce better results when the articular changes are in the initial stage of the degenerative process.
3. BMI less than 30. Obesity has a negative effect on the outcome of surgery in many orthopedic operations. Most orthopedists would agree that excess body weight could make a patient better candidate for osteotomy than for arthroplasty, but it is also true that obesity will represent a negative factor in view of the possible general postoperative complications.
4. Osteotomy would be best performed for primarily unicompartmental OA in knees with generally well-maintained range of motion at least 100° of flexion, less than 10° of flexion contracture.
5. An intact lateral joint compartment and intact soft tissue covering of the medial head of the tibia were further preconditions.
6. Osteotomy should preferably not be performed in patients with rheumatoid arthritis, very unstable knees, or knees with greater than 20° of varus deformity, because, according to Insall [6], these knees are complicated by an associated severe ligamentous laxity and subluxation. A patient who has varus deformity and anterior cruciate ligament insufficiency may be treated with an anterior cruciate ligament reconstruction in addition to proximal tibial osteotomy.
7. HTO should not be done in patients with severe bone loss (more than a few millimeters) of the medial tibia or medial femur. When medial compartment bony support is insufficient, congruent weight bearing on both tibial plateaus after the osteotomy is not possible.
8. The presence of severe varus deformity (>20°) may be associated with subluxation of the tibia. Subluxation greater than 1 cm is an absolute contraindication to osteotomy.
9. Poor general medical condition, chronic smoker, inflammatory disease, severe osteoporosis, and bad peripheral vascular status (no foot pulse) are among the general contraindications to HTO.

24.3 Pre-op Evaluation

24.3.1 Clinical Examination

The goal of knee osteotomy is to realign the mechanical axis of the limb, thereby shifting weight-bearing forces from a diseased compartment to a more normal compartment. The subjective pain intensity was determined by means of a visual analogue scale (VAS) from 0 to 10 (0 = no pain, 10 = unbearable pain). Knee range of motion should be evaluated because outcomes have been shown to deteriorate with diminished levels of knee flexion [12].

The Radiological Documentation Included

1. Double-leg-standing AP radiograph of the entire lower limb with patella facing forwards: To draw the mechanical axis and calculate the amount of varus correction needed (Fig. 24.1)
2. Standard supine AP and lateral view: To assess the lateral laxity by comparing the joint line convergent angle (Fig. 24.2) of the standing and supine films and calculate the posterior tibial slope in lateral view (Fig. 24.3)

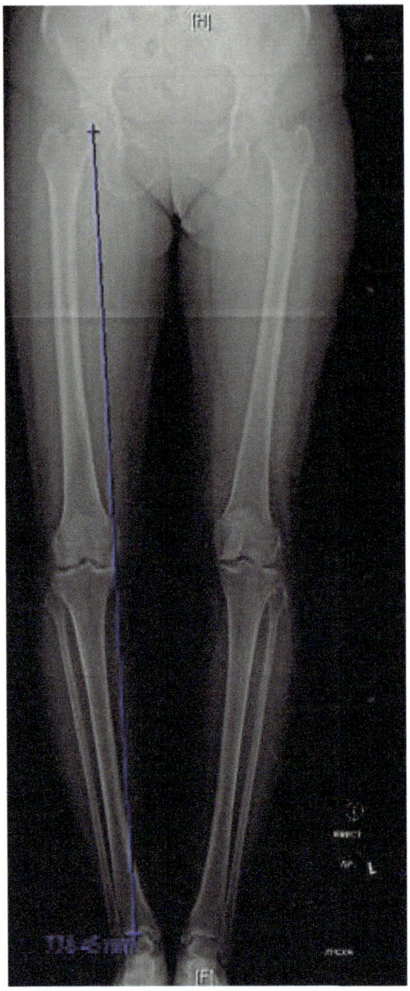

Fig. 24.1 Mechanical axis showing varus malalignment

3. Skyline view: Used to assess the patellofemoral articulation
4. MRI knee for cartilage sequence: To assess the size, area, and thickness of chondral lesion and to check the integrity of the other intra-articular structures.

24.3.2 Preoperative Planning

For the preoperative planning, we use an AP long-leg weight-bearing radiograph. The measurement of the mechanical axis is a line drawn from the center of the femoral head to the center of the ankle mortise. In normal knee the mechanical axis

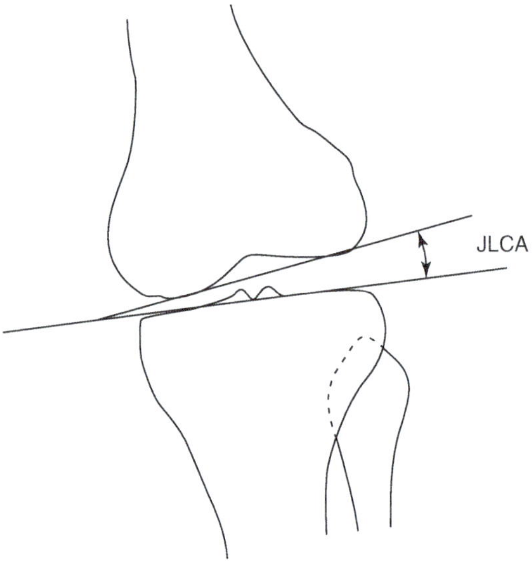

Fig. 24.2 The JLCA is formed by a line tangent to the distal femoral condyles and a line tangent to the tibial plateau

passes through the center of the joint or slightly varus (approximately 1° medially). In varus malalignment, the mechanical axis passes the tibial plateau more medially than the physiological mechanical axis deviation (MAD) of 10 mm. The anatomic axis is a line drawn through the center of the shaft of the femur and through the center of the shaft of the tibia. In the normal knee, the two lines cross each other in the center of the joint, making an angle of 5° (physiologic valgus). According to these parameters as the reference points of "normality," the deformity is measured. In the setting of the treatment of an isolated medial femoral chondral injury associated with malalignment, it is unclear whether knees will have better outcomes if overcorrected into valgus or simply corrected into physiologic alignment. Recent biomechanical work has shown that the medial compartment is completely unloaded with correction to between 6° and 10° of anatomic valgus and that the load is equalized between the medial and lateral compartments, with correction to between 0° and 4° of anatomic valgus. The study's authors recommended from these biomechanical data that treatment for varus gonarthrosis be overcorrection of the mechanical axis and that treatment for isolated medial femoral condyle chondral injuries

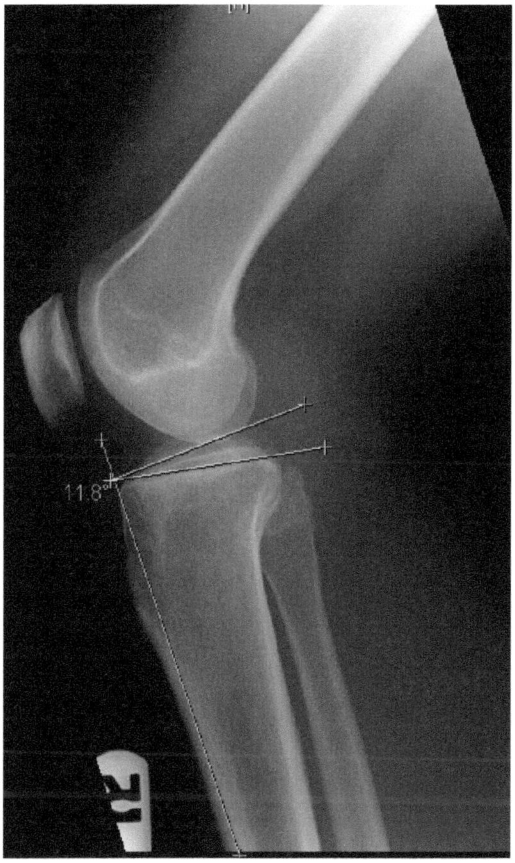

Fig. 24.3 Radiograph showing the angle of inclination of the tibial plateau according to the MH method using three lines. The *first green* is tangential to the tibial crest, the *second blue* is tangential to the proximal tibial articular surface, and the *third line* is perpendicular to the line of the tibial crest. The angle formed by the second and the third lines is equivalent to the posteroinferior slope of the plateau

involves only correction to physiologic alignment as opposed to overcorrection [13].

The first step is to draw the mechanical axis line from the center of the femoral head to the center of the talus. Next, a line that is parallel to the tibial plateau is drawn. A third line is drawn with the desired mechanical axis from the center of the femoral head to a point 62 % lateral on the transverse diameter of the tibial plateau [14]. The line of the desired mechanical axis is continued to the center of the ankle in its postoperative position. The center of rotation of angulation (CORA-D) lies in the lateral cortex at the tip of the fibula. Line DS connects CORA with the middle of the ankle joint. Line DS′ is drawn from CORA to the center of the ankle in its postoperative position and crosses the desired mechanical axis at the center of the ankle. The angle between lines DS and DS′ forms the correction angle (alpha). This correction angle (alpha) is transposed over the proposed osteotomy site (DO-DO′) which will give the amount of opening osteotomy (O-O′) (Fig. 24.4). The other way is to use the TomoFix bone spreader, which measures the angle of opening directly.

When there is severe ligamentous laxity, to plan the operation on radiographs made with the patient standing can lead to overcorrection, a potentially greater problem than undercorrection. If clinical examination showed ligamentous laxity, then calculate the joint line convergence angle, which is formed by a line tangent to the distal femoral condyles and a line tangent to the tibial plateau [15]. A single-leg weight-bearing full radiograph and a double-leg full radiograph, always in standing position, are obtained to measure the lower limb alignment. The difference in the joint line convergence angle between the two radiographs represents the component of malalignment due to ligamentous laxity. To prevent overcorrection, the soft tissue laxity is subtracted from the overall valgus correction.

24.3.3 Anesthesia

The operation is performed under spinal or general anesthesia with or without femoral block. Intravenous antibiotic prophylaxis is used according to hospital guidelines.

24.3.4 Positioning of the Patient

We prefer a normal operating table with the patient in a supine position and the C-arm of an image intensifier set up opposite the surgeon. Position the patient in such a way that the hip, knee, and ankle joint can be visualized with the image intensifier. The patient is draped as usual in knee surgery. The tourniquet is applied well proximal over the thigh (Fig. 24.5).

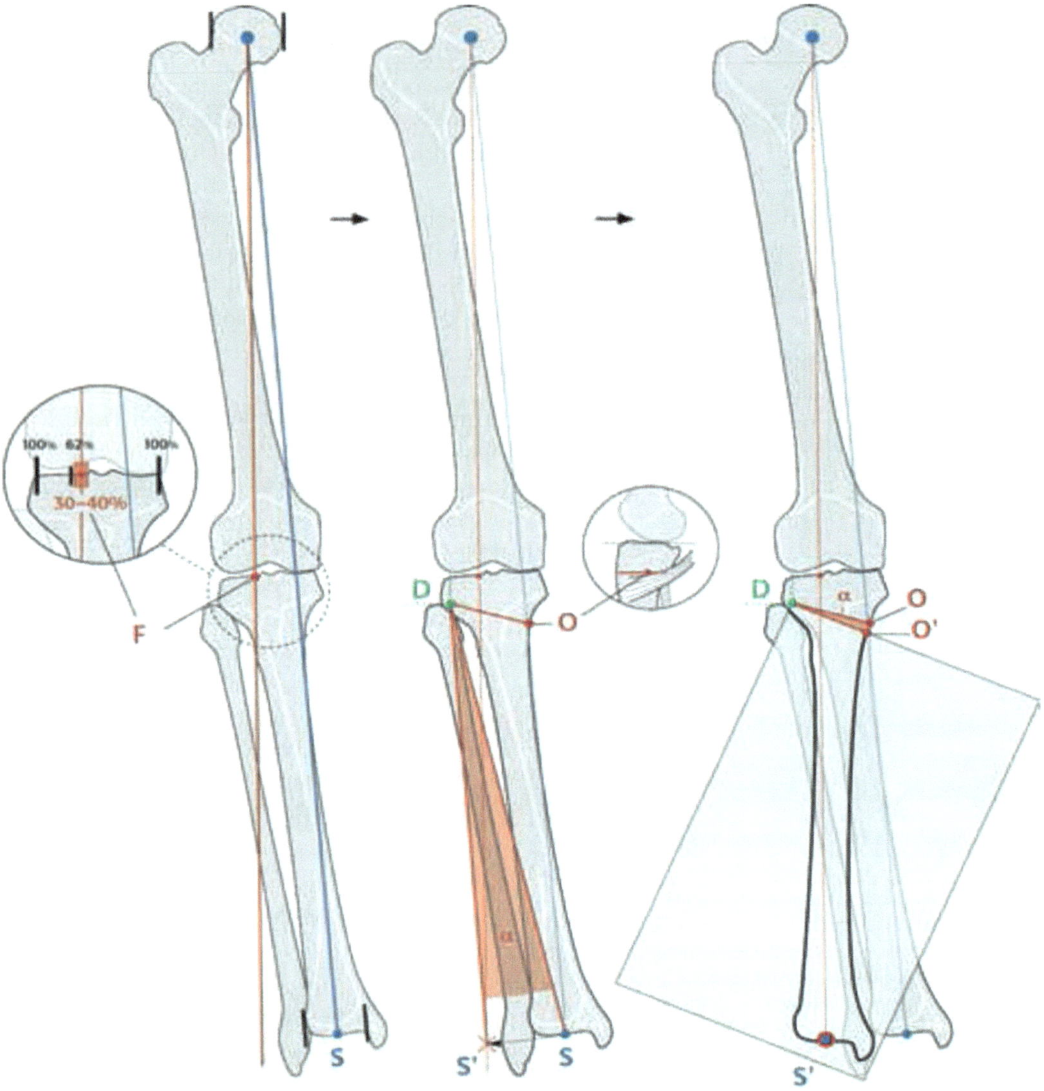

Fig. 24.4 Preoperative planning of the osteotomy. Overcorrection of the new mechanical axis according the work of Fujisawa (From AO folder p. 4)

24.3.5 Surface Markings

The surface markings of patella, patellar tendon, tibial tuberosity, medial joint line, and posteromedial border of proximal tibia are identified and marked with knee in 90° flexion (Fig. 24.6).

24.3.6 Techniques

The osteotomy we propose here is based on the opening wedge technique. We used new fixation device (TomoFix™) with an adapted surgical technique which allows stable fixation of the osteotomy. The procedure begins with examination under arthroscopy.

24.3.7 Arthroscopy

To ensure an intact lateral joint compartment and to treat additional intra-articular lesions, a knee arthroscopy is first performed on every patient to assess the cartilage lesion, degree of involvement of the other compartment, and the cruciate ligaments and meniscus. Debridement of the cartilage

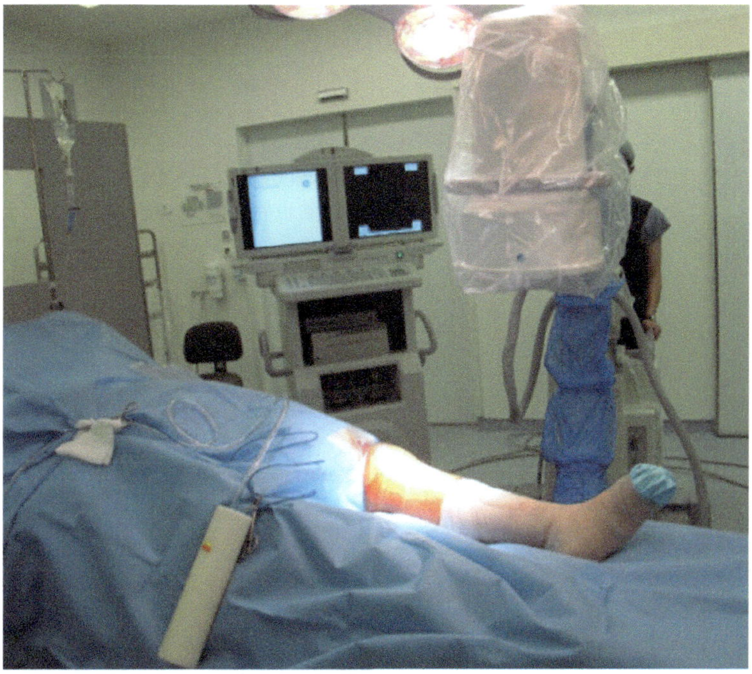

Fig. 24.5 Supine position and the C-arm of an image intensifier set up opposite the surgeon

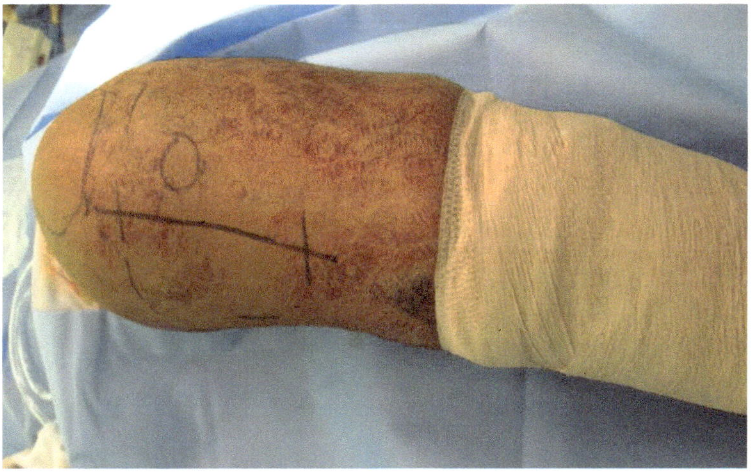

Fig. 24.6 Surface markings with knee in 90° flexion

lesion and microfracture is done in a standard way. Meniscal tears, loose bodies, osteophytes, and chondral flaps can cause mechanical symptoms that can be treated successfully with arthroscopy.

24.3.8 Incision and Exposure

After diagnostic knee arthroscopy, when indicated, a 5-cm vertical skin incision is made over the anteromedial aspect of the tibia, 2 cm medial to the tibial tuberosity starting from 1 cm below the joint line. The incision is performed directly down to the bone. A subperiosteal dissection is performed anteriorly under the patellar tendon and posteriorly deep to the pes anserinus tendons and superficial medial collateral ligament. Release of the more anterior fibers of the tibial attachment of the superficial medial collateral ligament is performed to place a Hohmann's retractor under the posterior surface of the tibia to protect the neurovascular bundle during osteotomy (Figs. 24.7 and 24.8). In a biomechanical study under reproducible dynamic loading conditions

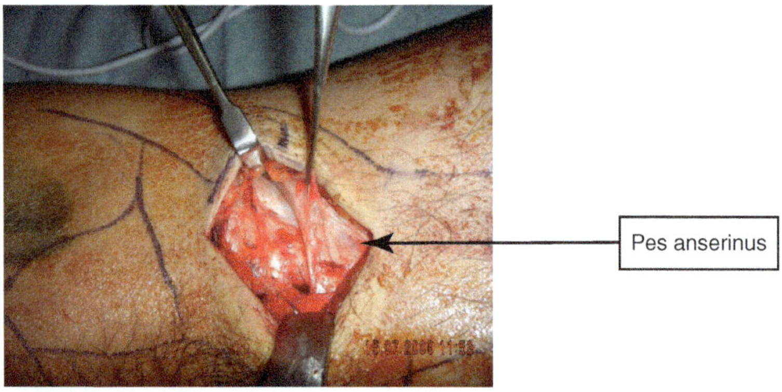

Fig. 24.7 Pes anserinus elevation

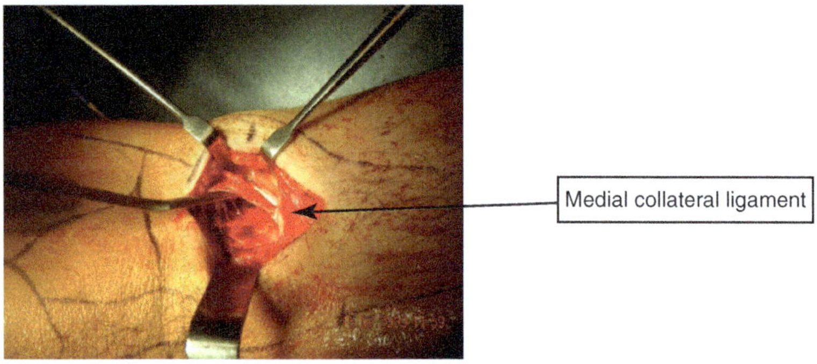

Fig. 24.8 Hohmann's retractor under the medial collateral ligament

using pressure-sensitive films with the corrected axis running through the "Fujisawa point," the load changed only after the complete release of the MCL from medial to lateral (64 %) [16].

24.4 Osteotomy

Position the knee in such a way to get the true AP view of the tibial plateau. This step is very crucial to do the osteotomy in the correct direction. The direction of the osteotomy in the frontal plane was marked with a 2.5-mm threaded K-wire under fluoroscopic control starting from 4 cm below the medial joint line, driven obliquely upward, laterally towards the tip of the fibular head (Fig. 24.9). There should be at least 1 cm of bone below the lateral tibial plateau to prevent intra-articular fracture during osteotomy [2]. Because the proximal tibia is sloped posteriorly, the osteotomy should be made in an oblique fashion to maintain an adequate bridge of bone along the posterior cortex of the tibia to facilitate the plate fixation [17].

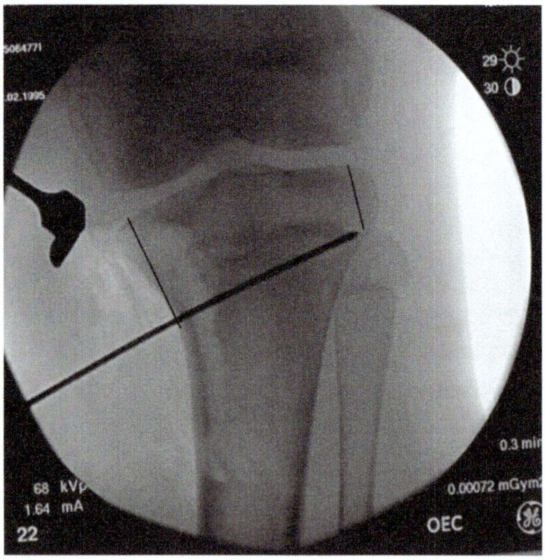

Fig. 24.9 Guidewire placement, 4 cm below the joint line, directed towards the tip of fibula

Mark the posterior 2/3 and anterior 1/3 of the medial surface of the tibia just below the guidewire. The first osteotomy is done in the posterior 2/3, parallel to the tibial slope, and ended 1 cm

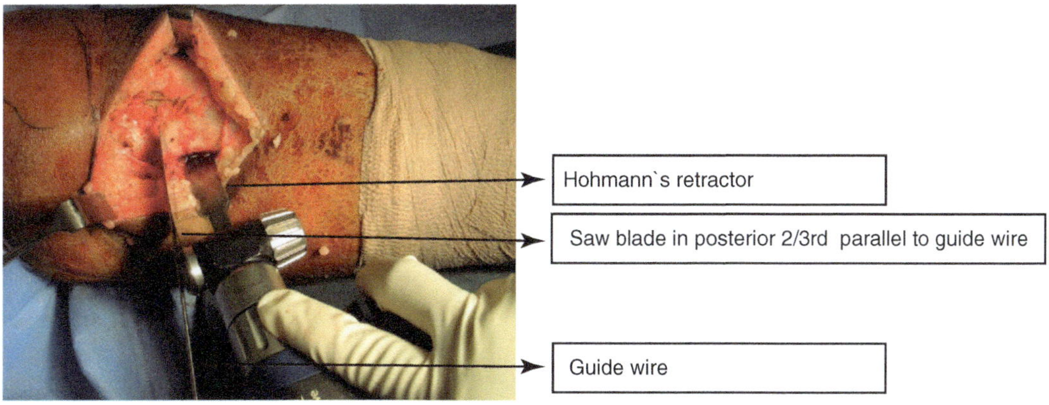

Fig. 24.10 Osteotomy blade below the guidewire, parallel to tibial slope, while Hohmann's retractor placed posteriorly

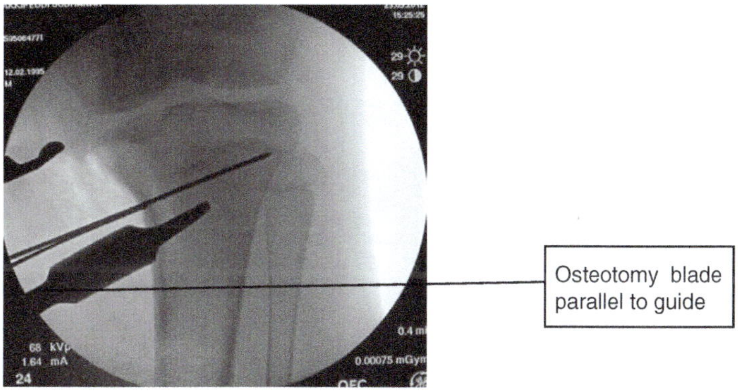

Fig. 24.11 End on view of the saw blade

from the lateral cortical margin at the level of the tip of the fibula. The saw blade is placed immediately below the guidewire to avoid proximal migration osteotomy into the joint. The saw blade should be adjusted to get an end on view in the image before starting the osteotomy (Figs. 24.10 and 24.11). This step is very important to make the posterior cut parallel to the tibial slope.

The neurovascular structures are protected with Hohmann's retractor until the completion of the posterior osteotomy. The parallelism between the saw blade and guidewire is checked intermittently under image. The saw is advanced slowly and intermittently with continuous cold-water irrigation to prevent thermal necrosis. The strong posteromedial cortex is osteotomized completely without violating the lateral tibial cortex as it is the hinge for correction. The osteotomy should be done within 1–1.5 cm from the lateral cortex to avoid loss of hinge which will lead to unstable situation (Figs. 24.12 and 24.13). This complication can be avoided by constantly checking under II (image intensifier).

The second anterior osteotomy is performed bicortically at 135° to the first osteotomy, angled upwards, proximal to tibial tuberosity, like a V shape. At least 1.5 cm thickness of tibial tuberosity should be maintained to prevent the fracture (Fig. 24.14)

24.4.1 Opening the Osteotomy Gap

Osteotomy gap should be opened gradually over several minutes in order to prevent the fracture of the lateral cortex. A chisel is inserted below the guidewire and advanced gradually up to the entire length of osteotomy, taking precautions not to

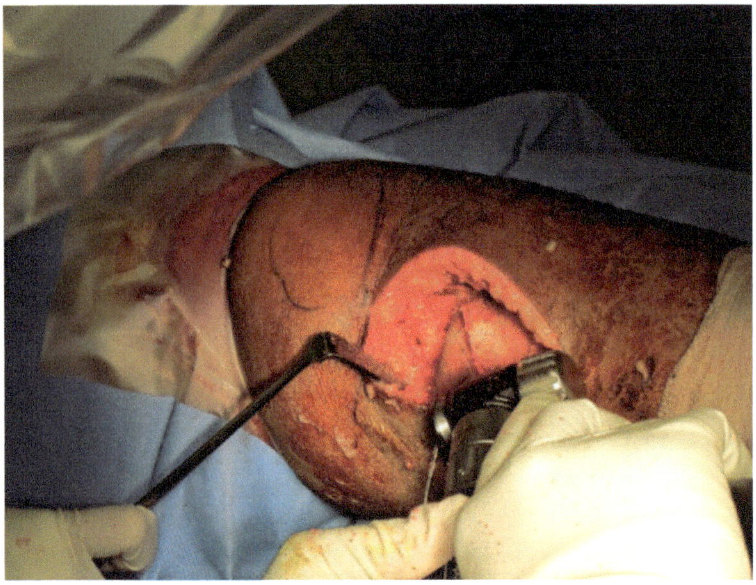

Fig. 24.12 Posterior 2/3 osteotomy

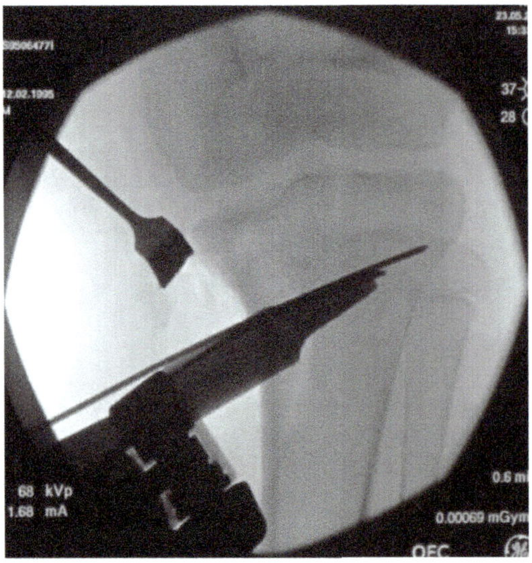

Fig. 24.13 Posterior 2/3 osteotomy to within 1–1.5 cm from the lateral cortex

fracture the lateral hinge. The second chisel is inserted in between the first one and the guidewire, advanced until it reaches few mm lesser length than the first one. Insert the third chisel between the other two but to a lesser length. This *stacking technique* gradually opens the osteotomy, leaving the lateral tibial cortex intact (Figs. 24.15 and 24.16).

Now, the chisels and guidewire are removed and the TomoFix bone spreader is inserted gradually until it reaches the lateral hinge. The spreader is opened slowly over a period until the desired opening angle is reached. The readings on the TomoFix bone spreader will directly give the angle of correction (Figs. 24.17, 24.18 and 24.19). Now, the alignment is checked with the leg in full extension and proper rotation using the cable method or alignment rod. The osteotomy gap is fine-tuned to get the mechanical axis through a point 62 % lateral on the transverse diameter of the tibial plateau.

The TomoFix bone spreader is removed and the lamina spreader is inserted anteriorly while the assistant is opening the osteotomy gently with valgus force (Fig. 24.20).The lamina spreader is opened gradually while maintaining the valgus force until the osteotomy gap opens sufficiently such that the chromos wedge can be inserted.

The selected chronOS bone wedge is inserted posteriorly to fill the osteotomy gap.

Placing the graft posteriorly is important to maintain the normal tibial slope (Fig. 24.21).

The bone spreader is removed and the prepared TomoFix plate is positioned 1 cm below the joint line on the medial surface of the tibia. Avoid placing the plate too anteriorly as doing so

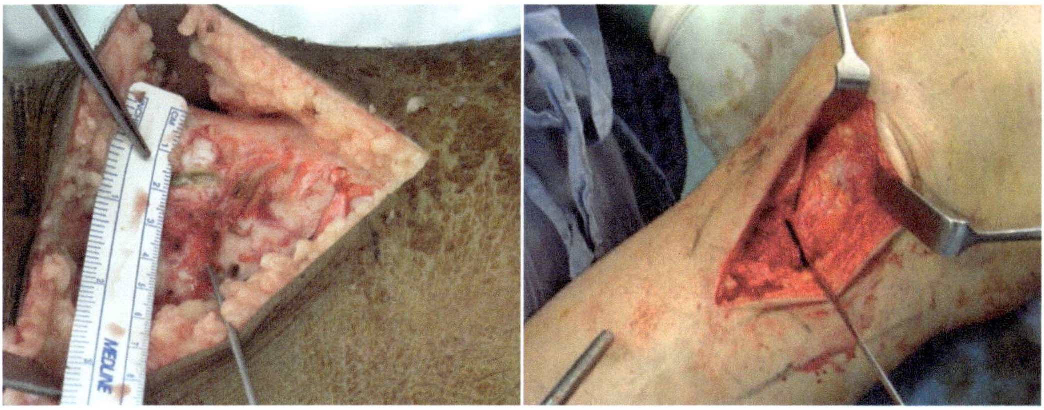

Fig. 24.14 Anterior osteotomy 135° to the posterior cut and 1.5 cm behind the tibial tuberosity, directed proximal to the tubercle

Fig. 24.15 Stacking technique with three chisels

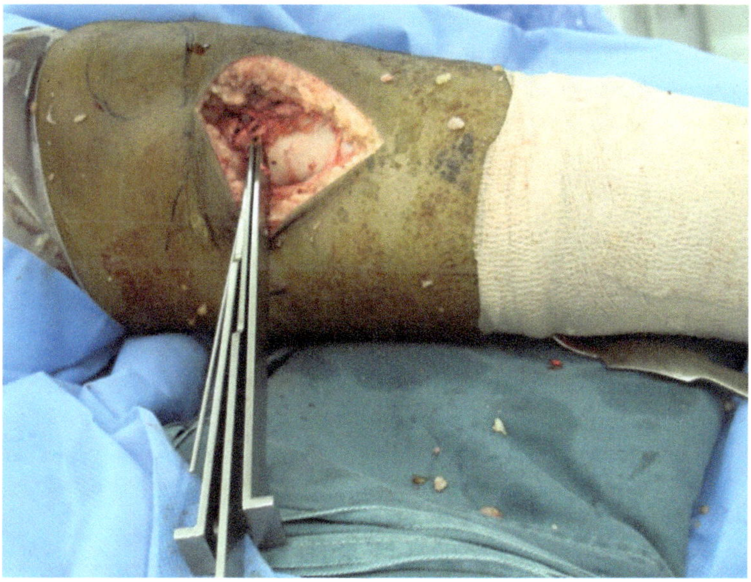

will increase the tibial slope. Likewise, placing the plate too posteriorly will decrease the slope. The plate is held temporarily with K-wires used proximally and distally. Locking screws are inserted according to the standard principles of locking plate. The final alignment is checked under image intensifier (Figs. 24.22 and 24.23). While the wound is irrigated, take care not to wash away the bone graft and the hematoma in the osteotomy gap. Then, it is closed over a drain without suction. Sterile compression dressings are applied.

24.4.2 Postoperative Follow-Up

After the operation, the knee is immobilized in a hinged knee brace in full extension or at flexion of approximately 10°, which allows full range of movements when unlocked. Passive flexion as well as extension in a continuous passive motion device is started the day after surgery. The drains are removed 48 h later. The patients are allowed to walk with touchdown weight bearing from second postoperative day and are discharged from the hospital in 4–5 days. Range of motion exercises and muscle strengthening exercises are encouraged. Plain X-rays are taken at 6 weeks postoperatively, and if healing is adequate, progressive weight bearing is allowed. Usually the bracing is discontinued at 6 weeks and weight bearing is increased gradually to full weight bearing. The weight-bearing radiographs are taken at the 6th, 12th week, and the 6th month to ensure maintenance of correction and healing (Fig. 24.24).

24.4.3 Complications and Troubleshooting

Intra-articular Fracture

Malpositioning of the guidewire closer to the lateral tibial plateau will lead to intra-articular fracture (Fig. 24.25). This can be avoided by perfect positioning of the guidewire not less than 1 cm

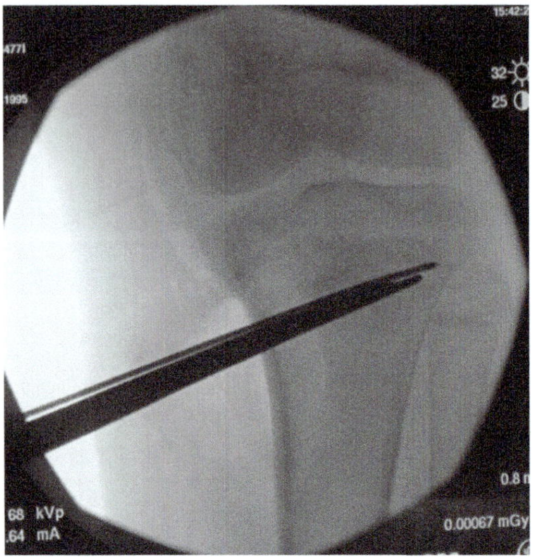

Fig. 24.16 Placement of the chisel

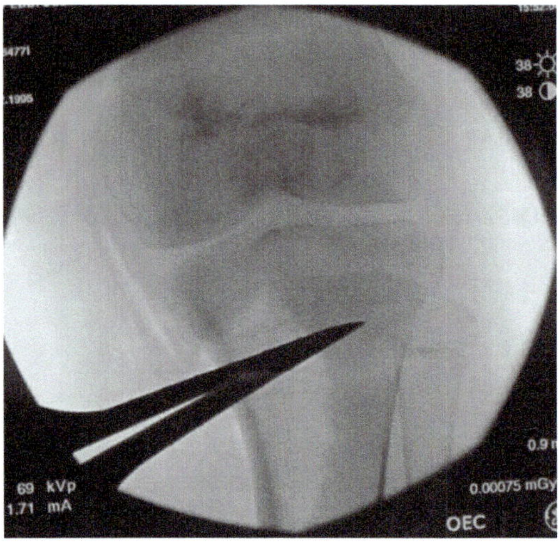

Fig. 24.18 The TomoFix bone spreader position checked with image

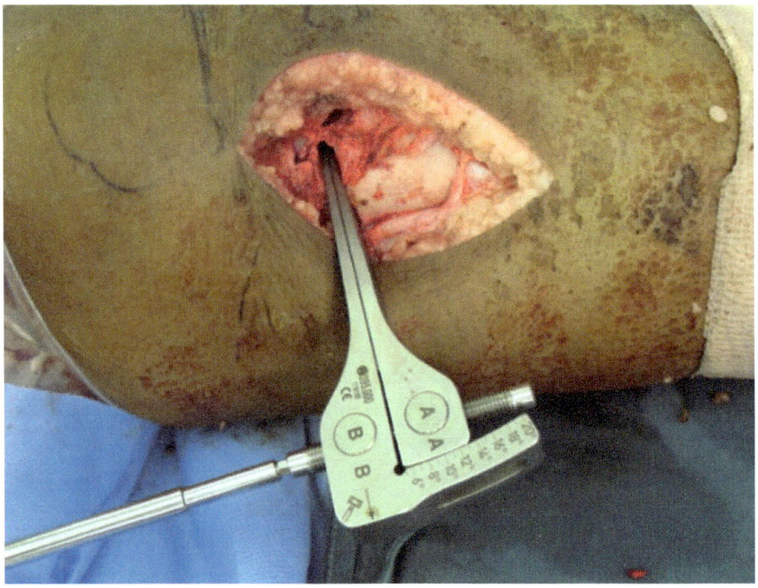

Fig. 24.17 TomoFix bone spreader

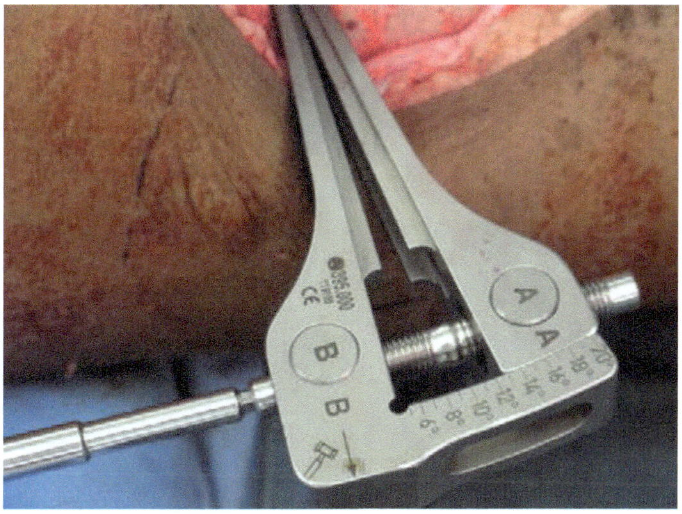

Fig. 24.19 The TomoFix bone spreader is calibrated to desired angle

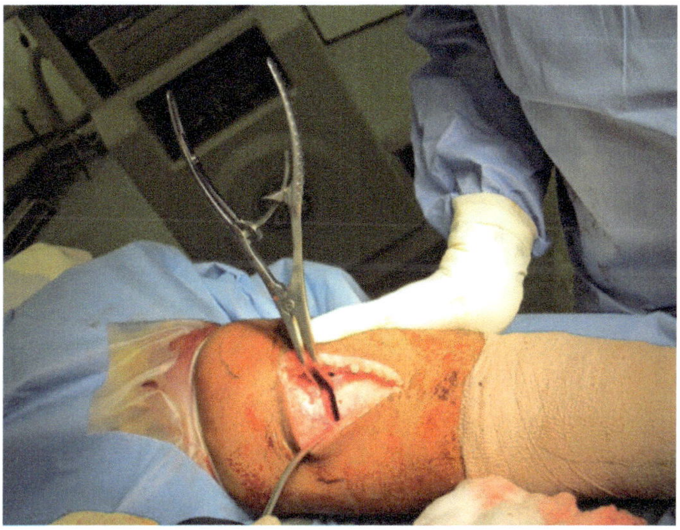

Fig. 24.20 Lamina spreader in place

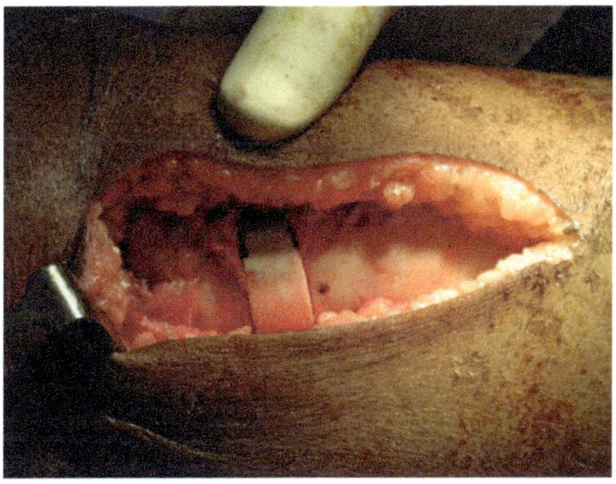

Fig. 24.21 Osteotomy gap filled with chronOS bone wedge posteriorly

below the lateral tibial plateau. The incidence of fracture is high if the wire is placed less than 1 cm away [18, 19]. Always do the osteotomy below the guidewire as the wire prevents the proximal migration of the osteotomy into the joint. Do not open the osteotomy without completely cutting the posteromedial tibial cortex. If fracture occurs, it can be managed by fixing through the proximal screws of the plate.

Loss of Lateral Hinge

An intact bony hinge is essential for the stability and when correctly preserved it prevents the osteotomy from any possible dislocation. If the hinge

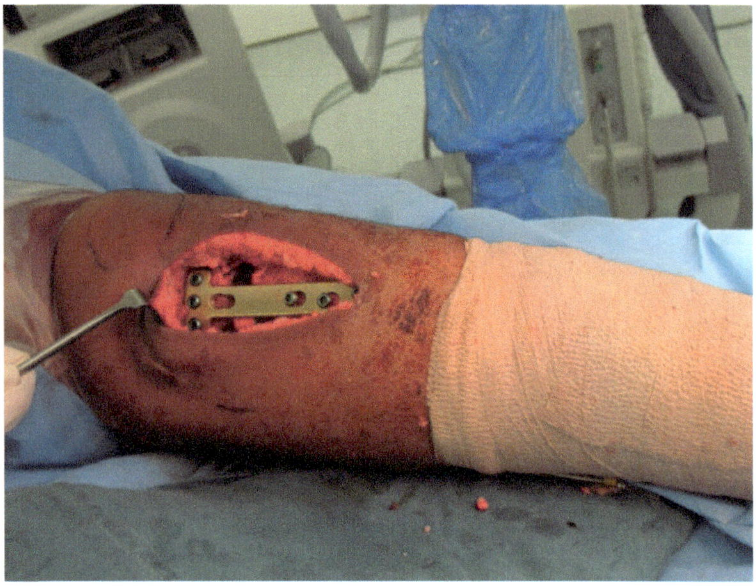

Fig. 24.22 TomoFix plate in place

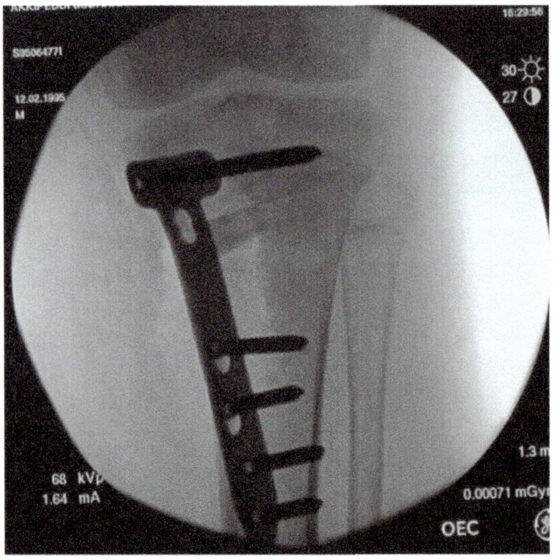

Fig. 24.23 Final image after fixation

is lost, then osteotomy becomes unstable. It needs staple fixation by another lateral incision or fixation through the proximal screws (Fig. 24.26).

This complication can be prevented by proper selection of the osteotomy site and careful monitoring under image during the osteotomy. The osteotomy should be proximal enough in the tibia to avoid maximum step-off of the bone profile and to address a more stable fixation.

Neurovascular Damage

Injuries to the vessels are not frequent. This could be safely protected by correct use of a Hohmann's retractor posteriorly or by keeping the knee flexed during the osteotomy. However, Zaidi et al. shows that flexion of the knee does not move the popliteal artery away from the tibia. It remains vulnerable to injury during high tibial osteotomy [20].

Delayed Union, Nonunion, and Loss of Angular Correction

This is a rare complication as the cancellous bone heals better. Heavy smokers and individuals with generalized bone disorders may be at risk. In comparison with closing wedge techniques, there is an increased potential for delayed union or nonunion, as well as for the loss of angular correction as the opening wedge osteotomy heals. By proper selection of the patients, this issue can be avoided.

Alteration of Tibial Slope

Tibial slope refers to the angle created by a line drawn from the anterior aspect to the posterior aspect of the proximal tibial plateau with a perpendicular line down the tibial diaphysis on a lateral radiograph. The normal posterior tibial slope is $10° \pm 3°$. During the operation, there was

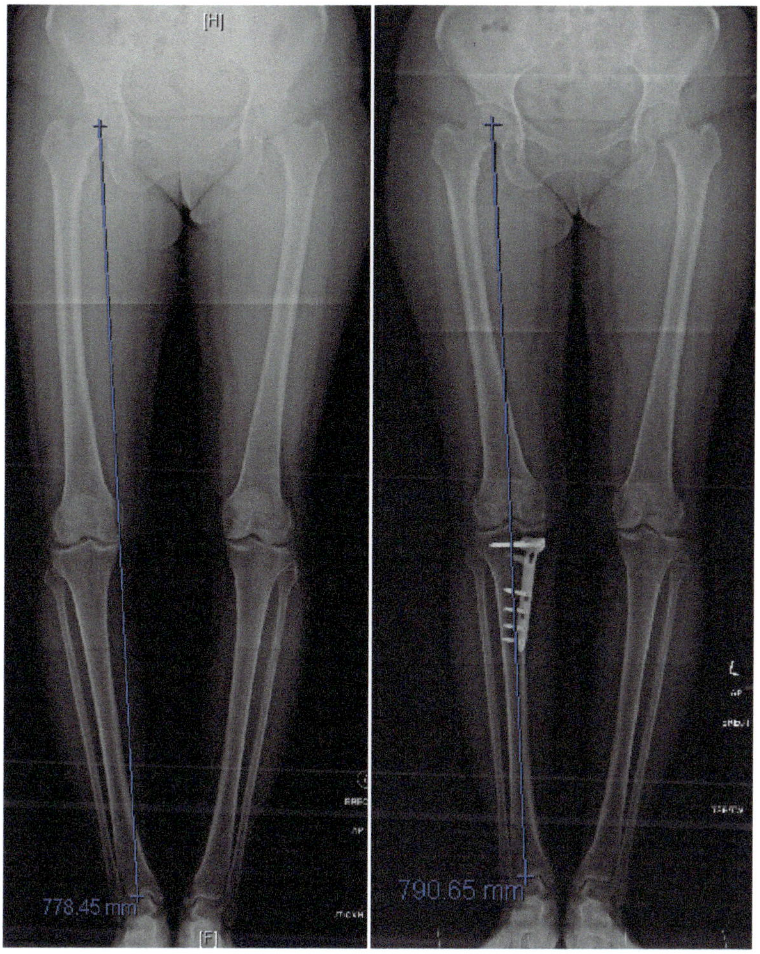

Fig. 24.24 Preoperative and 6 months postoperative X-ray showing mechanical axis

a tendency for the slope to enlarge, as the strong medio-dorsal ligaments and the pes anserinus act against the opening of the osteotomy (Fig. 24.27). To prevent flexion malalignment, soft tissue release should be carried out, especially in the case of contract medial capsule and ligaments. This complication can be avoided by making the posterior osteotomy parallel to posterior slope and placing the graft posteriorly. Positioning the plate too anteriorly will result in increased tibial slope and vice versa. The fixation system is the most stressed in the dorsal area of the osteotomy, as the plate lies anteromedial and there is no primary bone contact in the posterior aspect of the osteotomy. This relative instability was shown by a frequently visible formation of callus at the posterior cortex [17].

Patella Baja

In lateral closing wedge osteotomy, patella baja (decreased patellar height) may be caused by interstitial scarring of the patella ligament and new bone formation behind the patellar ligament in the site of the osteotomy, as well as contracture in and around the patellar ligament because of immobilization [21]. This can be minimized by rigid fixation early mobilization of knee joint [22]. In medial opening wedge osteotomy, distalization of the tibial tuberosity and a relative elevation of the joint line may lead to patella baja (Fig. 24.28). Patellar tracking may also be affected by HTO. This may result in anterior knee pain, and it may increase the risk of patellofemoral osteoarthritis due to increased contact stress across the patellofemoral joint. The effects

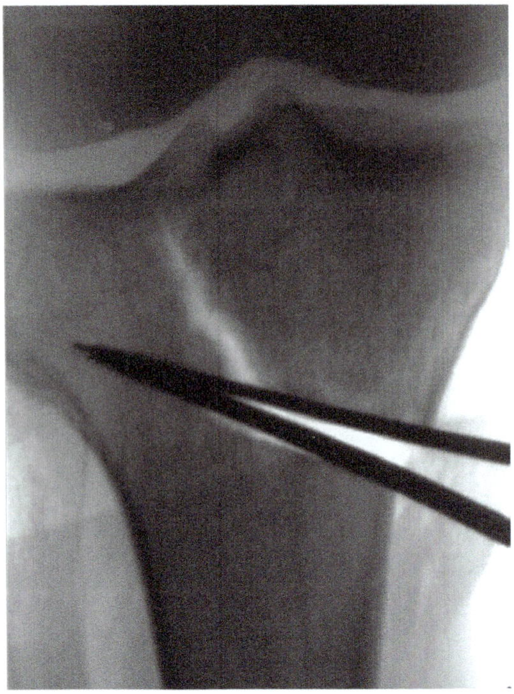

Fig. 24.25 Intra-articular fracture due to early opening up of osteotomy without cutting the posterior cortex

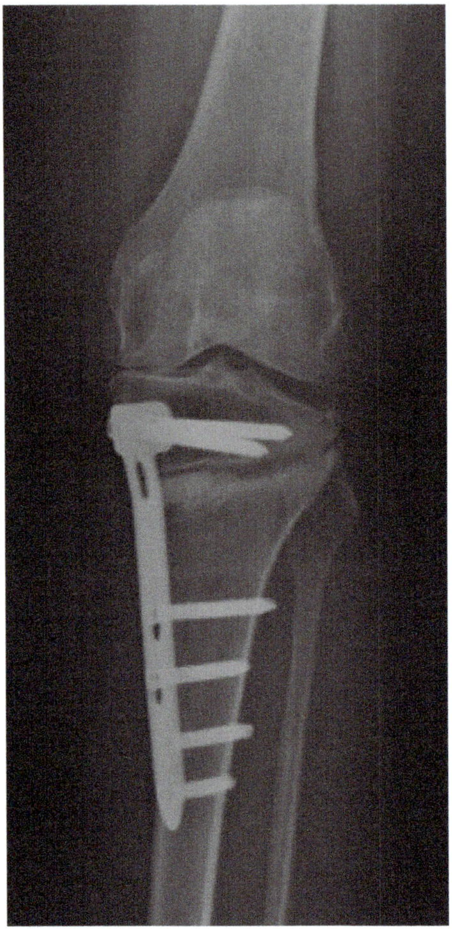

Fig. 24.26 Loss of lateral hinge, fixed with the proximal screws of the plate

of HTO on patellar height and patellar tracking may be of minimal clinical relevance, but in extensive opening wedge corrections, the effects may be quite large and adversely affect the patellofemoral joint [23]. Medial opening wedge osteotomy below the tibial tuberosity can be performed to avoid patella infera in varus knees, which may have a protective effect on the patellofemoral joint [24].

24.5 Adjuvant Tibial Tuberosity Osteotomy (TTO) for the Treatment of Patellofemoral Chondral Ulcer: Technical Details

24.5.1 Introduction

Patellofemoral cartilage lesions are due to different causes including sports trauma, traffic accidents, osteochondritis dissecans, patellofemoral malalignment and idiopathic chondromalacia. Patellofemoral malalignment encompasses a number of conditions, isolated or variously associated, such as increased Q-angle, high-riding patella (patella alta), trochlear dysplasia, increased femoral anteversion, excessive tension of lateral retinaculum, absence of medial patellofemoral ligament and vastus medialis obliquus hypotrophy [25–27]. Such disorders lead to altered articular congruence between patella and femoral trochlea that often progresses to severe cartilage damage of one or both patellar facets. Some cartilage defects are thought to be related to patellofemoral malalignment. In such cases the malalignment may be the source of knee pain and disability, and the cause of progression to patellofemoral osteoarthritis.

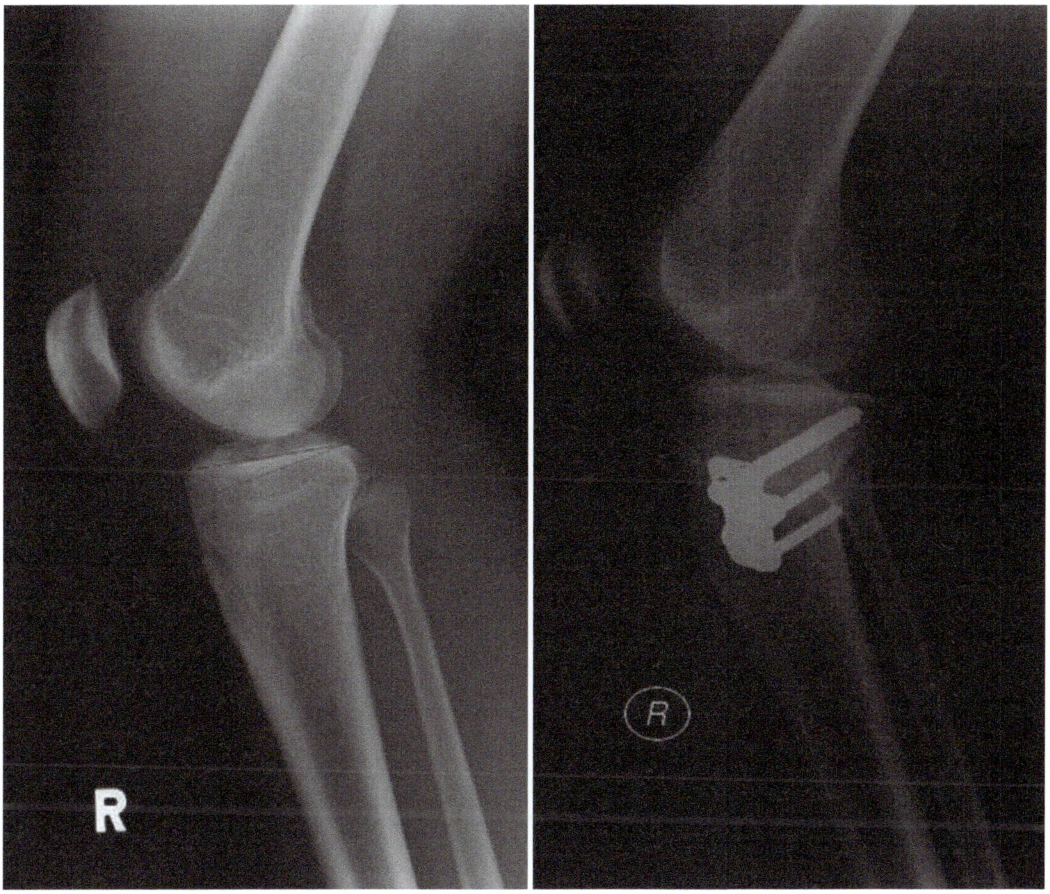

Fig. 24.27 Pre-op and post-op X-rays showing increase in tibial inclination which prevents the full extension

Realigning the extensor mechanism at the level of the tibial tubercle improves patellar tracking and unloads overloaded patellar articular surfaces [28, 29]. Numerous surgical techniques have been described in the literature to treat patellofemoral (PF) pain, chondrosis, and instability. The most notable include medialization, initially described by Roux and later popularized by Elmslie and Trillat, for the treatment of PF instability [30, 31] and anteriorization of the tibial tubercle described by Maquet [32] performed to treat PF pain associated with arthritis. Each of these procedures takes advantage of important technical alterations in patellar kinematics. Anteriorization of the tubercle elevates the distal extensor mechanism and serves to shift patellar contact forces proximally, while medialization results in a decrease of the lateral force vector. Fulkerson originally designed a tubercle osteotomy known as the anteromedialization (AMZ) to address patellofemoral chondrosis in conjunction with patellofemoral tilt and/or chronic patella sublaxation while avoiding complications of the Maquet technique [33]. This technique decrease in resultant force and increase in contact area would thus decrease joint surface stress, potentially decreasing the condition of overload contributing to pain [34].

The importance of anteromedialization technique for cartilage restoration procedure, which can optimize/minimize joint surface stress, was not realized initially. Brittberg et al. demonstrated poor result of autologous cultured chondrocyte implantation for treatment of patellofemoral cartilage defects when this joint surface stress factors was not taken into consideration [35].

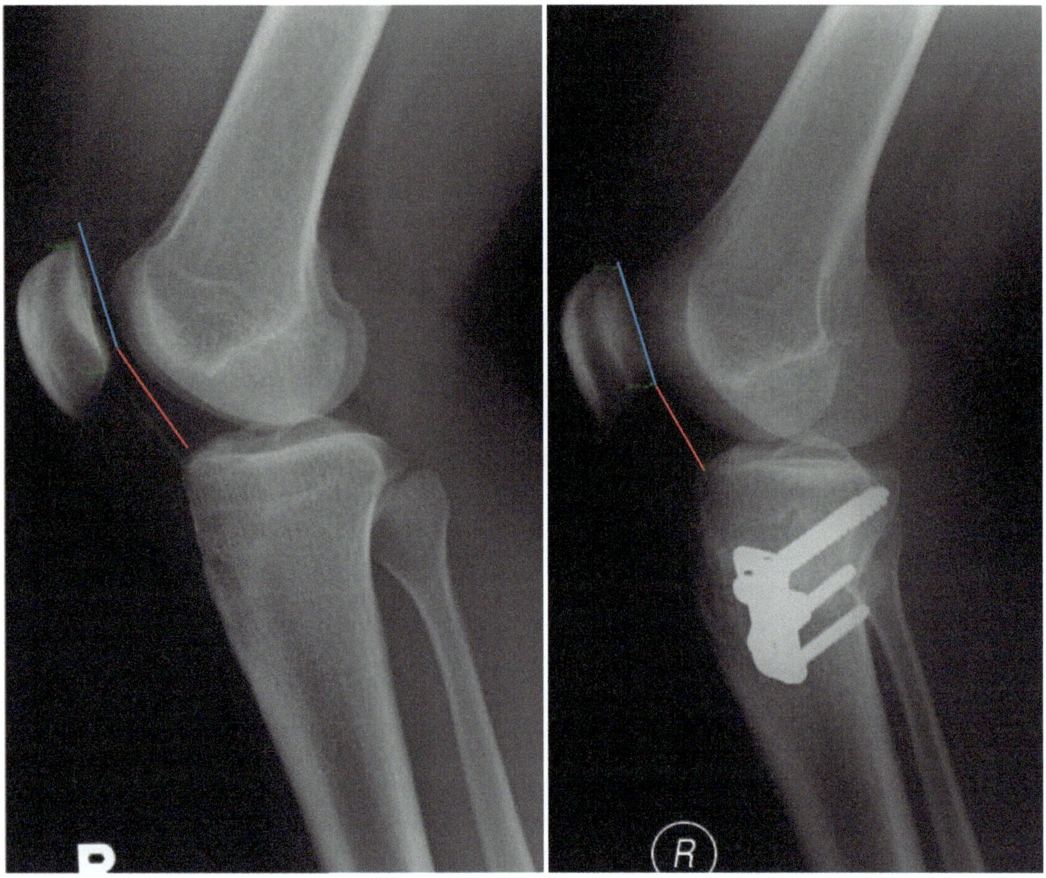

Fig. 24.28 Caton-Deschamps ratio (red/blue) showing patella baja after high tibial osteotomy

Although no randomized studies compared isolated AMZ to AMZ with cartilage restoration, the improved patient score of patellofemoral chondrosis treated with AMZ and cartilage restoration reported by Minas and Bryant are promising [36]. Other authors also have demonstrated superior results of combining AMZ with PF cartilage restorative procedures such as autologous chondrocyte implantation and osteoarticular grafting procedures within the PF compartment to either procedure performed independently [37–40]. According to Pidoriano et al., anteromedialization of the tibial tubercle improves knee function and relieves anterior knee pain in 90 and 85 % of type I and II patellar cartilage lesions (inferior pole and lateral facet), respectively, with lower success rates for type III (medial facet, 56 %) and type IV defects (proximal pole or diffuse lesions, 20 %) [41]. Gigante et al. also reported significant clinical improvement after 36 months of distal realignment and autologous chondrocyte implantation in treating large, isolated, patellar cartilage lesions associated with patellofemoral malalignment [42].

24.5.2 Patient Selection: Indications and Contraindications

Conservative treatment including rehabilitation program, bracing, and orthotics should be optimized before considering surgical intervention for patient with PF pain or maltracking. When standard conservative measures have failed, surgical intervention followed by careful rehabilitation often is successful if the underlying pathomechanics can be identified and addressed surgically. Patellofemoral chondral disease represents a spectrum with differing severities of altered loading, subluxation, chondrosis, or arthrosis. Indications for tibial tuberosity osteotomy (TTO) are primarily based upon mechanical and chondral pathologies specific to each individual knee. A TT–TG distance of 15 mm is considered normal; values of 20 mm are abnormal and should be considered for a tibial tubercle osteotomy [26, 43]. The optimal candidate for TTO are patients with isolated chondrosis of the distal or lateral patella, who have excessive lateral patellar tilt and/or subluxation associated with an increased TT–TG distance and minimal trochlear [35] chondrosis. This surgical technique also can be used as an adjunct procedure to patellofemoral cartilage restoration in an effort to improve the contact area and decrease PF forces to optimize the biomechanical environment of the new cartilage implant.

The contraindications include certain location of chondrosis as demonstrated by Pidoriano et al. [41]. Anteromedialization of tibial tubercle should be avoided in cases when the patellar chondrosis was medial, proximal, diffuse or with central trochlear or/and patellar involvement. It is also contraindicated in patients with a normal TT–TG distance and in patients who have symptoms not explained by an increased TT–TG distance. Standard contraindications to any osteotomy must also be considered, which includes smoking, infection, inflammatory arthropathy, marked osteoporosis inhibiting adequate fixation, complex regional pain syndrome, arthrofibrosis, inability to minimally weight-bear, and noncompliant patients.

24.5.3 Preoperative Preparation

The expected outcomes, risks, benefits, and potential complications are reviewed with the patient and his or her family by the surgeon. Proper history and thorough physical examination will be done by the surgeon. Patient imaging routinely begins by obtaining conventional radiographs as a screening tool: standing anteroposterior (AP), 45° flexion posteroanterior (PA "Rosenberg"), flexion lateral, shallow angle axial (Merchant), and long leg coronal alignment radiographs. To accurately assess patella subluxation, computed tomography (CT) of the patellofemoral joint is performed. It also allows calculation of desired anteromedialization based on the tibial tubercle to trochlear groove (TT–TG) distance. Anteriorization of between 10 and 15 mm decreases PF stress loads by approximately 20 % and results in minimal sagittal rotation of the patella, while medialization of 10–15 mm will normalize the TT–TG distance [26, 44]. For assessment of articular injury, MRI will provide information and will guide the type of cartilage repair; however, arthroscopy remains a gold standard procedure to assess chondral lesion.

24.5.4 Anaesthesia

The type of anesthesia used for the case is discussed with the patient and anesthesiologist. General or regional anaesthesia together with nerve blocks, including sciatic and femoral, will be decided by anesthesiologist. Co-morbidities and patient preference are taken into consideration. Patient without co-morbidities is scheduled for day surgery procedure and that will allow discharge on the same day. Prophylactic antibiotics are also given by anesthesia prior to the skin incision.

24.5.5 Patient Setup

Examination Under Anesthesia

The patient is positioned in the supine position with a side post and a gel-pad under the ipsilateral hemipelvis. This facilitates an initial arthroscopic evaluation of the knee and limits external rotation of the limb during the osteotomy. An examination under anaesthesia is initially performed to assess the Q angle, range of motion, patellar mobility, and tilt. It is imperative to compare to the contralateral knee exam. The procedure of choice is determined based on the

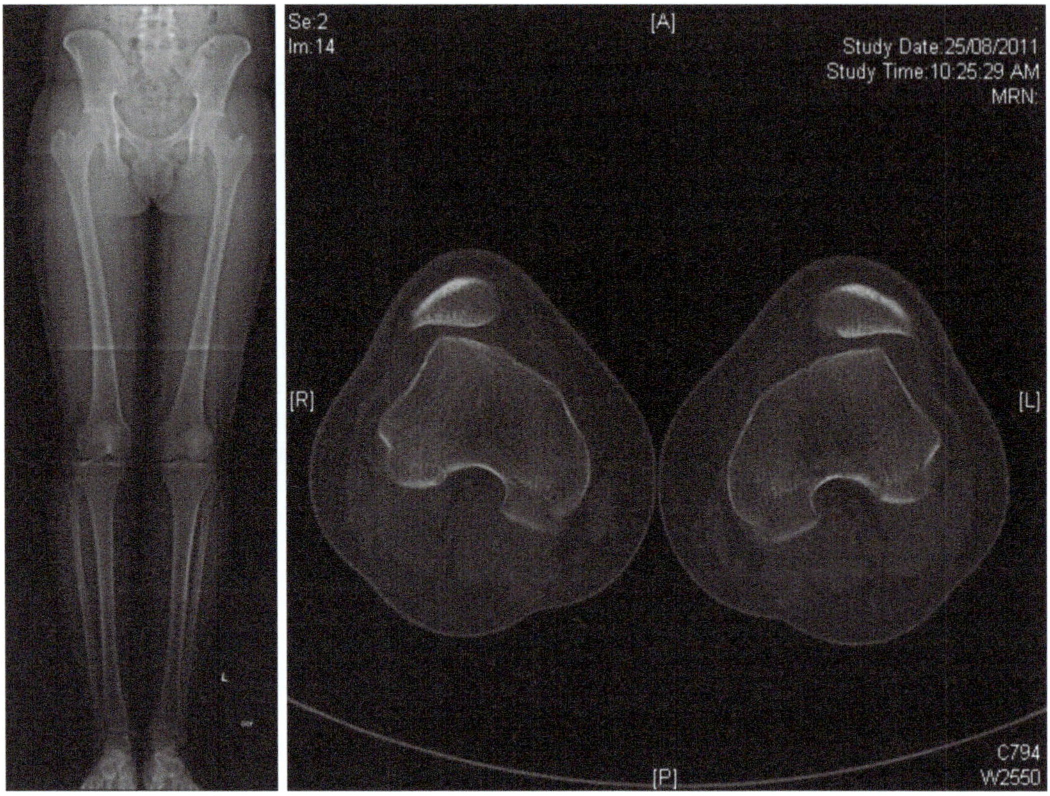

Fig. 24.29 Long lower limb radiograph and CT patella tracking shows bilateral patella subluxation

clinical examination and radiographic findings. The surgical area is shaved and wiped with alcohol. A tourniquet is then applied to the operative thigh and set to 250–300 mmHg. After prepping the operative extremity with betadine, the leg is draped in the standard sterile fashion.

24.5.6 Surgical Approach

Arthroscopic Evaluation

The surgery begins with identifying surface anatomy, including the patella, the borders of the patellar tendon, and the tibial tubercle. This surface anatomy is marked using marker pen. Initially, a diagnostic arthroscopy is performed. Through a superior lateral portal, using a 70-degree arthroscope, a complete assessment of the patellofemoral joint is possible. This portal allows for a safe evaluation of the joint, without risk of damaging the articular cartilage or the infrapatellar fat pad. The areas of chondrosis are regionally mapped using the ICRS region knee mapping system noting that significant patellar chondrosis may lead to termination of the procedure unless concomitant cartilage restoration has been planned. Arthroscopic lateral release will be done based on clinical and CT/MRI evaluation of patellar tilts if indicated. If the lateral retinaculum has been determined to be tight from the clinical examination, an open lateral release is performed.

Open surgery begins with a longitudinal incision just lateral to tibial crest, runs approximately 8–10 cm distally beginning at the patellar tendon insertion to the tibial tubercle (Fig. 24.29). The incision can be extended proximally to allow adequate exposure if concomitant cartilage restoration is being performed. If indicated, an open lateral release will be done. The lateral retinaculum is visualized. A nick is then made in the retinaculum with a no. 15 blade. Metzenbaum

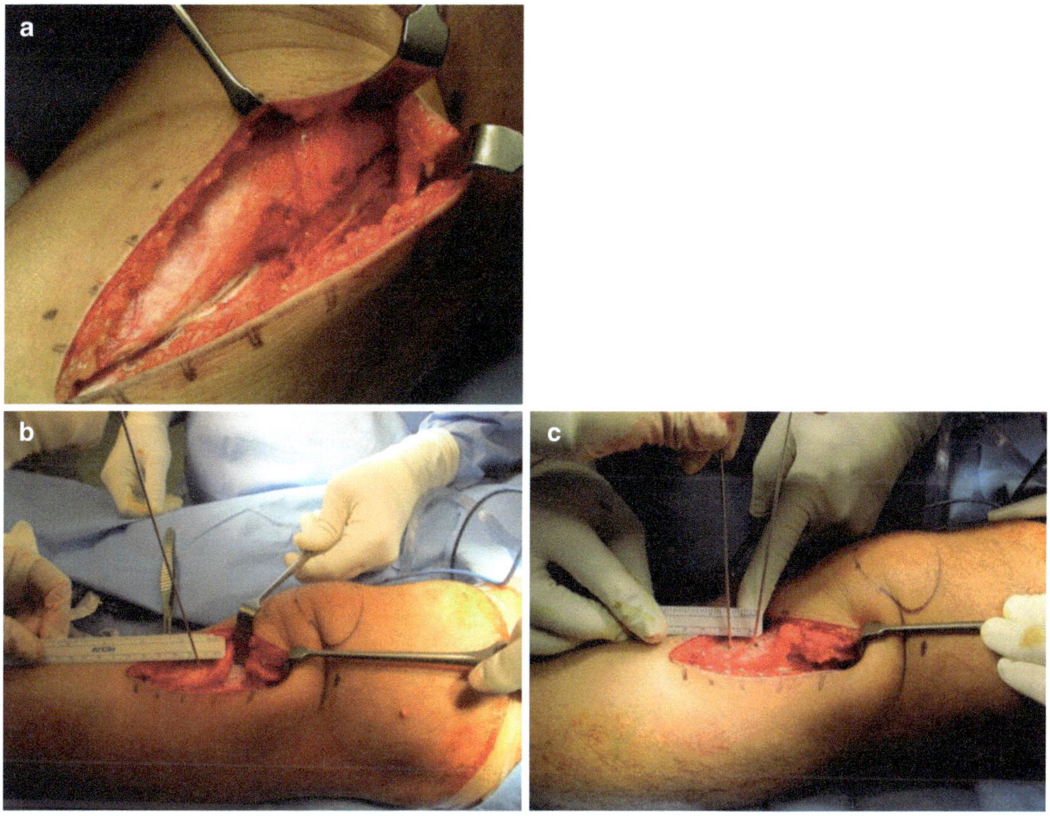

Fig. 24.30 (**a**) Lateral incision along lateral margin of tibial tuberosity and tibial crest. (**b**) The proximal screw should be placed 1.5 cm from patella tendon attachment. (**c**) The distal screw would be placed 1.5 cm apart

scissors are then used to complete the release proximally up to the vastus lateral obliquus (VLO) and distally through the patellotibial ligaments. The distal portion of the release is extended beyond the tibiofemoral joint, between the patellar tendon and the Gerdy tubercle. Care should be used to avoid injury to the lateral meniscus during the release. Proximally, the release is angled at about 45 ° at the level of the VLO to avoid injury to this structure, which can result in severe quadriceps weakness or medial patellar subluxation.

The patella tendon is identified and released from capsule medially and laterally to allow protection with a retractor and later tubercle elevation. The lateral incision is extended distally along the lateral margin of the tibial tuberosity and tibial crest allowing subperiosteal elevation of the anterior compartment musculature and thereby exposing the lateral wall of the tibia.

Anteromedialization can be performed using commercially available AMZ osteotomy systems (Tracker, DePuy Mitek, Inc, Raynham, New Jersey, and the T3 System, Arthrex, Inc, Naples, Florida). Fulkerson originally used an external fixator pin clamp to direct multiple pins in the osteotomy plane and then complete it with osteotomes [45]. The senior author performs osteotomy without using an external fixator pin clamp. The osteotomy begins with two pre-drilled hole over anterior cortex of the tibial, 1.5 cm distal to the patella tendon insertion and another 1.5 cm from the first hole (Fig. 24.30). This important step is essential to predetermine the site for fixation with the cortical screws after AMZ procedure.

A series of 3.2-mm drill bits are then used to guide the osteotomy angle. It begins proximal to the patella tendon insertion, 45° angle from anterolateral to posteromedial. Then, the drill bits are placed from posterolateral to anteromedial

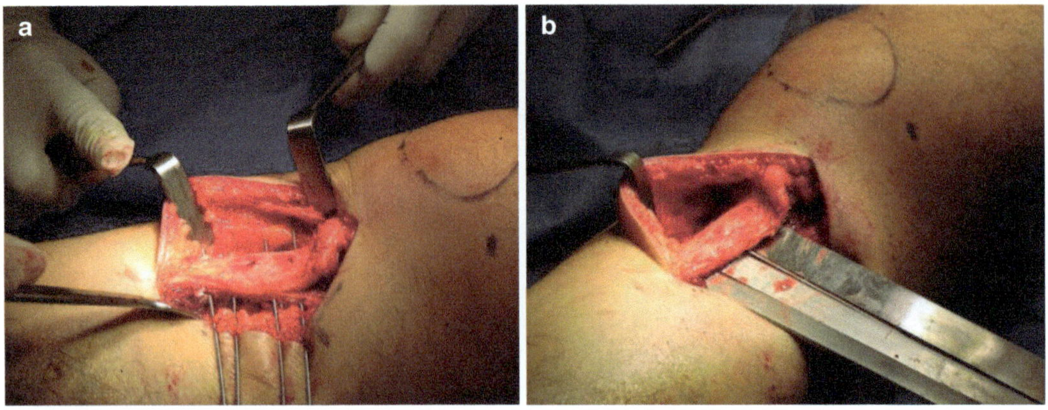

Fig. 24.31 (**a**) Four K-wires inserted through predrilled hole to guide the osteotomy. (**b**) A meticulous osteotomy is completed from lateral to medial tibial crest to create a 6–7 cm of tibial tuberosity pedicle

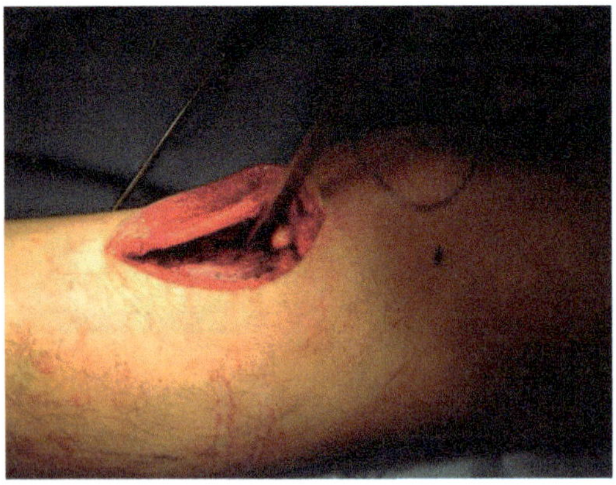

Fig. 24.32 A straight osteotome is used to pivot the tubercle preserving medial soft tissue sleever

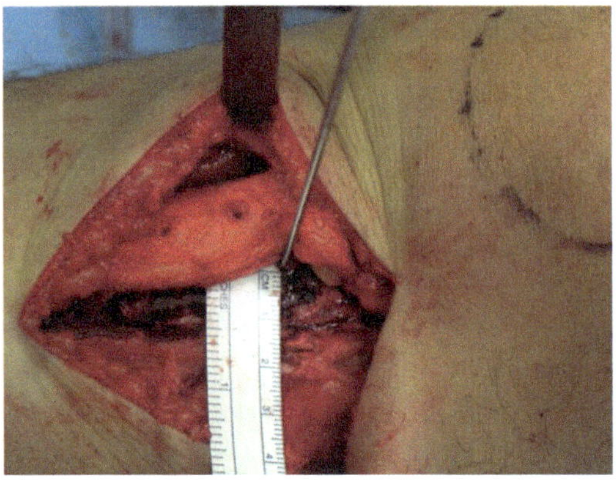

Fig. 24.33 A ruler is used to measure the required amount of anteriorization and medialization. Note the tubercle was transferred about 1.2 cm medially

direction to guide an anteromedialization of the osteotomy along 7–8 cm of tuberosity pedicle. They are placed under direct visualization of the lateral tibial crest. The drill is tapered distally to 2- to 3-mm anteriorly to hinge the osteotomy. Once the angle of the cut has been determined, the proximal portion of the osteotomy, just proximal to the patellar tendon insertion, is completed using a quarter-inch curved osteotome through a predrill holes. This proximal cut connects the medial and lateral edges of the osteotomy and prevents the osteotomy from extending into the tibial plateau. Using K-wires through a predrill hole as a guide, a meticulous osteotomy is completed from lateral to medial tibial crest to create a 6–7 cm of tibial tuberosity pedicle. Extra precaution is taken to ensure if the soft tissue over the medial and distal borders of the tuberosity pedicle remains intact to encourage healing of osteotomy and to avoid non-union (Figs. 24.31 and 24.32).

Once the osteotomy is complete, a half-inch straight osteotome is used to pivot the tubercle (Fig. 24.33). The bone pedicle is hinged distally and pushed up the inclined plane. Once the tubercle is hinged, it is transferred medially. A ruler is used to measure the required amount of anteriorization and medialization based on preoperative calculations. If required, the pedicles can be moved proximally or distally to address any underlying patella alta or infra. A Kirschner wire is used to temporarily secure the pedicle when correct positioning has been achieved (Fig. 24.34).

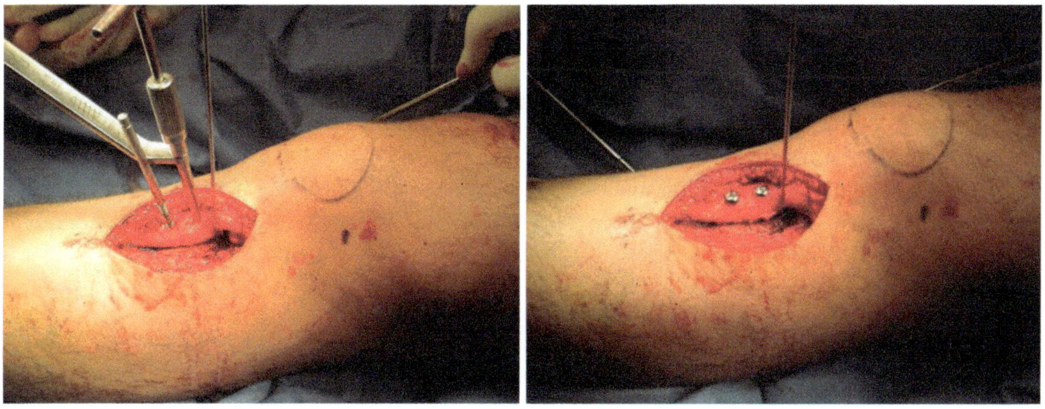

Fig. 24.34 A K-wire and 4.5 mm tap are used to maintain the pedicle before fix with two 4.5 mm cortical screws

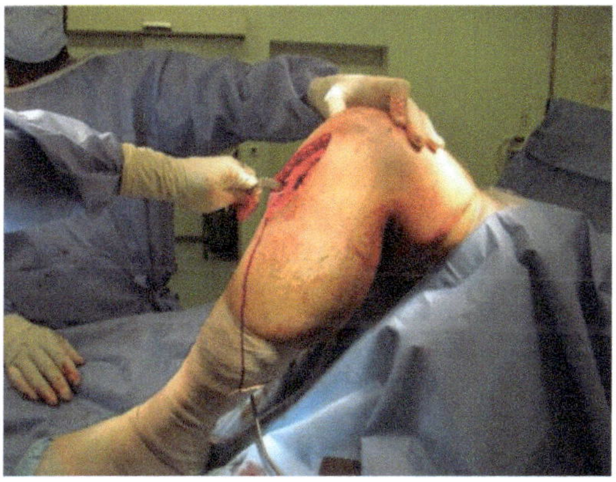

Fig. 24.35 Intra operative assessment of stability and position of transferred tubercle in both extension and flexion of the knee

The tuberosity pedicle is then drilled through a pre-drilled hole until the posterior cortex. Before the pedicle is fixed with cortical screw, 4.5 mm taps are used to maintain the pedicle to avoid it from "twisted" or moved while cortical screw is inserted on the pedicle at the transferred site. This extra step is important to maintain the precise location of the tubercle according to the pre-operative measurement. Two parallel 4.5-mm bicortical screws are then used to fix the tubercle (Fig. 24.35).

The position and stability is then confirmed by clinical examination, including range of motion, patellar tracking, glide, and tilt. After thorough irrigation, the surgical site is closed in a standard fashion.

Pearls and Pitfalls

Pearls

Excellent result of the procedure begins prior to the surgery.

1. Careful assessment of the underlying pathomechanics is critical for a successful outcome; these include malalignment of the extensor mechanism, trochlear dysplasia, soft-tissue imbalance, and chondral damage.
2. Preoperative counseling on patient expectation and rehabilitation is extremely important to prepare the patient for surgery and recovery.
3. The TT–TG measurement is an objective alternative to the Q-angle, quantifying the concept of tibial tuberosity malalignment. The mean TT–TG distance is 13 mm in asymptomatic patients and is considered excessive when above 20 mm.
4. Strengthening of proximal core muscles must be a focus of rehabilitation in conjunction with local musculature.
5. Meticulous osteotomy to ensure the medial site of tubercle remains intact to reduce risk of delayed union or non-union.
6. The use of K-wire and 4.5 mm tap to avoid the pedicle from twisting while insertion of screws.

Pitfalls

Common pitfalls exist through every phase of the treatment including patient selection, operative technique, and post-operative rehabilitation.

1. Poor patient selection. Diffuse or proximal patellar chondrosis should not be treated with anteromedialization. The increased joint reaction forces can exacerbate the symptoms and progression of the arthritis.
2. Increased medial patellofemoral and tibiofemoral stress can be detrimental due to over medialization of the tibial tubercle.
3. Pitfalls during the osteotomy include too shallow a cut, which results in little cancellous bone and mostly cortical bone to transfer. This pitfall can lead to a delayed union or nonunion. Another pitfall that can occur during the osteotomy includes not making the proximal cut behind the patellar tendon with the osteotome. This proximal cut connects the medial and lateral edges of the osteotomy and prevents the cut from extending proximally into the metaphysis or tibial plateau.
4. Weight bearing too early can lead to a fracture of the proximal tibia if the patient is returned to full weight bearing prior to radiographic healing.

24.5.7 Complications

Postoperative complications after TTO are similar to those encountered for other bony realignment including, fracture, malunion, nonunion,

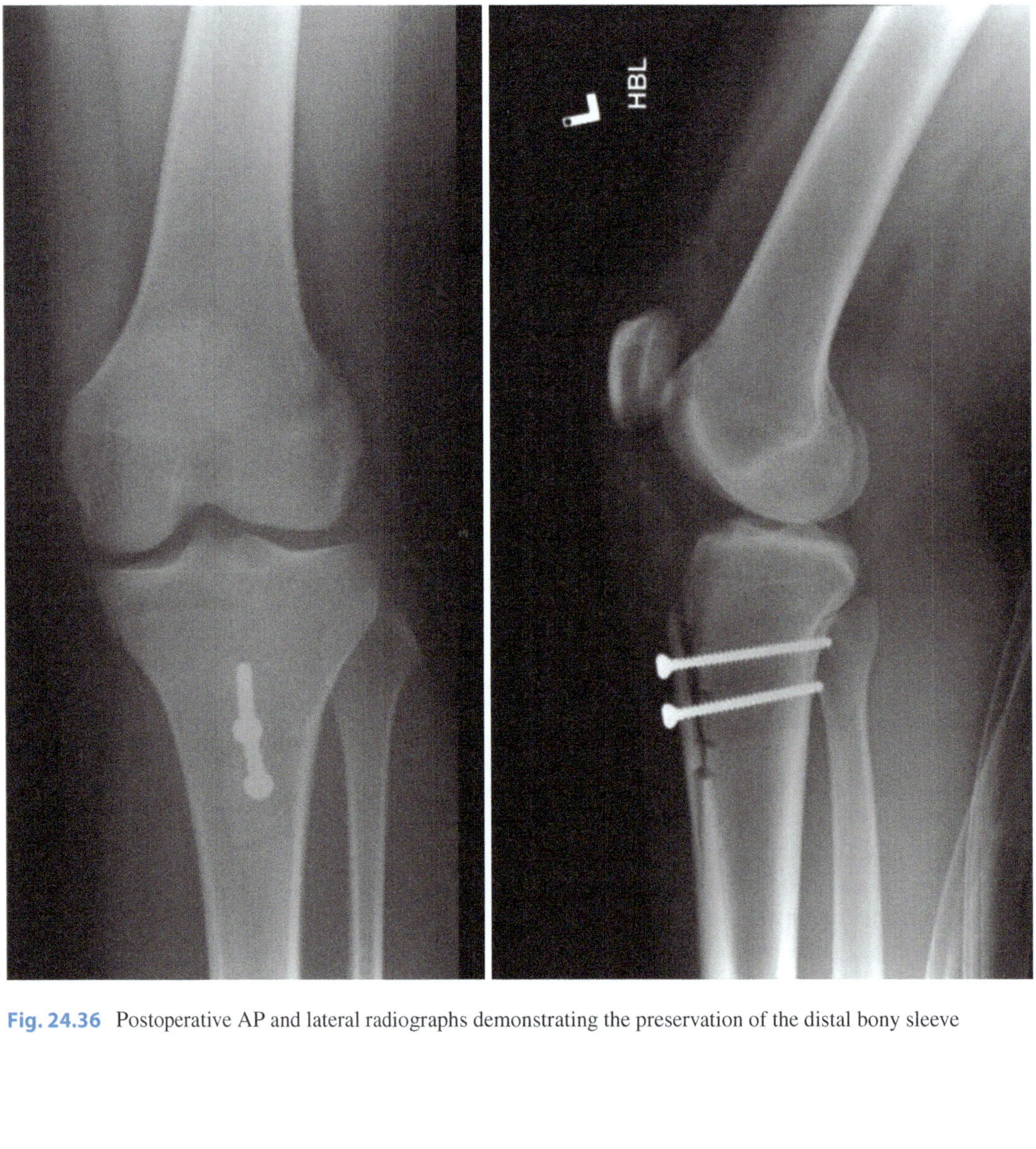

Fig. 24.36 Postoperative AP and lateral radiographs demonstrating the preservation of the distal bony sleeve

delayed union , loss of fixation, neurovascular injury, infection, compartment syndrome, deep venous thrombosis and rarely pulmonary embolism. Complications specific to TTO include symptomatic hardware, persistent pain, arthrofibrosis and stiffness, progressive chondral deterioration, complex regional pain syndrome, and intra-operative injury to the neurovascular structures including the popliteal artery and its trifurcation [46] and the deep peroneal nerve.

24.5.8 Rehabilitation

The postoperative rehabilitation actually begins before the elective procedure with a thorough discussion between the patient, surgeon, and a physical therapist to outline realistic expectations and anticipated progression to return to play. Postoperatively the patient is treated with standard compression dressings, protective bracing, and is monitored for immediate complications. The knee is protected with a hinged knee brace in extension which is unlocked at 2 weeks and discontinued when there is adequate lower extremity control (usually by 6 weeks). Range of motion is allowed up to 60 ° and will be modified throughout the rehabilitation process to accommodate for concomitant cartilage restorative procedures. Partial weight using crutches is allowed up to 6 weeks and will gradually full weight bearing is allowed once radiograph shows acceptable union of the osteotomy site.

24.5.9 Post-operative Follow-up

Routine radiograph in AP and lateral view to determine correct position of the screw will be done post-operatively. The follow-up will be conducted 2, 6 weeks, 3, 6 and 12 months after surgery, and once a year thereafter, and includes functional assessments, physical examinations and radiographic evaluations of the operated knee. If a concomitant cartilage restorative procedure was performed, a MRI with cartilage sequence will be reviewed at 1 year post-operatively. All patients are followed for a minimum of 2 years (range 2–13 years; median, 6.2 years) (Fig. 24.36).

References

1. Nagel A, Insall JN, Scuderi GR (1996) Proximal tibial osteotomy. A subjective outcome study. J Bone Joint Surg Am 78:1353–1358
2. Sprenger TR, Doerzbacher JF (2003) Tibial osteotomy for the treatment of varus gonarthrosis. Survival and failure analysis to twenty-two years. J Bone Joint Surg Am 85:469–474
3. Hernigou P, Medevielle D, Debeyre J, Goutallier D (1987) Proximal tibial osteotomy for osteoarthritis with varus deformity: a ten to thirteen year follow-up study. J Bone Joint Surg Am 69:332–354
4. Jackson JP, Waugh W (1961) Tibial osteotomy for osteoarthritis of the knee. J Bone Joint Surg Br 43:746–751
5. Coventry MB (1965) Osteotomy of the upper portion of the tibia for degenerative arthritis of the knee. J Bone Joint Surg Am 47:984–990
6. Insall JN, Joseph DM, Msika C (1984) High tibial osteotomy for varus gonarthrosis: a long-term follow-up study. J Bone Joint Surg Am 66:1040–1048
7. Coventry MB (1985) Upper tibial osteotomy for osteoarthritis. J Bone Joint Surg Am 67: 1136–1140
8. Verdonk PC, Verstraete KL, Almqvist KF, De Cuyper K, Veys EM, Verbruggen G, Verdonk R (2006) Meniscal allograft transplantation: long term clinical results with radiological and magnetic resonance imaging correlations. Knee Surg Sports Traumatol Arthrosc 14:694–706
9. Knutsen G, Drogset JO, Engebretsen L, Grøntvedt T, Isaksen V, Ludvigsen TC, Roberts S, Solheim E, Strand T, Johansen O (2007) A randomized trial comparing autologous chondrocyte implantation with microfracture. Findings at five years. J Bone Joint Surg Am 89(10):2105–2112
10. Knutsen G, Engebretsen L, Ludvigsen TC, Drogset JO, Grøntvedt T, Solheim E, Strand T, Roberts S, Isaksen V, Johansen O (2004) Autologous chondrocyte implantation compared with microfracture in the knee. A randomized trial. J Bone Joint Surg Am 86-A(3): 455–464
11. Sterett WI, Steadman JR (2004) Chondral resurfacing and high tibial osteotomy in the varus knee. Am J Sports Med 32:1243–1249
12. Weale AE, Lee AS, McEachern AG (2001) High tibial osteotomy using a dynamic axial external fixator. Clin Orthop 383:154–167
13. Mina C, Garrett WE, Pietrobon R, Glisson R, Higgins L (2008) High tibial osteotomy for unloading osteochondral defects in the medial compartment of the knee. Am J Sports Med 36:949–955
14. Fujisawa Y, Masuhara K, Shiomi S (1997) The effect of high tibial osteotomy o osteoarthritis of the knee. Orthop Clin North Am 10:585–608
15. Brown GA, Amendola A (2000) Radiographic evaluation and preoperative planning for high tibial osteotomies. Oper Tech Sports Med 1:2–14
16. Agneskirchner JD, Hurschler C, Stukenborg-Colsman C, Imhoff AB, Lobenhoffer P (2004) Effect of high

tibial flexion osteotomy on cartilage pressure and joint kinematics: a biomechanical study in human cadaveric knees. Winner of the AGA-DonJoy Award 2004. Arch Orthop Trauma Surg 124(9):575–584
17. Staubli AE, Jacob HA (2010) Evolution of open-wedge high-tibial osteotomy: experience with a special angular stable device for internal fixation without interposition material. Int Orthop (SICOT) 34:167–172
18. Rossi R, Bonasia DE, Amendola A (2011) The role of high tibial osteotomy in the varus knee. J Am Acad Orthop Surg 19:590–599
19. Poignard A, Flouzat Lachaniette CH, Amzallag J, Hernigou P (2010) Revisiting high tibial osteotomy: fifty years of experience with the opening wedge technique. J Bone Joint Surg Am 92:187–195
20. Zaidi SHA, Cobb AG, Bentley G (1995) Danger to the popliteal artery in high tibial osteotomy. J Bone Joint Surg Br 77-B:384–386
21. Brouwer RW, BiermaZeinstra SMA, van Koeveringe AJ, Verhaa J (2005) Patellar height and the inclination of the tibial plateau after opening-wedge tech high tibial osteotomy the open versus the closed-wedge technique. J Bone Joint Surg Br 87-B:1227–1232
22. Billings A, Scott DF, Camargo MP, Hofmann AA (2000) High tibial osteotomy with a calibrated osteotomy guide, rigid internal fixation, and early motion: long term follow-up. J Bone Joint Surg Am 82: 70–79
23. Gaasbeek R, Welsing R, Barink M, Verdonschot N, van Kampen A (2007) The influence of open and closed high tibial osteotomy on dynamic patellar tracking: a biomechanical study. Knee Surg Sports Traumatol Arthrosc 15:978–984
24. Stoffel K, Willers C, Korshid O, Kuster M (2007) Patellofemoral contact pressure following high tibial osteotomy: a cadaveric study. Knee Surg Sports Traumatol Arthrosc 15:1094–1100
25. Arendt EA, Fithian DC, Cohen E (2002) Current concepts of lateral patella dislocation. Clin Sports Med 21(3):499–519
26. Dejour H, Walch G, Nove-Josserand L, Guier C (1994) Factors of patellar instability: an anatomic radiographic study. Knee Surg Sports Traumatol Arthrosc 2(1):19–26
27. Desio SM, Burks RT, Bachus KN (1998) Soft tissue restraints to lateral patellar translation in the human knee. Am J Sports Med 26(1):59–65
28. Boden PB, Pearsall AW, Garrett WE Jr, Feagin JA Jr (1997) Patellofemoral instability: evaluation and management. J Am Acad Orthop Surg 5:47–57
29. Fulkerson JP (1994) Patellofemoral pain disorders: evaluation and management. J Am Acad Orthop Surg 2:124–132
30. Roux C (1888) Recurrent dislocation of the patella: operative treatment. Rev Chir 8:682–689
31. Goldthwait JE (1904) Slipping or recurrent dislocation of the patella: with the report of eleven cases. Boston Med Surg J 150:169–174
32. Maquet P (1978) Biomechanics of the patello-femoral joint. Acta Orthop Belg 44:41–54
33. Fulkerson JP, Becker GJ, Meaney JA et al (1990) Anteromedial tibial tubercle transfer without bone graft. Am J Sports Med 18(5):490–497
34. Beck PR, Thomas AL, Farr J, Lewis PB, Cole BJ (2005) Trochlear contact pressure following anteromedialization of tibial tubercle. AM J Sport Me 33:1710–1715
35. Brittberg M, Lindah A, Nilsson A, Ohlsson C, Isaksson O, Petersen L (1994) Treatment of deep cartilage defects in the knee with autologous chondrocyte transplantation. N Engl J Med 331:889–895
36. Minas T, Bryant T (2005) The role of autologous chondrocyte implantation in the patellofemoral joint. Clin Orthop Relat Res 436:30
37. Farr J (2007) Autologous chondrocyte implantation improves patellofemoral cartilage treatment outcomes. Clin Orthop Relat Res 463:187–194
38. Henderson IJP, Lavigne P (2006) Periosteal autologous chondrocyte implantation for patellar chondral defect in patients with normal and abnormal patellar tracking. Knee 13:274–279
39. Peterson L, Brittberg M, Kiviranta I et al (2002) Autologous chondrocyte transplantation. Biomechanics and long-term durability. Am J Sports Med 30:2–12
40. Steinwachs M, Kreuz PC (2007) Autologous chondrocyte implantation in chondral defects of the knee with a type I/III collagen membrane: a prospective study with a 3-year follow-up. Arthroscopy 23:381–387
41. Pidoriano AJ, Weinstein RN, Buuck DA, Fulkerson JP (1997) Correlation of patellar articular lesions with results from anteromedial tibial tubercle transfer. Am J Sports Med 25(4):533–537
42. Gigante A, Enea D, Greco F, Bait C, Denti M, Schonhuber H, Volpi P (2009) Distal realignment and patellar autologous chondrocyte implantation: mid-term results in a selected population. Knee Surg Sports Traumatol Arthrosc 17:2–10
43. Beaconsfield T, Pintore E, Maffulli N, Petri GJ (1994) Radiological measurements in patellofemoral disorders. A review. Clin Orthop 308:18–28
44. Cohen ZA, Henry JH, McCarthy DM et al (2003) Computer simulations of patellofemoral joint surgery. Patient-specific models for tuberosity transfer. Am J Sports Med 31:87–98
45. Fulkerson JP (1983) Anteromedialization of the tibial tuberosity for patellofemoral malalignment. Clin Orthop Relat Res 177:176–181
46. Kline AJ, Gonzales J, Beach WR et al (2006) Vascular risk associated with bicortical tibial drilling during anteromedial tibial tubercle transfer. Am J Orthop 35:30–32

Distal Femoral Varus Osteotomy for Correction of Valgus Deformity

25

William Bugbee

Contents

W. Bugbee, MD
Division of Orthopaedic Surgery, Scripps Clinic,
10666 North Torrey Pines Rd,
La Jolla, CA 92037, USA

Department of Orthopaedic Surgery,
University of California, San Diego, La Jolla, CA, USA
e-mail: bugbee.william@scrippshealth.org

25.1 Introduction

Lower extremity malalignment in association with arthritis or cartilage deficiency is a common clinical entity. Identification and management of limb malalignment, either alone or in conjunction with cartilage restoration, is increasingly recognized as an essential part of the treatment algorithm. Although osteotomies around the knee have been described extensively in the literature, most studies report on the use of proximal tibial valgus osteotomy for varus deformities. The use of varus-producing osteotomies for valgus deformity is less common and few clinical studies have been published. These studies generally report the outcome of small cohorts of patients undergoing medial closing wedge osteotomies for treatment of lateral compartment arthritis and have documented acceptable outcomes at intermediate term follow-up [1–7]. The use of opening wedge osteotomies on the tibial side for varus deformity has become well established as a favored alternative and is now used more commonly than closing wedge techniques [8]. However, little is known regarding the analogous opening wedge technique for femoral osteotomy used to correct valgus deformity. Our experience with the opening wedge distal femoral varus osteotomy has been favorable and is an integral component of our management of patients with cartilage or meniscal pathology of the lateral compartment of the knee.

A.A. Shetty et al. (eds.), *Techniques in Cartilage Repair Surgery*,
DOI 10.1007/978-3-642-41921-8_25,

25.2 Patient Selection

Candidates for distal femoral osteotomy include younger patients with established lateral compartment arthritis, usually secondary to meniscectomy, or individuals undergoing cartilage restoration procedures associated with valgus limb alignment. In practical terms, these are two distinct groups that share a similar valgus limb malalignment. Patients under 55 years of age, without significant medial compartment pathology, good range of motion, and stable ligaments, are considered candidates. Individuals with subjective symptoms of instability or mild clinical laxity but intact ligaments are appropriate candidates as this is a classic feature of valgus malalignment readily treatable by osteotomy. Patient evaluation includes observation of the patient, static stance to asses limb alignment, and gait analysis, because valgus deformity can be dynamic. Rotational deformities of the limb and patellofemoral dysplasia or malalignment are commonly associated with valgus deformity and should be carefully investigated.

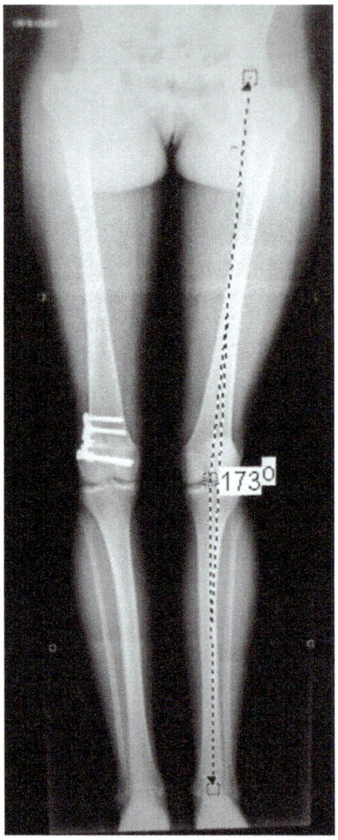

Fig. 25.1 Standing long alignment radiograph demonstrating mechanical valgus alignment of the left leg

Radiographic evaluation of potential candidates for distal femoral osteotomy includes full-length standing AP radiographs of bilateral lower extremities. In addition, standing AP views of the knees and a standing PA view of the knee with 45° of flexion, lateral view of the knee, and patellofemoral view are obtained. The long alignment radiograph is used to measure the overall anatomic and mechanical axes of the limb and to determine if the lateral compartment is experiencing overload due to overall genu valgum (Fig. 25.1). The standing AP and PA flexion views of the knee allow determination of the amount of joint space narrowing in the anterior and posterior portions of the lateral compartment, respectively. The lateral and patellofemoral views are helpful for determining the condition of the patellofemoral joint. If any concern remains, stress radiographs may be obtained to test for ligamentous stability and joint subluxation.

The decision to include varus osteotomy in the treatment program is highly individualized. Many surgeons and patients are reluctant to proceed with an operation that is perceived as technically challenging and requiring a long postoperative rehabilitation. However, any individual that has cartilage and/or meniscal deficiency should at least be evaluated for abnormalities in alignment. Malalignment may be one of the predisposing factors leading to the cartilage pathology or may accelerate joint degeneration subsequent to cartilage injury. The author's opinion is that what may have once been considered "physiologic" valgus in an individual with a healthy knee should subsequently be considered "pathologic" in the presence of lateral compartment cartilage or meniscal injury. We will often include a small (5–7°) varus correction in patients with little or no joint space narrowing. Once clear evidence of lateral compartment joint space loss is evident, particularly on the standing flexed knee radiograph, and mechanical alignment axis is clearly within the lateral compartment, the threshold for osteotomy should be low.

25.3 Surgical Technique

The author's preference is for a lateral opening wedge distal femoral osteotomy. On theoretical grounds, the opening wedge technique has advantages over medial closing wedge techniques that include (1) a single bone cut, (2) maintenance of axial and rotational stability with an intact medial hinge, (3) better control of the amount of correction, and (4) more anatomic correction of the typical patho-anatomy of excessive distal femoral valgus. Relative disadvantages include potential for delayed union and irritation of the sensitive lateral knee structures by hardware or surgical trauma. The amount of correction is determined as that necessary to restore the mechanical alignment to neutral, i.e., through the center of the knee. We use a simplified calculation that the millimeter value of the linear correction at the osteotomy site is equal to 1° of correction of axial alignment. The goal is to restore the mechanical axis to neutral. This is quite different than the overcorrection goal often associated with valgus tibial osteotomies. Not overcorrecting a femoral varus osteotomy is important.

The patient is placed supine on a radiolucent operating table to allow fluoroscopic imaging of the entire lower extremity from the hip to the ankle. Our anesthetic preference is general with regional nerve block, which can provide 24 h of postoperative pain control. If the osteotomy is to be combined with another procedure, the osteotomy is generally performed last.

The operated limb including the ipsilateral hip is prepped free (including the anterior iliac crest) and a small bump is placed under the hip to maintain the leg in neutral alignment on the table (Fig. 25.2). A sterile tourniquet is placed but only used if necessary. An 8–10 cm incision is made over the lateral aspect of the distal femur (Fig. 25.3). The iliotibial band is incised in line with the incision and the vastus lateralis is then dissected off the lateral intermuscular septum to expose the femoral shaft and the metaphysis distal to the lateral epicondyle. The joint can be entered, if necessary, but generally the capsule remains intact.

Using fluoroscopy, the starting point for the osteotomy is located approximately 2–3 cm proximal to the lateral femoral epicondyle. A guide pin is angled medially and distally such that it exits between the metaphyseal flare and the medial epicondyle (Figs. 25.4 and 25.5). The goal is to create the osteotomy in the metaphyseal bone without violating the patellofemoral joint. The superior most aspect of the trochlea should be palpated to ensure that the guide pin is not too distal. If the guide pin is too distal, the superior aspect of the joint will be violated during the osteotomy. After the guide pin has been placed in the appropriate position, the osteotomy can be performed. The surgeon should consider not only the angle of the osteotomy on the AP view but also in the lateral plane. In order to preserve the sagittal plane alignment of the femur, the osteotomy should be performed perpendicular to the axis of the femur in the lateral plane. Any deviation will create either excessive flexion or

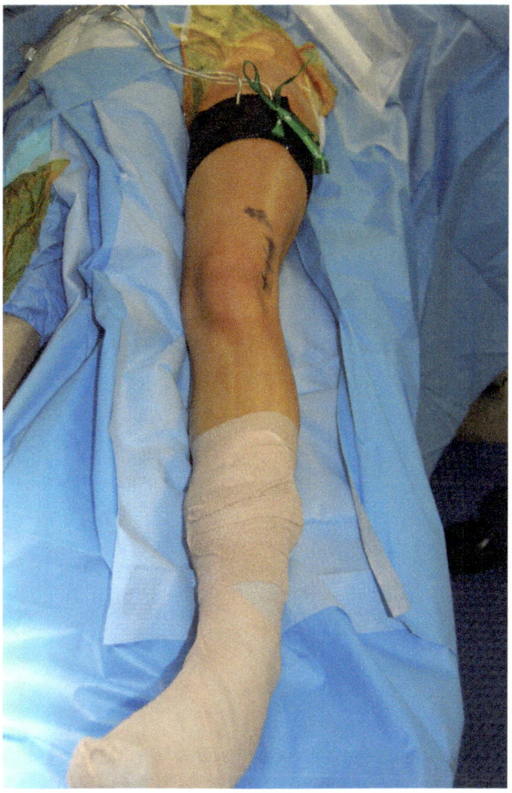

Fig. 25.2 Intraoperative photograph of surgical draping of the operative leg. Note exposure of anterior iliac crest for potential bone graft harvest

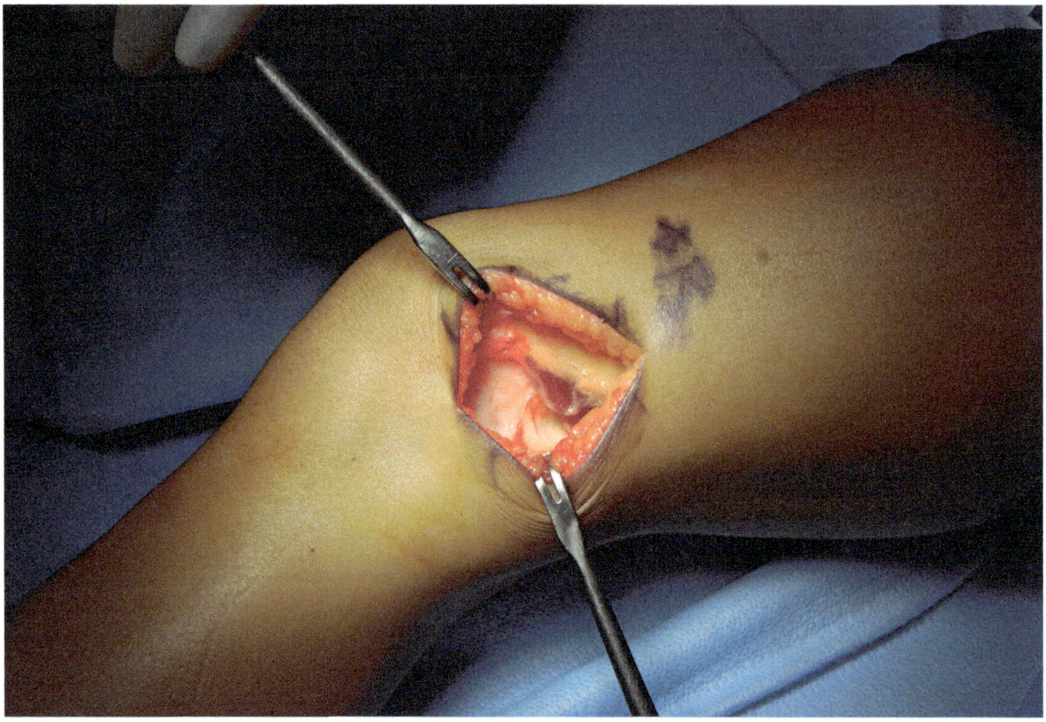

Fig. 25.3 Incision on the lateral side of the knee. Iliotibial band has been incised and retracted, vastus lateralis has been released, and distal femoral periosteum is exposed

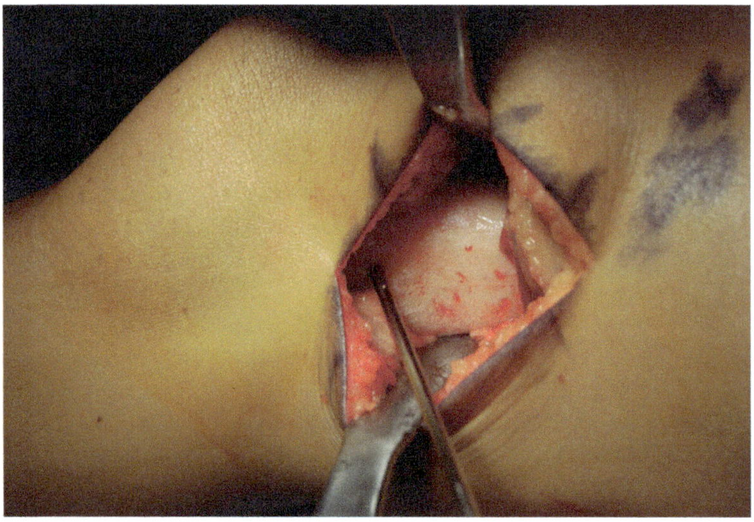

Fig. 25.4 Position of guide wire placed in the distal femur

extension of the femur depending on the angle of the osteotomy. This may be desirable, for example, if the patient has a fixed flexion contracture at the knee and a small amount of hyperextension of the distal femur is desired. More commonly, inadvertent flexion at the osteotomy site is a technical error that should be avoided. Once the first guide pin is accurately placed, a second guide pin can be placed either directly anterior or posterior in such a position that the second pin is not seen on an AP view of the distal femur. This ensures that an osteotomy created parallel to the plane of both guide pins will be perpendicular to the long axis of the femur in the lateral plane. The osteotomy can then be performed using both pins as a guide. An oscillating saw is used to start the osteotomy, either just above or below the guide pins, to create the proper plane (Fig. 25.6). Once this has been done, a series of sharp osteotomes are used to complete the osteotomy (Fig. 25.7). The goal is not to create a complete cut but instead to keep the medial cortex intact to act as a hinge. Intermittent manual varus stress can be used to judge the progress of the osteotomy. Once the majority of the cortex has been freed, the distraction device is placed in the osteotomy site and slowly opened (Figs. 25.8 and 25.9). The amount of opening correlates with the amount of correction attained. This is most easily determined preoperatively using digital radiographic tools or tracing paper cutouts of the proposed osteotomy on long-standing alignment films. Our goal is for the mechanical axis to pass between the knee center and the medial tibial spine. Once the desired amount of correction is obtained, fluoroscopy is used to evaluate the mechanical axis. If the mechanical axis is over or under-corrected, adjustments can be made at this time. We will also directly measure the millimeter correction at the osteotomy site. At this time the surgeon should ensure that the osteotomy is opened equally anterior and posterior. A lateral fluoroscopic image is critical to ensure proper sagittal alignment. Once the correction is felt to be appropriate, a plate is used to fix the osteotomy

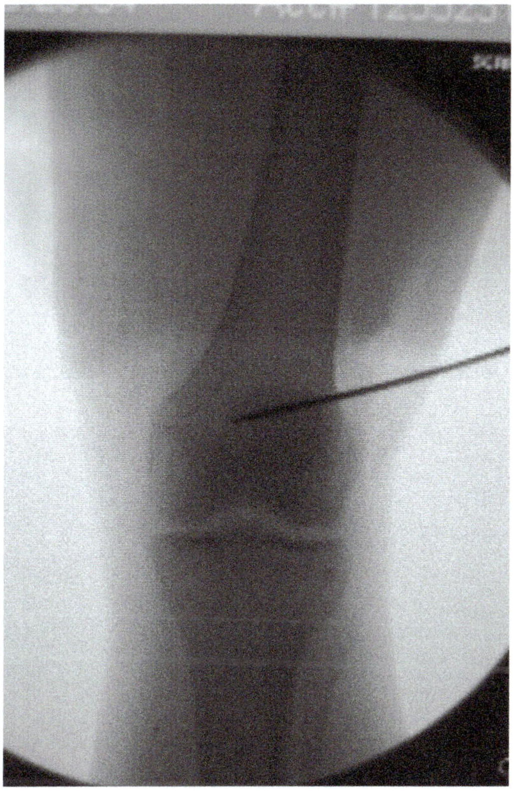

Fig. 25.5 Intraoperative fluoroscopic image confirming guidewire positioning

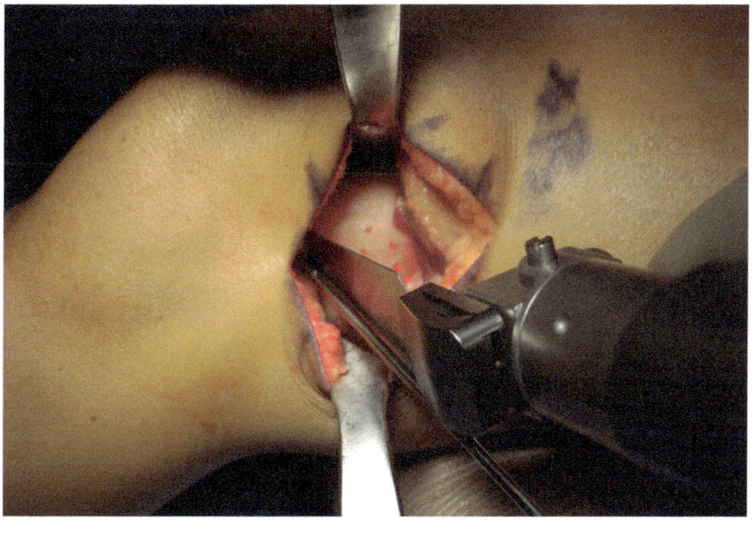

Fig. 25.6 Initiation of osteotomy with oscillating saw. Retractors are protecting soft tissue structures. Saw is perpendicular to the long axis of the femur

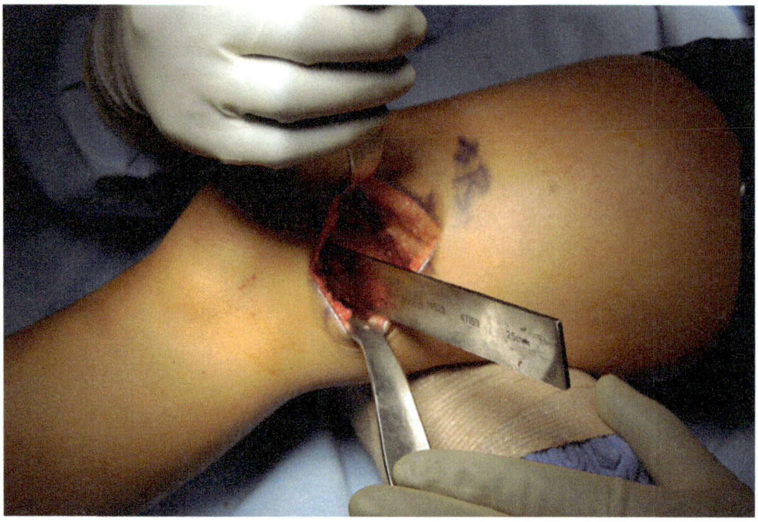

Fig. 25.7 Osteotomes are used for completion of the osteotomy in a controlled fashion

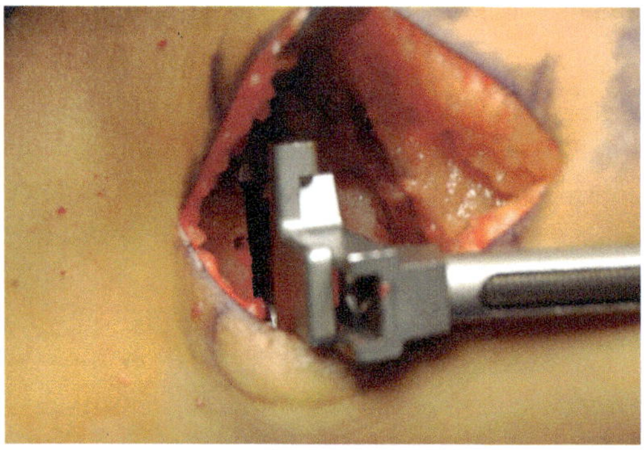

Fig. 25.8 The opening device is placed within the osteotomy site

(Fig. 25.10). A number of instrument and implant systems are available for use on the distal femur including the VS plates (Biomet, Warsaw, Indiana), Puddu plates (Arthrex, Naples, Florida), and TomoFix plates (Synthes, West Chester, Pennsylvania). Depending on the patient and size of correction, either iliac crest bone graft or allograft is utilized. Both methods of bone grafting have been equally successful. Final fluoroscopic images are obtained to confirm correction and hardware position (Figs. 25.11 and 25.12).

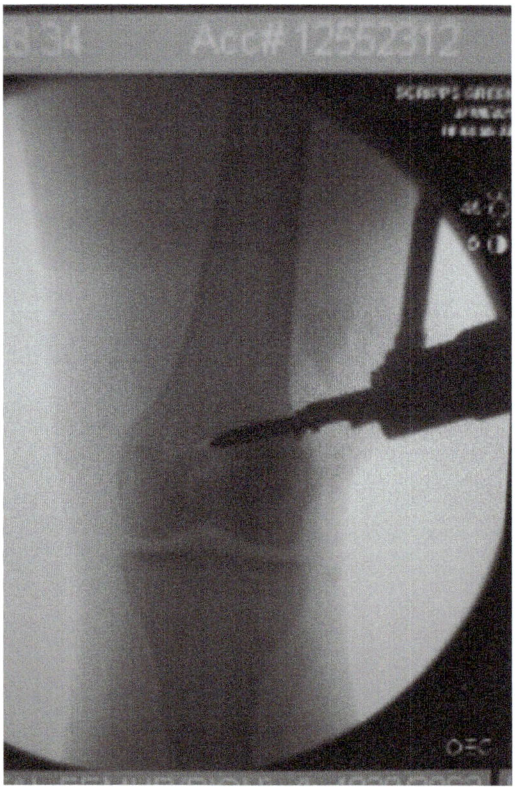

Fig. 25.9 Fluoroscopic image of the osteotomy opening device in place prior to initiating correction force

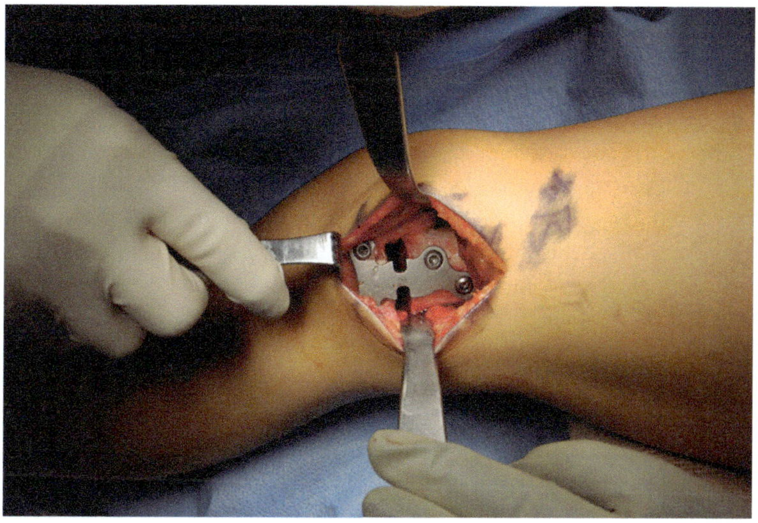

Fig. 25.10 The fixation plate is in place and fixed with four screws

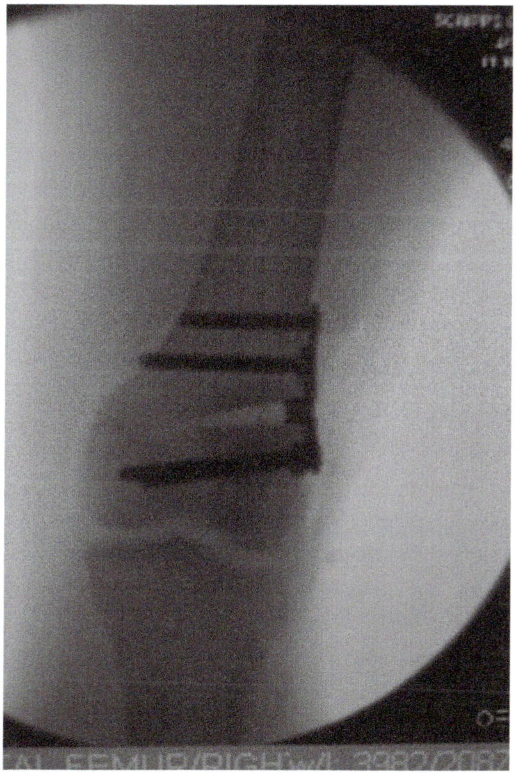

Fig. 25.11 Anteroposterior fluoroscopic image of the completed osteotomy prior to bone grafting

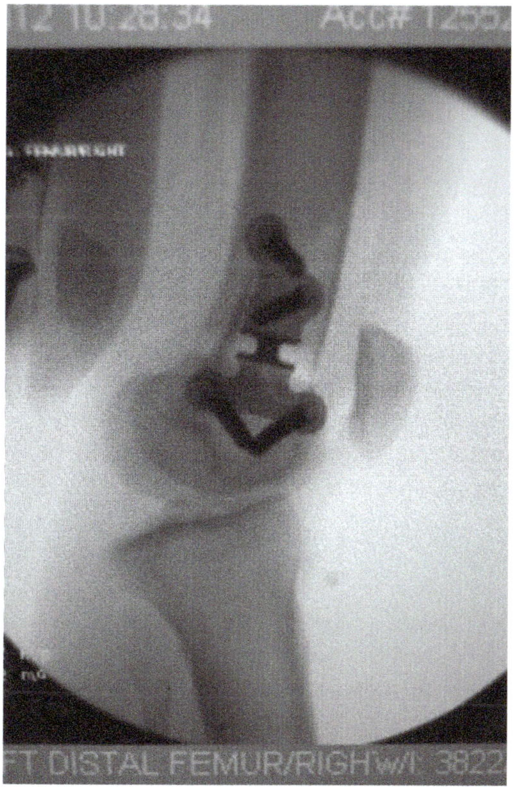

Fig. 25.12 Lateral fluoroscopic image of completed osteotomy confirming position of plate and screws and symmetric opening of the osteotomy site

25.4 Postoperative Care

The patient is placed in a knee immobilizer or locked range of motion (ROM) brace overnight for pain control and to protect against falls associated with the use of nerve blocks. The ROM brace is unlocked on postoperative day 1 to allow full motion. All patients are allowed to start range of motion exercises immediately and isometric strengthening when tolerated. Patients are kept touchdown weight bearing for 6–8 weeks or until radiographic healing is evident. Progressive weight bearing is allowed at 8 weeks, initially with the use of a single crutch or cane until 12–16 weeks. Low-resistance cycling exercises are started at 4 weeks, and resistance training begins after radiographic healing. Sporting activities may be resumed 6 months postoperatively. Patients generally demonstrate progressive pain relief and functional improvement up to 1 year after surgery.

25.5 Potential Complications

The complications reported for distal femoral osteotomy are similar to that reported for high tibial osteotomy. Usual concerns include loss of fixation, nonunion, and loss of correction. Great care should be taken to confirm that the medial metaphyseal bone is intact. If a fracture through the medial side is evident either intraoperatively or postoperatively, weight bearing should be restricted and closer radiographic follow-up obtained. Many of the fixation devices are not adequately designed for an unstable distal femoral fragment. Delayed or nonunion is also a potential problem. We routinely use iliac crest plugs in conjunction with allograft bone chips and have had no problems with bone healing. Stiffness is another potential problem due to the location of the osteotomy across the suprapatellar region leading to capsular or quadriceps adhesions. Early range of motion is critical and fixation of the osteotomy should be rigid enough to allow motion exercises. The most common postoperative issue with the lateral opening wedge osteotomy is symptomatic hardware. This may be secondary to the use of larger fixation devices or due to the fact that structures on the lateral side of the knee such as the iliotibial band are more sensitive to irritation. Patients should be counseled on the possibility of later hardware removal. Another concern that arises in patients who have undergone distal femoral osteotomy is the potential for increased difficulty in performing a subsequent knee arthroplasty. The literature is mixed on this subject with some authors claiming inferior outcome and need for increased constraint and others claiming the osteotomy improves patellar tracking after total knee arthroplasty.

25.6 Clinical Outcome

Re-fixation-femoral alignment was 3° varus (range, 8° varus to 4° valgus). All but two patients were within ±2° of intraoperative correction goals. Clinically and statistically significant improvements in KOOS, IKDC, and KS-F scores were noted postoperatively. One nonunion occurred and was treated with re-fixation and grafting. All other osteotomies demonstrated radiographic healing by 6 months. No postoperative infections, nerve palsies, or wound complications occurred. Eighteen of thirty-five knees (51 %) had a mean of 1.6 surgeries after osteotomy. Thirteen knees underwent hardware removal, five knees had an arthroscopy, five knees underwent revision osteochondral allograft transplantation, three knees had a manipulation, one knee had an anterior cruciate ligament reconstruction, and one knee had a meniscus repair. Five knees were converted to total knee arthroplasties and one knee was converted to unicompartmental knee arthroplasty at a median of 2.4 years (range, 1.7–7.2 years). Survivorship, using conversion to arthroplasty as an endpoint, was 81 % at 5 years.

We used the opening wedge distal femoral varus osteotomy procedure as a primary treatment for lateral compartment arthritis with valgus deformity or in conjunction with a joint-preserving procedure such as osteochondral allograft transplantation or meniscus transplantation. As a result of this patient selection, the average age of our cohort (36.7 years) is at least 10 years younger than other reported series of distal femoral osteotomy [1–7]. Nonetheless, the outcomes reported here are comparable to other reports. Dewilde et al. reported on the outcome of opening wedge distal femoral osteotomy for lateral arthritis of the knee [9]. Nineteen patients underwent opening wedge osteotomy using the Puddu plate and calcium phosphate. Knee scores improved from 43 to 78 and survivorship was 82 % at 7 years. Das et al. reported on 12 patients with an average age of 52 years also undergoing opening wedge distal femoral osteotomy (average correction 11°) with the Puddu plate [10]. At 74 months of follow-up, Lysholm scores improved from 64 to 77 points and two of the 12 knees were converted to total knee arthroplasty. Conversely, Jacobi observed delayed osteotomy healing and a high rate of symptomatic hardware in 14 patients undergoing lateral opening wedge osteotomy using the TomoFix plate [11]. The authors reported satisfactory outcomes once healing had occurred and the hardware was removed but abandoned the opening wedge technique in favor of the medial closing wedge. This experience may be due to the relatively large size and rigid fixation of the TomoFix plate.

25.7 Summary

The lateral opening wedge distal femoral varus osteotomy is a valuable procedure for managing young, active patients with knee pathology associated with valgus deformity. The opening wedge technique is technically less demanding than previously described techniques of medial closing wedge [12–14].

References

1. Edgerton BC, Mariani EM, Morrey BF (1993) Distal femoral varus osteotomy for painful genu valgum. A five-to-11-year follow-up study. Clin Orthop Relat Res 288:263–269
2. Finkelstein JA, Gross AE, Davis A (1996) Varus osteotomy of the distal part of the femur. A survivorship analysis. J Bone Joint Surg Am 78:1348–1352
3. Mathews J, Cobb AG, Richardson S, Bentley G (1998) Distal femoral osteotomy for lateral compartment osteoarthritis of the knee. Orthopedics 21:437–440
4. Aglietti P, Menchetti PP (2000) Distal femoral varus osteotomy in the valgus osteoarthritic knee. Am J Knee Surg 13:89–95
5. Wang JW, Hsu CC (2005) Distal femoral varus osteotomy for osteoarthritis of the knee. J Bone Joint Surg Am 87:127–133
6. Backstein D, Morag G, Hanna S, Safir O, Gross A (2007) Long-term follow-up of distal femoral varus osteotomy of the knee. J Arthroplasty 22:2–6
7. Kosashvili Y, Safir O, Gross A, Morag G, Lakstein D, Backstein D (2010) Distal femoral varus osteotomy for lateral osteoarthritis of the knee: a minimum ten-year follow-up. Int Orthop 34:249–254
8. Floerkemeier S, Staubli AE, Schroeter S, Goldhahn S, Lobenhoffer P (2013) Outcome after high tibial open-wedge osteotomy: a retrospective evaluation of 533 patients. Knee Surg Sports Traumatol Arthrosc 21:170–180
9. Dewilde TR, Dauw J, Vandenneucker H, Bellemans J (2013) Opening wedge distal femoral varus osteotomy using the Puddu plate and calcium phosphate bone cement. Knee Surg Sports Traumatol Arthrosc 21:249–254
10. Das D, Sijbesma T, Hoekstra HJ, Van Leuven W (2008) Distal femoral opening-wedge osteotomy for lateral compartment osteoarthritis of the knee. Open Access Surg 1:25–29
11. Jacobi M, Wahl P, Bouaicha S, Jakob RP, Gautier E (2011) Distal femoral varus osteotomy: problems associated with the lateral open-wedge technique. Arch Orthop Trauma Surg 131:725–728
12. Healy WL, Anglen JO, Wasilewski SA, Krackow KA (1988) Distal femoral varus osteotomy. J Bone Joint Surg Am 70:102–109
13. Stahelin T, Hardegger F, Ward JC (2000) Supracondylar osteotomy of the femur with use of compression. Osteosynthesis with a malleable implant. J Bone Joint Surg Am 82:712–722
14. Sternheim A, Garbedian S, Backstein D (2011) Distal femoral varus osteotomy: unloading the lateral compartment: long-term follow-up of 45 medial closing wedge osteotomies. Orthopedics 34:e488–e490

Meniscal Allograft Transplantation

26

M. Marcacci, S. Zaffagnini, A. Grassi,
G.M. Marcheggiani Muccioli, T. Bonanzinga,
M.P. Neri, A. Visani, M. Nitri, and D. Bruni

Contents

26.1 Introduction

Meniscal tears are the most common knee injuries, with a reported annual incidence of 61 per 100,000 people [1]. For years meniscectomy has been considered the gold standard treatment for meniscal lesions, due to the lack of knowledge regarding the role of the meniscus and the long-term effects of its deficiency. In fact nowadays, it is well known that even partial deficiency of the meniscus could be destructive for knee joint at long term. It is reported that meniscectomy increases the risk of developing knee osteoarthritis after 10 years of about 20 % for medial meniscus and 40 % for lateral meniscus [2] (Fig. 26.1). This is due to its important and irreplaceable functions, such as increasing congruity of the joint, reducing contact stresses, shock absorption, stabilization, proprioception, and cartilage lubrification and nutrition [3, 4]. For these reasons the management of meniscal tears changed

M. Marcacci • S. Zaffagnini (✉) • A. Grassi
G.M.M. Muccioli • T. Bonanzinga • M.P. Neri
A. Visani • M. Nitri • D. Bruni
II Orthopaedic and Traumathologic Clinic - Biomechanics Lab, Rizzoli Orthopaedic Institute, Via di Barbiano 1/10, 40136 Bologna, Italy
e-mail: stefano.zaffagnini@biomec.ior.it

A.A. Shetty et al. (eds.), *Techniques in Cartilage Repair Surgery*,
DOI 10.1007/978-3-642-41921-8_26, © ESSKA 2014

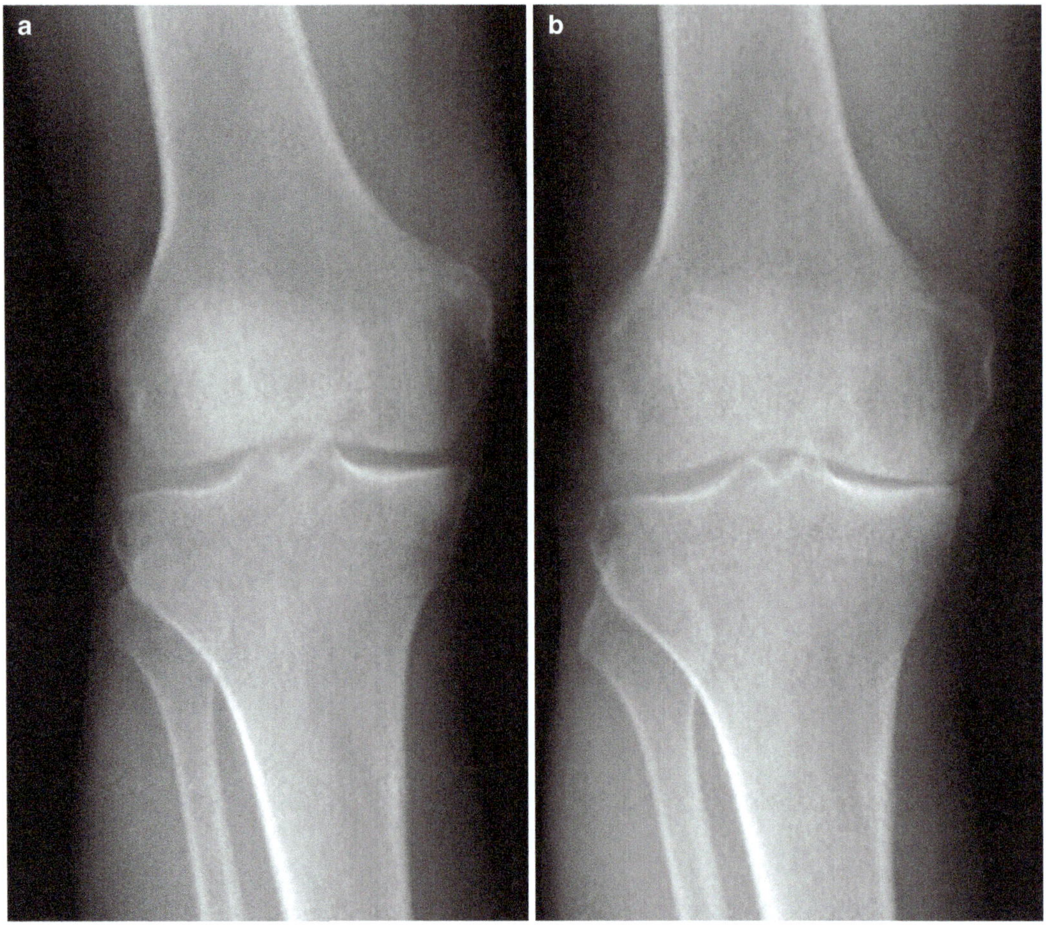

Fig. 26.1 Anteroposterior radiographs of the knee before (**a**) and 10 years after a medial meniscectomy (**b**). Reducing of medial joint space is evident

dramatically over the years, from aggressive toward more conservative strategies. In this background meniscal substitution with allograft and more recently with scaffolds has been proposed in case of irreparable lesions.

The first meniscal allograft transplantation (MAT) was performed in 1984 by Milachivski, who reported after 5 years the results of 23 MAT associated with anterior cruciate ligament (ACL) reconstruction [5].

Since then, huge progresses have been made regarding techniques, graft processing, patient selection, and evaluation, and thousands of patients have been treated with MAT in about 30 years [6]. Although there are a high number of studies reporting good outcomes and acceptable incidence of minor complications of this treatment, there is still controversy in considering MAT as experimental or gold standard treatment for postmeniscectomy symptomatic patient, as recently proposed [6].

Moreover, there is not a standard technique to perform MAT, and various authors supported by experimental and in vitro studies proposed different options to process, size, and fix the graft. Most of the authors proposed also different indications to MAT, associating or not associating concomitant surgeries.

As we can see the meniscal allograft transplantation is still a controversial issue that needs more accurate and high-quality studies in order to clarify its real benefits and its potential chondroprotective effect.

26.2 Patient Selection and Preoperative Evaluation

Surgery for the meniscus-deficient knee should be considered only after exhausting all nonsurgical measures. Nonsurgical treatments of patients who have undergone meniscectomy include unloading braces, encouraging nonimpact activities, and medications. When these measures fail to provide relief of symptoms or to prevent joint space narrowing, MAT may be considered [7].

Accurate selection of patients and both clinical and radiological evaluation are mandatory in order to obtain a good result and prevent early failure.

26.2.1 Indications

The indication for meniscal allograft transplantation has yet to be comprehensively defined. There is no consensus regarding inclusion or exclusion criteria; therefore, MAT could be suggested in a patient that meets all the following features:

- Young age (<55 years)
- History of meniscectomy
- Pain localized to the meniscus-deficient compartment
- Stable knee joint
- No malalignment (<2° of deviation toward affected compartment, as compared with the contralateral mechanical axis)
- Articular cartilage with minor evidence of degenerative changes (<grade 3 according to International Cartilage Repair Society classification or <III° according to Outerbridge classification) (Table 26.1)

MAT could also be performed in ACL-deficient patient with history of medial meniscectomy in conjunction with concomitant ACL reconstruction, as it has been reported that associated MAT improves laxity when compared to isolated ACL reconstruction [8].

Table 26.1 Description of Outerbridge grading for cartilage damage

Grade	Description
Grade 0	Normal cartilage
Grade 1	Cartilage with softening and swelling;
Grade 2	Partial thickness that do not reach subchondral bone
Grade 3	Fissuring to the level of subchondral bone
Grade 4	Exposed subchondral bone

26.2.2 Contraindications

Generally the most common contraindication to MAT is advanced chondral degeneration, characterized by cartilage wear and radiographic evidence of osteophytes or femoral condyle flattening. It is reported that a better outcome is achieved in patient with mild unicompartmental arthritic changes, while higher risk of graft extrusion and rupture in knees with advanced osteoarthritis. Localized chondral defects may be addressed concomitantly with chondrocyte transplantation, osteochondral grafting, or synthetic scaffolds.

Also malalignment is reported to cause abnormal pressure on the meniscal allograft resulting in impaired revascularization that could lead to degeneration and loosening of the graft. Therefore, a corrective osteotomy should be considered in case of greater than 2° of deviation toward the involved compartment, as compared to contralateral mechanical axis [9].

Obesity, synovial disease, inflammatory arthritis, untreated instability of knee joint, and previous joint infections represent other contraindications to take into account. The lack of symptoms remains a controversial issue, as prophylactic meniscal transplantation is not routinely recommended. In fact MAT is not without risks and current evidence has yet to demonstrate long time prevention of arthrosis. On the other hand, meniscal transplantation could be performed prior to symptom onset in young, athletic patients with complete meniscectomy, as better outcomes are reported in knees with less degenerative changes.

26.2.3 Clinical Evaluation

In order to satisfy the inclusion criteria, an accurate history of knee trauma, injuries, and surgical procedure should be obtained. Knee pain, swelling, and mechanical symptoms exacerbated by physical

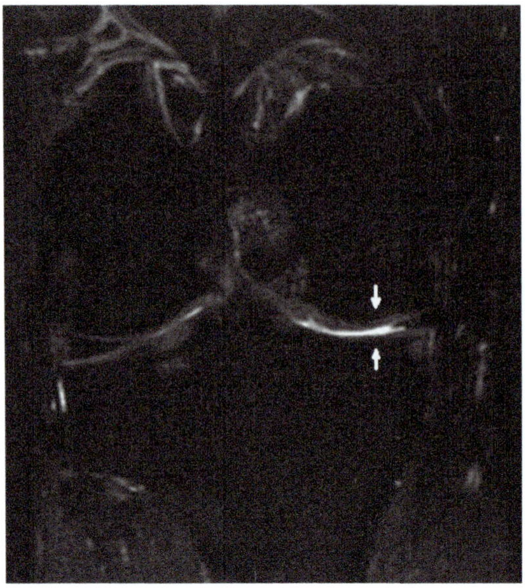

Fig. 26.2 MRI appearance of medial meniscus-deficient knee (*white arrows*)

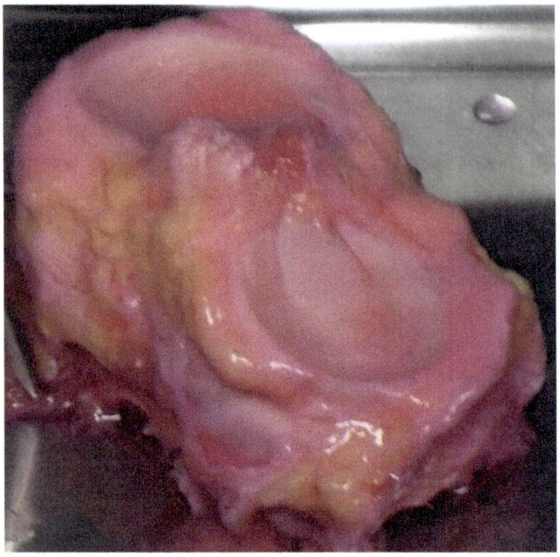

Fig. 26.3 Fresh meniscal allograft

activity are often complained after several years of adequate knee function after a meniscectomy.

A targeted physical examination should be performed and height, weight, and BMI collected as well. With the patient standing, lower limb alignment is evaluated. Then range of motion and ligamentous stability are assessed both for affected and contralateral knee. Pain and tenderness should be reported exclusively to the affected compartment and ipsilateral quadriceps strength, and circumference reduction could be noted as consequence of knee pain.

26.2.4 Radiological Evaluation

An accurate radiological planning is mandatory to correctly address the surgery. Weight-bearing AP radiographs of bilateral knees in full extension and a non-weight bearing 45° of flexion lateral radiography are required. Rosenberg view (45° flexion weight-bearing PA radiograph) could be helpful to detect subtle joint space narrowing, while long-view mechanical axis radiography is necessary in case of low limb malalignment. MRI should be performed whenever possible, as it allows to evaluate the meniscal defect (Fig. 26.2), ligament lesions, subchondral bone pathologies, and cartilage status.

26.3 Graft Choice

The correct choice of the graft plays a crucial role in the good results of the procedure. In particular, the type of preservation and the sizing method could highly influence the outcomes of the transplantation, even causing early failure or rupture.

26.3.1 Graft Preservation

After the harvesting, different methods for graft preservation are available, with specific biologic implications, risks, and results.

Fresh Allograft

This preservation technique is obtained, keeping the graft at 4 °C in sterile tissue culture medium for 7 days without loss of viability (Fig. 26.3). Fresh allografts are thought to be the ideal type of transplant, because fresh tissue contains large number of cells. However, despite the viable chondrocyte population may have a beneficial effect in maintaining the mechanical integrity of the graft after the transplantation [10], the replacement of 95 % of donor cells by host cells is reported at 1 year after the transplantation [11], making the cell's viability a questionable issue. Furthermore, due to the short time of viability, it is quite impossible to match the meniscal size of donor and receiver. The lack of the sterilization process that would damage the cell's viability increases the risk of disease transmission, contributing to the restricted use of this method of graft preservation.

Lyophilization

It consists of a dehydration process that destroys all viable cells of the graft and denatures histocompatibility antigens as well. These features make the graft less likely to provoke immune response. On the other hand, lyophilized allografts are reported to have high risk of shrinkage, disruption, synovitis, and effusion [5]. These findings suggest that lyophilization may not be an appropriate processing method for meniscal allografts [12].

Cryopreservation

It is accomplished by storing the graft at −180 °C, usually with dimethyl sulfoxide or glycerol. This method partially allows the cell membrane integrity, but the percentage of viable cells is reported to decrease with storage time [13]. Furthermore, sterilization techniques that affect cells viability cannot be performed. As similar results have been described with normal and cryopreserved menisci, no evidences support the additional cost of this method.

Deep-Frozen (Fresh-Frozen)

This method consists in the graft storage at −80 °C (Fig. 26.4). Similar to lyophilization, deep-freezing destroys viable cells and denatures histocompatibility antigens, and sterilization is allowed as well. However, in this case, mechanical proprieties are not significantly altered by freezing process. The lower costs and the lack of evidences of inferior outcomes of deep-frozen allografts make this method the most commonly used [9].

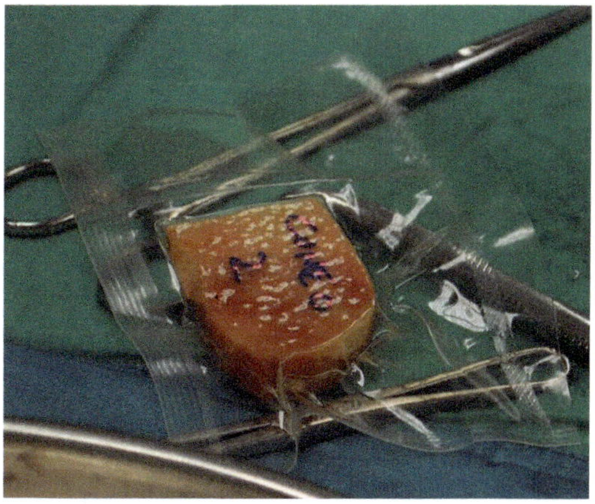

Fig. 26.4 Fresh-frozen meniscal allograft

26.3.2 Graft Sizing

Sizing of the graft plays a crucial role in the success or failure of the implant. In fact undersized grafts result in poor congruity with the femoral condyle and may produce excessive load [14], while oversized grafts may be predisposed to extrude from the compartment, causing inadequate load transmission [9]. The tolerance for size mismatch is estimated to be within 5 % of the original meniscus [15].

Various sizing methods have been proposed in order to obtain the correct size and maximize the graft's successful healing and functionality.

Intraoperative Sizing

In the first meniscal transplantation studies, allografts were shaped with the scalpel and then placed on the tibial plateau [5]. However, this procedure destroys the collagenous network and alters the graft mechanical proprieties [16].

MRI and CT Sizing

Several studies reported MRI as more accurate than radiography in preoperative sizing of the menisci for allograft transplantation [17, 18]. On the other hand, MRI and CT have been shown to underestimate the size of menisci [12]. MRI and CT have been used to estimate the graft size considering the contralateral meniscus as well, even if considerable

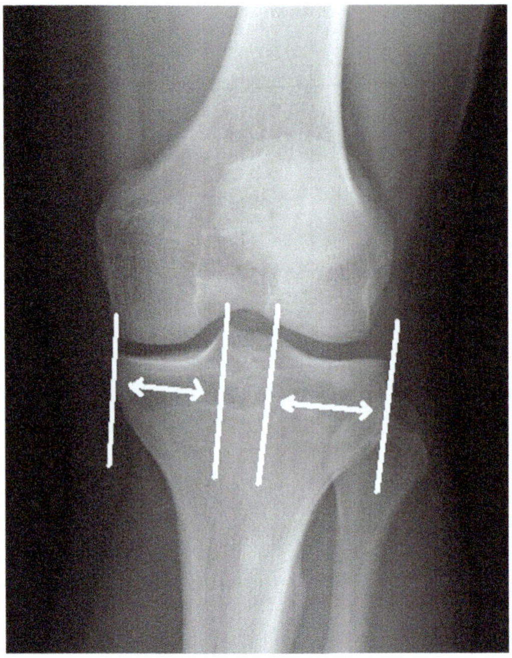

Fig. 26.5 The meniscal width is obtained measuring the distance from the peak of the tibial eminence to the periphery of the tibial metaphysis on anteroposterior films

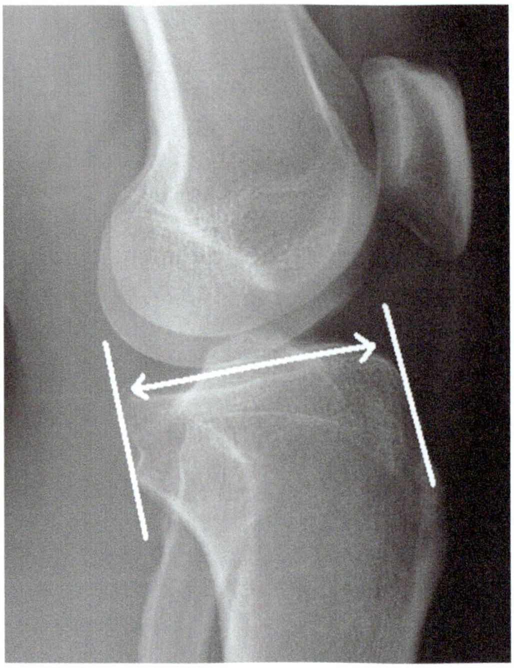

Fig. 26.6 The meniscal length is the 70 % of and the distance measured at the joint line between a line running parallel to the tibia's anterior and posterior margins on lateral films from the lateral meniscus and 80 % for medial meniscus

anatomical variability and asymmetry between right and left meniscus have been described [19].

Radiographic Sizing

Plain radiographies have been widely used as gold standard of preoperative graft sizing [9]. The common method has been developed by Pollard [20]. The correct graft size is obtained from plain films corrected for magnification, measuring the distance from the peak of the tibial eminence to the periphery of the tibial metaphysis on anteroposterior films and measuring the distance at the joint line between a line running parallel to tibia's anterior and posterior margin on lateral films. The first measure represents the meniscal width (Fig. 26.5), while meniscal length is the 70 % of the second measure for lateral meniscus and 80 % for medial meniscus (Fig. 26.6). Width matching using plain radiographs has been reported to be more reliable than length matching when it is sought to assure adequate positioning of meniscal transplants, and width mismatch has showed to predict graft subluxation [21]. Recently a modified Pollard method, consisting of reducing the total size of the graft by 5 %, has been proposed in order to decrease the percentage of meniscal extrusion [22].

Anthropometric-Based Sizing

As height, weight, and gender have been found to correlate to meniscal tissue dimensions [23], Van Thiel proposed a validated regression model that uses these variables to accurately predict required allograft meniscal size, with slightly more accuracy compared to radiographic and magnetic resonance imaging sizing techniques [24].

26.4 Techniques

A large number of techniques of meniscal allograft transplantation have been proposed by various authors, ranging from open, arthroscopically assisted, and arthroscopic techniques, each one with its own pros and cons. Although a wide range of options are available, a primary issue of each technique is the graft fixation. Two types are distinguished: bony fixation of the meniscal horns to the tibia and capsular fixation of the peripheral margin of the allograft.

- *Meniscal Horns Fixation.* This objective can be achieved with the use of soft tissue attachments, bone plugs or bridge, and suture anchors. Evidences are controversial regarding which method guarantees adequate fixation, as cadaver studies showed how bone-to-bone fixation is required to restore optimally normal contact mechanics of the transplant [25, 26], while clinical practice showed how difficult it could be achieving the perfect size match of donor and recipient and obtaining an optimal position of the graft, reporting altered contact pressure distribution in cases of nonanatomic placement of the graft [27]. Furthermore, histological evaluation showed significantly better results in bone-plug free transplants, and animal studies reported less immunogenic effect as well [28]. Besides bone-plug fixation, good clinical results have been reported also suturing meniscal horns to the ligamentous tibial bone attachment [29] and using transosseous sutures tied over a bony bridge over the anterior aspect of the proximal tibia [30]. Recently, posterior horn fixation with transosseous suture and anterior horn fixation to the capsule with an out-in stitch has been described [31].
- *Capsular Fixation.* The graft must be securely sutured to the capsule using standard meniscal repair techniques, as peripheral capsular fixation is an indispensable requisite for graft healing and vascularization. The lack of clinical controlled studies comparing different fixation techniques does not allow to determine the best suture method; thus, nonasorbable or nonasorbable sutures, vertical stitches, or all-inside devices could be used on the base of surgeon preferences [12].

26.4.1 Open Techniques

Open techniques for meniscal allograft transplantation are first described in the late 1980s. Nowadays, these have been almost completely replaced by arthroscopical or arthroscopically assisted techniques because of less soft tissue disruption, the possibility to avoid collateral detachment, decreased morbidity, and early rehabilitation. However, some believe that an open surgical procedure may enable more secure peripheral suturing or bony fixation of the graft allowing greater precision and stability [9].

Double Bone-Plug Technique

The open approach to meniscal transplantation is performed with knee at 80° of flexion. A paramedial parapatellar incision is made in case of medial meniscus transplantation. Using a curved 1 in. osteotome, the origin of medial collateral ligament on the femoral epicondyle is removed. The medial compartment is exposed using valgus stress. Two 10 mm holes are prepared directly at the anatomic site of each horn's bony insertion. The graft, prepared leaving two bone blocks attached to meniscal horns, is placed on the tibial plateau. The middle of each of the graft's bone plugs is secured with 20 mm long, 4 mm cancellous screw, or in alternative a bioabsorbable 7 mm diameter interference screw is inserted alongside the bone block. Then the meniscal edge is sutured to the joint capsule. Finally reattachment of the medial epicondyle to the femur is achieved by a staple or screw [15].

A lateral double bone-plug technique could be performed in a similar manner, although the "trough" technique is preferred because of the closeness of the anterior and posterior lateral meniscus insertions.

Trough (Bridge-in-Slot) Technique

This technique could be performed for both meniscal transplantations, although it is almost exclusively reserved to lateral meniscus transplantation, because the distance between the anterior and posterior horns of lateral meniscus is often 1 cm or less. For this reason the graft is prepared incorporating both insertions on a single bone bridge. Then a paramedial parapatellar incision is made and a rectangular bone trough is prepared at the lateral meniscal anterior and posterior tibial attachment sites to match the dimensions of the prepared lateral meniscal transplant. Then the allograft is inserted into the trough and secured using a no. 2 braided suture [15].

This technique could be used for combination of medial and lateral meniscal transplantation, implanting the allograft with a common bone bridge that contains both menisci attachments [14].

Soft Tissue Fixation

Medial or lateral parapatellar incision is performed depending on the interested compartment. The collateral ligament is released with a bone plug from the epicondyle to open up the compartment and allowing the suture fixation of all the allograft to meniscal rim. In addition, the meniscal soft tissue at the anterior and posterior horns may be fixed with transosseous suture [32].

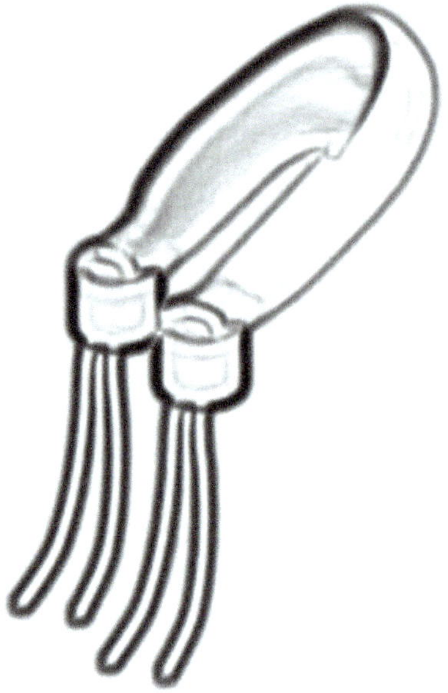

Fig. 26.7 The allograft is prepared leaving two bone plugs at the posterior and anterior horns, with sutures passing trough each bone plug

26.4.2 Arthroscopically Assisted

With the advent of arthroscopic era, open techniques were modified and adapted in order to be partially assisted form arthroscopy, reducing the extent of accesses and soft tissue disruption and trying to improve surgical outcomes.

Double Bone-Plug Technique

Due to menisci anatomy, this technique is reserved to medial meniscal transplantation. The patient is placed in the supine position on the operating room table with a tourniquet applied with a leg holder, and the table was adjusted to allow 90° of knee flexion. Diagnostic arthroscopy is done to confirm the preoperative diagnosis and articular cartilage changes. Then the allograft is prepared leaving two bone plugs as follows: the posterior bone plug was 8 mm in diameter and 12 mm in length. The anterior bone plug was 12 mm in diameter and 12 mm in length. Three 2-0 nonabsorbable sutures were passed retrograde trough each bone plug, with two additional locking sutures for secure fixation of the bone plugs within the tibial tunnel (Fig. 26.7). A 4-cm skin incision was made on the anterior aspect of the tibia adjacent to the tibial tubercle and patellar tendon. A second 3-cm posteromedial incision was made. A guide pin was placed adjacent to the tibial tubercle and was directed to the anatomic posterior meniscal attachment, and a tibial tunnel was drilled over the guidewire to a diameter of 8 mm. At least 8 mm of opening was required adjacent to the posterior cruciate ligament in the femoral notch to pass the posterior osseous portion of the graft . In tight knees, a subperiosteal release of the long fibers of the tibial attachment of the medial collateral ligament could be required.

The meniscal bed is prepared by removing any remaining meniscal tissue while preserving a 3-mm rim when possible. A 3-cm medial arthrotomy was used to pass the posterior bone portion of the graft. The posterior attachment guidewire is retrieved, and the sutures attached to the posterior bone are passed. Then the optimal location for the anterior meniscal bone attachment was identified and a 12-mm rectangular bone attachment was fashioned to correspond to the anterior bone portion of the meniscal graft. A 4-mm bone tunnel is placed at the base of this bone trough. The sutures are passed trough the bone tunnel, and the anterior horn is seated (Fig. 26.8). Tension is applied to the anterior bone sutures and inside-out suture repair is per-

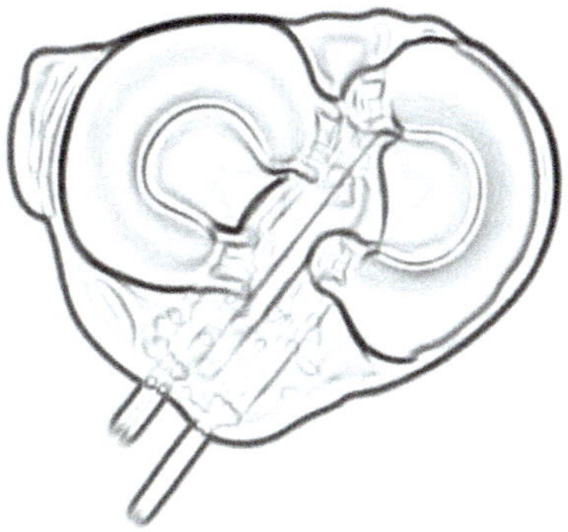

Fig. 26.8 The sutures locked in the bone plugs are passed trough the corresponding tibial tunnels and the graft is positioned on the tibial plateau

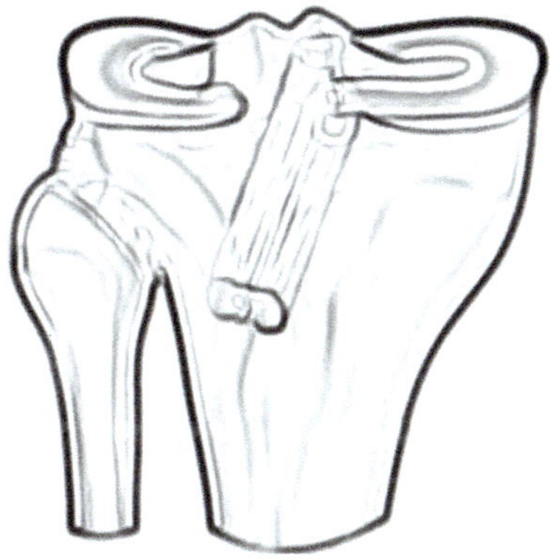

Fig. 26.9 Once the graft is in the correct position, it is secured tying the sutures on the anterior aspect of the tibia

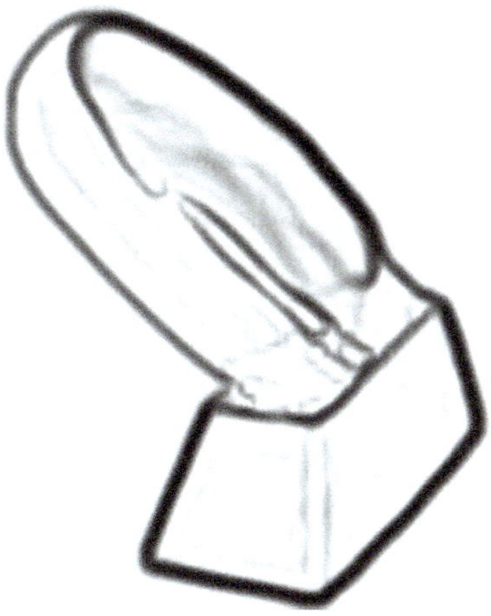

Fig. 26.10 The graft is prepared with the central bone portion incorporating the anterior and posterior meniscal attachments

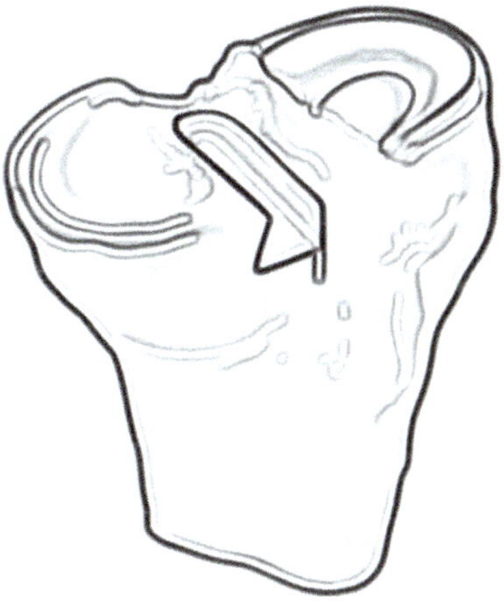

Fig. 26.11 A rectangular bone trough is prepared at the lateral meniscal anterior and posterior tibial attachment sites to match the dimensions of the prepared lateral meniscal transplant

formed after closing the anterior arthrotomy. Finally sutures are tied on the anterior aspect of proximal tibia [33] (Fig. 26.9).

Trough (Bridge-in-Slot) Technique

This technique is almost exclusively reserved for lateral meniscus transplantation. The graft is prepared with the central bone portion incorporating the anterior and posterior meniscal attachments and measuring 8–9 mm in width and 35 mm in length (Fig. 26.10). A limited 3-cm lateral arthrotomy is made just adjacent to the patellar tendon. A similar 3-cm posterolateral longitudinal approach is performed. A rectangular bone trough is prepared at the lateral meniscal anterior and posterior tibial attachment sites to match the dimensions of the prepared lateral meniscal transplant (Fig. 26.11). A 4-mm anterior tibial tunnel is drilled into the bone trough, exiting just distal to the joint line, and two sutures are passed over the central bone area of the transplant for fixation of the graft to the tibial trough. The allograft was inserted into the trough (Fig. 26.12) and the knee is flexed, extended, and rotated to confirm correct allograft placement. Finally the central bone attachment sutures are tied, the arthrotomy closed, and the inside-out meniscal repair performed [33].

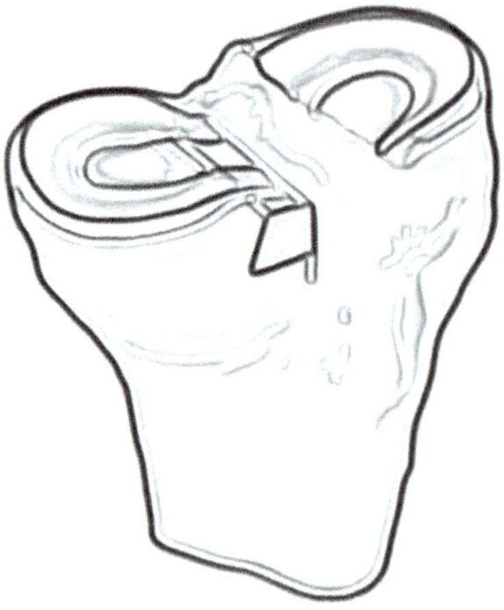

Fig. 26.12 The bone plug is inserted into the trough and the meniscal graft is placed in the correct position

Keyhole Technique

This technique can be considered as a variation of the trough technique performed creating a round trough that narrows at the surface of the tibial plateau, allowing the bone bridge to lock into the tibial bone trough. This method should be reserved to lateral meniscal transplantation. The technique is performed making a 3–4-cm parapatellar incision with dissection to the joint capsule. The tibial guide from the keyhole instrument set is used for guide pin placement parallel to the horn attachments. An 11-mm reamer is drilled over the guide pin and subsequently a rongeur or burr is used to make a 6-mm-wide slot connecting the superior aspect of the 11-mm tunnel to the tibial eminence groove. It is necessary to perform an arthrotomy when making the keyway slot, but when preparing the slot posteriorly, a dry arthroscopic technique is very helpful for visualization. The tibial slot sizer is used to assure the keyway is completely prepared, and then the preparation of the allograft can be performed. The graft is mounted on the workstation and anchored by 2 posts and the cylindrical section of the graft is prepared by advancing the handheld, slotted, coring reamer over one half of the graft and subsequently completed from the opposite end. An oscillating saw is used to make vertical cuts down the long axis of the graft to prepare the slot portion of the graft. A "reduction" suture is placed in the posterior corner of the allograft and passed trough the knee at a position approximating that of the graft, and with light tension on the suture to assist in graft reduction, the graft is inserted using a collared pin. Initially, horizontal sutures should be placed in the superior aspect of the graft, starting from the posterior and then the middle section of the graft. Once the preliminary sutures are placed, the capsule is closed and the repair is completed using arthroscopic techniques. Vertical mattress sutures are commonly used due to their greater strength, while all-inside methods are often used at the most posterior aspect to avoid neurovascular injury. Routinely, 8–10 sutures are all that are needed to secure the graft [34].

26.4.3 Arthroscopic Techniques

The most recent techniques described in the field of meniscal allograft transplantation are performed completely arthroscopically. To allow graft fixation without performing arthrotomic accesses, bone-plug free grafts are used. This offers advantage as less morbidity, early rehabilitation, and easier matching to compartment size [30, 31, 35].

Double Tibial Tunnel

After a complete diagnostic arthroscopy, debridement of meniscal remnants is done to achieve a good bleeding bed. Then, two 6-mm bone tunnels are drilled at the anatomic sites of meniscal insertion. The allograft is prepared placing sutures with Krackow mattress at both horns. One additional vertical mattress suture is placed from 1.5 cm of the posterior horn in order to aid in situating the graft. The posterior horn suture is used to pull the meniscal allograft in place. Then an inside-out technique with vertical mattress sutures is used to fix the graft to the rim. Finally the sutures placed in the anterior and posterior horns are tied together over the tibia cortical surface [35] (Fig. 26.13).

Single Tibial Tunnel

After removing the remnant of the native meniscus and creating a bleeding bed at the periphery, the graft is prepared by removing bone plugs and fixing one nonabsorbable suture to the posterior meniscal horn in a modified Mason-Allen fashion and an absorbable one to the anterior meniscal horn in a modified Kessler fashion (Fig. 26.14). The superior portion of the meniscus is marked with radial signs with a surgical marker to prevent mismatching and twisting during arthroscopic insertion. A 3-mm drill is used to prepare one tibial tunnel with the entrance on the medial side of the tibia. For medial meniscal transplantation, the posterior tunnel is placed behind the medial tibial spine and in front of the PCL tibial insertion site. For lateral meniscal transplantation, the tunnel is placed behind the ACL tibial insertion. A knot pusher was used to pass a "shuttle suture" trough the posterior tibial tunnel. The "shuttle suture" was tied to the nonabsorbable suture placed into the posterior horn and passed trough the posterior tunnel, acting as a transport suture from inside to outside (Fig. 26.15). The graft is introduced in the joint space with a fine, smooth Klemmer forceps trough the arthroscopic portal (enlarged to 1 cm) and located correctly by pulling the suture fixed to the posterior meniscal horn. Then, the graft is fixed to the capsule with a mean of 5 "all-inside" stitches, keeping under desired tension the 2 meniscal horn-fixing sutures (Fig. 26.16). The anterior meniscal horn is then fixed to the capsule by the previously placed absorbable suture trough the corresponding working arthroscopic portal

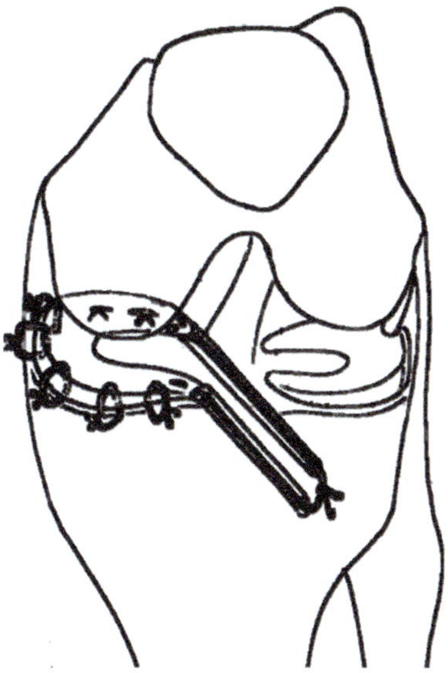

Fig. 26.13 Final aspect of the double-tunnel arthroscopic MAT. The graft is secured to the tibia trough two sutures and to the capsule with inside-out vertical mattress sutures

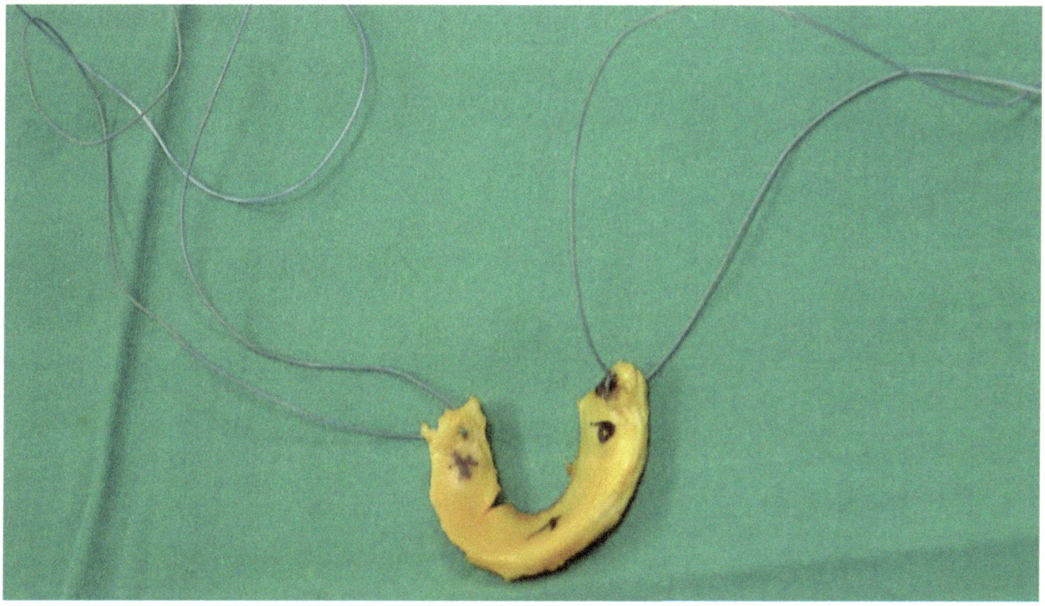

Fig. 26.14 The graft is prepared by removing the bone plugs and fixing one nonabsorbable suture to the posterior meniscal horn in a modified Mason-Allen fashion and an absorbable one to the anterior meniscal horn in a modified Kessler fashion

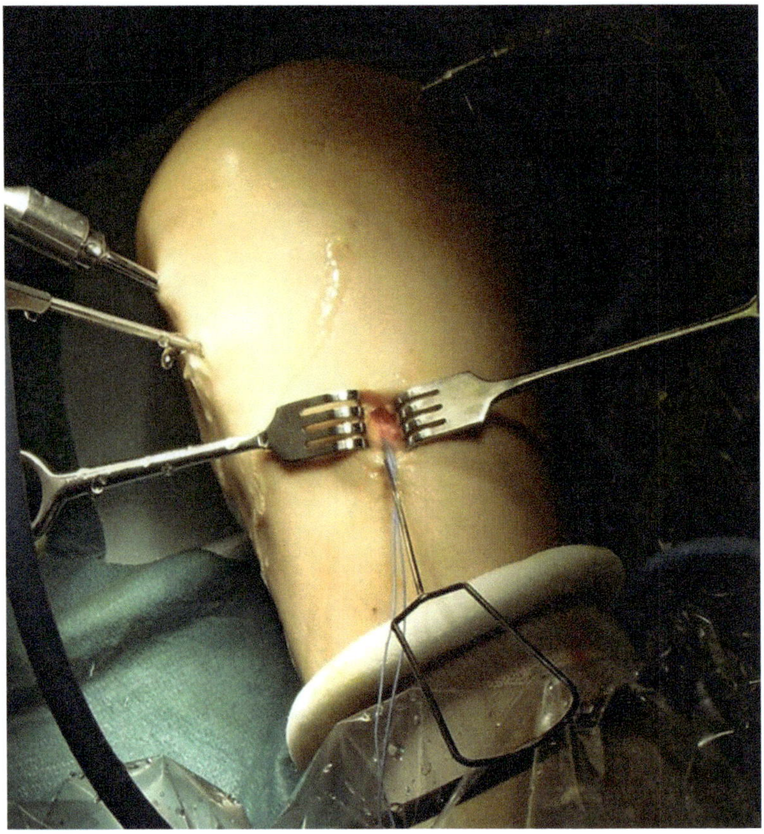

Fig. 26.15 A knot pusher is used to pass a "shuttle suture" trough the posterior tibial tunnel. The "shuttle suture" is tied to the nonabsorbable suture placed into the posterior horn and passed trough the posterior tunnel, acting as a transport suture from inside to outside

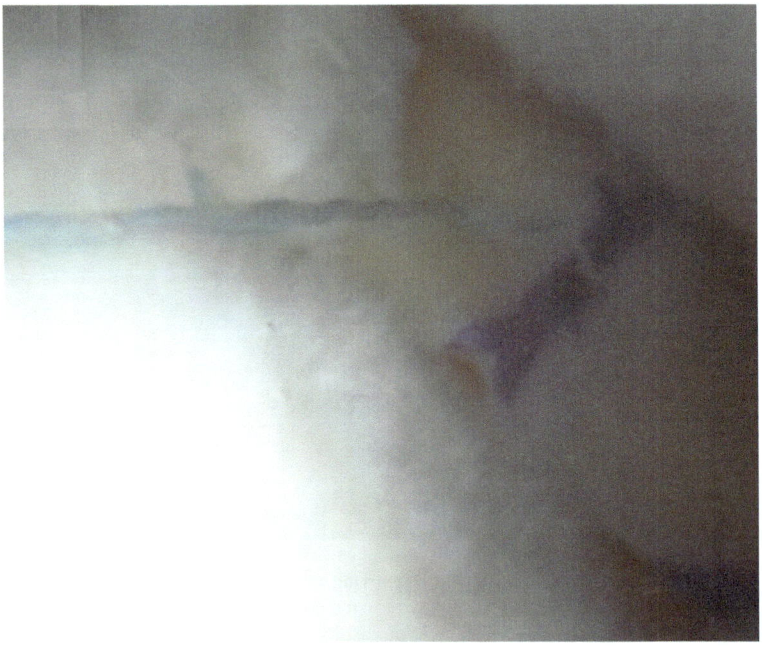

Fig. 26.16 Arthroscopic capture of single-tunnel MAT. The graft is fixed to the capsule with a mean of 5 "all-inside" stitches, keeping under desired tension the 2 meniscal horn-fixing sutures

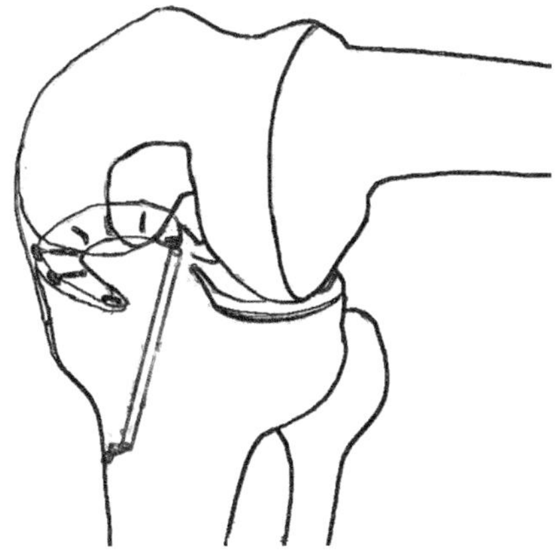

Fig. 26.17 Final aspect of the single-tunnel arthroscopic MAT

(Fig. 26.17). Finally, after the transplanted meniscus is checked for stability and matching, skin suture, a compressive bandage, and a full extension brace are placed [31].

26.5 Associated Procedures

Associated procedures are very common when MAT is performed, as only 36 % of all transplantations described in literature are isolated and only three trials present data of isolated MAT [36–38]. The percentage most commonly performed in association with MAT is ACL reconstruction (42 % of associated procedures and 30 % of cases), while the second most common concomitant surgery is cartilage treatment (31 %). Also corrective osteotomy is performed frequently, in 19 % of MAT. Other procedures performed rarely comprise osteotomies of the tibial tuberosity, retinacular releases, adhesiolysis, capsular placation, hardware, and loose body removals [6].

26.5.1 MAT and ACL

Meniscal transplantation combined with ACL reconstruction is performed in knees with ACL insufficiency and meniscal deficiency. In fact it is reported better KT-1000 arthrometer results in patients treated with ACL reconstruction and medial MAT compared to ACL reconstruction alone [8]. Different techniques of ACL reconstruction are used, comprising single or double bundle and hamstrings, patellar tendon, or allogeneic grafts. Usually ACL tunnels are performed before meniscal allograft insertion. Then MAT is completed. When performing MAT with bone plug or trough technique, special care is required because the ACL tibial tunnel often encroaches on the bone trough. To avoid this problem, the ACL graft passage and femoral fixation should be done before placing lateral meniscal allograft bone bridge [7]. Graf et al. [39] reported good clinical results at mean 9.7-year follow-up, with stable knees and patient satisfaction. Radiographic evaluation showed abnormal IKDC grade in 88 % of patients, due to significant degenerative arthritis at the time of transplantation.

26.5.2 MAT and Cartilage Treatment

As chondral damage is considered a negative prognostic factor in meniscal allograft transplantation, cartilage repair and restoration techniques are becoming a necessary adjunct to meniscus transplant for optimal biological joint preservation. The combination of these two surgical techniques has been shown to have the same outcomes as either technique was performed individually [40]. The options available include autologous chondrocyte implantation (ACI), microfractures, osteochondral allograft, and bioengineered scaffolds. Improving in clinical objective and subjective scores is reported at 1–4.5 years follow-up. Although 50 % of patients is reported to require 1 or more subsequent surgeries from 2 to 4 years after combined MAT and cartilage treatment (most of which was debridement of ACI hypertrophy), failure rate is 12 %. Most of the failures are due to MAT (85 %) versus the cartilage techniques [40].

26.5.3 MAT and Osteotomies

Even if osteotomy is a very common procedure associated to MAT, no studies report the results of these two procedures alone. Most of the time the treatment with osteotomy and MAT represents the subgroup of a wider group of patients treated with the combination of different techniques. The high number of osteotomies performed is due to the necessity to correct the axial malalignment in order to prevent the overload on the graft and avoid early failure. Usually closing wedge high tibial osteotomy is performed with medial MAT in case of varus malalignment, while open wedge distal femoral osteotomy is performed with lateral MAT in case of valgus malalignment [31]. In fact axial malalignment is frequently present in patients treated with total or subtotal meniscectomy several years before the onset of symptoms; in this scenario MAT and osteotomy appear the only biological solution available in order to correctly address the meniscus deficiency. The debate of which of the two procedures really improve pain and symptoms is unknown, unless controlled trial comparing osteotomy alone and MAT plus osteotomy in homogeneous groups of patients is performed.

26.6 Rehabilitation

Rehabilitation after MAT is a still debated and controversial issue, as the effects of loading on the new meniscal graft are not well understood. Different rehabilitation regimens have been proposed in clinical practice, but there is still lack of consensus, similarly to meniscal repair [9]. Good results have been reported with immediate full range of motion and unlimited weight bearing, while other studies recommended full extension and non-weight bearing even for 6 weeks [41]. A prudent approach to rehabilitation after MAT is represented by initially limiting flexion, as after 60° anterior translation of the meniscus and increased stress on posterior repair begin. Also weight-bearing restriction is suggested, to not compromise the graft healing and fixation during the early postoperative revascularization. Isometric exercises are recommended to prevent muscle atrophy. The expected time to sport activity resumption ranges from 4 to 12 months [9].

As a sample, the rehabilitative protocol proposed by Marcacci et al. [31] (Table 26.2) consists of 4 weeks with a full extension knee brace. The brace immobilizer is removed two times a day to perform knee mobilization with motorized hardware. Starting the day after surgery, patients begin progressive range of motion from 0° to 45° over the first 2 weeks and 0° to 90° over the next 2 weeks, after which full motion is progressively allowed. At week 6 postoperatively, patients are allowed to fully bend the knee involved in transplantation. Over the first 4 weeks, patients are allowed to walk without weight bearing with 2 crutches. At week 4 postoperatively, patients start to bear weight as tolerated and wean off 1 crutch. At week 6 postoperatively, full weight bearing is started. Quadriceps-setting exercises and straight-leg raises begin from the second day after surgery. After 2 weeks, patients start stationary bike exercises and are allowed to perform swimming pool exercises (after stitches are removed). Only at week 4 the rehabilitation of the musculature trough isotonic exercises is initiated. Return to noncontact sports is not allowed until the fourth month, and patients are advised not to resume contact sports until 8 months postoperatively.

Table 26.2 Rehabilitation protocol after MAT proposed by Marcacci et al. [31]

Time	Motion	Weight bearing	Exercise
Weeks 1–2	Full extension (brace), passive mobilization 0–45°	No weight bearing (2 crutches)	Quadriceps strengthening (isometric)
Weeks 3–4	Full extension (brace), passive mobilization 0–90°	No weight bearing (2 crutches)	Cyclette, water gym
Weeks 5–6	Complete	Partial weight bearing (1 crutch)	Quadriceps strengthening (isotonic)
Week 7–month 4	Complete	Full weight bearing	Progressive return to sport (noncontact)
Month 5–8	Complete	Full weight bearing	Progressive return to sport (contact)

Otherwise, standardized rehabilitation protocols are not applicable in every patient, as the rehabilitative programs are often determined by the very frequent concomitant procedures performed at the time of MAT, in particular cartilage treatment. Thus, a correct one should be tailored considering age, expectation, and associated surgeries.

26.7 Risks and Complication

Although meniscal allograft transplantation is considered a safe procedure, it is not totally free of risks. In addition to the usual potential complications of surgery and anesthesia, other risks are related to the allograft tissue and to the surgical technique.

26.7.1 Immunological Reaction

Although meniscal allografts have been demonstrated to express class I and II histocompatibility antigens and to present the possibility to produce host immune response (in particular regarding bone-plug grafts) [42], it is reported only one case of frank immunologic rejection of a cryopreserved graft, based on histologic and clinical evidence [43]. Furthermore, fresh meniscal allografts are reported to not elicit significant immune response at mean 4.5-year follow-up [9]. Only subclinical immunoreactivity is demonstrated in deep-frozen allografts [44], with unknown effects on graft health and outcomes.

Considering these findings, in general MAT is considered safe, with no evidence of failure or rejection due to immunological response [12].

26.7.2 Disease Transmission

The use of meniscal allograft creates a risk of transmission of diseases. As MAT is not a life-saving measure, this risk is justified only if it is exceedingly small. The different methods of preservation and processing do not present the same risks of disease transmission. In fact, as deep-freezing and lyophilization cannot destroy human immunodeficiency virus (HIV), grafts treated with these methods present a risk of HIV transmission of 1 in 8 million. HIV and other transmissible life-threatening viral diseases like hepatitis B made sterilization techniques a crucial issue in the graft management. Gamma irradiation is the most common secondary sterilization method. The dosage of 3.6 mrad, necessary to inactivate all but 1/1,000,000 HIV-infected bone cells, is reported to produce significant changes in the mechanical proprieties of meniscal tissue, compromising its survival [45]. Regarding fresh and cryopreserved allograft, nonsterilization methods are possible without compromising the cells viability and the potential advantage of these conservation methods. Nevertheless, controversies are present regarding cell viability issues and the advantage of nonsterilized meniscal allografts.

Given the pitfalls associated with graft processing techniques, stringent donor selection and screening are mandatory in order to make graft processing techniques as safe as possible [12].

26.7.3 Failure

A common definition of failure is (sub)total destruction/removal of the graft with or without conversion to arthroplasty. Using this definition, the failure rate is reported to be 10.6 %. If the need for partial meniscectomy or a subsequent procedure is considered as a failure criteria, the percentage rises. The most commonly reported cause of failure is the tearing of the graft [6]. The reasons of graft rupture are various.

Uncorrect Position of the Graft

Hoop stress transmission and functional load transmission across the knee depend upon correct position and fixation of the anterior and posterior horn attachment sites. When the allograft's posterior horn is fixed in an excessively anterior position, proper load sharing is not reestablished, while an excessively anterior position of medial meniscal transplant may result in excessive compressive forces and meniscal damage [25].

Uncorrect Size of the Graft

Also the sizing of the graft plays a crucial role in the success or failure of the implant. Undersized grafts result in poor congruity with the femoral condyle and may produce excessive loads [14], while oversized grafts may be predisposed to extrude from the compartment, resulting in inadequate transmission of compressive loads across the knee [14]. Furthermore, improper sizing may exacerbate biological or immune responses, which could potentially compromise the outcome of the allograft.

Graft Extrusion

Meniscal allograft extrusion (Fig. 26.18) could be caused by preoperative sizing mismatch due to technical problems in examining radiography, over-tensioning of the meniscal suture during surgery, overstuffing with expulsion of part of the meniscal body out of the knee joint cavity, loss of fixation of both horns of the transplanted meniscus, nonanatomical position of the insertion site of the graft, and resection of too much native tissue [31]. Marcacci et al. [31] reported a 72 % of partially extruded grafts after a minimum FU of 3 years, while Verdonk [46] found a similar percentage at 10-year minimum FU. Lee et al. [47] founded a 40 % extruded allografts, but they also reported that the extruded grafts tend to be stable over the long term. Gonzales-Lucena et al. [35] reported an extrusion of 36.3 % with regard to the global allograft size in a series of 33 grafts from 5 to 8 years FU. Although these findings, no significant correlations are reported between meniscal extrusion and various clinical and radiologic outcomes at 3-year FU [31, 48]. Even if the extrusion phenomenon does not appear to influence the clinical results, it could compromise the long-term outcome and beneficial effect since an extruded graft has different biomechanical effect and predicts the increase of subchondral bone lesions and tibial plateau bone expansion [49].

26.8 Results

At the state of the art, the knowledge of MAT outcome is confounded by patient- and surgeon-specific variables, like degree of preoperative arthrosis, graft processing, surgical technique, associated procedures, and clinical and

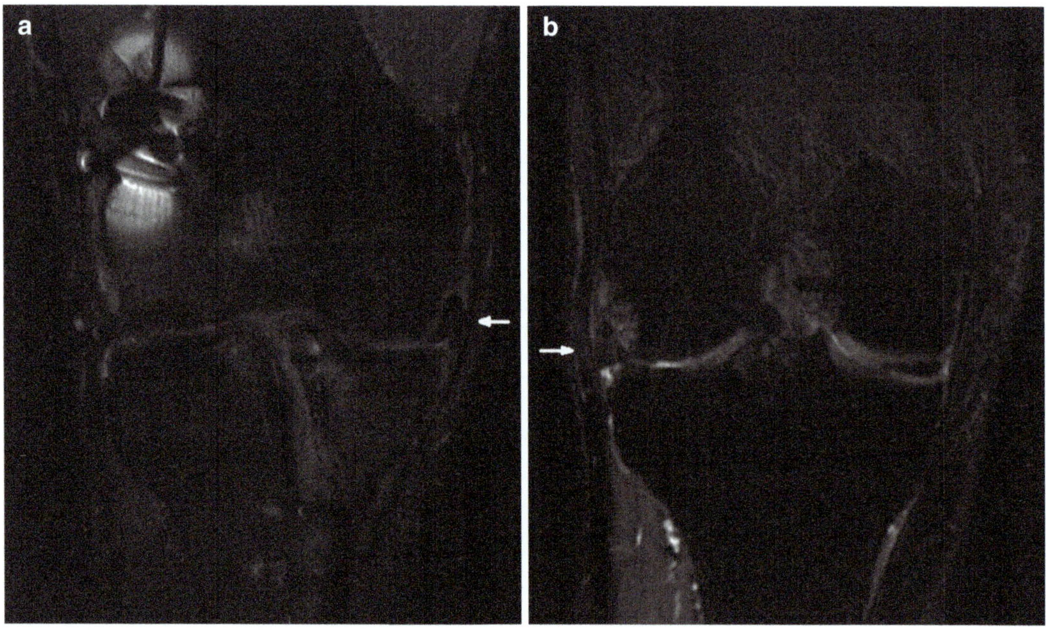

Fig. 26.18 MRI showing extrusion (*white arrows*) of medial (**a**) and lateral (**b**) meniscal allograft

radiological outcome measures. Furthermore, the quality of the studies on this controversial topic is poor, as stated in a recent meta-analysis [6]. Thus, the real effect of MAT, especially regarding long-term outcomes and chondroprotective effect, is yet to be defined.

The most important finding of more than 20 years of MAT is that this procedure is safe and reliable and should no longer be considered experimental [6].

Most of the trails present short- or medium-term outcomes, showing excellent/good results in 84 % of patients; however, the improvement of clinical scores showed a tendency to slowly decrease over time [6]. The long-term results of a case series of 100 MAT show that pain relief and functional improvement persist in approximately 70 % of patients at 10-year follow-up [50]. Generally, similar results have been reported both for medial and lateral MATs and also when the transplantation is performed alone or with concomitant procedures.

Regarding chondroprotective effect of MAT, the lack of control group consisting of conservatively treated symptomatic postmeniscectomy patients limits the power to detect it. Currently it has not yet been shown that MAT prevents or delays the degenerative process derived from meniscal deficiency over time, although various findings suggest a trend in this way.

No progression of joint space narrowing in a considerable number of patients has been reported at long-term follow-up [46]. Some authors even showed joint space gain in some patients, especially with lateral MAT [38, 39]. These promising findings obtained with radiographic evaluation seem supported by MRI evaluation as well. In fact improvement in cartilage status at 3-year follow-up [31] and potential chondroprotective effects over 10 years in a subgroup of patients [46] have been reported. On the other hand, shrinkage, extrusion, rupture, and altered signal of the graft were reported as well, both with MRI and second-look arthroscopy. Several authors documented arthroscopically good healing and incorporation of the graft and normal appearance of cartilage [6], while others reported histological evidence of viable cells in the graft periphery, neovascularization from the synovial lining and variable collagenous architecture. No evidence of immunologic rejection was documented [6].

Considering the removal of the graft or conversion to TKA as failure criteria, the overall mean failure rate is 10.6 %. If extended to MRI evidence of rupture or the need for subsequent procedures as wall, the rate increases [6]. Giving the complexity of this kind of surgery, in particular when MAT is associated to other procedures, the overall complication rate is 21.3 % and includes manipulation under anesthesia and graft rupture [6].

In conclusion, MAT is a safe and reliable procedure that enables the symptomatic patient after a meniscectomy to resume high levels of activity and works as a long-term "bridging" procedure before arthroplasty.

References

1. Baker BE, Peckham AC, Pupparo F, Sanborn JC (1985) Review of meniscal injury and associated sports. Am J Sports Med 13(1):1–4
2. Chatain F, Adeleine P, Chambat P, Neyret P, Société Française d'Arthroscopie (2003) A comparative study of medial versus lateral arthroscopic partial meniscectomy on stable knees: 10-year minimum follow-up. Arthroscopy 19(8):842–849
3. McDevitt CA, Webber RJ (1990) The ultrastructure and biochemistry of meniscal cartilage. Clin Orthop Relat Res 252:8–18
4. McBride ID, Reid JG (1988) Biomechanical considerations of the menisci of the knee. Can J Sport Sci 13(4):175–187
5. Milachowski KA, Weismeier K, Wirth CJ (1989) Homologous meniscus transplantation. Experimental and clinical results. Int Orthop 13(1):1–11
6. Elattar M, Dhollander A, Verdonk R, Almqvist KF, Verdonk P (2011) Twenty-six years of meniscal allograft transplantation: is it still experimental? A meta-analysis of 44 trials. Knee Surg Sports Traumatol Arthrosc 19(2):147–157
7. Sekiya JK, Ellingson CI (2006) Meniscal allograft transplantation. J Am Acad Orthop Surg 14(3):164–174
8. Garrett JC (1992) Meniscal transplantation. In: Aichroth PC, Canon WD, Patel DV (eds) Knee surgery: current practice. Raven, New York, pp 95–103
9. Lubowitz JH, Verdonk PC, Reid JB 3rd, Verdonk R (2007) Meniscus allograft transplantation: a current concepts review. Knee Surg Sports Traumatol Arthrosc 15(5):476–492

10. Siegel MG, Roberts CS (1993) Meniscal allografts. Clin Sports Med 12(1):59–80
11. Debeer P, Decorte R, Delvaux S, Bellemans J (2000) DNA analysis of a transplanted cryopreserved meniscal allograft. Arthroscopy 16(1):71–75
12. Rijk PC (2004) Meniscal allograft transplantation – part I: background, results, graft selection and preservation, and surgical considerations. Arthroscopy 20(7):728–743
13. Arnoczky SP, McDevitt CA, Schmidt MB, Mow VC, Warren RF (1988) The effect of cryopreservation on canine menisci: a biochemical, morphologic, and biomechanical evaluation. J Orthop Res 6(1):1–12
14. Rodeo SA (2001) Meniscal allografts – where do we stand? Am J Sports Med 29(2):246–261
15. Wilcox TR, Goble EM, Doucette SA (1996) Goble technique of meniscus transplantation. Am J Knee Surg 9(1):37–42
16. Kohn D (1994) Meniscus transplantation. In: Fu FH (ed) Advance in operative orthopaedics, vol 2. Mosby-Year Book, Chicago, pp 49–76
17. Shaffer B, Kennedy S, Klimkiewicz J, Yao L (2000) Preoperative sizing of meniscal allografts in meniscus transplantation. Am J Sports Med 28(4):524–533
18. Haut TL, Hull ML, Howell SM (2000) Use of roentgenography and magnetic resonance imaging to predict meniscal geometry determined with a three-dimensional coordinate digitizing system. J Orthop Res 18(2):228–237
19. Johnson DL, Swenson TM, Livesay GA, Aizawa H, Fu FH, Harner CD (1995) Insertion-site anatomy of the human menisci: gross, arthroscopic, and topographical anatomy as a basis for meniscal transplantation. Arthroscopy 11(4):386–394
20. Pollard ME, Kang Q, Berg EE (1995) Radiographic sizing for meniscal transplantation. Arthroscopy 11(6):684–687
21. Lee BS, Chung JW, Kim JM, Kim KA, Bin SI (2012) Width is a more important predictor in graft extrusion than length using plain radiographic sizing in lateral meniscal transplantation. Knee Surg Sports Traumatol Arthrosc 20(1):179–186
22. Jang SH, Kim JG, Ha JG, Shim JC (2011) Reducing the size of the meniscal allograft decreases the percentage of extrusion after meniscal allograft transplantation. Arthroscopy 27(7):914–922
23. Stone KR, Freyer A, Turek T, Walgenbach AW, Wadhwa S, Crues J (2007) Meniscal sizing based on gender, height, and weight. Arthroscopy 23(5): 503–508
24. Van Thiel GS, Verma N, Yanke A, Basu S, Farr J, Cole B (2009) Meniscal allograft size can be predicted by height, weight, and gender. Arthroscopy 25(7): 722–727
25. Alhalki MM, Howell SM, Hull ML (1999) How three methods for fixing a medial meniscal autograft affect tibial contact mechanics. Am J Sports Med 27(3):320–328
26. Paletta GA Jr, Manning T, Snell E, Parker R, Bergfeld J (1997) The effect of allograft meniscal replacement on intraarticular contact area and pressures in the human knee. A biomechanical study. Am J Sports Med 25(5):692–698
27. Sekaran SV, Hull ML, Howell SM (2002) Nonanatomic location of the posterior horn of a medial meniscal autograft implanted in a cadaveric knee adversely affects the pressure distribution on the tibial plateau. Am J Sports Med 30(1):74–82
28. Bos GD, Goldberg VM, Zika JM, Heiple KG, Powell AE (1983) Immune responses of rats to frozen bone allografts. J Bone Joint Surg Am 65(2):239–246
29. Verdonk R (1997) Alternative treatments for meniscal injuries. J Bone Joint Surg Br 79(5):866–873
30. Alentorn-Geli E, Seijas Vázquez R, García Balletbó M, Alvarez Díaz P, Steinbacher G, Cuscó Segarra X, Rius Vilarrubia M, Cugat Bertomeu R (2011) http://www.ncbi.nlm.nih.gov/pubmed/20390252 Arthroscopic meniscal allograft transplantation without bone plugs. Knee Surg Sports Traumatol Arthrosc. 19(2):174–182
31. Marcacci M, Zaffagnini S, Muccioli GM, Grassi A, Bonanzinga T, Nitri M, Bondi A, Molinari M, Rimondi E (2012) Meniscal allograft transplantation without bone plugs: a 3-year minimum follow-up study. Am J Sports Med 40(2):395–403
32. Verdonk PC, Demurie A, Almqvist KF, Veys EM, Verbruggen G, Verdonk R (2006) Transplantation of viable meniscal allograft. Surgical technique. J Bone Joint Surg Am 88(Suppl 1 Pt 1):109–118
33. Noyes FR, Barber-Westin SD, Rankin M (2004) Meniscal transplantation in symptomatic patients less than fifty years old. J Bone Joint Surg Am 86-A(7):1392–1404
34. Carter TR (2002) Meniscal allograft: key-hole technique. Oper Tech Sports Med 10:144–149
35. González-Lucena G, Gelber PE, Pelfort X, Tey M, Monllau JC (2010) Meniscal allograft transplantation without bone blocks: a 5- to 8-year follow-up of 33 patients. Arthroscopy 26(12):1633–1640
36. Sekiya JK, West RV, Groff YJ, Irrgang JJ, Fu FH, Harner CD (2006) Clinical outcomes following isolated lateral meniscal allograft transplantation. Arthroscopy 22(7):771–780
37. Stollsteimer GT, Shelton WR, Dukes A, Bomboy AL (2000) Meniscal allograft transplantation: a 1- to 5-year follow-up of 22 patients. Arthroscopy 16(4):343–347
38. van Arkel ER, de Boer HH (1995) Human meniscal transplantation. Preliminary results at 2 to 5-year follow-up. J Bone Joint Surg Br 77(4):589–595
39. Graf KW Jr, Sekiya JK, Wojtys EM (2004) Long-term results after combined medial meniscal allograft transplantation and anterior cruciate ligament reconstruction: minimum 8.5-year follow-up study. Arthroscopy 20(2):129–140
40. Harris JD, Cavo M, Brophy R, Siston R, Flanigan D (2011) Biological knee reconstruction: a systematic review of combined meniscal allograft transplantation and cartilage repair or restoration. Arthroscopy 27(3):409–418
41. Fritz JM, Irrgang JJ, Harner CD (1996) Rehabilitation following allograft meniscal transplantation: a review

of the literature and case study. J Orthop Sports Phys Ther 24(2):98–106
42. Khoury MA, Goldberg VM, Stevenson S (1994) Demonstration of HLA and ABH antigens in fresh and frozen human menisci by immunohistochemistry. J Orthop Res 12(6):751–757
43. Hamlet W, Liu SH, Yang R (1997) Destruction of a cryopreserved meniscal allograft: a case for acute rejection. Arthroscopy 13(4):517–521
44. Rodeo SA, Seneviratne A, Suzuki K, Felker K, Wickiewicz TL, Warren RF (2000) Histological analysis of human meniscal allografts. A preliminary report. J Bone Joint Surg Am 82-A(8):1071–1082
45. Yahia L, Zukor D (1994) Irradiated meniscal allotransplants of rabbits: study of the mechanical properties at six months postoperation. Acta Orthop Belg 60(2):210–215
46. Verdonk PC, Verstraete KL, Almqvist KF, De Cuyper K, Veys EM, Verbruggen G, Verdonk R (2006) Meniscal allograft transplantation: long-term clinical results with radiological and magnetic resonance imaging correlations. Knee Surg Sports Traumatol Arthrosc 14(8):694–706
47. Lee DH, Kim TH, Lee SH, Kim CW, Kim JM, Bin SI (2008) Evaluation of meniscus allograft transplantation with serial magnetic resonance imaging during the first postoperative year: focus on graft extrusion. Arthroscopy 24(10):1115–1121
48. Ha JK, Shim JC, Kim DW, Lee YS, Ra HJ, Kim JG (2010) Relationship between meniscal extrusion and various clinical findings after meniscus allograft transplantation. Am J Sports Med 38(12):2448–2455
49. Wang Y, Wluka AE, Pelletier JP, Martel-Pelletier J, Abram F, Ding C, Cicuttini FM (2010) Meniscal extrusion predicts increases in subchondral bone marrow lesions and bone cysts and expansion of subchondral bone in osteoarthritic knees. Rheumatology (Oxford) 49(5):997–1004, Epub 2010 Feb 24
50. Verdonk PC, Demurie A, Almqvist KF, Veys EM, Verbruggen G, Verdonk R (2005) Transplantation of viable meniscal allograft. Survivorship analysis and clinical outcome of one Hundred cases. J Bone Joint Surg Am 87(4):715–724

Part IX

Rehabilitation, Pain Management and Follow-Up

Rehabilitation After Cartilage Repair Surgery: Part II Practical Issues

27

Knut Beitzel, Ludwig Kohn, and Andreas B. Imhoff

Contents

27.1 Introduction

The primary aim of any rehabilitative procedure after cartilage repair is to reach the optimal recovery of daily activities and sportive level. It is commonly accepted that most surgical procedures for cartilage repair demand a prolonged rehabilitation period of up to 6 or more months [25, 37]. To support the healing process and optimize the postoperative result, this period should be seen equally important as the operative procedure itself [54, 63]. Although high level of evidence data is limited, basic principles are commonly accepted to direct the postoperative rehabilitation [25, 33]. These should be oriented on each individual patient and his/her specific injury/lesion, the specifics of the surgical procedure, and the particularities of each individual rehab process. This allows for choosing the correct exercises and training methods. Overall, such a process requires an interdisciplinary team of all involved therapists (surgeon, physiotherapist, primary care physicians, etc.).

General principles for the rehabilitation phase after cartilage repair surgery should be:

- Respect the characteristics of the cartilage repair construct and the characteristics of wound/tissue healing.
- Continuously assess for signs of overloading or inflammation and base the progression on functional criteria.
- Utilize the joint as a bioreactor by adequate joint loading and motion as well as optimizing the joint homeostasis.

K. Beitzel
Department of Trauma and Orthopedic Surgery, Berufsgenossenschaftliche Unfallklinik Murnau, Murnau, Germany

L. Kohn • A.B. Imhoff (✉)
Department of Orthopaedic Sports Medicine, Technical University Munich, Munich, Germany
e-mail: imhoff@tum.de

A.A. Shetty et al. (eds.), *Techniques in Cartilage Repair Surgery*,
DOI 10.1007/978-3-642-41921-8_27, © ESSKA 2014

- Respect the functional chains of motion and emphasize adequate core stability.
- Continuously communicate within the interdisciplinary rehabilitation team.

27.2 Basic Principles

A steady progression without jeopardizing or harming the repair construct is needed to achieve the primary goal of the optimal recovery up to the pre-injury level of sports and daily activities [14, 25, 66, 71]. Factors like age, weight, sportive activity, and size, localization, and type of the repaired construct should be regarded in its progression [25]. Respecting the basic principles will help to coordinate the rehab process [31].

The *first principle* is to coordinate the rehabilitation process according to the specific remodeling time required by the surgical treatment/repair and the common characteristics of wound/tissue healing. Therefore it is imperative to choose adequate loads for allowing growth and regeneration to be obtained without damaging or overloading the cartilage tissue [65, 66]. The regeneration progress after cartilage therapy can be grossly divided into four phases (time based rehabilitation) [22–28]:

1. Proliferation
2. Transition
3. Remodeling
4. Maturation [8, 9, 17, 19, 44, 48, 49]

It has to be noted that the time previous to the surgical procedure should also be respected, since adequate exercises can be applied to improve muscular strength and coordination for the postsurgical phase.

The *second principle* should be seen in continuous assessment for signs of overload or inflammation, which could indicate possible postoperative complications (such as infection and delamination of graft) or an inadequate load progression. This also includes the continuous evaluation of criterions, which should be regarded as imperative to the progression into the next level/phase of rehabilitation (criterion-based rehabilitation) [25, 31].

As the *third principle* we recommend the focus on the functional chains of motion and an optimization of core stability. These mechanisms help the patient to adequately load the repaired joint and facilitate a "physiological" function. Optimized neuromuscular functions help the joint to effectively distribute loads and protect the passive structures from reinjury. Although not finally proven in prospective studies, core stability has to be regarded as a basis for the adequate development of these tasks. Exercises and training methods within the rehabilitation procedure should therefore permanently focus on the improvement of these functions.

The *fourth principle* is to use the joint as a bioreactor for optimizing the healing of the cartilage construct. Therefore it is essential to optimize the joint homeostasis with adequate joint loading and motion. Effusion and hyperthermia may have a negative effect on cartilage regeneration and should be avoided. Furthermore a mobilization of the affected joint under moderate loading is also important for the nutrition of the cartilage and cartilage construct as well as for the healing.

The *fifth principle* is the continuous communication within the interdisciplinary rehabilitation team. Rehabilitation after cartilage therapy continues over a long period, and the patient has to be motivated throughout this time to optimize his/her compliance. Additionally possible overload or failure of the graft must be detected at an early stage to adequately change the procedure. This finally allows the patient to securely proceed through the different phases of rehabilitation.

27.3 Rehabilitation Phase (I): "Protection Phase"

The first 4–6 weeks after surgery are regarded as the early phases of rehabilitation, which are focused on protection of the implant. Additional goals are modulation of the joint homeostasis, improvement of joint motion, and patient education. The aim is to decrease inflammatory reactions of the joint and to restore range of motion. Successfully finishing this phase, the patient should be able to handle daily activities, realize the importance of continuous passive motion, and use crutches correctly to match the acceptable weight-bearing restrictions.

27.3.1 Restoring Joint Homeostasis

Effusions as well as a temperature increase due to an inflammatory reaction frequently occur after cartilage interventions. This may lead to an induction of proteolytic enzymes, which have a destructive effect on cartilage. Furthermore, intra-articular effusion in the knee joint leads to a reduced activity of the quadriceps tendon [24, 30, 35, 36, 46]. Therefore it is necessary to decrease the joint temperature with sufficient postoperative cryotherapy in order to reduce swelling/effusion. On the other hand diminished joint effusion decreases the arthrogenic quadriceps muscle inhibition [29, 38, 50, 53]. Moreover the affected limb should be positioned above heart level, and compression can be added to reduce the effusion in the initial postoperative period.

27.3.2 Improvement of Range of Motion

Detonization of hypertonic and shortened muscles may additionally increase joint mobility and decrease pain – especially, if the operated extremity is immobilized for a prolonged time. Immobilization has several negative effects on cartilage [10]. It leads to a reduction of cartilage metabolism, proteoglycan, and water content and thus results in a lower overall stiffness of the cartilage and reduced cartilage thickness [20, 22, 39]. Salter as well as Williams et al. could demonstrate the positive effect of continuous passive motion (CPM) on the cartilage regeneration in several animal studies [57–59, 70]. CPM is seen to protect as well as stimulate cartilage regeneration and differentiation. The effectiveness of CPM therapy for treatment of cartilage defects with periosteal flaps (1. Generation) could be verified in several studies [1, 41]. Positive effects of the CPM were demonstrated in comparison to isolated active training [1, 45, 60].

Overall CPM represents an important issue in the rehabilitation after cartilage repair. According to recent literature, the use of CPM for approximately 6–8 h a day for a minimum of 6 weeks postoperative is recommended (starting within 12–18 postoperative hours) [7, 25, 32, 34, 43, 56, 62]. A combination of CPM with adequate neuromuscular training is important to prevent muscular disbalance or dysfunctions [13, 32, 69]. If sufficient unloading can be assured, alternative devices like a stationary bicycle can be used.

27.3.3 Improvement of Neuromuscular Function

Studies demonstrated that a reduction of proprioception and muscle atrophy occur after trauma, surgery, or even just due to osteoarthritis [2–4, 6, 7, 15, 16, 18, 61]. In open surgical procedures, the disruption of mechanoreceptors may even lead to a greater degree of proprioceptive loss than observed in arthroscopic procedures [15, 26].

A proper neuromuscular and proprioceptive function as well as muscle strength is important for the stabilization of the joint and subsequent position and motion sequence. It is interesting to note that the reduction of proprioception may affect not only the ipsilateral but also the contralateral joint [18, 52, 55, 61]. Besides classic active assisted and active exercises, electromuscle stimulation (EMS) can be applied training of the extremities and the trunk. Thus the NMES is a good additional tool to correct a decreased muscle activity as well as to cause a muscle building [40, 47]. Contrary to this an improvement of muscular activity by the use of transcutaneous electrical nerve stimulation (TENS) is not effective according to the latest literature [29].

The retraining of coordination patterns via feedback and feedforward control systems in a functional, dynamic, and progressive manner is an important issue in postoperative neuromuscular control. In the early phases of the rehabilitation process, feedback-controlled coordination patterns consisting of slow movements should be performed. Proprioception should be trained on the affected and non-affected sides and throughout the full available range of motion [18, 52, 55, 61].

27.3.4 Weight Bearing and Gait Training

It was shown that a non-weight bearing or only partial weight bearing may lead to a decrease in proteoglycan content and gradual atrophy of the cartilage [5, 23, 27, 67]. Nevertheless it is imperative to consider localization, size, and type of surgical procedure to define the allowed weight-bearing limits. A gradual increase of weight bearing with consideration of these factors may help to facilitate the production of cartilage matrix and increase the mechanical qualities of the repair construct [11, 12, 68].

To effectively apply the allowed load limits, it is essential for the patient to learn how to walk (on plane, rough grounds, and stairs) correctly with the help of crutches. Including feedback mechanisms into specific gait exercises helps the patient to regulate their weight bearing and become familiar with the allowed weight limitations. The use of a kino-therapeutic bath may be a very useful tool in this stage.

27.4 Rehabilitation Phase II: "Transitional Phase"

The second phase includes weeks 7–12. The progressive stability of the cartilage tissue allows for progressive weight bearing as well as an increase in strength training. Weight bearing should be progressed until full weight bearing is reached, and a total recovery of the range of motion should be accomplished. Furthermore an improvement of the proprioception and of the neuromuscular as well as functional skills should be aspired. However an overloading which might result in harming the repair construct has to be strictly avoided. Exercise progression must not cause pain, which should be taken as a serious sign of overload. Furthermore swelling, effusion, hyperthermia, and regression/stagnation of range of motion may represent signs of overloading.

27.4.1 Improvement in Range of Motion

Progressive relaxing and stretching of the muscles, tendons, and fascias should further emphasize improvement of range of motion. Relaxing of muscles can be accomplished by the use of strain-counterstrain exercises, muscle energy techniques, or functional massages. Patella mobilization as well as loosening adhesions of muscles, ligaments, and neurovascular structures additionally facilitates range of motion. However, full stretching exercises should only be performed at the end of this phase, since stretching could lead to a hyper-compression of the repair tissue (Fig. 27.1a, b).

Physiological range of motion should be restored in this phase. Active assisted exercises using, e.g., a roller board wiping should be emphasized.

27.4.2 Improvement of Sensomotoric Function, Endurance, and Strength

Functional exercises can be enhanced to increase sensomotoric functions, endurance, and strength with the progression of weight bearing. Cardiovascular endurance is improved with endurance training against low resistance (e.g., stationary bicycle). Isometric strengthening and proprioceptive neuromuscular exercises utilizing resistance proximal to the affected joint are progressed (Fig. 27.2a–c).

It is important to differ open kinetic chain exercises (OKC) and closed kinetic chain exercises (CKC). Biomechanical studies have shown

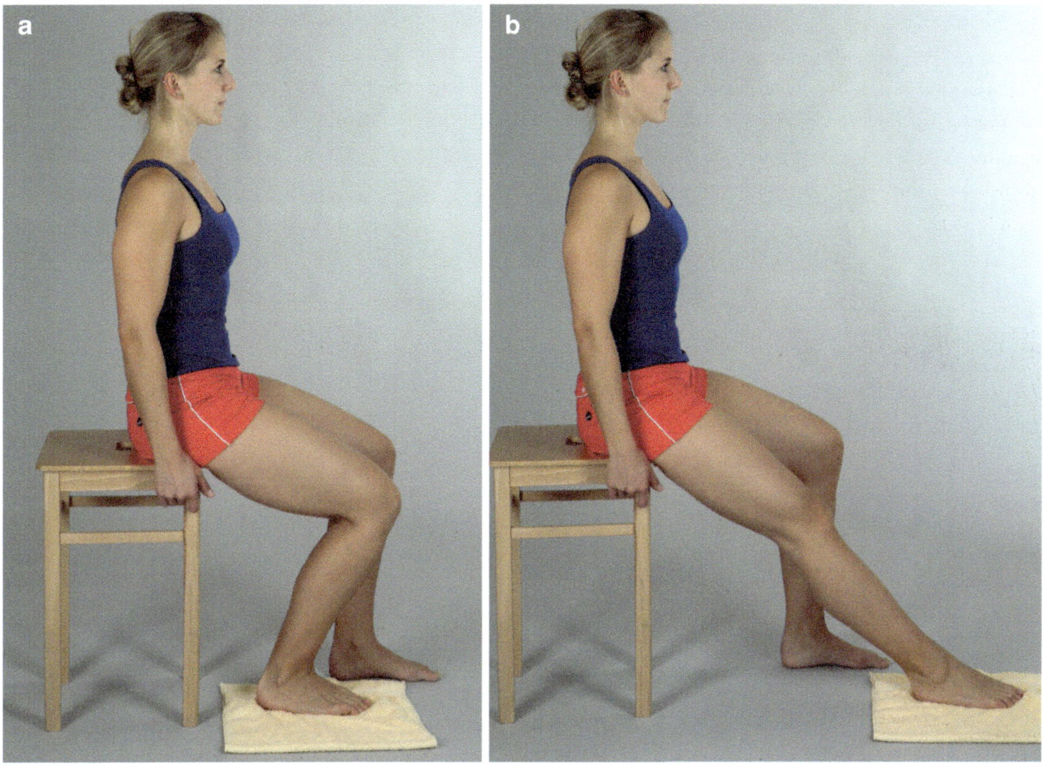

Fig. 27.1 (**a**, **b**) Active sliding exercise with partial weight bearing for improvement of ROM [31]

that OKC exercise may cause increased shear forces, while CKC exercises may increase contact pressures in the knee according to different joint positions [21, 42, 51, 64] (Fig. 27.3a, b).

In total, CKC exercises are seen superior to OKC exercises in functional terms, because the motion sequence is more physiologic. Hence an improved proprioceptive training and a synergetic muscle contraction are caused [25]. Besides exercises focusing only on the affected joint, training for core stabilization should be further emphasized.

27.4.3 Gait Training

Full weight bearing and a normal gait pattern should be achieved throughout phase II. Requirements for walking without crutches are that there is no evasion movement of the gait pattern and the patient has to be able to stabilize his/her pelvis and mechanical axis. The patient should learn to climb stairs and practice the physical rolling motion of the foot and also activities of daily living like getting in and out of a vehicle. Walking on different grounds and also on inclined plains helps achieving a normal gait pattern and improves stabilizing functions of the knee (Fig. 27.4a, b).

27.5 Rehabilitation Phase III: "Remodeling Phase"

Remodeling of the tissue repair will further progress to an organized structure with improved load-bearing capacity within weeks 12–26. The main goals of this phase are the complete return to the activities of daily living and the enhancement of a gradual return to sports (cycling, jogging, unidirectional sports-specific training). This is accomplished by a progressive increase of the intensity in cardiovascular strength and sensomotoric training.

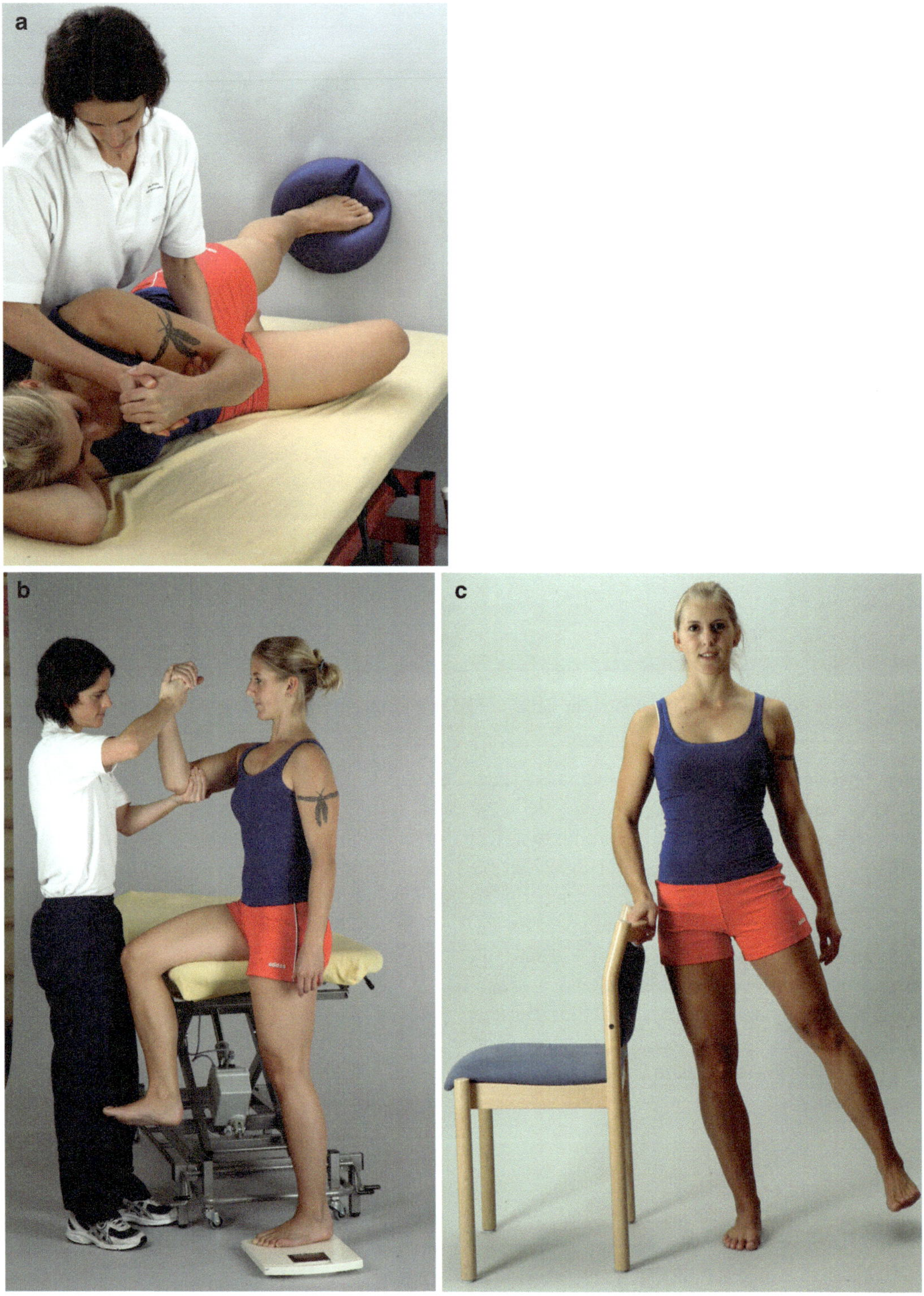

Fig. 27.2 (**a**–**c**) Different exercises for sensomotoric training using increased weight bearing [31]

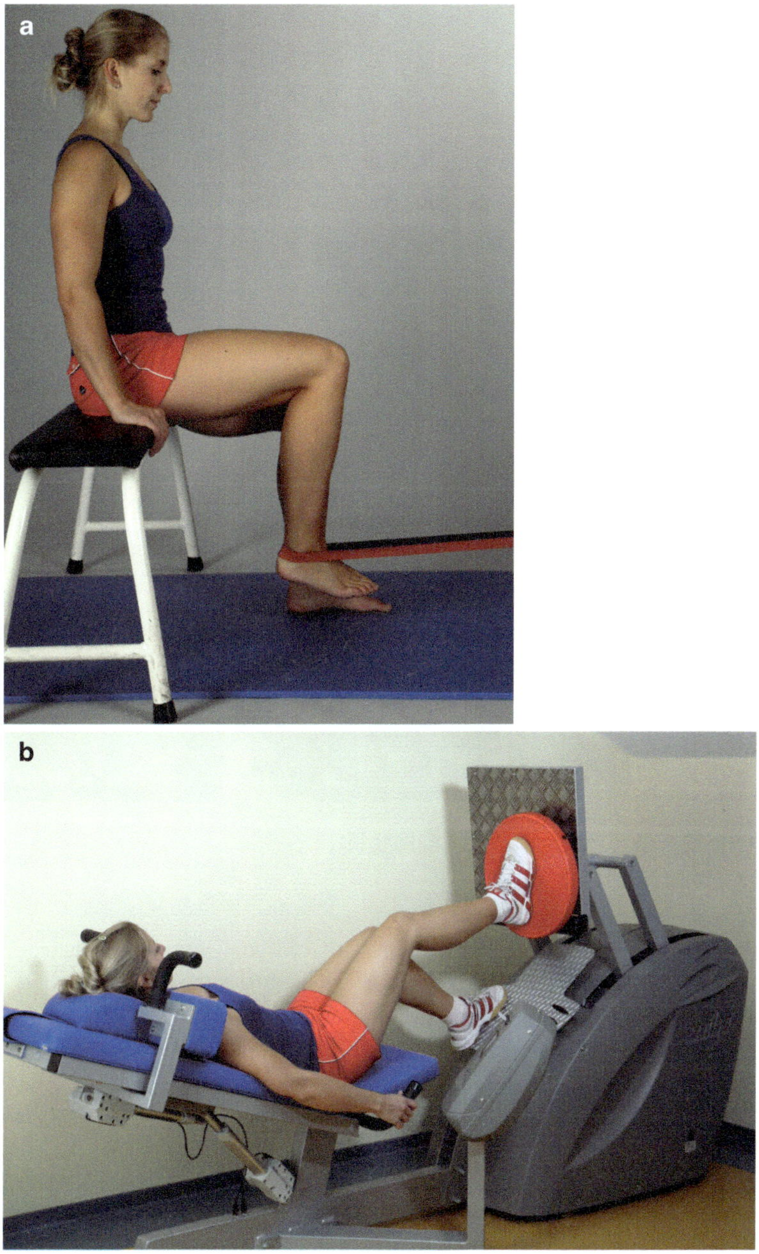

Fig. 27.3 Strengthening in open (**a**) and closed (**b**) kinetic chain exercises [31]

27.5.1 Improvement in Range of Motion

Active and passive exercises to further improve the joint's motion are continued, and stretching is further progressed. Patients should be aware that a full and pain-free range of motion is a key criterion for return to sportive activity (Fig. 27.5a, b).

27.5.2 Improvement of Sensomotoric Function, Endurance, and Strength

Sensomotoric training is further progressed using higher loads and increasing stimulation with the help of different assistive equipment (e.g., instability devices). Additional tasks

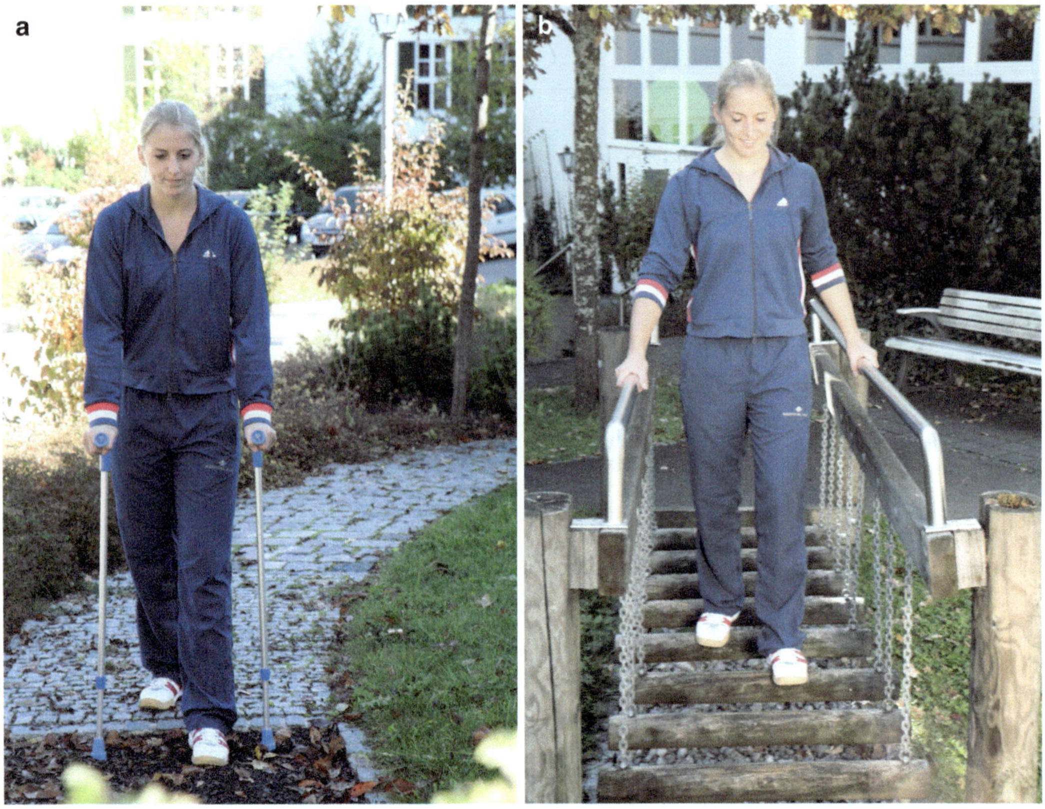

Fig. 27.4 (**a**, **b**) Variations in gait training [31]

such as one-leg stand, exercises with closed eyes, or incorporated juggling tasks are useful. Further exercises to increase sensomotoric function are practicing excentric tasks, "stop and go" movements, and quick direction changes (Fig. 27.6a–c).

Loading on the affected joint should be adapted to the patient's individual progression. Exercises to restore muscle power are, e.g., step-ups, wall slides, squats, and one-leg stabilization. An elastic band or different weights can be useful additional tools. Core stabilization is still seen as an important issue for the stabilization of the peripheral joints and should be further improved in this phase (Fig. 27.7a, b).

The intensity and amount of endurance training is progressively increased according to the patient's abilities. In the end of phase III, given an adequate stabilization and strengthening is accomplished and rotation movement is permitted, static climbing exercises on a wall (boulder training) can be very effective to increase the sensomotoric function, stabilization, and muscle growth of the whole body.

27.6 Rehabilitation Phase IV: "Maturation (Sports-Specific Recovery)"

Studies have shown that an active and sportive "lifestyle" might be helpful to achieve better results after cartilage therapy [37]. Therefore the patient/athlete should be encouraged to regain an active life including sportive activity.

The cartilage tissue reaches full maturation in phase IV ranging from 6 months after surgery up to about 18 months postoperatively. Complete maturation of the repaired tissue allows for full participation in impact sports. The final goal of

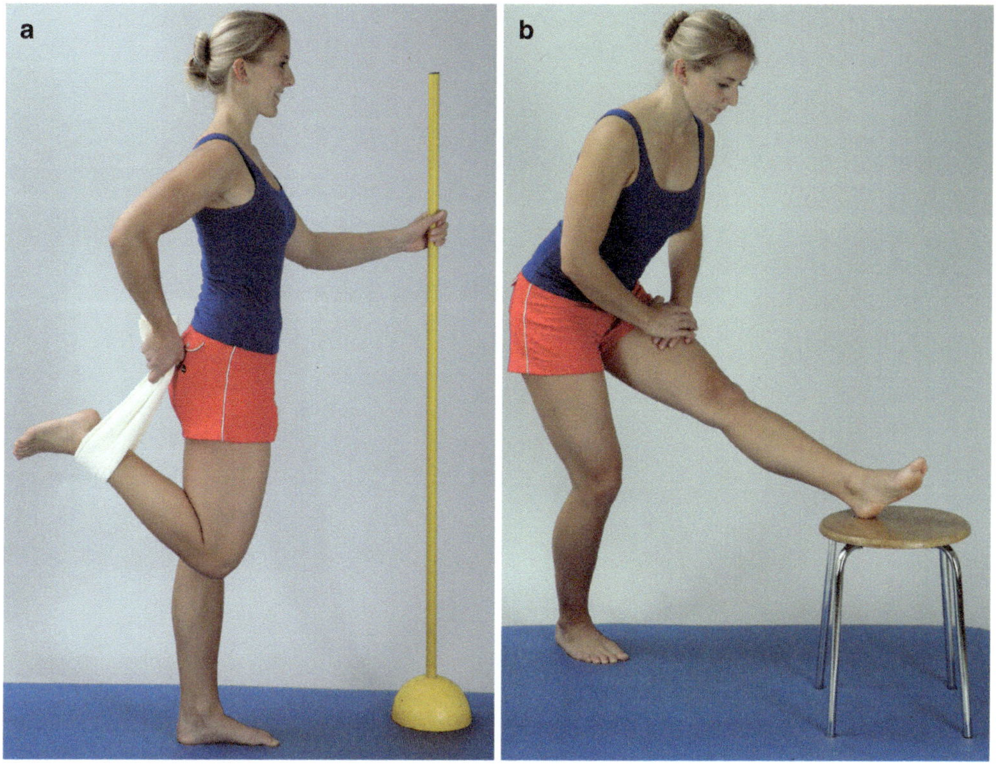

Fig. 27.5 (**a**, **b**) Variations of stretching exercises as self-training [31]

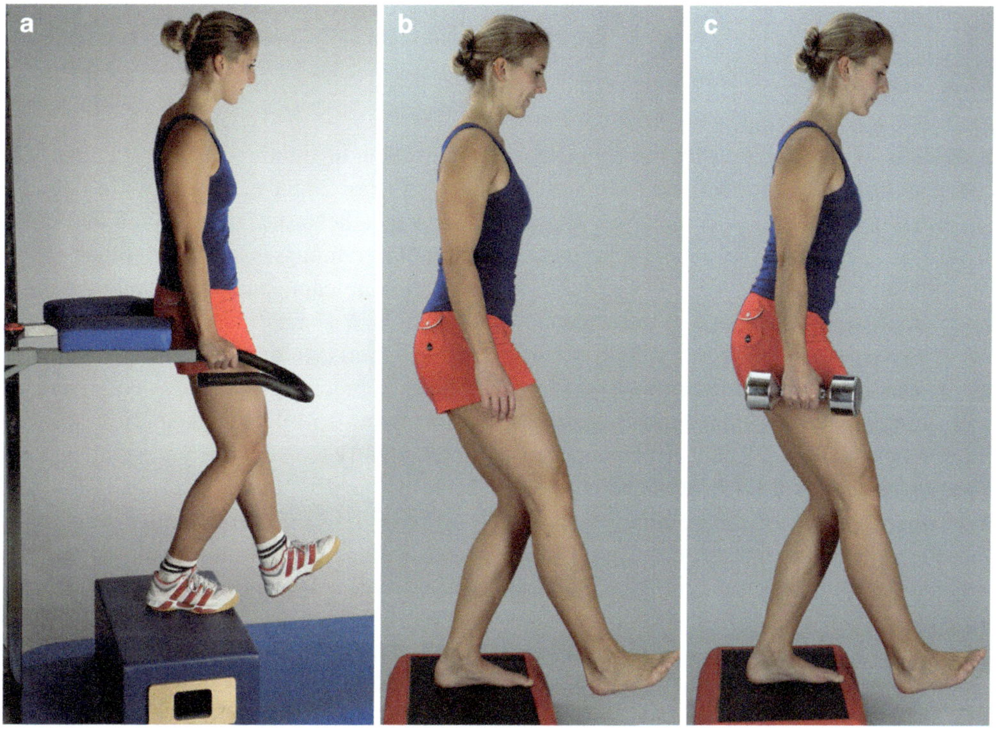

Fig. 27.6 Excentric training with (**a**) less than body weight, (**b**) body weight, and (**c**) additional weight [31]

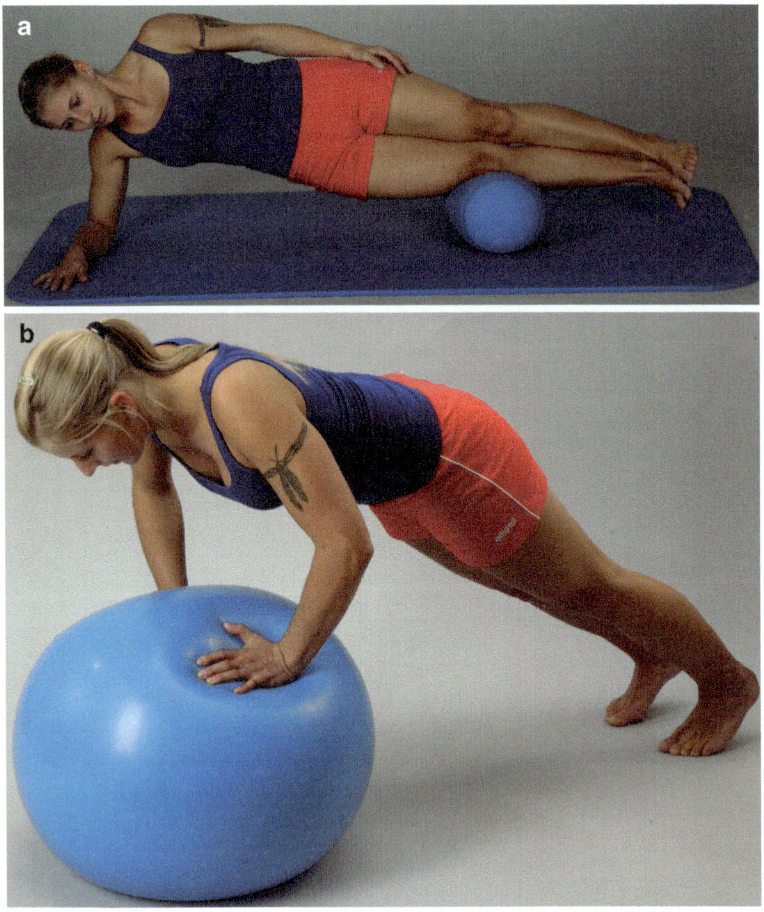

Fig. 27.7 (**a**, **b**) Improvement of core stability [31]

this phase is to enable the patient to compete at the level of former sportive activity.

Criteria for the return to competitive athletic activities are based on the patient's individual evaluation and experience (e.g., "beginner" vs. "expert"). There is still a lack of evidence concerning this question. However minimal basic requirements for the return to competitive sports are a pain-free joint with full range of motion and adequate ligamentous stability. Isokinetic measurements can be used for quantification of the athlete's performance, and more complex testing setups may be helpful to determine overall functional abilities such as sensomotoric function and core stability [28, 31].

To allow an optimized joint function and provide protection from reinjury, a gradual progression of training intensity should be performed (Fig. 27.8a–c). This should begin with sports-specific tasks, training for participation in regular training sessions, and training for participation in team games and finally end in participation in competitive games. Especially in contact sports, the first sports-specific training should be practiced with slow tempo and without tackling to relearn the motion sequences. Subsequently the tempo is increased, and opponents are added to the situation. This allows practicing in a safe "competitive" environment and finally preparing for competitions. Even having reached the highest level, the athlete should be emphasized to further continue with sensomotoric and core training in order to prevent reinjury.

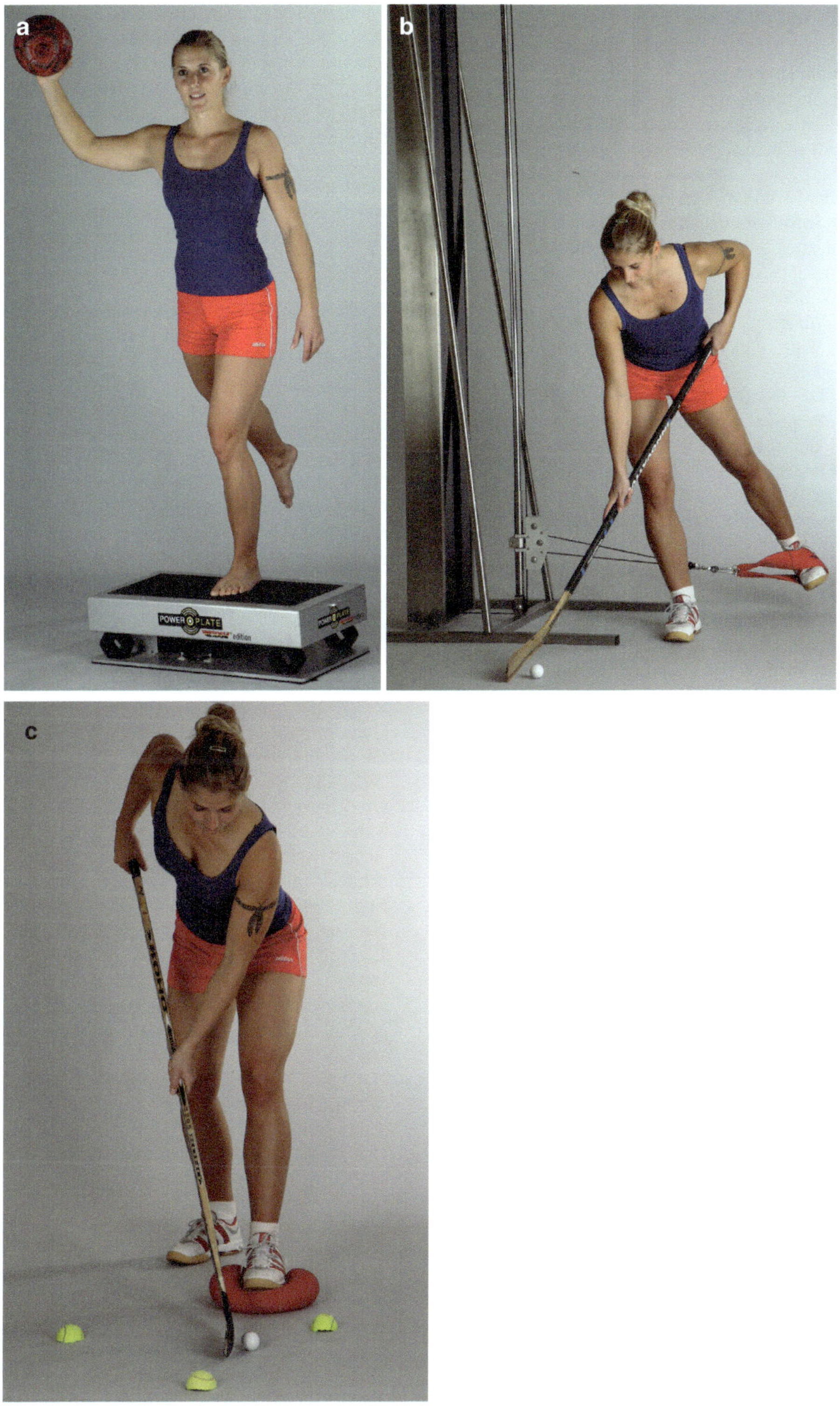

Fig. 27.8 (**a–c**) Functional exercises with increased instability and additional sports-specific tasks [31]

References

1. Alfredson H, Lorentzon R (1999) Superior results with continuous passive motion compared to active motion after periosteal transplantation. A retrospective study of human patella cartilage defect treatment. Knee Surg Sports Traumatol Arthrosc 7(4):232–238
2. Attfield SF, Wilton TJ, Pratt DJ, Sambatakakis A (1996) Soft-tissue balance and recovery of proprioception after total knee replacement. J Bone Joint Surg Br 78(4):540–545
3. Baker V, Bennell K, Stillman B, Cowan S, Crossley K (2002) Abnormal knee joint position sense in individuals with patellofemoral pain syndrome. J Orthop Res 20(2):208–214
4. Beard DJ, Dodd CA, Trundle HR, Simpson AH (1994) Proprioception enhancement for anterior cruciate ligament deficiency. A prospective randomised trial of two physiotherapy regimes. J Bone Joint Surg Br 76(4):654–659
5. Behrens F, Kraft EL, Oegema TR Jr (1989) Biochemical changes in articular cartilage after joint immobilization by casting or external fixation. J Orthop Res 7(3):335–343
6. Bennell KL, Hinman RS, Metcalf BR, Crossley KM, Buchbinder R, Smith M, McColl G (2003) Relationship of knee joint proprioception to pain and disability in individuals with knee osteoarthritis. J Orthop Res 21(5):792–797
7. Bowen TR, Feldmann DD, Miller MD (2004) Return to play following surgical treatment of meniscal and chondral injuries to the knee. Clin Sports Med 23(3):381–393, viii–ix
8. Brittberg M, Lindahl A, Nilsson A, Ohlsson C, Isaksson O, Peterson L (1994) Treatment of deep cartilage defects in the knee with autologous chondrocyte transplantation. N Engl J Med 331(14):889–895
9. Brittberg M, Nilsson A, Lindahl A, Ohlsson C, Peterson L (1996) Rabbit articular cartilage defects treated with autologous cultured chondrocytes. Clin Orthop Relat Res 326:270–283
10. Buckwalter JA (1995) Activity vs. rest in the treatment of bone, soft tissue and joint injuries. Iowa Orthop J 15:29–42
11. Buckwalter JA (1998) Articular cartilage: injuries and potential for healing. J Orthop Sports Phys Ther 28(4):192–202
12. Buckwalter JA, Lohmander S (1994) Operative treatment of osteoarthrosis. Current practice and future development. J Bone Joint Surg Am 76(9):1405–1418
13. Cohen NP, Foster RJ, Mow VC (1998) Composition and dynamics of articular cartilage: structure, function, and maintaining healthy state. J Orthop Sports Phys Ther 28(4):203–215
14. Ebert JR, Ackland TR, Lloyd DG, Wood DJ (2008) Accuracy of partial weight bearing after autologous chondrocyte implantation. Arch Phys Med Rehabil 89(8):1528–1534
15. Fremerey RW, Lobenhoffer P, Zeichen J, Skutek M, Bosch U, Tscherne H (2000) Proprioception after rehabilitation and reconstruction in knees with deficiency of the anterior cruciate ligament: a prospective, longitudinal study. J Bone Joint Surg Br 82(6):801–806
16. Friden T, Roberts D, Ageberg E, Walden M, Zatterstrom R (2001) Review of knee proprioception and the relation to extremity function after an anterior cruciate ligament rupture. J Orthop Sports Phys Ther 31(10):567–576
17. Frisbie DD, Oxford JT, Southwood L, Trotter GW, Rodkey WG, Steadman JR, Goodnight JL, McIlwraith CW (2003) Early events in cartilage repair after subchondral bone microfracture. Clin Orthop Relat Res 407:215–227
18. Fuchs S, Thorwesten L, Niewerth S (1999) Proprioceptive function in knees with and without total knee arthroplasty. Am J Phys Med Rehabil 78(1):39–45
19. Grande DA, Pitman MI, Peterson L, Menche D, Klein M (1989) The repair of experimentally produced defects in rabbit articular cartilage by autologous chondrocyte transplantation. J Orthop Res 7(2): 208–218
20. Gray ML, Pizzanelli AM, Grodzinsky AJ, Lee RC (1988) Mechanical and physiochemical determinants of the chondrocyte biosynthetic response. J Orthop Res 6(6):777–792
21. Grelsamer RP, Klein JR (1998) The biomechanics of the patellofemoral joint. J Orthop Sports Phys Ther 28(5):286–298
22. Grodzinsky AJ, Roth V, Myers E, Grossman WD, Mow VC (1981) The significance of electromechanical and osmotic forces in the nonequilibrium swelling behavior of articular cartilage in tension. J Biomech Eng 103(4):221–231
23. Haapala J, Arokoski J, Pirttimaki J, Lyyra T, Jurvelin J, Tammi M, Helminen HJ, Kiviranta I (2000) Incomplete restoration of immobilization induced softening of young beagle knee articular cartilage after 50-week remobilization. Int J Sports Med 21(1): 76–81
24. Halmovici N (1982) Three years experience in direct intraarticular temperature measurement. Biomed Therm 2:453–473
25. Hambly K, Bobic V, Wondrasch B, Van Assche D, Marlovits S (2006) Autologous chondrocyte implantation postoperative care and rehabilitation: science and practice. Am J Sports Med 34(6):1020–1038
26. Hess T, Gleitz M, Hopf T, Olfs S, Mielke U (1995) Changes in muscular activity after knee arthrotomy and arthroscopy. Int Orthop 19(2):94–97
27. Hinterwimmer S, Krammer M, Krotz M, Glaser C, Baumgart R, Reiser M, Eckstein F (2004) Cartilage atrophy in the knees of patients after seven weeks of partial load bearing. Arthritis Rheum 50(8): 2516–2520

28. Hirschmuller A, Baur H, Braun S, Kreuz PC, Sudkamp NP, Niemeyer P (2011) Rehabilitation after autologous chondrocyte implantation for isolated cartilage defects of the knee. Am J Sports Med 39(12):2686–2696
29. Hopkins J, Ingersoll CD, Edwards J, Klootwyk TE (2002) Cryotherapy and transcutaneous electric neuromuscular stimulation decrease arthrogenic muscle inhibition of the vastus medialis after knee joint effusion. J Athl Train 37(1):25–31
30. Horvath SM, Hollander JL (1949) Intra-articular temperature as a measure of joint reaction. J Clin Invest 28(3):469–473
31. Imhoff AB, Beitzel K, Stamer K, Klein E (2010) Rehabilitation in Der Orthopadischen Chirurgie: Op-Verfahren Im Uberblick – Physiotherapie – Sporttherapie. Springer, Berlin/Heidelberg/New York
32. Irrgang JJ, Pezzullo D (1998) Rehabilitation following surgical procedures to address articular cartilage lesions in the knee. J Orthop Sports Phys Ther 28(4):232–240
33. Jakobsen RB, Engebretsen L, Slauterbeck JR (2005) An analysis of the quality of cartilage repair studies. J Bone Joint Surg Am 87(10):2232–2239
34. Jones DG, Peterson L (2006) Autologous chondrocyte implantation. J Bone Joint Surg Am 88(11):2502–2520
35. Kern H (1980) Zur Anwendung der Kryotherapie in der Praxis. Physiotherapie 71:823–825
36. Kern H, Fessl L, Trnavsky G, Hertz H (1984) Das Verhalten der Gelenkstemperatur unter Eisapplikation-Grundlage fur die praktische Anwendung. Wien Klin Wochenschr 96:832–837
37. Kreuz PC, Steinwachs M, Erggelet C, Lahm A, Krause S, Ossendorf C, Meier D, Ghanem N, Uhl M (2007) Importance of sports in cartilage regeneration after autologous chondrocyte implantation: a prospective study with a 3-year follow-up. Am J Sports Med 35(8):1261–1268
38. Kuenze C, Hart JM (2010) Cryotherapy to treat persistent muscle weakness after joint injury. Phys Sportsmed 38(3):38–44
39. Lee RC, Frank EH, Grodzinsky AJ, Roylance DK (1981) Oscillatory compressional behavior of articular cartilage and its associated electromechanical properties. J Biomech Eng 103(4):280–292
40. Lieber RL, Silva PD, Daniel DM (1996) Equal effectiveness of electrical and volitional strength training for quadriceps femoris muscles after anterior cruciate ligament surgery. J Orthop Res 14(1):131–138
41. Lorentzon R, Alfredson H, Hildingsson C (1998) Treatment of deep cartilage defects of the patella with periosteal transplantation. Knee Surg Sports Traumatol Arthrosc 6(4):202–208
42. McGinty G, Irrgang JJ, Pezzullo D (2000) Biomechanical considerations for rehabilitation of the knee. Clin Biomech (Bristol, Avon) 15(3):160–166
43. Minas T, Peterson L (1999) Advanced techniques in autologous chondrocyte transplantation. Clin Sports Med 18(1):13–44, v–vi
44. Nam EK, Makhsous M, Koh J, Bowen M, Nuber G, Zhang LQ (2004) Biomechanical and histological evaluation of osteochondral transplantation in a rabbit model. Am J Sports Med 32(2):308–316
45. O'Driscoll SW, Keeley FW, Salter RB (1986) The chondrogenic potential of free autogenous periosteal grafts for biological resurfacing of major full-thickness defects in joint surfaces under the influence of continuous passive motion. An experimental investigation in the rabbit. J Bone Joint Surg Am 68(7):1017–1035
46. Osbahr DC, Cawley PW, Speer KP (2002) The effect of continuous cryotherapy on glenohumeral joint and subacromial space temperatures in the postoperative shoulder. Arthroscopy 18(7):748–754
47. Paternostro-Sluga T, Fialka C, Alacamlioglu Y, Saradeth T, Fialka-Moser V (1999) Neuromuscular electrical stimulation after anterior cruciate ligament surgery. Clin Orthop Relat Res 368:166–175
48. Peterson L, Brittberg M, Kiviranta I, Akerlund EL, Lindahl A (2002) Autologous chondrocyte transplantation. Biomechanics and long-term durability. Am J Sports Med 30(1):2–12
49. Peterson L, Minas T, Brittberg M, Nilsson A, Sjogren-Jansson E, Lindahl A (2000) Two- to 9-year outcome after autologous chondrocyte transplantation of the knee. Clin Orthop Relat Res 374:212–234
50. Pietrosimone BG, Hart JM, Saliba SA, Hertel J, Ingersoll CD (2009) Immediate effects of transcutaneous electrical nerve stimulation and focal knee joint cooling on quadriceps activation. Med Sci Sports Exerc 41(6):1175–1181
51. Powers CM, Ward SR, Fredericson M, Guillet M, Shellock FG (2003) Patellofemoral kinematics during weight-bearing and non-weight-bearing knee extension in persons with lateral subluxation of the patella: a preliminary study. J Orthop Sports Phys Ther 33(11):677–685
52. Reider B, Arcand MA, Diehl LH, Mroczek K, Abulencia A, Stroud CC, Palm M, Gilbertson J, Staszak P (2003) Proprioception of the knee before and after anterior cruciate ligament reconstruction. Arthroscopy 19(1):2–12
53. Rice D, McNair PJ, Dalbeth N (2009) Effects of cryotherapy on arthrogenic muscle inhibition using an experimental model of knee swelling. Arthritis Rheum 61(1):78–83
54. Robert H (2002) Techniques for repair of chondral and osteochondral lesions in the knee. Principles of rehabilitation. Ann Readapt Med Phys 45(2):62–68
55. Roberts D, Friden T, Stomberg A, Lindstrand A, Moritz U (2000) Bilateral proprioceptive defects in patients with a unilateral anterior cruciate ligament reconstruction: a comparison between patients and healthy individuals. J Orthop Res 18(4):565–571
56. Rodrigo JJ, Steadman JR, Silliman JF (1994) Improvement in full- thickness chondral defect healing in the human knee after debridement and

microfracture using continuous passive motion. Am J Knee Surg 7:109–116
57. Salter RB (1989) The biologic concept of continuous passive motion of synovial joints. The first 18 years of basic research and its clinical application. Clin Orthop Relat Res 242:12–25
58. Salter RB (1994) The physiologic basis of continuous passive motion for articular cartilage healing and regeneration. Hand Clin 10(2):211–219
59. Salter RB (1996) History of rest and motion and the scientific basis for early continuous passive motion. Hand Clin 12(1):1–11
60. Salter RB, Simmonds DF, Malcolm BW, Rumble EJ, MacMichael D, Clements ND (1980) The biological effect of continuous passive motion on the healing of full-thickness defects in articular cartilage. An experimental investigation in the rabbit. J Bone Joint Surg Am 62(8):1232–1251
61. Sharma L, Pai YC, Holtkamp K, Rymer WZ (1997) Is knee joint proprioception worse in the arthritic knee versus the unaffected knee in unilateral knee osteoarthritis? Arthritis Rheum 40(8):1518–1525
62. Shimizu T, Videman T, Shimazaki K, Mooney V (1987) Experimental study on the repair of full thickness articular cartilage defects: effects of varying periods of continuous passive motion, cage activity, and immobilization. J Orthop Res 5(2):187–197
63. Steadman JR, Rodkey WG, Rodrigo JJ (2001) Microfracture: surgical technique and rehabilitation to treat chondral defects. Clin Orthop Relat Res 391(Suppl):S362–S369
64. Stiene HA, Brosky T, Reinking MF, Nyland J, Mason MB (1996) A comparison of closed kinetic chain and isokinetic joint isolation exercise in patients with patellofemoral dysfunction. J Orthop Sports Phys Ther 24(3):136–141
65. Van Assche D, Staes F, Van Caspel D, Vanlauwe J, Bellemans J, Saris DB, Luyten FP (2010) Autologous chondrocyte implantation versus microfracture for knee cartilage injury: a prospective randomized trial, with 2-year follow-up. Knee Surg Sports Traumatol Arthrosc 18(4):486–495
66. Van Assche D, Van Caspel D, Vanlauwe J, Bellemans J, Saris DB, Luyten FP, Staes F (2009) Physical activity levels after characterized chondrocyte implantation versus microfracture in the knee and the relationship to objective functional outcome with 2-year follow-up. Am J Sports Med 37(Suppl 1):42S–49S
67. Vanwanseele B, Lucchinetti E, Stussi E (2002) The effects of immobilization on the characteristics of articular cartilage: current concepts and future directions. Osteoarthritis Cartilage 10(5):408–419
68. Waldman SD, Spiteri CG, Grynpas MD, Pilliar RM, Hong J, Kandel RA (2003) Effect of biomechanical conditioning on cartilaginous tissue formation in vitro. J Bone Joint Surg Am 85-A(Suppl 2): 101–105
69. Walker JM (1998) Pathomechanics and classification of cartilage lesions, facilitation of repair. J Orthop Sports Phys Ther 28(4):216–231
70. Williams JM, Moran M, Thonar EJ, Salter RB (1994) Continuous passive motion stimulates repair of rabbit knee articular cartilage after matrix proteoglycan loss. Clin Orthop Relat Res 304:252–262
71. Wondrasch B, Zak L, Welsch GH, Marlovits S (2009) Effect of accelerated weightbearing after matrix-associated autologous chondrocyte implantation on the femoral condyle on radiographic and clinical outcome after 2 years: a prospective, randomized controlled pilot study. Am J Sports Med 37(Suppl 1): 88S–96S

28 Orthobiologics

Clint Soppe, Sara Jurek, Matthew Wichman, and Bert Mandelbaum

Contents

C. Soppe, MD (✉) • S. Jurek, MD
M. Wichman, MD • B. Mandelbaum, MD
Santa Monica Orthopaedic and Sports Medicine Group, Santa Monica, CA, USA

28.1 Hyaluronic Acid

28.1.1 Basic Science

Hyaluronic acid is a polysaccharide chain composed of repeating disaccharide units of *N*-acetylglucosamine and glucuronic acid. Articular hyaluronic acid is made mostly of approximately 12,500 disaccharide units, which yields an average molecular weight of five million daltons (d). Type B synoviocytes or fibroblasts produce endogenous hyaluronic acid and secrete it into the joint space [63]. Endogenous hyaluronic acid provides joint shock absorption and lubrication, in addition to promoting chondrocyte differentiation and proliferation [30, 34, 65]. A healthy knee contains approximately 2 mL of synovial fluid with a concentration of hyaluronic acid of 2.5–4.0 mg/mL. The concentration of hyaluronic acid in an osteoarthritic knee is reduced by up to 50 %. Additionally, there is less interaction between the hyaluronic acid molecules, and the molecular size of the hyaluronic acid is reduced; both cause much lower dynamic, elastic, and viscous properties of the synovial fluid as well as diminished barrier and filter effects. These changes within an osteoarthritic knee constitute a loss of lubrication. This loss of lubrication causes increased stress forces; these increased stress forces further disturb the collagen network, a vital contributor to articular surface integrity. A compromised articular surface with resultant loss of barrier integrity negatively influences nutrient availability and impedes articular cartilage waste removal [63].

A.A. Shetty et al. (eds.), *Techniques in Cartilage Repair Surgery*,
DOI 10.1007/978-3-642-41921-8_28, © ESSKA 2014

28.1.2 Viscosupplementation

The term "viscosupplementation" refers to the intra-articular injection of exogenous hyaluronic acid (HA) as a treatment for osteoarthritis of the knee. The purpose of HA injection is to attempt to recreate the joint's normal homeostatic environment both by replacing lost HA and possibly stimulating the production of endogenous hyaluronic acid [11]. The majority of the earlier forms of clinical HA were made with rooster combs, and while most of the currently available forms of viscosupplementation are still avian-derived (rooster combs), Euflexxa and Orthovisc are bacterial derivatives [4, 14]. These non-avian-derived products may be useful in patients with a poultry allergy and those who are strict vegans [63]. Studies have demonstrated that exogenous HA inhibits tissue nociceptors, stimulates endogenous HA formation, and has both anti-inflammatory and chondroprotective effects [25, 61]. The anti-inflammatory effects result from downregulation of IL-8, TNF-α, and iNOS in synoviocytes [25]. The chondroprotective effects result from gene expression downregulation of OA-associated cytokines and enzymes [62]. Augmenting the findings of in vitro and animal studies, a clinical study has shown HA-induced human chondroprotection on both radiographic and high-magnification arthroscopic evaluation [66]. One study notes evidence that HA has the ability to preserve chondrocyte density and vitality, as well as joint space [24]. This chondroprotective property has led some researchers to advocate the use of viscosupplementation for small articular cartilage defects in athletes, as well as an in-season, postinjury treatment of patients with MRI-proven bone bruises. While these researchers acknowledge the need for further study to validate the efficacy of these suggested indications, they argue that the low morbidity associated with the use of HA supports its use for these situations [66].

Viscosupplementation has gained acceptance as a treatment modality in the postoperative knee due to the chondroprotective effects of HA. The injection of HA in the postoperative period can reduce persistent knee pain following arthroscopy. Additionally, HA has been shown to reduce joint swelling and to be NSAID sparing [39]. An animal study has demonstrated the disease-modifying effects of HA; these include a reduction in cartilage degeneration as well as promotion of tissue repair after microfracture through the inhibition of nitric oxide and the stabilization of proteoglycan structure [19, 24, 29, 56].

28.1.3 Clinical Use

Multiple hyaluronic acid products are now widely available, with an estimated annual expenditure of $725 million in the USA [5]. Most preparations of HA require a series of injections, but a recent randomized, double-blinded, placebo-controlled trial comparing a single injection of hylan G-F 20 (Synvisc) to placebo in the treatment of knee OA demonstrated the efficacy of a single injection of HA in treating knee OA [13]. An additional study showed that a single 6 mL injection of hylan G-F 20 (Synvisc-One) was equally effective and as well tolerated clinically as three 2 mL injections performed 1 week apart from each other [16]. A meta-analysis of 20 randomized, placebo-controlled trials concluded that HA was most effective in the treatment of patients with pain associated with knee OA who were in the mild to moderate stages of OA and who were under the age of 65 [48]. The overall incidence of HA side effects is approximately 1 % per injection, with the most common side effects consisting of local reactions in the treated knee (pain, local swelling, and warmth) and usually lasting no more than 1–2 days [46, 63].

Proponents of HA use as a first-line nonoperative treatment for osteoarthritis and pain associated with cartilage degeneration/damage point to the high incidence of gastrointestinal complications with oral NSAID therapy as well as the increased risk of infection and enhanced progression of cartilage breakdown associated with frequent intra-articular steroid injections [4, 14, 58]. These proponents argue that the expense of HA injections is justified therapeutically by the claimed prolonged duration of clinical effect. A recent meta-analysis sought to evaluate the post-intervention time course of the effect of HA (the "therapeutic trajectory") to shed additional light on the true clinical impact of HA and its overall efficacy. This meta-analysis evaluated 54 trials with a total of 7,545 participants and found a therapeutic trajectory of HA for knee OA pain over 6 months following the intervention. Specifically, the patient experiences the clinical impact at 4 weeks, with a peak effectiveness reached at 8 weeks, and a residual detectable clinical effect in reduction of pain experienced until 24 weeks [5]. The magnitude of effect was noted in this analysis to be modest, up to four times better than the peak effect size of acetaminophen, better than NSAIDs, and equivalent to COX-2 inhibitors [35, 60, 67]. An additional review of the literature looking at 76 placebo-controlled trials concluded that HA was effective in the treatment of patients with knee OA and that the maximal benefit was achieved within the week 5 to week 13 range. The authors also noted varying degrees of benefit, depending on the various types of HA used [7]. Another study noted that higher molecular weight HA was likely to be more efficacious than lower molecular weight HA [38]. A multicenter, blinded study comparing the efficacy of HA (hylan G-F 20, Synvisc) with corticosteroid (triamcinolone hexacetonide (TH, Aristospan)) for knee OA found that HA was superior to steroid injection in terms of pain relief and that the maximal efficacy of steroid occurred at week 2, while the maximal efficacy of HA occurred at week 12, leading researchers to suggest a possible synergistic effect by using both corticosteroid for its early onset of action and HA for its better overall efficacy and prolonged benefits [14, 62].

Not every study or review of the use of intra-articular HA in the treatment of knee OA is entirely supportive of this intervention. A meta-analysis published in JAMA in 2003 looked at all blinded, randomized controlled trials comparing HA to placebo injection for the treatment of knee OA and concluded that while a majority of the studies reviewed did find a significant benefit with HA injection, this benefit might be an overestimation of effect due to publication bias [38]. Similarly, a review published in the Journal of American Academy of Orthopaedic Surgeons looking at six meta-analyses and one additional randomized controlled trial concluded that in general, the results of the studies demonstrated a positive effect, but the authors declined to make a recommendation for or against the use of HA in the treatment of knee OA, citing the potential for publication bias, lack of quality trials, and unclear clinical significance [48]. A study comparing Hylan G-F 20 (Synvisc) and the corticosteroid betamethasone sodium phosphate-betamethasone acetate (Celestone Soluspan) found that both interventions provided patients with modest improvements in function, but did not detect a difference between the two with respect to pain relief or function at 3 or 6 months of follow-up. The authors note the additional pain and potential risk associated with the three-injection course of Hylan G-F 20 and the approximately 100-fold difference in pharmacy cost as reasons for not utilizing HA as a first-line treatment for patients with knee OA [36].

28.2 Platelet-Rich Plasma

28.2.1 Basic Science

PRP has previously been defined as a twofold or greater increase in platelet concentration above baseline levels or a greater than 1.1×10^6 platelet/μL [41]. But in reality, there is no exact definition of PRP because there are many different formulations. Depending on what company is used, the amount of platelets and, white and red blood cells and the ratios of these factors may differ quite significantly affecting healing in ways we do not fully understand. That is why comparing studies using different centrifuge systems is challenging [20, 26, 41]. The theory of clinical benefit with cartilage healing using PRP is based on platelet wound healing properties [44]. Platelets can enhance and modify tissue healing by the release of growth factors from the α-granules from the platelets. These growth factors include platelet-derived growth factor (PDGF), insulin-like growth factor (IGF-I, IGF-II), fibroblast growth factor (FGF), vascular endothelial growth factor

(VEGF), as well as many other cytokines and bioactive factors that contribute to healing [2, 8, 9, 20, 21, 47, 50, 53]. This section will review the current scientific and clinical literature involving cartilage repair and restoration as well as in treatment for osteoarthritis.

28.2.2 PRP and Articular Cartilage Injury

Due to the reparative properties of PRP, it has been used to augment the repair and regeneration of focal cartilage injuries as well as in the osteoarthritic patient. In vitro experiments have shown that PRP exposed to mesenchymal stem cells (MSCs) increased the proliferation of MSCs as well as chondrogenic differentiation [42]. Akeda et al. showed that PRP increased proteoglycans and type II collagen in porcine articular cartilage [1]. More basic science research has shown that PRP may enhance and stimulate progenitor cells from human subchondral bone after microfracture [33]. Milano et al. demonstrated improvement in sheep osteochondral defects treated with microfracture and PRP compared to microfracture alone [40]. Taking these studies to humans, Wu et al. theorized using a PRP/fibrin clot with a scaffold in isolated cartilage defects could allow an autologous source of cells with a minimally invasive technique [64]. Gobbi presented unpublished data from the 2009 International Cartilage Repair Society meeting of 20 patients undergoing articular cartilage repair using a sticky clot of PRP/thrombin with average IKDC scores improving from 48.27 to 68.58 at 20-month follow-up. At 1 year, second-look arthroscopies showed hyaline-like tissue with good surrounding integration [21]. Siclari et al. reviewed 52 patients with 1-year follow-up who underwent placement of a collagen scaffold immersed in PRP with bone marrow stimulation. KOOS scores rose from 55 to 91, and histologic specimens from five patients showed hyaline-like cartilage repair tissue [52]. This study showed promising results; however, a prior study of five patients using a similar technique had disappointing outcomes on MRI [18]. Sun et al. saw improvement in healing of osteochondral defects in rabbits using PRP in a PLGA compared to PLGA alone [57]. Treatment with PRP in athletes with chondral lesions has been found to be safe and effective for the recovery of some articular cartilage injuries [17]. More research is needed to further define the role of PRP in articular cartilage repair.

28.2.3 PRP and Osteoarthritis

PRP has also shown to have an effect on overall degeneration of cartilage and osteoarthritis of the knee. Affecting joint homeostasis and decreasing catabolic processes by augmenting interleukins and metalloproteinases may be another way PRP can modulate the osteoarthritic joint [22]. Hyaluronic acid has proven beneficial for treatment of cartilage degeneration [7], and Anitua et al. showed the PRP may increase the production of HA by synovial cells [3]. PRP has been shown to be effective and safe in the treatment of OA [31, 49]. Compared to HA in patients with degenerative cartilage lesions and OA, PRP proved more efficacious and gave longer relief of symptoms. The beneficial effects seem to be increased in younger patients with more mild disease [32, 37, 55]. It is not known if these changes are temporary or if there is a more permanent effect on the joint by modulating the intra-articular environment. Blinded, randomized controlled trials are needed to further elucidate the results of these studies.

28.3 Corticosteroids

There have been many substances that have been injected intra-articularly over the years. These include formalin, glycerol, and even petroleum jelly [45]. Many of these did not withstand the test of time. Since the 1950s, clinicians have regularly been using corticosteroids to treat cartilage lesions ranging from focal cartilage defects to diffuse osteoarthritis. In 1951, Thorne was the first clinician to inject steroids into the knee joint of a patient with rheumatoid arthritis. He noticed a significant relief of symptoms and was the first to relate the anti-inflammatory nature of this substance [59, 60]. There is a wide range of preparations of corticosteroids that differ only by chemical structure, which affects the lipophilic nature and therefore solubility of each preparation. The mechanism of action however does not vary.

28.3.1 Basic Science

The mechanism of action of corticosteroids is based on their lipophilic nature. They bind to the cell's nucleus and alter mRNA transcription resulting in reduction of macrophages, lymphocytes, and mast cells [12, 15]. This indirectly reduces inflammation by secondary reduction of lysosomal enzyme release, decreased phagocytosis, and reduction of inflammatory mediators including IL-1, leukotrienes, and prostaglandins [54]. This reduction in inflammatory mediators is believed to be responsible for the associated pain relief.

28.3.2 Efficacy

Review of the literature demonstrates multiple meta-analyses. The Cochrane Musculoskeletal Group reviewed ten studies. They concluded that week 1 was the only time point with a statistically significant difference that was found between corticosteroid and placebo [6]. This was supported by the meta-analysis by Hepper et al., who found similar findings with week 1 as the only time point with significant differences [27]. While the literature supports only short-term relief in osteoarthritis, for focal articular cartilage lesions, they may serve to help reduce effusions and associated inflammation and synovitis.

28.3.3 Negative Effects

One cannot discuss intra-articular steroids without the mention of potential negative effects. While steroids inhibit the early phases of inflammation (edema, capillary dilatation, and leukocyte migration), they also inhibit the later, restorative phases (fibroblastic proliferation and collagen deposition) [23]. A carefully designed animal study compared the effects of steroids to placebo in rabbit knees. It was identified that the knees injected with steroids showed thinning of the articular cartilage, loss of hyaline appearance, increased cartilage fibrillation, and loss of the ability to repair itself [51]. These negative effects have repeatedly been shown to be dose dependent and in moderation may be limited.

28.3.4 Summary

Clearly the use of intra-articular corticosteroids has withstood the test of time. The literature has shown the reproducible effects to be short-lived; however, many clinicians use it as a first line in the treatment of either symptomatic articular cartilage lesions or osteoarthritis. In moderation, these are safe injections meant to treat symptoms and not to promote cartilage repair or healing. If overused, there exists evidence that steroids may be harmful, and their use should be taken seriously.

28.4 Bone Marrow Aspirate Concentrate

Cell-based therapies are the newest wave of treatments for cartilage injury. While bone marrow cells have been used clinically for more than a decade, a more recently introduced therapeutic option is the use of bone marrow aspirate concentrate (BMAC) which is a one-step method of maximizing both pluripotent mesenchymal stem cells (MSCs) and growth factors (GFs). This can be harvested and injected in a single surgical setting. A study by Hernigou et al. demonstrated that the efficacy of stem cell therapy is dependent on the number of progenitor cells available [28]. The unconcentrated number of cells in native bone marrow aspirate harvested from the iliac crest seems to be less than ideal to promote cartilage repair; however, with newer techniques, the levels of MSCs and GFs can be significantly increased by concentrating the sample. In a sample of ten patients, the number of total nucleated cells in bone marrow aspirate was 19×10^6. In a series of 200 patients who underwent BMAC procedure, that number increased to 72×10^6 [10, 43]. This clearly demonstrates a greater than 3.5-fold increase in nucleated cells.

This is a newer cell-based technology that has promising early clinical results; however, well-controlled studies are still lacking. There are many potential uses for BMAC, and it holds much promise as a future tool in the armamentarium for treatment of articular cartilage injury.

References

1. Akeda K, An HS, Okuma M, Attawia M, Miyamoto K, Thonar EJ, Lenz ME, Sah RL, Masuda K (2006) Platelet-rich plasma stimulates porcine articular chondrocyte proliferation and matrix biosynthesis. Osteoarthritis Cartilage 14(12):1272–1280
2. Alsousou J, Thompson M, Hulley P, Noble A, Willett K (2009) The biology of platelet-rich plasma and its application in trauma and orthopaedic surgery: a review of the literature. J Bone Joint Surg Br 91(8):987–996
3. Anitua E, Sánchez M, Nurden AT, Zalduendo MM, de la Fuente M, Azofra J, Andía I (2007) Platelet-released growth factors enhance the secretion of hyaluronic acid and induce hepatocyte growth factor production by synovial fibroblasts from arthritic patients. Rheumatology (Oxford) 46(12):1769–1772
4. Ayral X (2001) Injections in the treatment of osteoarthritis. Best Pract Res Clin Rheumatol 15:609–626
5. Bannuru RR, Natov NS, Dasi UR, Schmid CH, McAlindon TE (2011) Therapeutic trajectory following intra-articular hyaluronic acid injection in knee osteoarthritis – meta-analysis. Osteoarthritis Cartilage 19(6):611–619
6. Bellamy N, Campbell J, Robinson V, Gee T, Bourne R, Wells G (2006) Intra-articular corticosteroid for treatment of osteoarthritis of the knee. Cochrane Database Syst Rev (19):CD005328
7. Bellamy N, Campbell J, Robinson V et al (2006) Viscosupplementation for the treatment of osteoarthritis of the knee. Cochrane Database Syst Rev (2):CD005321
8. Bennett NT, Schultz GS (1993) Growth factors and wound healing: biochemical properties of growth factors and their receptors. Am J Surg 165(6):728–737
9. Blaney Davidson EN, van der Kraan PM, van den Berg WB (2007) TGF-beta and osteoarthritis. Osteoarthritis Cartilage 15(6):597–604, Epub 2007 Mar 27
10. BMAC2 Product Guide. Harvest Technologies Corp., Plymouth, MA, USA
11. Buckwalter JA, Saltzman C, Brown T (2004) The impact of osteoarthritis: implications for research. Clin Orthop Relat Res 427(suppl):S6–S157
12. Centeno LM, Moore ME (1994) Preferred intra-articular corticosteroids and associated practice: a survey of members of the American College of Rheumatology. Arthritis Care Res 7(3):151–155
13. Chevalier X, Jerosch J, Goupille P, van Dijk N, Luyten FP, Scott DL, Bailleul F, Pavelka K (2010) Single, intra-articular treatment with 6 ml hylan G-F 20 in patients with symptomatic primary osteoarthritis of the knee: a randomised, multicentre, double-blind, placebo controlled trial. Ann Rheum Dis 69(1): 113–119
14. Clegg TE, Caborn D, Mauffrey C (2013) Viscosupplementation with hyaluronic acid in the treatment for cartilage lesions: a review of current evidence and future directions. Eur J Orthop Sur Traumatol 23:119–24
15. Cole BJ, Schumacher HR Jr (2005) Injectable corticosteroids in modern practice. J Am Acad Orthop Surg 13(1):37–46
16. Conrozier T, Jerosch J, Beks P, Kemper F, Euller-Ziegler L, Bailleul F, Chevalier X (2009) Prospective, multi-centre, randomized evaluation of the safety and efficacy of five dosing regimens of viscosupplementation with hylan G-F 20 in patients with symptomatic tibio-femoral osteoarthritis: a pilot study. Arch Orthop Trauma Surg 129(3):417–423
17. Cugat R, Carrillo JM, Serra I, Soler C (2006) Articular cartilage defects reconstruction by plasma rich in growth factors. In: Brittberg M, Marcacci M, Zanasi S (eds) Basic science, clinical repair and reconstruction of articular cartilage defects: current status and prospects. Timeo Editore, Bologna, pp 801–807
18. Dhollander AA, De Neve F, Almqvist KF, Verdonk R, Lambrecht S, Elewaut D, Verbruggen G, Verdonk PC (2011) Autologous matrix-induced chondrogenesis combined with platelet-rich plasma gel: technical description and a five pilot patients report. Knee Surg Sports Traumatol Arthrosc 19(4):536–542
19. Diaz-Gallego L, Prieto JG, Coronel P, Gamazo LE, Gimeno M, Alvarez AI (2005) Apoptosis and nitric oxide in an experimental model of osteoarthritis in rabbit after hyaluronic acid treatment. J Orthop Res 23(6):1370–1376
20. Fortier LA, Barker JU, Strauss EJ, McCarrel TM, Cole BJ (2011) The role of growth factors in cartilage repair. Clin Orthop Relat Res 469(10):2706–2715
21. Foster TE, Puskas BL, Mandelbaum BR, Gerhardt MB, Rodeo SA (2009) Platelet-rich plasma: from basic science to clinical applications. Am J Sports Med 37(11):2259–2272
22. Frisbie DD, Kawcak CE, Werpy NM, Park RD, McIlwraith CW (2007) Clinical, biochemical, and histologic effects of intra-articular administration of autologous conditioned serum in horses with

experimentally induced osteoarthritis. Am J Vet Res 68(3):290–296
23. Gilman A (1985) The pharmacological basis of therapeutics, 7th edn. Macmillan Publishing Company, New York
24. Goldberg VM, Buckwalter JA (2005) Hyaluronans in the treatment of osteoarthritis of the knee: evidence for disease-modifying activity. Osteoarthritis Cartilage 13(3):216–224
25. Greenberg DD, Stoker A, Kane S, Cockrell M, Cook JL (2006) Biochemical effects of two different hyaluronic acid products in a co-culture model of osteoarthritis. Osteoarthritis Cartilage 14(8):814–822
26. Hall MP, Band PA, Meislin RJ, Jazrawi LM, Cardone DA (2009) Platelet-rich plasma: current concepts and application in sports medicine. J Am Acad Orthop Surg 17(10):602–608
27. Hepper CT et al (2009) The efficacy and duration of intra-articular corticosteroid injection for knee osteoarthritis: a systematic review of level I studies. J Am Acad Orthop Surg 17:638–646
28. Hernigou P et al (2002) Treatment of osteonecrosis with autologous bone marrow grafting. Clin Orthop Relat Res 405:14–23
29. Hulmes DJ, Marsden ME, Strachan RK, Harvey RE, McInnes N, Gardner DL (2004) Intra-articular hyaluronate in experimental rabbit osteoarthritis can prevent changes in cartilage proteoglycan content. Osteoarthritis Cartilage 12(3):232–238
30. Kawasaki K, Ochi M, Uchio Y, Adachi N, Matsusaki M (1999) Hyaluronic acid enhances proliferation and chondroitin sulfate synthesis in cultured chondrocytes embedded in collagen gels. J Cell Physiol 179(2): 142–148
31. Kon E, Buda R, Filardo G, Di Martino A, Timoncini A, Cenacchi A, Fornasari PM, Giannini S, Marcacci M (2010) Platelet-rich plasma: intra-articular knee injections produced favorable results on degenerative cartilage lesions. Knee Surg Sports Traumatol Arthrosc 18(4):472–479
32. Kon E, Mandelbaum B, Buda R, Filardo G, Delcogliano M, Timoncini A, Fornasari PM, Giannini S, Marcacci M (2011) Platelet-rich plasma intra-articular injection versus hyaluronic acid viscosupplementation as treatments for cartilage pathology: from early degeneration to osteoarthritis. Arthroscopy 27(11):1490–1501
33. Krüger JP, Hondke S, Endres M, Pruss A, Siclari A, Kaps C (2012) Human platelet-rich plasma stimulates migration and chondrogenic differentiation of human subchondral progenitor cells. J Orthop Res 30(6):845–852. doi:10.1002/jor.22005
34. Kujawa MJ, Caplan AI (1986) Hyaluronic acid bonded to cell culture surfaces stimulates chondrogenesis in stage 24 limb mesenchyme cell cultures. Dev Biol 114(2):504–518
35. Lee C, Hunsche E, Balshaw R, Kong SX, Schnitzer TJ (2005) Need for common internal controls when assessing the relative efficacy of pharmacologic agents using a meta-analytic approach: case study of cyclooxygenase 2-selective inhibitors for the treatment of osteoarthritis. Arthritis Rheum 53:510e8
36. Leopold SS, Redd BB, Warme WJ, Wehrle PA, Pettis PD, Shott S (2003) Corticosteroid compared with hyaluronic acid injections for the treatment of osteoarthritis of the knee. A prospective, randomized trial. J Bone Joint Surg Am 85-A(7):1197–1203
37. Li M, Zhang C, Ai Z, Yuan T, Feng Y, Jia W (2011) Therapeutic effectiveness of intra-knee-articular injection of platelet-rich plasma on knee articular cartilage degeneration. Zhongguo Xiu Fu Chong Jian Wai Ke Za Zhi 25(10):1192–1196
38. Lo GH, LaValley M, McAlindon T, Felson DT (2003) Intra-articular hyaluronic acid in treatment of knee osteoarthritis: a meta-analysis. JAMA 290(23):3115–3121
39. Mathies B (2006) Effects of Viscoseal, a synovial fluid substitute, on recovery after arthroscopic partial meniscectomy and joint lavage. Knee Surg Sports Traumatol Arthrosc 14(1):32–39
40. Milano G, Sanna Passino E, Deriu L, Careddu G, Manunta L, Manunta A, Saccomanno MF, Fabbriciani C (2010) The effect of platelet rich plasma combined with microfractures on the treatment of chondral defects: an experimental study in a sheep model. Osteoarthritis Cartilage 18(7):971–980
41. Miller Y, Bachowski G, Benjamin R, Eklund DK, Hibbard AJ, Lightfoot T (2007) Practice guidelines for blood transfusions: a compilation from recent peer-reviewed literature, 2nd edn. American Red Cross, Washington, DC, p 56
42. Mishra A, Tummala P, King A, Lee B, Kraus M, Tse V, Jacobs CR (2009) Buffered platelet- rich plasma enhances mesenchymal stem cell proliferation and chondrogenic differentiation. Tissue Eng Part C Methods 15(3):431–435
43. Muschler G et al (2006) Comparison of bone marrow aspiration and bone core biopsy as methods for harvest and assay of human connective tissue progenitor. In: Scientific paper 41; presented at 58th Association of Bone and Joint Surgeons Meeting, Buenos Aires, Argentina
44. Nurden AT, Nurden P, Sanchez M, Andia I, Anitua E (2008) Platelets and wound healing. Front Biosci 13:3532–3548
45. Pemberton R (1935) Arthritis and rheumatoid conditions. Their nature and treatment. JAMA, Philadelphia 105(16):1295.
46. Peyron JG (1993) Intraarticular hyaluronan injections in the treatment of osteoarthritis: state-of-the-art review. J Rheumatol 20(suppl 39):3–9
47. Qureshi AH, Chaoji V, Maiguel D, Faridi MH, Barth CJ, Salem SM, Singhal M, Stoub D, Krastins B, Ogihara M, Zaki MJ, Gupta V (2009) Proteomic and phospho-proteomic profile of human platelets in basal, resting state: insights into integrin signaling. PLoS One 4(10):e7627
48. Richmond J, Hunter D, Irrgang J, American Academy of Orthopaedic Surgeons et al (2009) Treatment of osteoarthritis of the knee (nonarthroplasty). J Am Acad Orthop Surg 17(9):591–600

49. Sampson S, Reed M, Silvers H, Meng M, Mandelbaum B (2010) Injection of platelet-rich plasma in patients with primary and secondary knee osteoarthritis: a pilot study. Am J Phys Med Rehabil 89(12):961–969
50. Senzel L, Gnatenko DV, Bahou WF (2009) The platelet proteome. Curr Opin Hematol 16(5):329–333
51. Shaw NE et al (1973) The influence of corticosteroids on normal and papain-treated articular cartilage in the rabbit. J Bone Joint Surg Br 55B:197–205
52. Siclari A, Mascaro G, Gentili C, Cancedda R, Boux E (2012) A cell-free scaffold-based cartilage repair provides improved function hyaline-like repair at one year. Clin Orthop Relat Res 470(3):910–919
53. Smyth SS, McEver RP, Weyrich AS, Morrell CN, Hoffman MR, Arepally GM, French PA, Dauerman HL, Becker RC, 2009 Platelet Colloquium Participants (2009) Platelet functions beyond hemostasis. J Thromb Haemost 7(11):1759–1766
54. Snibbe JC, Gambardella RA (2005) Use of injections for osteoarthritis in joints and sports activity. Clin Sports Med 24(1):83–91
55. Spaková T, Rosocha J, Lacko M, Harvanová D, Gharaibeh A (2012) Treatment of knee joint osteoarthritis with autologous platelet-rich plasma in comparison with hyaluronic acid. Am J Phys Med Rehabil 91(5):411–417
56. Strauss E, Schachter A, Frenkel S, Rosen J (2009) The efficacy of intra-articular hyaluronan injection after the microfracture technique for the treatment of articular cartilage lesions. Am J Sports Med 37(4):720–726
57. Sun Y, Feng Y, Zhang CQ, Chen SB, Cheng XG (2010) The regenerative effect of platelet-rich plasma on healing in large osteochondral defects. Int Orthop 34(4):589–597, Epub 2009 May 12
58. Tehranzadeh J, Booya F, Root J (2005) Cartilage metabolism in osteoarthritis and the influence of viscosupplementation and steroid: a review. Acta Radiol 3:288–296
59. Thorn, quoted by Hollander JL et al (1951) Hydrocortisone injected into arthritic joints. J Am Med Assoc 147:1629–1635
60. Towheed TE, Maxwell L, Judd MG, Catton M, Hochberg MC, Wells G (2006) Acetaminophen for osteoarthritis. Cochrane Database Syst Rev (1): CD004257
61. Waddell DD, Bert JM (2010) The use of hyaluronan after arthroscopic surgery of the knee. Arthroscopy 26(1):105–111
62. Wang CT, Lin YT, Chiang BL, Lin YH, Hou SM (2006) High molecular weight hyaluronic acid downregulates the gene expression of osteoarthritis-associated cytokines and enzymes in fibroblast-like synoviocytes from patients with early osteoarthritis. Osteoarthritis Cartilage 14(12):1237–1247
63. Watterson JR, Esdaile JM (2000) Viscosupplementation: therapeutic mechanisms and clinical potential in osteoarthritis of the knee. J Am Acad Orthop Surg 8(5):277–284
64. Wu WJ, Dong Q, Liu Y, Mao T, Chen F (2009) Platelet-rich plasma: a promising cell carrier for micro-invasive articular cartilage repair. Med Hypotheses 72(4):455–457
65. Yagishita K, Sekiya I, Sakaguchi Y, Shinomiya K, Muneta T (2005) The effect of hyaluronan on tendon healing in rabbits. Arthroscopy 21(11):1330–1336
66. Zaslav K, McAdams T, Scopp J, Theosadakis J, Mahajan V, Gobbi A (2012) New frontiers for cartilage repair and protection. Cartilage 3(1): 77S–86S
67. Zhang W, Nuki G, Moskowitz RW, Abramson S, Altman RD, Arden NK et al (2010) OARSI recommendations for the management of hip and knee osteoarthritis part III: changes in evidence following systematic cumulative update of research published through January 2009. Osteoarthritis Cartilage 18(4):476e99

Anaesthesia in Cartilage Repair Surgery

29

Paul Hayden

Contents

P. Hayden, BSc, MRCP, FRCA, DICM, FFICM
Department of Anaesthesia and Critical Care, Medway NHS Foundation Trust, Kent, UK
e-mail: paulhayden@nhs.net

29.1 Introduction

The main priority of anaesthesia for knee cartilage repair surgery is the maintenance of patient safety with high-quality analgesia. With the emergence and growing popularity of "fast track" surgery, reducing hospital length of stay has become an additional priority and has influenced the conduct of anaesthesia for the variety of surgical procedures that can be undertaken to repair knee cartilage.

As with all operations, the type of anaesthetic administered is individualised to the patient depending on the type of surgery and the patient's co-morbidities. For minor operations such as knee arthroscopy, micro-fracture and meniscal repairs, most patients are suitable for general anaesthesia with supplemental intravenous analgesia. For major knee surgery, regional anaesthetic techniques such as neuraxial techniques and lower limb nerve blocks have become routine, providing excellent, safe, intra-operative and post-operative analgesia.

29.2 General Anaesthesia

For short-duration knee arthroscopy, in patients with no or minor chronic health problems, a general anaesthetic is commonly administered with intravenous analgesia and anti-emetics. Simple oral analgesics are usually sufficient to control post-operative discomfort. Most anaesthetists prescribe a multimodal analgesic regime including

A.A. Shetty et al. (eds.), *Techniques in Cartilage Repair Surgery*,
DOI 10.1007/978-3-642-41921-8_29, © ESSKA 2014

regular paracetamol and nonsteroidal anti-inflammatory drugs such as ibuprofen or diclofenac with additional weak opioids such as dihydrocodeine if required. For the vast majority of patients, this is usually sufficient as pain is generally mild and of a short duration. In fact, repeated doses of intravenous paracetamol have been demonstrated in randomised trials to be effective even in major lower limb orthopaedic surgery [1].

For major knee surgery, several intravenous adjuncts have been investigated such as high-dose methylprednisolone, administered preoperatively, and pregabalin, which may show benefit in reducing the severity and incidence of chronic post-operative pain [2, 3]. These drugs, however, have not been investigated in large multicentre trials, and as such, they require further investigation before their routine use can be recommended.

The injection of local anaesthetics, such as bupivacaine or ropivacaine, into the knee joint at the end of surgery is a controversial topic with the concern that they may be chondrotoxic [4]. Although this has been demonstrated in both animal models and human subjects, there are a variety of confounding factors including the individual joint, dose and duration of local anaesthetic injected, co-administration of epinephrine, use of bone cement and inadvertent injection of chlorhexidine and other bioabsorbable materials [5–7]. It seems that there may also be variability in the risk of chondrotoxicity based on the individual type of local anaesthetic used with lidocaine particularly implicated [8]. Therefore, a causative relationship between local anaesthetics and chondrotoxicity in humans has not been clearly established. Whilst a recent randomised controlled study reported that intra-articular local anaesthetic provided beneficial short-term pain control compared with placebo, given the potential risk of chondrotoxicity, they advocated that intra-articular injection of local anaesthetic should not be used [9].

29.3 Regional Anaesthesia

Neuraxial techniques such as local anaesthetic injected into either the subdural space or epidural space have become popular for lower limb surgery, particularly in patients at increased risk from general anaesthesia such as those with significant cardiac or respiratory disease. Neuraxial anaesthetics may be administered in combination with general anaesthesia, or sedation, or the patient may remain awake during the operation. In the case of prolonged surgery, sedation or general anaesthesia is usually recommended as prolonged immobility whilst surgery takes place can become uncomfortable for patients.

In addition to their excellent analgesic properties, neuraxial techniques are associated with reduced perioperative blood loss, reduced incidence of venous thromboembolism post-operatively, anti-inflammatory effects and possibly reduced incidence of surgical site infection [10]. The reduction in blood loss is thought to be due to relative intra-operative hypotension and veno-dilatation, whilst the reduction in venous thromboembolism is probably due to attenuation of the perioperative stress response. Similarly, attenuation of the stress response, inhibition of c-fibre activation and sympathetic blockade are thought to be the mechanisms for the anti-inflammatory effects of regional anaesthetics compared with systemic analgesics alone [11].

Recent studies have demonstrated improved quality of post-operative analgesia and patient satisfaction when using spinal anaesthesia, compared with intravenous analgesia alone, and reduced time to mobilise post-operatively when compared to epidural anaesthetics. Furthermore, the safety of spinal anaesthesia is improved compared with epidural anaesthesia with the incidence of significant complications (including paraplegia and death) estimated at 1.6–2.6 per 100,000 patients with spinal anaesthesia versus 8.2–17.4 per 100,000 patients having epidural anaesthesia [12].

29.3.1 Epidural Anaesthesia

Whilst epidural anaesthesia is still a routinely used technique for major lower limb surgery, its use has waned over the past decade due primarily to the success of spinal anaesthesia and a resurgence in the use of lower limb nerve block techniques.

Although epidural techniques undoubtedly produce excellent pain relief, reduced mobility after surgery, raised likelihood of urinary retention and an increased risk of significant neurological complications such as nerve damage have limited their use. A Cochrane review published in 2003 also concluded that the analgesic benefit of epidural anaesthesia was only superior to intravenous opiates for the first 4–6 h, at the expense of an increased incidence of hypotension and urinary retention [13].

29.3.2 Spinal Anaesthesia

Spinal anaesthesia provides rapid-onset, predictable and safe analgesia and anaesthesia for lower limb surgery. The duration of regional anaesthesia provided by a spinal block is approximately 2–4 h, depending on the type, volume and concentration of local anaesthetic used, although adjuncts, including opiates such as morphine, diamorphine or fentanyl, are often added to increase the duration of analgesia provided. This is at the expense of an increased incidence of nausea and vomiting and pruritus. As with epidural anaesthesia, the incidence of urinary retention and hypotension is increased, compared with intravenous opiates.

29.3.3 Spinal Anaesthesia for Ambulatory Surgery

The success of spinal anaesthesia for major lower limb surgery has led to its increased use for minor lower limb surgery such as knee arthroscopy. Historically, the potential side effects of spinal anaesthesia such as urinary retention and reduced post-operative mobility on the day of surgery have limited the widespread use of the technique for ambulatory surgery. However, with the introduction of short-duration local anaesthetics such as low-dose hyperbaric bupivacaine and prilocaine, the use of spinal anaesthesia for ambulatory surgery is now increasing with the duration of motor block limited to 2–3 h and reduction in time to spontaneous voiding compared with spinal anaesthetics using conventional doses of bupivacaine [14–16].

29.3.4 Peripheral Nerve Blockade

Sensory innervation to the knee is transmitted via the femoral, sciatic and obturator nerves. Therefore, ideally all of these nerves should be targeted for effective analgesia. In practice, femoral and sciatic nerve blocks are the most common techniques used. As anaesthetists have developed their skills using high-resolution ultrasound to guide the insertion of nerve blocks, a variety of approaches to anaesthetise the relevant nerves for knee surgery have developed, using lower total doses of local anaesthetic and enhancing safety by minimising inadvertent neural injury.

Femoral nerve blocks are technically straightforward to perform with a low incidence of complications and produce analgesia for up to 24 h although this can be prolonged with the use of continuous local anaesthetic delivery systems. The incidence of motor blockade is reduced with the use of low concentrations of local anaesthetic, and the higher volumes used with these techniques provide some local anaesthetic spread into the lumbar plexus to provide obturator nerve anaesthesia.

Sciatic nerve blockade prevents posterior knee pain post-operatively but is technically more challenging to perform and associated with an increased incidence of motor block.

Lumbar plexus blocks are a suitable alternative to femoral and sciatic blocks with more reliable blockade of the obturator nerve. Complications are significantly higher than femoral nerve blocks however primarily due to inadvertent epidural and vascular spread of local anaesthetic [17].

29.3.5 Continuous Femoral Nerve Blockade

For prolonged post-operative analgesia, epidurals are commonly used but are associated with prolonged bilateral motor weakness, therefore limiting post-operative mobility and delaying hospital discharge. With the advent of several commercially available peripheral nerve catheters, continuous peripheral nerve blockade has become a popular technique, providing several benefits for patients such as an improved quality of analgesia compared with opiates, reduced nausea and vomiting and improved rates of functional recovery. The techniques however require increased technical skill compared with "single shot" techniques and take longer to perform. Several commercially available local anaesthetic delivery systems have been developed, allowing patients to be managed on the general ward and even discharged home with the devices in situ.

29.4 Carbon Dioxide Arthroscopy

As surgical techniques for cartilage repair surgery have developed, the requirement for fluid-free knee arthroscopy has arisen to allow the injection of stem cells into bony surfaces. As with abdominal laparoscopic surgery, there is the possibility for subcutaneous emphysema and venous gas embolism, the latter potentially leading to fatal circulatory collapse [18]. This may be minimised with gases that readily dissolve in the circulation, such as carbon dioxide, rather than air, whilst case reports have suggested that a lower limb tourniquet is essential to help minimise its incidence [19, 20].

In summary, there are several methods to provide effective, safe anaesthesia and analgesia for knee cartilage repair surgery, the choice of which must be determined by the anaesthetist after careful consideration of the relevant surgical and patient-specific requirements and the procedure planned whilst appreciating the patient's preferences.

References

1. Sinatra RS et al (2012) Intravenous acetaminophen for pain after major orthopedic surgery: an expanded analysis. Pain Pract 12(5):357–365
2. Lunn TH et al (2011) Effect of high-dose preoperative methylprednisolone on pain and recovery after total knee arthroplasty: a randomized, placebo-controlled trial. Br J Anaesth 106(2):230–238
3. Buvanendran A et al (2010) Perioperative oral pregabalin reduces chronic pain after total knee arthroplasty: a prospective, randomized, controlled trial. Anesth Analg 110(1):199–207
4. Webb ST, Ghosh S (2009) Intra-articular bupivacaine: potentially chondrotoxic? Br J Anaesth 102(4): 439–441
5. Gomoll AH et al (2006) Chondrolysis after continuous intra-articular bupivacaine infusion: an experimental model investigating chondrotoxicity in the rabbit shoulder. Arthroscopy 22(8):813–819
6. Hansen BP et al (2007) Postarthroscopic glenohumeral chondrolysis. Am J Sports Med 35(10): 1628–1634
7. Dragoo JL et al (2010) Chondrotoxicity of low pH, epinephrine, and preservatives found in local anesthetics containing epinephrine. Am J Sports Med 38(6):1154–1159
8. Dragoo JL et al (2012) The in vitro chondrotoxicity of single-dose local anesthetics. Am J Sports Med 40(4):794–799
9. Campo MM et al (2012) A randomised controlled trial for the effectiveness of intra-articular Ropivacaine and Bupivacaine on pain after knee arthroscopy: the DUPRA (DUtch Pain Relief after Arthroscopy)-trial. Knee Surg Sports Traumatol Arthrosc 20(2):239–244
10. Chang CC, Lin HC, Lin HW (2010) Anesthetic management and surgical site infections in total hip or knee replacement: a population-based study. Anesthesiology 113(2):279–284
11. Kettner SC, Willschke H, Marhofer P (2011) Does regional anaesthesia really improve outcome? Br J Anaesth 107(Suppl 1):i90–i95
12. Cook TM, Counsell D, Wildsmith JA (2009) Major complications of central neuraxial block: report on the Third National Audit Project of the Royal College of Anaesthetists. Br J Anaesth 102(2):179–190
13. Choi PT et al (2003) Epidural analgesia for pain relief following hip or knee replacement. Cochrane Database Syst Rev (3):CD003071
14. Nair GS et al (2009) Systematic review of spinal anaesthesia using bupivacaine for ambulatory knee arthroscopy. Br J Anaesth 102(3):307–315
15. Hendriks MP et al (2009) Plain articaine or prilocaine for spinal anaesthesia in day-case knee arthroscopy: a double-blind randomized trial. Br J Anaesth 102(2): 259–263
16. Black AS et al (2011) Spinal anaesthesia for ambulatory arthroscopic surgery of the knee: a comparison of low-dose prilocaine and fentanyl with bupivacaine and fentanyl. Br J Anaesth 106(2):183–188
17. Auroy Y et al (2002) Major complications of regional anesthesia in France: the SOS Regional Anesthesia Hotline Service. Anesthesiology 97(5):1274–1280
18. Habegger R, Siebenmann R, Kieser C (1989) Lethal air embolism during arthroscopy. A case report. J Bone Joint Surg Br 71(2):314–316
19. Riddell RR (1990) CO2 arthroscopy of the knee. Clin Orthop Relat Res 252:92–94
20. Lotman DB (1987) Pneumoperitoneum and acidosis during arthroscopy with CO2. Arthroscopy 3(3): 185–186

Preoperative and Postoperative Radiological Assessment

30

M.O. Brix, S. Domayer, P. Bilagi, and S. Trattnig

Contents

M.O. Brix, MD (✉)
Department of Orthopaedics, Medical University of Vienna, Vienna, Austria
e-mail: martin.brix@meduniwien.ac.at

S. Domayer, MD, PhD
Orthopaedic Rehabilitation Center SKA Zicksee, St. Andrä am Zicksee, Austria

P. Bilagi, MD
Kent Knee Unit, Spire Alexandra Hospital, Impton Lane, Chatham, Kent, UK

S. Trattnig, MD
High Field MR Centre, Department of Biomedical Imaging and Image-guided Therapy, Medical University of Vienna, Vienna, Austria

30.1 Introduction

All surgical cartilage repair techniques require valid, reproducible, and widely applied diagnostics, which provide a basis for staging and for follow-up of the cartilage repair tissue as well as the adjacent cartilage.

Histology is the gold standard, but the availability is limited, due to the invasiveness of biopsy harvest. In addition, there is difficulty in choosing an appropriate biopsy site within the transplant area and state of the subchondral bone.

Magnetic resonance imaging (MRI) has become the method of choice in articular cartilage imaging. MRI not only offers the possibility of preoperative assessment regarding defect size and localization of the defect, but it is also a noninvasive, safe, and reproducible tool for the follow-up, helps to evaluate the quality and success of tissue repair processes after surgery, and provides also information about degenerative changes in the joint after cartilage repair. The usage of cartilage-specific sequences provides information about the morphological state of the cartilage, including the early stages of disease process. Furthermore, there exist several more demanding techniques, which provide information about biochemical properties such as the glycosaminoglycan (GAG) content or the integrity of the collagen network. Additionally, there are also scoring systems, which offer clinicians the opportunity to evaluate the cartilage in a semiquantitative way.

A.A. Shetty et al. (eds.), *Techniques in Cartilage Repair Surgery*,
DOI 10.1007/978-3-642-41921-8_30, © ESSKA 2014

Table 30.1 Effect of several parameters on signal-to-noise ratio (SNR)

Parameter	Effect on SNR
Slice thickness	↑ ↑
Field of view	↑ ↑
Repetition time	↑ ↑
Echo time	↑ ↓
Matrix size	↑ ↓
Power of the magnetic field	↑ ↑
Bandwidth	↑ ↓
Usage of dedicated coils	↑ ↑

30.2 Basic Requirements and Cartilage-Specific Sequences

Due to the complex, zonally anisotropic internal structure of cartilage resulting in a short T2 relaxation time and because of its inherent lack of depth, MRI of articular cartilage is still challenging. Therefore, the highest spatial resolution with an acceptable signal-to-noise ratio (SNR) is required. Parameters influencing the signal-to-noise ratio, like the slice thickness or the field strength, are shown in Table 30.1. Imaging of the articular cartilage is possible at most clinically available MR systems, but it has been shown that a voxel size lower than 300 μm is required to reveal fraying of the cartilage [1]. High-field MRI, like 1.5 Tesla (T) or 3 T systems, is able to provide such resolutions in reasonable scan times. These systems provide also the opportunity of 3-D acquisition with high resolution, high SNR and high contrast-to-noise ratio [2].

30.2.1 Morphological MRI

The usage of cartilage-specific sequences with a high resolution allows the demonstration of damaged cartilage at an early stage. For the evaluation of the repair tissue, the same standard morphological MR imaging acquisition techniques can be performed as those used for native cartilage [3]. The most widespread cartilage-specific MRI techniques are:

- Intermediate-weighted fast spin echo (FSE)
- 3-D fat-suppressed T1-weighted gradient-echo (GRE) acquisition
- isotropic 3-D sequences (3-D DESS, d-D FSE SPACE)

Each technique has particular properties that complement each other.

The intermediate-weighted FSE sequence, which uses differences in T2 weighting, is more sensitive for assessment of the internal cartilage structure. The reason is that collagen fibers with a highly regular structure are interacting with water molecules and immobilize them, which leads to an interaction between their protons and consecutively to an acceleration of T2 relaxation. Another advantage of this technique is the low susceptibility to metal artifacts with regard to diagnostics after surgery. This technique provides results with high accuracy, an overall sensitivity of 87 %, specificity 94 %, and accuracy of 92 % [4, 5]. It produces dark cartilage against bright synovial fluid and therefore a high contrast (Fig. 30.1a, b).

On the other side, the 3-D fat-suppressed GRE technique visualizes cartilage defects attributable to T1 differences between cartilage and fluid. The technique is able to provide thinner sections, which is beneficial in identifying lesions and for 3-D analysis. The strength of this technique is the visualization of the thickness and the surface of the cartilage [2]. The technique provides similar results with overall sensitivity of 86 %, specificity of 97 %, and accuracy of 91 % for the detection of cartilage lesions of the knee [6]. The cartilage signal is higher than fluid in T1-weighted fat-suppressed images (Fig. 30.1c, d).

Currently, 3-D sequences are getting more and more into routine protocols. The big advantage of those sequences is, that they can be reformatted in any plane. Therefore only one sequence, for example in sagittal plane, is necessary and the reformatting into coronal and axial plane cane be done without any loose of signal or resolution. This is beneficial for the scan time. The voxel dimension can be as small as 0.4 mm^3 which allows a very detailed resolution [2]. The 3-D DESS (double-echo steady state) sequence is a gradient echo based sequence, which was introduced many years ago [7], but improved magnet systems were necessary for adequate measurement [8]. The benefits of this sequence are a high SNR, a high cartilage-to-fluid contrast and low partial volume artifacts. A negative aspect is the high sensitivity to susceptibility

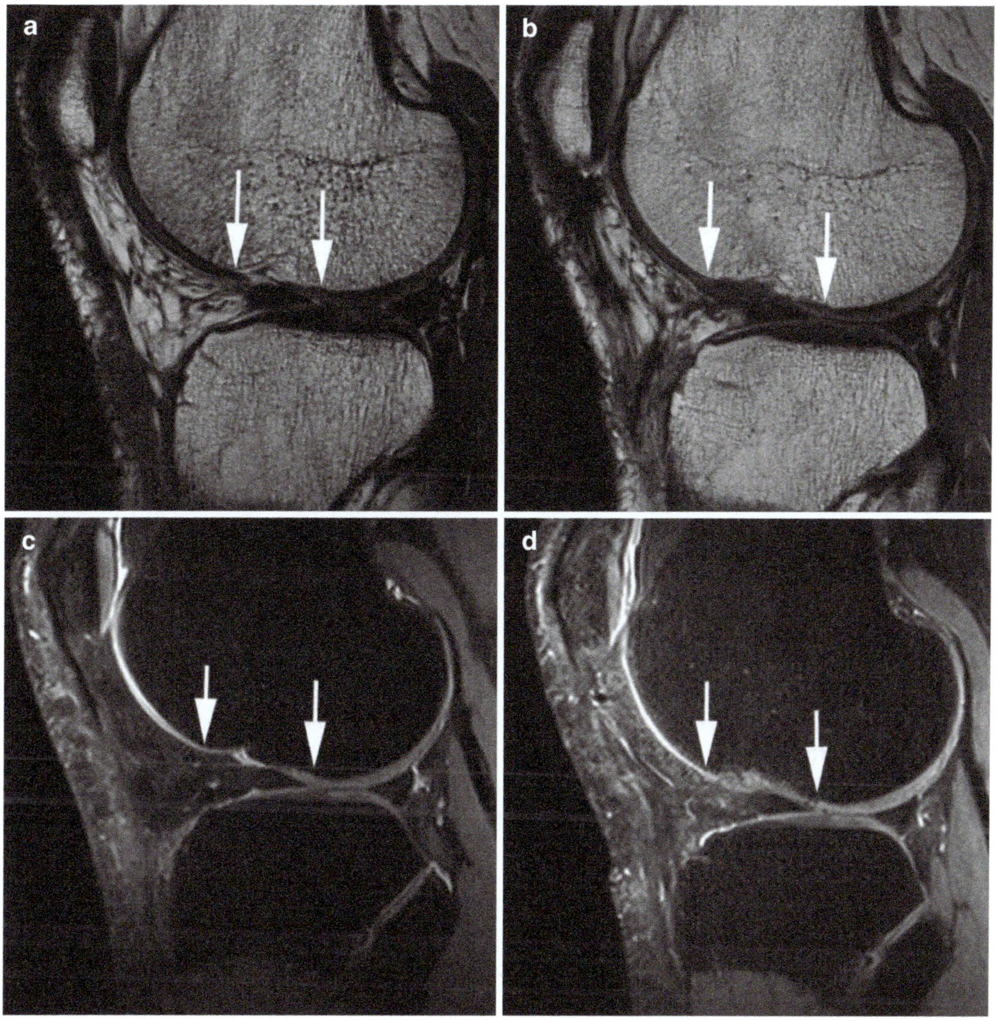

Fig. 30.1 The images demonstrate a defect on the lateral femoral condyle (**a**, **c**) and the repair tissue 1 year after MACT procedure (**b**, **d**). The defect, respectively the borders of the implant, is marked with the *arrows*. (**a**, **b**) Sagittal T2-FSE image, with dark cartilage against bright synovial fluid. (**c**, **d**) Sagittal T1-weighted, fat-saturated GRE image, with bright cartilage against low signal

artifacts [9]. The 3-D FSE SPACE (sampling perfection with application-optimized contrasts using different flip-angle evolutions) provides the highest SNR in comparison to other isotropic 3-D sequences [10], however this results in longer acquisition times [9].

30.2.2 Usage of Coils

In addition to adequate field strength and cartilage-specific sequences, dedicated surface coils are important preconditions to achieve good image quality. Currently, surface coils for the wrist, shoulder, knee, and ankle are standard. Most of them are multichannel phased-array coils. Lutterbey et al. demonstrated that using a standard body coil at 3 T for imaging of the knee gave a lower image quality than achieved using a 1.5 T scanner with a dedicated knee coil [11].

30.2.3 Preoperative Assessment

The importance of the preoperative assessment lies in the identification of the defect, its size, and

Table 30.2 MRI classification of articular chondral lesions [9]

Grade I	Abnormal intrachondral signal with a normal chondral surface
Grade II	Mild surface irregularity and/or focal loss of less than 50 % of the cartilage thickness
Grade III	Severe surface irregularity and/or focal loss of 50–100 % of the cartilage thickness
Grade IV	Complete loss of articular cartilage, with exposure of the subchondral bone

localization. The status of the subchondral bone is also of importance. The preoperative MRI is furthermore used to rule out meniscal tears as well as stability issues. A very important parameter is the joint alignment; therefore, the long leg view is used to discover varus or valgus deformity.

30.3 Cartilage Classification Systems Based on Morphology

Clinical scores remain the basis for the comparison of different surgical techniques and the outcome. For morphological MRI there are several classifications to describe articular cartilage and its repair tissue. One commonly used classification is the one published by Yulish et al. who first adapted the pathological changes described by Shahriaree [12, 13]. The classification uses four different grades based on the cartilage thickness and is very similar to the Outerbridge grading system or the ICRS classification, which are widely used in clinical practice and based on arthroscopic findings. The Yulish classification is shown in Table 30.2.

The persistent improvement in cartilage repair techniques in the last few years has prompted the need for comparable parameters. In general, the repair tissue should be compared with the adjacent native cartilage. On morphological MRI, the cartilage repair tissue should have a smooth surface, which continues the original articular contour at the same level as the adjacent articular cartilage. Ideally, the signal intensity of the repair tissue should be isointense compared to the adjacent native cartilage, but it is well known that in the first months after surgical treatment, there is a difference in the signal intensity, due to storage of water. The investigator should however not only pay attention on the repair tissue and the filling of the defect but also consider the subchondral plate, the subchondral bone marrow, and other parameters of the joint (such as effusion or adjacent soft tissue).

The MOCART score (magnetic resonance observation of cartilage repair tissue) published by Marlovits et al. [14, 15] is currently the most comprehensive MRI score for the particular assessment of cartilage repair. The score is based on following parameters as shown in Table 30.3:

- Degree of defect repair and filling of the defect
- Integration to border zone
- Surface of the repair tissue
- Structure of the repair tissue
- Signal intensity of the repair tissue
- Subchondral lamina
- Subchondral bone
- Adhesions
- Effusion

The use of the MOCART score is simple and allows for a high interobserver variability with an intraclass correlation coefficient (ICC) of >0.81 in eight of nine variables, indicating almost perfect agreement according to Landis and Koch [15–17]. Only the variable "structure of repair tissue" has an ICC of 0.765 which means a substantial agreement [15]. The recommended morphological sequences are both used in the MOCART score, which allows for the assessment of different cartilage lesions and can be done without significant change in imaging time [18]. The MOCART score is widely used in clinics, which has been demonstrated in a recent review by de Windt et al. [19].

With the implementation of new 3-D techniques into routine diagnostics, the score has been further modified to a 3-D MOCART score [20]. The 3-D MOCART score used all variables of the original score, and new variables were additionally included with the aims to use the capabilities of isotropic MRI, to include results of recent studies, and to adapt to the needs of

Table 30.3 MRI classification of articular cartilage repair tissue: MOCART score [14, 15]

Variables	Points
1. Degree of defect repair and filling of the defect	
O Complete	20
O Hypertrophy	15
Incomplete	
O >50 % of the adjacent cartilage	10
O <50 % of the adjacent cartilage	5
O Subchondral bone exposed	0
2. Integration to border zone	
O Complete	15
Incomplete	
O Demarcating border visible	10
Defect visible	
O <50 % of the length of the repair tissue	5
O >50 % of the length of the repair tissue	0
3. Surface of repair tissue	
O Surface intact	10
Surface damaged	
O <50 % of repair tissue depth	5
O >50 % of repair tissue depth or total degeneration	0
4. Structure of repair tissue	
O Homogenous	5
O Inhomogeneous or cleft formation	0
5. Signal intensity	
Dual-T2-FSE	
O Isointense	15
O Moderately hyperintense	5
O Markedly hyperintense	0
3-D-GE-FS	
O Isointense	15
O Moderately hypointense	5
O Markedly hypointense	0
6. Subchondral lamina	
O Intact	5
O Not intact	0
7. Subchondral bone	
O Intact	5
O Not intact (edema, granulation tissue, cysts, sclerosis)	0
8. Adhesion	
O No	5
O Yes	0
9. Effusion	
O No	5
O Yes	0
Maximal sum	**100**

patients and physicians in a clinical routine examination [20]. The correlation between the standard MOCART score and the newer 3-D score depicted a highly significant correlation ($p<0.001$) in eight of nine variables with a Pearson coefficient between 0.566 and 0.932 (variable "bone marrow edema: $p<0.05$; Pearson coefficient 0.257)[20]. The 3-D MOCART score is shown in Table 30.4.

30.4 Biochemical Imaging

In the last years, several biochemical MRI techniques have been developed for clinical use in order to characterize quantitative properties of articular cartilage and repair tissue. The loss of GAGs and increased water content occur in the earliest stage of cartilage of cartilage degeneration. Furthermore, articular cartilage repair techniques aim to create a hyaline-like repair tissue. The most important biochemical MRI techniques will be described in the following and are shown in Table 30.5. One has to consider that the particular techniques are able to evaluate different properties of the articular cartilage and are therefore of particular value to define repair tissue quality: dGEMRIC, sodium imaging and gagCEST visualize the GAG content, T2 mapping the integrity of the collagen network. Furthermore there are differences in clinical application. dGEMRIC and T2 mapping are more or less clinical applicable techniques, whereas gagCEST is in the initial stage, although it shows promising results. Sodium imaging seems to stay limited to a 7T MRI, therefore is a clinical application not relevant.

30.4.1 Delayed Gadolinium-Enhanced MRI of Cartilage (dGEMRIC)

dGEMRIC is currently the most widely used method for analyzing the depletion of GAG in the articular cartilage. In particular, dGEMRIC allows to assess the GAG content of articular

Table 30.4 MRI classification of articular cartilage repair tissue: 3-D MOCART score [20]

Variables				
1. Defect fill (*degree of defect repair and filling of the defect in relation to the adjacent cartilage*)				
O	0 %			
O	0–25 %			
O	25–50 %			
O	50–75 %			
O	75–100 %			
O	100 %			
O	100–125 %			
O	125–150 %			
O	150–200 %			
O	>200 %			
Localization				
O Whole area of cartilage repair			O>50 %	O<50 %
O Central	O Peripheral	O Weight bearing		O Non-weight bearing
2. Cartilage Interface (*integration with adjacent cartilage to border zone in two planes*)				
Sagittal (femur, patella, trochlea, tibia)				
O	Complete			
O	Demarcating border visible (split-like)			
O	Defect visible<50 %			
O	Defect visible >50 %			
Coronal (femur, tibia), axial (patella, trochlea)				
O	Complete			
O	Demarcating border visible (split-like)			
O	Defect visible <50 %			
O	Defect visible >50 %			
Localization				
O Whole area of cartilage repair			O>50 %	O<50 %
O Weight bearing		O Non-weight bearing		
3. Bone Interface (*integration of the transplant to the subchondral bone, integration of a possible periosteal flap*)				
O	Complete			
O	Partial delamination			
O	Complete delamination			
O	Delamination of periosteal flap			
Localization				
O Weight bearing		O Non-weight bearing		
4. Surface (*constitution of the surface of the repair tissue*)				
O	Surface intact			
O	Surface damaged<50 % depth			
O	Surface damaged>50 % depth			
O	Adhesions			
Localization				
O Whole area of cartilage repair			O>50 %	O<50 %
O Central	O Peripheral	O Weight bearing		O Non-weight bearing
5. Structure (*constitution of the repair tissue*)				
O	Homogeneous			
O	Inhomogeneous or cleft formation			

Table 30.4 (continued)

Variables				
Localization				
O Whole area of cartilage repair			O>50 %	O<50 %
O Central	O Peripheral	O Weight bearing		O Non-weight bearing
6. Signal intensity (*intensity of MR signal in the repair tissue in comparison to the adjacent cartilage*)				
O	Normal (identical to adjacent cartilage)			
O	Nearly normal (slight areas of signal alteration)			
O	Abnormal (large areas of signal alteration)			
Localization				
O Central	O Peripheral	O Weight bearing		O Non-weight bearing
7. Subchondral lamina (*constitution of the subchondral lamina*)				
O	Intact			
O	Non Intact			
Localization				
O Whole area of cartilage repair			O>50 %	O<50 %
O Central	O Peripheral	O Weight bearing		O Non-weight bearing
8. Chondral osteophytes (*osteophytes within the cartilage repair area*)				
O	Absent			
O	Osteophytes <50 % of the thickness of the cartilage transplant			
O	Osteophytes >50 % of the thickness of the cartilage transplant			
Localization				
Size: _____ mm (plane: _____) × _____ mm (plane: _____)				
O Central	O Peripheral	O Weight bearing		O Non-weight bearing
9. Bone marrow edema (*maximum size and localization in relation to the cartilage repair tissue and other alterations assessed in the 3-D MOCART score*)				
O	Absent			
O	Small (<1 cm)			
O	Medium (<2 cm)			
O	Large (<4 cm)			
O	Diffuse			
Localization				
Size: _____ mm (plane: _____) × _____ mm (plane: _____)				
O Central	O Peripheral	O Weight bearing		O Non-weight bearing
O Relation to other alterations within this score of variable No. _____				
10. Subchondral bone (*constitution of the subchondral bone*)				
O	Intact			
O	Granulation tissue			
O	Cyst			
O	Sclerosis			
Localization				
O Whole area of cartilage repair			O>50 %	O<50 %
O Central	O Peripheral	O Weight bearing		O Non-weight bearing
11. Effusion (*approximately size of joint effusion visualized in all planes*)				
O	Absent			
O	Small			
O	Medium			
O	Large			

Table 30.5 Features of selected biochemical MRI techniques

Type of MR examination	Cartilage component	Contrast agent	Acquisition time	Protocol complexity	Spatial resolution
dGEMRIC	GAG specific	Yes	≈5 min	High	0.2×0.2
T2 mapping	Collagen network and water content specific	No	≈5 min	Low	0.6×0.6
Sodium MRI	GAG specific	No	≈20 min	Medium	1.5×1.5 (7 T)
gagCEST	GAG specific	No	≈15 min	Low	0.6×0.6

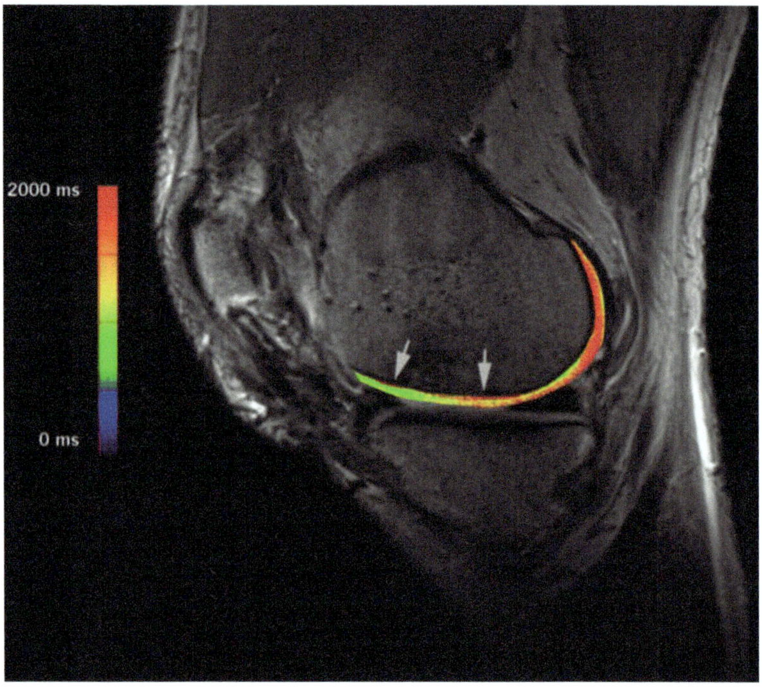

Fig. 30.2 Sagittal color-coded contrast-enhanced T1 map of a 35-year-old male patient, 3 years after MACT procedure. The borders of the implant are marked with the *arrows*

cartilage and has proven its feasibility in many studies, in vitro and in vivo [21–25]. The principle of dGEMRIC relies on the negative fixed charge density (FCD) of the GAG side chains. Maroudas et al. have demonstrated that there is a strong correlation between FCD and GAG content [26]. The administered negatively charged contrast agent (gadolinium diethylenetriamine pentaacetate anion, Gd-DTPA2-) accumulates in an inverse distribution into the cartilage [27, 28]. Therefore T1, which is determined by Gd-DTPA2- concentration, can be used as a specific measure for the GAG concentration and the contrast agent will equilibrate in an area with a lower GAG content in a higher concentration. An area with a focal cartilage lesion and consequently a loss of GAG results in lower T1 values compared to healthy cartilage (Fig. 30.2). Trattnig et al. demonstrated that only the measurement of postcontrast T1 values is necessary for the evaluation [24]. Therefore, the protocol recommended by Burstein et al. should be used [21]: after an intravenous administration of 0.2 mmol gadolinium per kilogram body weight (double dose), the patients should exercise the knee moderately for 20 min, which means, for example, walking up and down the stairs. Ninety minutes after application of the contrast agent, the MRI should be performed. This period of time is necessary to allow the contrast agent to fully diffuse into

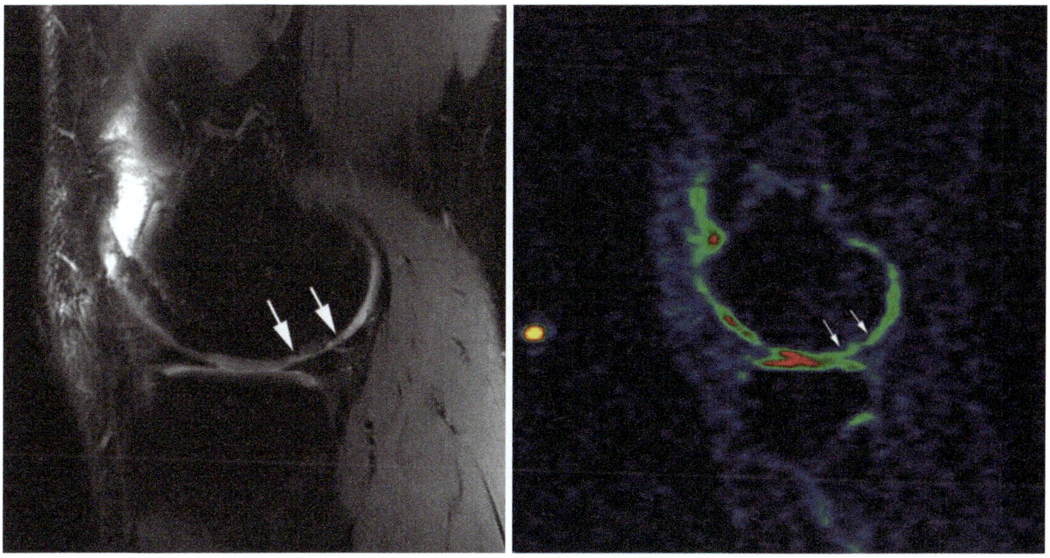

Fig. 30.3 Sagittal T1-weighted, fat-saturated GRE image (*left*) and corresponding color-coded sagittal sodium 3-D GRE image in a 43-year-old woman obtained 42 months after MFX procedure. The repair tissue is situated between the *arrows*

the cartilage, before the images are acquired. However, because cartilage thickness is variable between different regions in the knee and different joints, the time delay to reach the equilibrium should be modified, as appropriate for the region the investigator is interested in [21]. The dGEMRIC technique has also been optimized for the hip, the ankle, and the wrist joints [29–33]. The technique is reported to have a fair reproducibility ranging from 5 to 15 % [34, 35].

One disadvantage of dGEMRIC is the potential but extremely rare adverse event of nephrogenic systemic fibrosis. It is described that the contrast agent is a possible trigger in patients with renal failure [36–38]. Consequently, before the investigation, normal renal function must be verified via serum creatinine level.

30.4.2 Sodium Imaging

The principle of sodium imaging is similar to that of dGEMRIC. Once again the negative FCD of the GAG side chains play a major role. These negative charged ions attract positive counter ions (e.g., sodium) and water molecules. Shapiro et al. depicted the feasibility of calculating FCD by sodium imaging [39]. Based on the fact that GAG molecules are counterbalanced by sodium ions, sodium imaging was successfully introduced for the assessment of healthy articular cartilage and cartilage repair tissue after surgical repair [40–44]. The major advantage of sodium imaging over dGEMRIC is the high specificity to GAG without the need of a contrast agent. The technique has demonstrated to be capable to detect even small changes in the GAG content [45, 46]. Furthermore, the low sodium content of adjacent tissues allows a good contrast to the surrounding structures of articular cartilage (Fig. 30.3).

The disadvantage of sodium imaging is that it requires ultrahigh-field MRI (7 T and above), because a smaller gyromagnetic ratio, a significantly shorter T2 relaxation time, a lower resonance frequency, and a lower concentration of sodium nuclei result in a sodium MR signal of articular cartilage that is 1/4,000–1/5,000 smaller than the proton MR signal [47]. Currently there exist roughly 50 7 T MRI units worldwide, which demonstrates the very low accessibility for sodium MRI. Nevertheless, sodium imaging offers an excellent evaluation tool for the introduction of new GAG-specific MRI techniques.

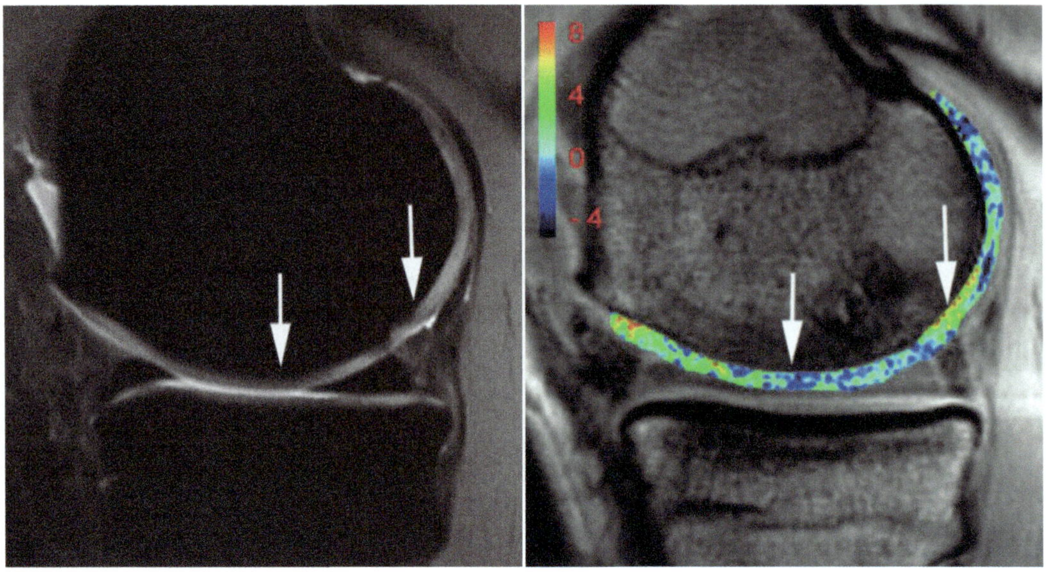

Fig. 30.4 Sagittal T1-weighted, fat-saturated GRE image (*left*) and corresponding color-coded gagCEST image of a 21-year-old female patient, 2 years after MACT procedure. The implant is located on the medial femoral condyle and marked by the *arrows*. The implant is demonstrating a lower signal than the surrounding cartilage

30.4.3 GAG-Specific Chemical Exchange Saturation Transfer (gagCEST)

gagCEST is one of the most promising techniques for the future. The technique was first described by Ling et al. who identified the dependence of CEST imaging on GAG through hydrogen 1(^{1}H) and carbon 13 (^{13}C) [48]. The technique is specific for the cartilage GAG content and has already been used for the assessment of GAG after cartilage repair [49]. The basic principle of gagCEST is a reduction of bulk water MR signal after off-resonant spins are selectively presaturated by radiofrequency irradiation and then undergo chemical exchange with bulk water protons [48, 50]. CEST uses the possibility to accumulate molecule-specific saturation information on bulk water protons for the indirect detection particular metabolites [51]. The potential to evaluate the GAG content in intervertebral discs at 3 T has already been demonstrated [52]. It therefore seems to be possible that the technique can be used to measure the GAG content in articular cartilage (Fig. 30.4).

30.4.4 T2 Mapping

Opposed to the previously described techniques, which are related to the GAG content, T2 mapping is able to describe the composition of articular cartilage on the basis of collagen structure and hydration [53]. Due to the orientation of collagen fibers in healthy cartilage, T2 shows an increase from the deep to the superficial layer (Fig. 30.5). In the deep layer, collagen fibers run anisotropically perpendicular to subchondral bone; therefore, there is a reduced mobility of water and lower T2 relaxation time values. In the superficial layer, the collagen fibers are randomly oriented, which leads to higher T2 values [54]. Consequently, zonal evaluation of articular cartilage is important in T2 analysis. Free water leads to a prolongation of T2 in general. The loss of proteoglycans will lead to increased water and to higher T2 values.

T2 mapping has found widespread application for the evaluation of the repair tissue after surgical repair [55–58]. White et al. proved in a horse model study that zonal T2 mapping is able to distinguish between normal hyaline cartilage and cartilage repair tissue [59].

The gold standard for T2 mapping would be spin echo imaging with separate acquisitions for each echo time, but this is not possible in clinical routine, due to the long measurement time. Therefore, multislice multiecho spin echo (MESE) sequences are often used, providing faster imaging, but there are some aspects to be considered with regard to accuracy. For multislice imaging, slice-selective refocusing pulses are necessary, which produce transitional regions at slice boundaries. As a result, the imperfect refocusing pulses and hence stimulated echo contribution in fast spin echo introduce mixed T1 and T2 contrast to the image. Maier et al. demonstrated in agarose phantom measurements that a substantial inaccuracy is introduced with 10–13 % longer T2 values [60]. Additional parameters, which may affect T2 quantification, are field inhomogeneities and insufficient sampling of the T2 decay curve, and magnetization transfer contrast created by refocusing pulses for other slices diminishes the signal intensity in cartilage [60, 61].

Another possible pitfall is the magic angle effect, which is a T2-related artifact. This phenomenon depends on the orientation of the collagen fibrils to the static magnetic field. An orientation of the collagen fibers to the static magnetic field in an angle of 55° could lead to an artificial increase of signal intensity (Fig. 30.5).

In conclusion, a certain error of absolute T2 values has to be expected when using different T2 mapping protocols. Nevertheless, the strength of the technique is the assessment of the zonal collagen network organization of cartilage and cartilage repair tissue.

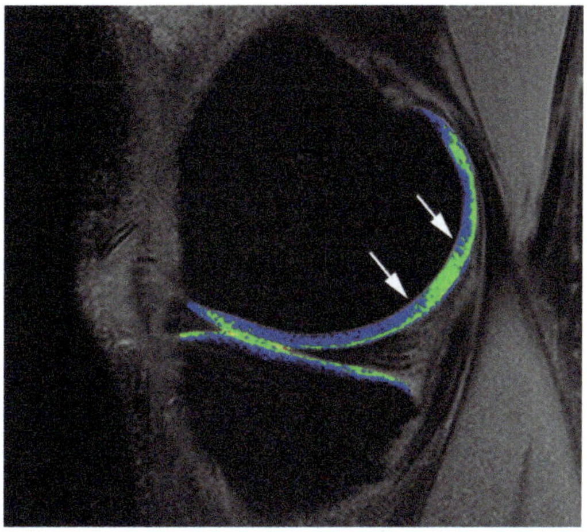

Fig. 30.5 Sagittal T2 map of the medial condyle of a healthy 32-year-old male volunteer. The image demonstrates the typical zonal variation resulting in lower signal in the deep zone and higher signal in the superficial zone. The *arrows* depict the magic angle effect with an artificial increase of signal intensity

Conclusion

With MRI, orthopedic surgeons have a powerful tool for the identification of the number, size, and depth of cartilage lesions at the time of initial injury, and they are able to assess the morphological status of cartilage repair tissue. Furthermore, with the ongoing development of biochemical imaging techniques, surgeons can get information about the biochemical composition of articular cartilage and its repair tissue. This information may help to guide decision-making by providing surgeons with novel information about repair tissue quality and its behavior.

References

1. Rubenstein JD, Li JG, Majumdar S, Henkelman RM (1997) Image resolution and signal-to-noise ratio requirements for MR imaging of degenerative cartilage. AJR Am J Roentgenol 169:1089–1096
2. Trattnig S, Winalski C, Marlovits S, Jurvelin J (2011) Magnetic resonance imaging of cartilage repair a review. Cartilage 2(1):5–26
3. Recht M, Bobic V, Burstein D, Disler D, Gold G, Gray M, Kramer J, Lang P, McCauley T, Winalski C (2001) Magnetic resonance imaging of articular cartilage. Clin Orthop Relat Res 391(Suppl):S379–S396
4. Kramer J, Recht MP, Imhof H, Stiglbaüer R, Engel A (1994) Postcontrast MR arthrography in assessment of cartilage lesions. J Comput Assist Tomogr 18:218–224
5. Kramer J, Scheurecker A, Mohr E, Engel A, Recht M (1997) Magnetic resonance arthrography: benefits and indication. In: MRI innovations contrast-enhancing agents clinical impact. Advances in MRI contrast, Wolters Kluwer Academic Publishers, The Netherlands. pp 104–109
6. Disler DG, McCauley TR, Kelman CG, Fuchs MD, Ratner LM, Wirth CR, Hospodar PP (1996)

Fat-suppressed three-dimensional spoiled gradient-echo MR imaging of hyaline cartilage defects in the knee: comparison with standard MR imaging and arthroscopy. AJR Am J Roentgenol 167:127–132
7. Hardy PA, Recht MP, Piraino D, Thomasson D (1996) Optimization of a dual echo in the steady state (DESS) free-precession sequence for imaging cartilage. J Magn Reson Imaging 6:329–335
8. Eckstein F, Kunz M, Schutzer M, Hudelmaier M, Jackson RD, Yu J, Eaton CB, Schneider E (2007) Two year longitudinal change and test-retest-precision of knee cartilage morphology in a pilot study for the osteoarthritis initiative. Osteoarthr. Cartil 15:1326–1332
9. Roemer FW, Crema MD, Trattnig S, Guermazi A (2011) Advances in imaging of osteoarthritis and cartilage. Radiology 260:332–354
10. Friedrich KM, Reiter G, Kaiser B, Mayerhöfer M, Deimling M, Jellus V, Horger W, Trattnig S, Schweitzer M, Salomonowitz E (2011) High-resolution cartilage imaging of the knee at 3T: basic evaluation of modern isotropic 3D MR-sequences. Eur J Radiol 78:398–405
11. Lutterbey G, Behrends K, Falkenhausen MV, Wattjes MP, Morakkabati N, Gieseke J, Schild H (2007) Is the body-coil at 3 Tesla feasible for the MRI evaluation of the painful knee? A comparative study. Eur Radiol 17:503–508
12. Yulish BS, Montanez J, Goodfellow DB, Bryan PJ, Mulopulos GP, Modic MT (1987) Chondromalacia patellae: assessment with MR imaging. Radiology 164:763–766
13. Shahriaree H (1985) Chondromalacia. Contemp Orthop 67B:42–43
14. Marlovits S, Striessnig G, Resinger CT, Aldrian SM, Vecsei V, Imhof H, Trattnig S (2004) Definition of pertinent parameters for the evaluation of articular cartilage repair tissue with high-resolution magnetic resonance imaging. Eur J Radiol 52:310–319
15. Marlovits S, Singer P, Zeller P, Mandl I, Haller J, Trattnig S (2006) Magnetic resonance observation of cartilage repair tissue (MOCART) for the evaluation of autologous chondrocyte transplantation: determination of interobserver variability and correlation to clinical outcome after 2 years. Eur J Radiol 57:16–23
16. Landis JR, Koch GG (1977) The measurement of observer agreement for categorical data. Biometrics 33:159–174
17. Koch GG, Landis JR, Freeman JL, Freeman DH, Lehnen RC (1977) A general methodology for the analysis of experiments with repeated measurement of categorical data. Biometrics 33:133–158
18. Trattnig S, Mlynárik V, Huber M, Ba-Ssalamah A, Puig S, Imhof H (2000) Magnetic resonance imaging of articular cartilage and evaluation of cartilage disease. Invest Radiol 35:595–601
19. de Windt TS, Welsch GH, Brittberg M, Vonk LA, Marlovits S, Trattnig S, Saris DBF (2013) Is magnetic resonance imaging reliable in predicting clinical outcome after articular cartilage repair of the knee?: a systematic review and meta-analysis. Am J Sports Med 41:1695–1702
20. Welsch GH, Zak L, Mamisch TC, Resinger C, Marlovits S, Trattnig S (2009) Three-dimensional magnetic resonance observation of cartilage repair tissue (MOCART) score assessed with an isotropic three-dimensional true fast imaging with steady-state precession sequence at 3.0 Tesla. Invest Radiol 44:603–612
21. Burstein D, Velyvis J, Scott KT, Stock KW, Kim YJ, Jaramillo D, Boutin RD, Gray ML (2001) Protocol issues for delayed Gd(DTPA)(2-)-enhanced MRI (dGEMRIC) for clinical evaluation of articular cartilage. Magn Reson Med 45:36–41
22. Gillis A, Bashir A, McKeon B, Scheller A, Gray ML, Burstein D (2001) Magnetic resonance imaging of relative glycosaminoglycan distribution in patients with autologous chondrocyte transplants. Invest Radiol 36:743–748
23. Trattnig S, Marlovits S, Gebetsroither S, Szomolanyi P, Welsch GH, Salomonowitz E, Watanabe A, Deimling M, Mamisch TC (2007) Three-dimensional delayed gadolinium-enhanced MRI of cartilage (dGEMRIC) for in vivo evaluation of reparative cartilage after matrix-associated autologous chondrocyte transplantation at 3.0T: preliminary results. J Magn Reson Imaging 26:974–982
24. Trattnig S, Burstein D, Szomolanyi P, Pinker K, Welsch GH, Mamisch TC (2009) T1(Gd) gives comparable information as Delta T1 relaxation rate in dGEMRIC evaluation of cartilage repair tissue. Invest Radiol 44:598–602
25. Mayerhoefer ME, Welsch GH, Mamisch TC, Kainberger F, Weber M, Nemec S, Friedrich KM, Dirisamer A, Trattnig S (2010) The in vivo effects of unloading and compression on T1-Gd (dGEMRIC) relaxation times in healthy articular knee cartilage at 3.0 Tesla. Eur Radiol 20:443–449
26. Maroudas A, Muir H, Wingham J (1969) The correlation of fixed negative charge with glycosaminoglycan content of human articular cartilage. Biochim Biophys Acta 177:492–500
27. Bashir A, Gray ML, Burstein D (1996) Gd-DTPA2- as a measure of cartilage degradation. Magn Reson Med 36:665–673
28. Bashir A, Gray ML, Boutin RD, Burstein D (1997) Glycosaminoglycan in articular cartilage: in vivo assessment with delayed Gd(DTPA)(2-)-enhanced MR imaging. Radiology 205:551–558
29. Kim Y-J, Jaramillo D, Millis MB, Gray ML, Burstein D (2003) Assessment of early osteoarthritis in hip dysplasia with delayed gadolinium-enhanced magnetic resonance imaging of cartilage. J Bone Joint Surg Am 85-A:1987–1992
30. Tiderius CJ, Jessel R, Kim Y-J, Burstein D (2007) Hip dGEMRIC in asymptomatic volunteers and patients with early osteoarthritis: the influence of timing after contrast injection. Magn Reson Med 57:803–805
31. Domayer SE, Mamisch TC, Kress I, Chan J, Kim YJ (2010) Radial dGEMRIC in developmental dysplasia of the hip and in femoroacetabular impingement: preliminary results. Osteoarthritis Cartilage 18:1421–1428

32. Domayer SE, Trattnig S, Stelzeneder D, Hirschfeld C, Quirbach S, Dorotka R, Nehrer S, Pinker K, Chan J, Mamisch TC, Dominkus M, Welsch GH (2010) Delayed gadolinium-enhanced MRI of cartilage in the ankle at 3 T: feasibility and preliminary results after matrix-associated autologous chondrocyte implantation. J Magn Reson Imaging 31:732–739
33. Bittersohl B, Miese FR, Dekkers C, Senyurt H, Kircher J, Wittsack H-J, Antoch G, Krauspe R, Zilkens C (2013) T2* mapping and delayed gadolinium-enhanced magnetic resonance imaging in cartilage (dGEMRIC) of glenohumeral cartilage in asymptomatic volunteers at 3 T. Eur Radiol 23:1367–1374
34. Multanen J, Rauvala E, Lammentausta E, Ojala R, Kiviranta I, Häkkinen A, Nieminen MT, Heinonen A (2009) Reproducibility of imaging human knee cartilage by delayed gadolinium-enhanced MRI of cartilage (dGEMRIC) at 1.5 Tesla. Osteoarthritis Cartilage 17:559–564
35. Siversson C, Tiderius C-J, Neuman P, Dahlberg L, Svensson J (2010) Repeatability of T1-quantification in dGEMRIC for three different acquisition techniques: two-dimensional inversion recovery, three-dimensional look locker, and three-dimensional variable flip angle. J Magn Reson Imaging 31:1203–1209
36. Marckmann P, Skov L, Rossen K, Dupont A, Damholt MB, Heaf JG, Thomsen HS (2006) Nephrogenic systemic fibrosis: suspected causative role of gadodiamide used for contrast-enhanced magnetic resonance imaging. J Am Soc Nephrol 17:2359–2362
37. Grobner T (2006) Gadolinium – a specific trigger for the development of nephrogenic fibrosing dermopathy and nephrogenic systemic fibrosis? Nephrol Dial Transplant 21:1104–1108
38. Thomsen HS (2006) Nephrogenic systemic fibrosis: a serious late adverse reaction to gadodiamide. Eur Radiol 16:2619–2621
39. Shapiro EM, Borthakur A, Gougoutas A, Reddy R (2002) 23Na MRI accurately measures fixed charge density in articular cartilage. Magn Reson Med 47:284–291
40. Reddy R, Insko EK, Noyszewski EA, Dandora R, Kneeland JB, Leigh JS (1998) Sodium MRI of human articular cartilage in vivo. Magn Reson Med 39:697–701
41. Borthakur A, Shapiro EM, Akella SVS, Gougoutas A, Kneeland JB, Reddy R (2002) Quantifying sodium in the human wrist in vivo by using MR imaging. Radiology 224:598–602
42. Borthakur A, Mellon E, Niyogi S, Witschey W, Kneeland JB, Reddy R (2006) Sodium and T1rho MRI for molecular and diagnostic imaging of articular cartilage. NMR Biomed 19:781–821
43. Trattnig S, Welsch GH, Juras V, Szomolanyi P, Mayerhoefer ME, Stelzeneder D, Mamisch TC, Bieri O, Scheffler K, Zbyn S (2010) 23Na MR imaging at 7 T after knee matrix-associated autologous chondrocyte transplantation preliminary results. Radiology 257:175–184
44. Zbýň S, Stelzeneder D, Welsch GH, Negrin LL, Juras V, Mayerhoefer ME, Szomolanyi P, Bogner W, Domayer SE, Weber M, Trattnig S (2012) Evaluation of native hyaline cartilage and repair tissue after two cartilage repair surgery techniques with (23)Na MR imaging at 7 T: initial experience. Osteoarthritis Cartilage 20:837–845
45. Insko EK, Kaufman JH, Leigh JS, Reddy R (1999) Sodium NMR evaluation of articular cartilage degradation. Magn Reson Med 41:30–34
46. Borthakur A, Shapiro EM, Beers J, Kudchodkar S, Kneeland JB, Reddy R (2000) Sensitivity of MRI to proteoglycan depletion in cartilage: comparison of sodium and proton MRI. Osteoarthritis Cartilage 8:288–293
47. Trattnig S, Zbyn S, Schmitt B, Friedrich K, Juras V, Szomolanyi P, Bogner W (2012) Advanced MR methods at ultra-high field (7 Tesla) for clinical musculoskeletal applications. Eur Radiol 22:2338–2346
48. Ling W, Regatte RR, Navon G, Jerschow A (2008) Assessment of glycosaminoglycan concentration in vivo by chemical exchange-dependent saturation transfer (gagCEST). Proc Natl Acad Sci U S A 105:2266–2270
49. Krusche-Mandl I, Schmitt B, Zak L, Apprich S, Aldrian S, Juras V, Friedrich KM, Marlovits S, Weber M, Trattnig S (2012) Long-term results 8 years after autologous osteochondral transplantation: 7 T gagCEST and sodium magnetic resonance imaging with morphological and clinical correlation. Osteoarthritis Cartilage 20:357–363
50. Singh A, Haris M, Cai K, Kassey VB, Kogan F, Reddy D, Hariharan H, Reddy R (2012) Chemical exchange saturation transfer magnetic resonance imaging of human knee cartilage at 3 T and 7 T. Magn Reson Med 68:588–594
51. Schmitt B, Zbyn S, Stelzeneder D, Jellus V, Paul D, Lauer L, Bachert P, Trattnig S (2011) Cartilage quality assessment by using glycosaminoglycan chemical exchange saturation transfer and (23)Na MR imaging at 7 T. Radiology 260:257–264
52. Kim M, Chan Q, Anthony M-P, Cheung KMC, Samartzis D, Khong P-L (2011) Assessment of glycosaminoglycan distribution in human lumbar intervertebral discs using chemical exchange saturation transfer at 3 T: feasibility and initial experience. NMR Biomed 24:1137–1144
53. Mosher TJ, Dardzinski BJ (2004) Cartilage MRI T2 relaxation time mapping: overview and applications. Semin Musculoskelet Radiol 8:355–368
54. Smith HE, Mosher TJ, Dardzinski BJ, Collins BG, Collins CM, Yang QX, Schmithorst VJ, Smith MB (2001) Spatial variation in cartilage T2 of the knee. J Magn Reson Imaging 14:50–55
55. Domayer SE, Kutscha-Lissberg F, Welsch G, Dorotka R, Nehrer S, Gäbler C, Mamisch TC, Trattnig S (2008) T2 mapping in the knee after microfracture at 3.0 T: correlation of global T2 values and clinical outcome – preliminary results. Osteoarthritis Cartilage 16:903–908

56. Trattnig S, Mamisch TC, Welsch GH, Glaser C, Szomolanyi P, Gebetsroither S, Stastny O, Horger W, Millington S, Marlovits S (2007) Quantitative T2 mapping of matrix-associated autologous chondrocyte transplantation at 3 Tesla: an in vivo cross-sectional study. Invest Radiol 42:442–448
57. Welsch GH, Mamisch TC, Domayer SE, Dorotka R, Kutscha-Lissberg F, Marlovits S, White LM, Trattnig S (2008) Cartilage T2 assessment at 3-T MR imaging: in vivo differentiation of normal hyaline cartilage from reparative tissue after two cartilage repair procedures – initial experience. Radiology 247:154–161
58. Mamisch TC, Trattnig S, Quirbach S, Marlovits S, White LM, Welsch GH (2010) Quantitative T2 mapping of knee cartilage: differentiation of healthy control cartilage and cartilage repair tissue in the knee with unloading – initial results. Radiology 254:818–826
59. White LM, Sussman MS, Hurtig M, Probyn L, Tomlinson G, Kandel R (2006) Cartilage T2 assessment: differentiation of normal hyaline cartilage and reparative tissue after arthroscopic cartilage repair in equine subjects. Radiology 241:407–414
60. Maier CF, Tan SG, Hariharan H, Potter HG (2003) T2 quantitation of articular cartilage at 1.5 T. J Magn Reson Imaging 17:358–364
61. Pai A, Li X, Majumdar S (2008) A comparative study at 3 T of sequence dependence of T2 quantitation in the knee. Magn Reson Imaging 26:1215–1220

Part X

The Future

The Future of Cartilage Repair Surgery

31

Alberto Gobbi, Anup Kumar, Georgios Karnatzikos, and Norimasa Nakamura

Contents

A. Gobbi, MD (✉) • G. Karnatzikos, MD
Orthopaedic Arthroscopic Surgery International, OASI Bioresearch Foundation Gobbi NPO, via Amadeo 24, Milan 20133, Italy
e-mail: gobbi@cartilagedoctor.it; giokarnes@gmail.com

A. Kumar, MD
Department of Orthopaedics, India Institute of Medical Sciences, Patna, Bihar 801505, India
e-mail: dr.anup@gmail.com

N. Nakamura, MD, PhD, FRCS
Institute for Medical Science in Sports, Osaka Health Science University, 1-9-27 Tenma, Kita-ku, Osaka City, Osaka 530-0043, Japan

Center for Advanced Medical Engineering and Informatics, Osaka University, 2-2 Yamadaoka, Suita, Osaka 565-0871, Japan
e-mail: n-nakamura@ort.med.osaka-u.ac.jp

31.1 Introduction

Cartilage has long been recognized as having limited healing potential, which is multifactorial in nature [1]. It is avascular (and thus less able to transport new cells to the injury site), hypocellular, aneural, and alymphatic. When cartilage injury occurs, surgical intervention may be necessary to achieve repair of the resulting focal chondral defects and obtain good functional outcome.

Articular cartilage injuries are not uncommon; large studies have shown chondral lesions to be present in approximately 60 % of knee arthroscopies [2, 3]. Chondral injuries may be isolated defects but are frequently found in association with other internal derangements such as meniscal tears, cruciate ligament damage (in approximately 25 % acute and over 50 % chronic), patellar dislocation, or osteochondritis dissecans.

Numerous options exist in the treatment of cartilage lesions. Any form of planned treatment should be based on patient characteristics and expectations, clinical symptoms, and parameters such as lesion size, depth, and associated issues like leg axis alignment, ligamentous and meniscal integrity, and the presence of bone deficiencies. All coexisting pathologies should be treated before or in a concomitant procedure [4–6].

A.A. Shetty et al. (eds.), *Techniques in Cartilage Repair Surgery*, DOI 10.1007/978-3-642-41921-8_31, © ESSKA 2014

31.2 Surgical Options for Cartilage Repair

Traditional palliative techniques or newer reparative treatment options have been utilized to improve the healing of cartilage lesions and have demonstrated variable results. Arthroscopic debridement and cartilage abrasion can provide symptomatic pain relief but with no actual hyaline tissue formation. These techniques remove superficial cartilage layers, which include collagen fibers that are responsible for the tensile strength, creating a less functional cartilage tissue [7]. However, they are often used as first-line treatment for small cartilage defects in order to remove unstable cartilage flaps.

Bone marrow stimulation techniques, such as subchondral plate drilling or microfracture [8], have been reported to stimulate production of hyaline-like tissue with variable properties and durability compared to normal cartilage, in some cases decreasing pain and disability [9]. However, recent studies demonstrated that these techniques produce fibrocartilaginous tissue, which degenerates with time [10–13].

Osteochondral autologous transplantation (OATS) and mosaicplasty can restore normal cartilage tissue, but they can be applied only to small defects (10–12 mm) and there are some concerns regarding donor site morbidity [10, 14].

Autologous chondrocyte implantation (ACI) [15] has been proven to be capable of restoring normal hyaline-like cartilage tissue, which is mechanically and functionally stable even in athletes at long-term follow-up. However, this two-step procedure showed local morbidity for periosteal harvest and uncertain distribution of chondrocyte solution [16–19]. Additionally, the possible complication of periosteal patch hypertrophy prompted the scientific community to develop new techniques including second-generation ACI. The use of a three-dimensional scaffold for autologous chondrocyte culture was developed with the aim to both improve the biologic performance of chondrogenic autologous cells and render the surgical technique easier. Surgeons have now been enabled to perform this procedure arthroscopically [20–23]. Second-generation ACI should be suggested in young athletes with large superficial cartilage defects; furthermore, it shows favorable results in lesions located at the patellofemoral joint [24]. However, this is still a two-step procedure with arthroscopic evaluation and biopsy followed by implantation, either arthroscopically or by mini-arthrotomy [20, 23–26].

31.3 Mesenchymal Stem Cells

Recent directions in cartilage repair are moving towards the possibility of performing one-step surgery; several groups are analyzing the possibility of using mesenchymal stem cells (MSCs) with chondrogenic potential and growth factors (GF), thus avoiding the first surgery for cartilage biopsy and subsequent chondrocyte cell cultivation, with a significant reduction of the cost of the total procedure [27–30]. MSCs have a self-renewal capacity and multi-lineage differentiation potential, and they can be characterized by their cultivation behavior and their differentiation potential into adipogenic, osteogenic, and chondrogenic cells; therefore, once MSCs are cultured in the appropriate microenvironment, they can differentiate to chondrocytes and form cartilage [31–34].

Many authors have shown in animal and laboratory studies the use of MSCs with chondrogenic potential but only few clinical studies have been done [30, 31, 35–37]. The micromass culture or pellet culture system is generally considered a good in vitro model of chondrogenesis; Johnstone et al. [31] cultured MSCs as pellets at the bottom of a tube for 2 weeks in a specific serum-free cocktail medium; under these conditions cells organize a cartilaginous matrix by secreting proteoglycans and type II collagen, and cells appear as real chondrocytes embedded in their own matrix lacunae. Nixon et al. [30] showed early enhanced chondrogenesis in cartilage defects in an equine model; they concluded that MSCs arthroscopic implantation in horses improved cartilage healing response.

Research are currently exploring the possibility of implanting stem cells in the laboratory to differentiate into chondrocytes and which can then be utilized with a synthetic scaffold [35] or scaffold free [36] for implantation. Ochi et al. [37] observed that in a rat model the injection of cultured MSCs combined with bone marrow stimulation can accelerate the regeneration of articular cartilage; they noted that this cell therapy was a less-invasive treatment for cartilage injury. In their other animal study [38], they introduced a MSCs delivery system with the help of an electromagnetic field, enhancing the proliferation of cartilage inside the chondral defect after intra-articular injection, decreasing ectopic cartilage formation. Fortier et al. [39] concluded in their animal studies that development of patient-side configuration techniques for intraoperative stem cell isolation and purification for immediate grafting have significant advantages in time savings and immediate application of an autogenous cell for cartilage repair.

Wakitani et al. [40] used autologous culture of expanded bone marrow for repair of cartilage defects in osteoarthritic knees; they chose 24 knees of 24 patients with knee OA who underwent a high tibial osteotomy; patients were divided into cell-transplanted group and cell-free group. After 16-month follow-up, they concluded that MSCs were capable of regenerating a repair tissue for large chondral defects. Giannini et al. [41] presented their one-step surgery procedure using MSCs and scaffold.

31.4 One-Step Surgery: Bone Marrow Aspirate Concentrate and a Collagen I/III-Based Matrix

Once MSCs are cultured in the appropriate microenvironment, they can differentiate to chondrocytes and form cartilage. In this regard, the use of bone marrow aspirate concentrated cells (BMAC), which contain multipotent MSCs and growth factors, can represent a possible alternative for regenerating cartilage tissue.

We prospectively followed up for 2 years a group of 15 nonprofessional athlete patients with 15 knees operated on for grade IV cartilage lesions of the knee [42]; all have been implanted using BMAC covered with a collagen I/III-based matrix in a one-step procedure. Bone marrow was harvested from ipsilateral iliac crest and subjected to concentration and activation with Batroxobin solution in order to produce a sticky clot, which was implanted into the prepared cartilage defect. Coexisting knee pathologies such as tibiofemoral axial alignment, patellofemoral alignment, and ligamentous insufficiency were treated during the same surgery in 12 patients. The patients followed the same specific rehabilitation protocol, which is similar to rehabilitation after second-generation ACI, for a minimum of 6 months (Table 31.1).

31.4.1 Surgical Technique

All the procedures are performed under spinal anesthesia and routine sterile preparation and draping; 60 mL of bone marrow aspirate is harvested from the ipsilateral iliac crest (Fig. 31.1a) using a dedicated aspiration kit and centrifuged using a commercially available system (BMAC Harvest Smart PreP2 System, Harvest Technologies, Plymouth, MA). In order to concentrate the baseline value of the bone marrow cells four to six times, we follow the method recommended by the manufacturer. Using a Batroxobin enzyme (Plateltex®act-Plateltex SRO Bratislava, SK), the bone marrow concentrate is activated in order to produce a sticky clot material (Fig. 31.1b), which is implanted into the prepared cartilage defect.

After arthroscopic evaluation, the knee is approached with a mini-arthrotomy, and the chondral defect is prepared and debrided with the use of curettes (Fig. 31.1c). Specific attention is

Table 31.1 Rehabilitation phases, objectives, and criteria to progress between phases

Phase	Objectives	Criteria to progress
1. Protection of the implant (0–6 weeks)	Protect the transplant from excessive loads/shearing forces Decrease pain and effusion Gain full extension and gradual recovery of knee flexion Retard muscle atrophy	Full active knee extension Knee flexion >120° No or minimum pain and swelling No pain during weight bearing Adequate muscle recruitment (quadriceps)
2. Transition and recovery of gait (6–12 weeks)	Return to normal gait pattern Progressive recovery in daily functional activities Increase the strength of the quadriceps and flexors Recovery of full range of motion	Normal gait Recovery of nearly full ROM (full extension, flexion >135°) Adequate muscle tone and neuromuscular control No pain or swelling
3. Maturation and recovery of running (12–24 weeks)	Return to a correct running pathway Further increase in strength of quadriceps and flexor muscles Further increase in functional activities level	Running without pain/swelling at 8 km/h for 10′ Adequate recovery of coordination/neuromuscular control Recovery of strength >80 % contralateral limb Single leg hop test: >80 % contralateral limb
4. Turnover and sport specific recovery (24–52 weeks)	Sustain high loads and impact activities Recovery sport specific skills Prepare athlete for a return to team and competition with good recovery of the aerobic endurance Maintain a good quality of life, avoiding excess of body fat and preventing risk of reinjury	Running without pain/effusion at 10 km/h for 15′ Recovery of strength >90 % contralateral limb Single leg hop test: >90 % contralateral limb Recovery of sport specific skills

paid to remove the calcified layer if present, while avoiding penetration of the subchondral bone and reducing the bleeding, as much as possible, from the bottom of the lesion. Damaged cartilage is removed until contained, shouldered defect remains, which is necessary in order to facilitate suturing the scaffold. The defect is templated and the collagen membrane (Chondro-Gide®-Geistlich Wolhusen, CH) fashioned according to the defect size. Finally, the prepared clot is pasted into the lesion (Fig. 31.1d). In order to protect MSCs, the defect is covered with a collagen-based membrane scaffold (Fig. 31.1e). The membrane is anchored to the surrounding cartilage using PDS 6-0 and sealed with fibrin glue (Tissucol, Baxter, Rome, Italy); the knee was then ranged through flexion and extension in order to check the stability of the implanted membrane.

31.4.2 Results

All the patients showed improvements in evaluation scores. Mean pre-op values were VAS 5, IKDC subjective 41.73, KOOS scores *P* = 66.6/*S* = 68.3/ADL = 70/SP = 41.8/QOL = 37.2, Lysholm 65, and Tegner 2.07. At final follow-up mean scores were VAS 0.8, IKDC subjective 75.5, KOOS *P* = 89.8/*S* = 83.6/ADL = 89.6/SP = 58.9/QOL = 68, Lysholm 87.9, and Tegner 4.1. No adverse reactions or post-op complication were noted. MRI showed good coverage of the lesions (Fig. 31.2a, b). Four patients gave their consent for second-look arthroscopy (Fig. 31.1f) but only 3 for a concomitant biopsy. Good histological findings were reported for all the specimens analyzed which presented many hyaline-like features [42] (Fig. 31.3a–c).

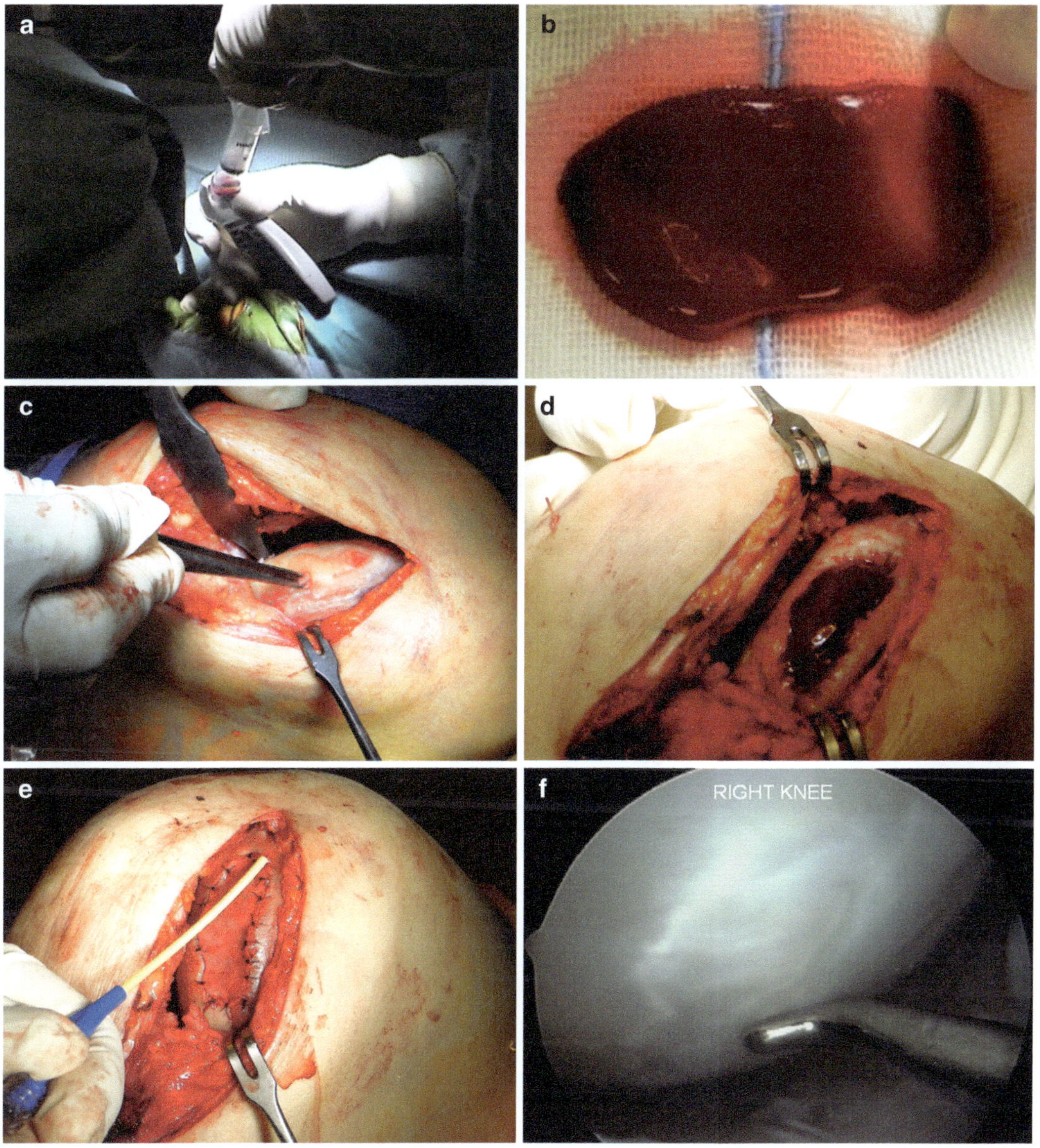

Fig. 31.1 (**a**) Bone marrow aspiration from iliac crest, (**b**) bone marrow aspirate concentrate (BMAC) clot after activation, (**c**) femoral condyle grade IV lesion, (**d**) pasting BMAC clot into the lesion, (**e**) covering the lesion with a collagen-based matrix, and (**f**) second-look arthroscopy at 1-year follow-up

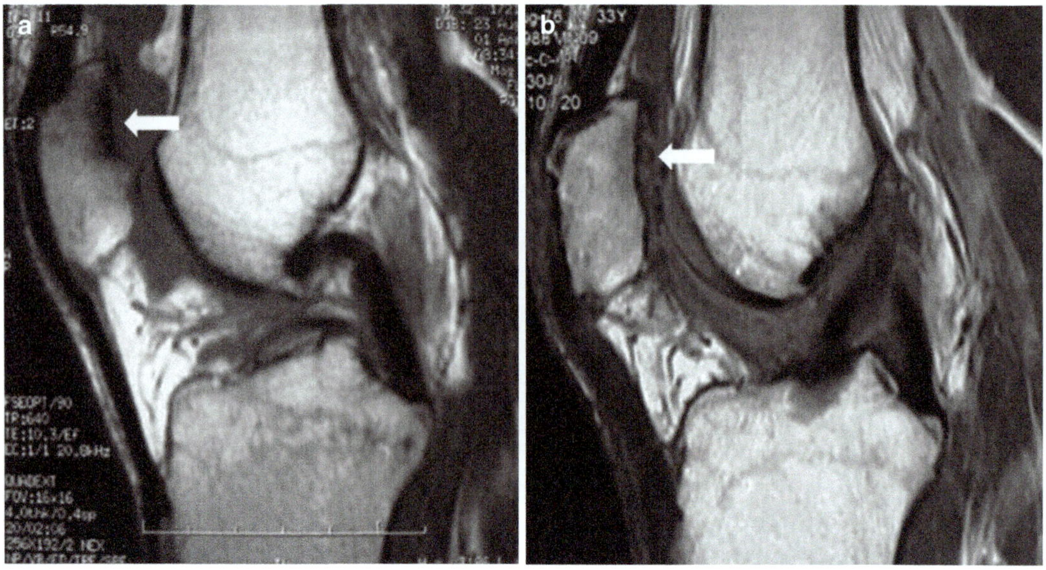

Fig. 31.2 "MRI in a 33-year-old amateur soccer player: (**a**) preoperative T1 sequence in sagittal plane showing a grade IV patellar lesion(*white arrow*) and (**b**) T1 sequence in sagittal plane at 2-year follow-up showing good coverage of the lesion

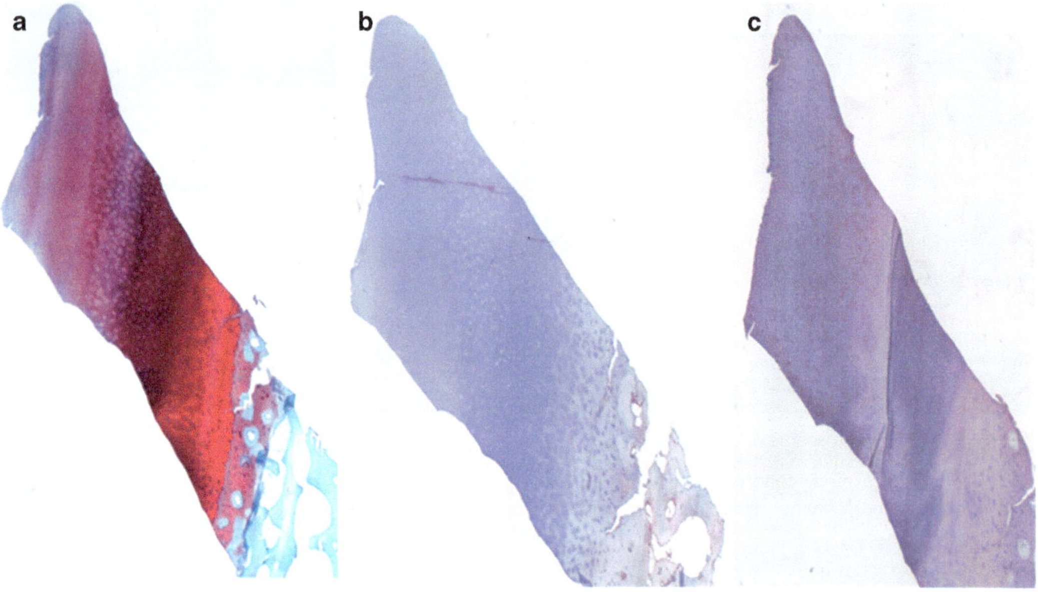

Fig. 31.3 Biopsy of a 48-year-old patient, with a 6.75 cm^2 patellar lesion, obtained after 24 months (original magnification, 40×). (**a**) Safranin O staining reveals a well-organized cartilage tissue with the typical features of normal articular cartilage. The superficial layer is regular. The tidemark is well evident. The proteoglycan component is well represented, and the cells show regular distribution along the extracellular matrix. The subchondral bone tissue is in a remodeling process. (**b**) Immunohistochemical analysis results of collagen type I are almost negative with only a few positive cells at the superficial layer. (**c**) Type II collagen is slightly positive in the extracellular matrix and at the cellular level

Conclusion

A number of viable options have been made available over the years to address problems concerning cartilage damage. The use of MSCs presents several positive features: its one-step nature, the use of a collagen I/III-based matrix, which favors cell concentration in the defect area and also allows early mobilization of the operated knee, and its lower cost if compared to standard two-step ACI procedures. Recently we published data on 25 patients treated with MSCs, at medium-term follow-up (average 41.3 ± 7 months), that confirmed the preliminary findings [43]. Preliminary and medium-term data are encouraging; however, further studies on clinical efficacy will clarify if simultaneous use of MSCs could represent a viable solution for regenerative medicine in cartilage repair. These studies showed less morbidities and complications inherent to cartilage surgical techniques by lessening surgical procedures translating to lower cost for the patient. However, long-term prospective randomized studies are suggested to confirm these preliminary results.

References

1. Hunter W (1743) On the structure and diseases of articulating cartilage. Philos Trans Rsoc Lond B Biol Sci 9:277
2. Curl WW, Krome J, Gordon E, Rushing J, Smith BP, Poehling GG (1997) Cartilage injuries: a review of 31516 knee arthroscopies. Arthroscopy 13:456–460
3. Flanigan DC, Harris JD, Trinh TQ, Siston RA, Brophy RH (2010) Prevalence of chondral defects in athletes' knees: a systematic review. Med Sci Sports Exerc 42(10):1795–1801, Review
4. Fulkerson JP (2002) Diagnosis and treatment of patients with patellofemoral pain. Am J Sports Med 30(3):447–456, Review
5. Gomoll A, Farr J (2009) Future developments in cartilage repair. In: Cole B, Gomoll A (eds) Biologic joint reconstruction. SLACK Incorporated, Thorofare
6. Minas T (2004) Autologous chondrocyte implantation in the osteoarthritic knee. In: Cole B, Malek M (eds) Articular cartilage lesions. Springer, New York
7. McKinley BJ, Cushner FD, Scott WN (1999) Debridement arthroscopy. 10-year follow-up. Clin Orthop 367:190–194
8. Steadman JR, Rodkey WG, Briggs KK (2002) Microfracture to treat full thickness chondral defects: surgical technique, rehabilitation, and outcomes. J Knee Surg 15:170–176
9. Steadman JR, Briggs KK, Rodrigo JJ, Kocher MS, Gill TJ, Rodkey WG (2003) Outcomes of microfracture for traumatic chondral defects of the knee: average 11-year follow-up. Arthroscopy 19:477–484
10. Gobbi A, Francisco R, Allegra F et al (2006) Arthroscopic treatment of osteochondral lesions of the talus: a prospective study of three different techniques. Arthroscopy 22(10):1085–1092
11. Gobbi A, Karnatzikos G, Kumar A (2013) Long-term results after microfracture treatment for full-thickness knee chondral lesions in athletes. Knee Surg Sports Traumatol Arthrosc. [Epub ahead of print] PubMed PMID: 24051505
12. Minas T, Gomoll AH, Rosenberger R, Royce RO, Bryant T (2009) Increased failure rate of autologous chondrocyte implantation after previous treatment with marrow stimulation techniques. Am J Sports Med 37(5):902–908
13. Saris DBF, Vanlauwe J, Victor J et al (2008) CCI results in better structural repair when treating symptomatic cartilage defects of the knee in a randomised clinical trial versus microfracture. Am J Sports Med 36(2):235–246
14. Hangody L, Fules P (2003) Autologous osteochondral mosaicplasty for the treatment of full-thickness defects of weight-bearing joints. J Bone Joint Surg Am 85-A(Suppl 3):25–32
15. Brittberg M, Lindahl A, Nilsson A, Ohlsson C, Isaksson O, Peterson L (1994) Treatment of deep cartilage defects in the knee with autologous chondrocyte transplantation. N Engl J Med 331(14):889–895
16. Minas T, Peterson L (1999) Advanced techniques in autologous chondrocyte transplantation. Clin Sports Med 18(1):13–44
17. Henderson I, Francisco R, Oakes B, Cameron J (2005) Autologous chondrocyte implantation for treatment of focal chondral defects of the knee – a clinical, arthroscopic, MRI and histologic evaluation at 2 years. Knee 12(3):209–216
18. Henderson IJ, Tuy B, Oakes B et al (2003) Prospective clinical study of autologous chondrocyte implantation and correlation with MRI at three and 12 months. J Bone Joint Surg Br 85:1060–1066
19. Peterson L, Vasiliadis HS, Brittberg M, Lindahl A (2010) Autologous chondrocyte implantation: a long-term follow-up. Am J Sports Med 38(6):1117–1124
20. Gobbi A, Bathan L (2009) Minimal invasive second-generation autologous chondrocyte implantation. In: Cole B, Gomoll A (eds) Biologic joint reconstruction. SLACK Incorporated, Thorofare

21. Kon E, Filardo G, Delcogliano M et al (2007) Arthroscopic second-generation autologous chondrocyte implantation at 48 months follow up. Osteoarthritis Cartilage 15(Suppl B, 22.1):44–45
22. Kon E, Gobbi A, Filardo G et al (2009) Arthroscopic second-generation A.C.I. Compared with microfractures for chondral lesions of the knee. Am J Sports Med 37:33
23. Marcacci M, Zaffagnini S, Kon E et al (2002) Arthroscopic autologous chondrocyte transplantation: technical note. Knee Surg Sports Traumatol Arthrosc 10:154–159
24. Gobbi A, Kon E, Filardo G et al (2009) Patellofemoral full-thickness chondral defects treated with second generation ACI: a clinical review at 5 years follow-up. Am J Sports Med 37(6):1083–1092
25. Marcacci M, Berruto M, Gobbi A, Kon E et al (2005) Articular cartilage engineering with Hyalograft C: 3-year clinical results. Clin Orthop Relat Res 435:96–105
26. Nehrer S, Domayer S, Dorotka R et al (2006) Three-year clinical outcome after chondrocyte transplantation using a hyaluronan matrix for cartilage repair. Eur J Radiol 57:3–8
27. Mackay AM, Beck SC, Murphy JM et al (1998) Chondrogenic differentiation of cultured human mesenchymal stem cells from marrow. Tissue Eng 4(4):415–428
28. Fortier LA, Balkman CE, Sandell LJ et al (2001) Insulin-like growth factor-I gene expression patterns during spontaneous repair of acute articular cartilage injury. J Orthop Res 19(4):720–728
29. Fortier LA, Mohammed HO, Lust G et al (2002) Insulin-like growth factor-I enhances cell-based repair of articular cartilage. J Bone Joint Surg Br 84(2):276–288
30. Nixon AJ, Wilke MM, Nydam DV (2007) Enhanced early chondrogenesis in articular defects following arthroscopic mesenchymal stem cell implantation in an equine model. J Orthop Res 25(7):913–925
31. Johnstone B, Hering TM, Caplan AI et al (1998) In vitro chondrogenesis of bone marrow-derived mesenchymal progenitor cells. Exp Cell Res 238(1): 265–272
32. Muraglia A, Cancedda R, Quarto R (2000) Clonal mesenchymal progenitors from human bone marrow differentiate in vitro according to a hierarchical model. J Cell Sci 113(Pt 7):1161–1166
33. Nakagawa Y, Nakamura T et al (2001) Osteochondral grafting and arthroplasty for end-stage osteochondritis dissecans of the capitellum-a case report and review of the literature. Am J Sports Med 29(5):650–655
34. Grigolo B, Lisignoli G, Desando G, Cavallo C, Marconi E, Tschon M et al (2009) Osteoarthritis treated with mesenchymal stem cells on hyaluronan-based scaffold in rabbit. Tissue Eng Part C Methods 15(4):647–658
35. Ando W, Frank CB, Nakamura DA et al (2009) Comparison of mesenchymal progenitor cells derived from different porcine tissues for lineage specific potential. ICRS Abstract Book. Miami, p 75
36. Ando W, Tateishi K, Katakai D, Hart DA, Higuchi C, Nakata K, Hashimoto J, Fujie H, Shino K, Yoshikawa H, Nakamura N (2008) In vitro generation of a scaffold-free tissue-engineered construct (TEC) derived from human synovial mesenchymal stem cells: biological and mechanical properties and further chondrogenic potential. Tissue Eng Part A 14(12):2041–2049
37. Ochi M, Kanaya A, Nishimori M Cell therapy for promotion of cartilage regeneration after drilling and ACL healing. 6TH Biennial ISAKOS Congress, Florence, Italy, 2007
38. Ochi M, Adachi N, Nobuto H, Agung M, Kawamata S, Yanada S (2006) Effects of CD44 antibody- or RGDS peptide – immobilized magnetic beads on cell proliferation and chondrogenesis of mesenchymal stem cells. J Biomed Mater Res A 77(4):773–784
39. Fortier L, Potter H, Rickey E, Schnabel L, Foo L, Chong L et al (2010) Concentrated bone marrow aspirate improves full-thickness cartilage repair combined to microfracture in an equine model. J Bone Joint Surg Am 92:1927–1937
40. Wakitani S, Imoto K, Yamamoto T et al (2002) Human autologous culture expanded bone marrow mesenchymal cell transplantation for repair of cartilage defects in osteoarthritic knees. Osteoarthritis Cartilage 10(3):199–206
41. Giannini S, Buda R, Vannini F et al (2009) One-step bone marrow-derived cell transplantation in talar osteochondral lesions. Clin Orthop Relat Res 467:3307–3320
42. Gobbi A, Karnatzikos G, Scotti C, Mahajan V, Mazzucco L, Grigolo B (2011) One-step cartilage repair with bone marrow aspirate concentrated cells and collagen matrix in full-thickness knee cartilage lesions: results at 2 year follow up. Cartilage 2(3): 286–299
43. Gobbi A, Karnatzikos G, Sankineani SR (2014) Treatment of Large Full-thickness Chondral Defects of the Knee in One-Step Surgery with Multipotent Stem Cells Am J Sports Med DOI: 10.1177/0363546513518007 (In Press)

Erratum to: Mesenchymal Stem Cell Induced Chondrogenesis (MCIC™)

Asode Ananthram Shetty, Seok-Jung Kim,
and Vishvas A. Shetty

Erratum to:
Chapter 10 in: A.A. Shetty et al. (eds.), *Techniques in Cartilage Repair Surgery*,
DOI 10.1007/978-3-642-41921-8_10

Figure 10.18 erroneously shows an ACIC patient. It has been replaced by an image of an MCIC patient (see next page).

The updated online version of this chapter can be found at
10.1007/978-3-642-41921-8_10

A.A. Shetty, MD, PhD, MCh, FRCS Ed., FRCS Eng., FRCS Orth (✉)
Department of Minimally Invasive Surgery,
Faculty of Health and Social Sciences,
Canterbury Christ Church University,
Pembroke Court 30, ME4 4UF
Chatham Maritime, Kent, UK

Faculty of Stem Cell Research and Regenerative Medicine, NITTE University, Mangalore, India
e-mail: aashetty@hotmail.com

S.-J. Kim, MD, PhD, FRCS
Department of Orthopedic Surgery,
Uijeongbu St. Mary's Hospital, College of Medicine,
The Catholic University of Korea, 480-717
Gyeonggi-do, Republic of (South Korea)

Faculty of Stem Cell Research and Regenerative Medicine, NITTE University, Mangalore, India
e-mail: orthopland@naver.com

V.A. Shetty
Department of Minimally Invasive Surgery,
Faculty of Health and Social Sciences,
Canterbury Christ Church University,
Pembroke Court 30, ME4 4UF,
Chatham Maritime, Kent, UK

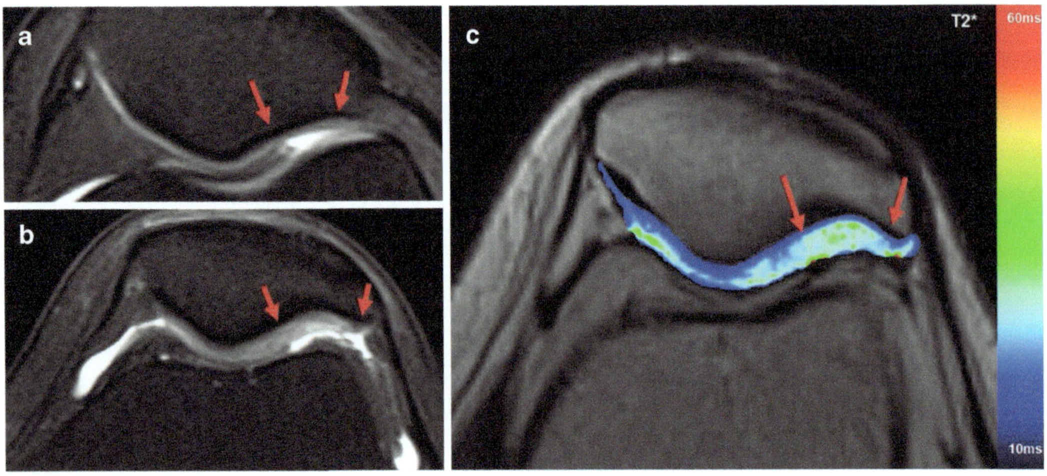

Fig. 10.18 MRI images for patellar femoral joint lesions. The area between the two red arrows indicate area of repaired cartilage lesions. (**a**) Morphological MRI scan pre-operatively. (**b**) Morphological MRI scan post-operatively. (**c**) MRI T2* mapping post-operatively

Index

A.A. Shetty et al. (eds.), *Techniques in Cartilage Repair Surgery*,
DOI 10.1007/978-3-642-41921-8, © ESSKA 2014

O

R

S

T

GPSR Compliance

The European Union's (EU) General Product Safety Regulation (GPSR) is a set of rules that requires consumer products to be safe and our obligations to ensure this.

If you have any concerns about our products, you can contact us on ProductSafety@springernature.com

In case Publisher is established outside the EU, the EU authorized representative is:

Springer Nature Customer Service Center GmbH
Europaplatz 3
69115 Heidelberg, Germany

Batch number: 10732756

Printed by Printforce, the Netherlands